THE CONDUCTION SYSTEM OF THE HEART

THE CONDUCTION SYSTEM OF THE HEART

STRUCTURE, FUNCTION AND CLINICAL IMPLICATIONS

edited by

H.J.J. WELLENS, M.D.,
K.I. LIE, M.D. AND M.J. JANSE, M.D.

Second printing

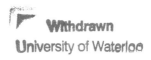
1978
MARTINUS NIJHOFF MEDICAL DIVISION - THE HAGUE

ACKNOWLEDGEMENTS

Many people assisted during the preparation of this book. We especially want to thank Dr. Robert H. Anderson for translating some of the manuscripts, and Miss N. Lambriex and Mrs. Y. Roels for their secretarial assistance. Astra Nederland made the organization of the workshop financially possible.

First printing 1976. (Published by H. E. Stenfert Kroese, Leiden).
Second printing 1978.

ISBN 90.247.2080.X

Photoset by Interprint (Malta) Ltd. Printed in The Netherlands.

PREFACE

This monograph had its genesis in a workshop on the specific conduction held in the spring of 1975.

The meeting was organized to discuss present knowledge on structure and function of the cardiac specialized tissues with emphasis on their clinical implications. Since much new information was presented, the participants agreed to prepare manuscripts and make their material available for publication. This has resulted in a book in which the cardiac specialized tissues are discussed by different specialists: the electron-microscopist, anatomist, pathologist, physiologist, physicist and clinician. Apart from their interest in the cardiac conduction system the participants shared the opinion that their contribution should be relevant to the understanding and treatment of patients with cardiac arrhythmias. The book should be useful for the clinician, the morphologist and the physiologist.

The workshop took place at the University Department of Cardiology, Wilhelmina Gasthuis, Amsterdam, The Netherlands. This is the home ground of one of the most outstanding electrocardiologists of our time, Dr. Dirk Durrer. By pairing genius and originality with endless fund of energy and dogged persistence he made several important contributions to modern cardiac electrophysiology. In recent years he created a cardiological institute where workers from various disciplines cooperate in the study and treatment of cardiac disease. Several of his pupils participated in the workshop and contributed to this volume.

In appreciation and thankfulness we want to dedicate this book to Dr. Dirk Durrer.

Hein J. J. Wellens
K. I. Lie
Michiel J. Janse

CONTENTS

Sinus node and atrium

The atrioventricular junction, the bundle branches and the ventricle

The Wolff-Parkinson-White syndrome

Myocardial infarction

LIST OF CONTRIBUTORS

Masood Akhtar, M.D., Cardiovascular Program, U.S. Public Health Service Hospital, Staten Island, N.Y.

Maurits A. Alessie, Department of Physiology, University of Amsterdam.

Robert H. Anderson, M.D., Cardiothoracic Institute, Brompton Hospital, London.

Irany de Azevedo, M.D., Cardiopulmonary Department, The Lankenau Hospital, Philadelphia, Pa.

Arthur L. Bassett, Ph.D., Department of Pediatrics and Pharmacology, University of Miami Hospitals and Clinics, Miami, Fla.

Anton E. Becker, M.D., Department of Pathology, Wilhelmina Gasthuis, Amsterdam.

Jacques Billette, M.D., Department of Physiology, University of Montreal, Montreal.

Felix I. M. Bonke, Department of Physiology, University of Amsterdam.

Frans J. L. van Capelle, Ph.D., Department of Cardiology and Clinical Physiology, Wilhelmina Gasthuis, Amsterdam.

Antonio Caracta, M.D., Cardiovascular Program, U.S. Public Health Service Hospital, Staten Island, N.Y.

Agustin Castellanos, Jr., M.D., Department of Cardiology, University of Miami School of Medicine, Miami, Fla.

Philippe Coumel, M.D., Hôpital Lariboisière, Paris.

R. Coutte, M.D., Hôpital de la Salpêtrière, Paris.

Paul F. Cranefield, M.D., Ph.D., Department of Pharmacology. College of Physicians and Surgeons of Columbia University, New York, N.Y.

Rudolf Th. van Dam, M.D., Department of Cardiology and Clinical Physiology, Wilhelmina Gasthuis, Amsterdam.

Anthony N. Damato, M.D., Cardiovascular Program, U.S. Public Health Service Hospital, Staten Island, N.Y.

J. Cl. Demoulin, M.D., Hôpital Universitaire de Bavière, Liège.

Pablo Denes, M.D., Cardiology Section, Abraham Lincoln School of Medicine, University of Illinois College of Medicine, Chicago, Ill.

Ramesh C. Dhingra, M.D., Abraham Lincoln School of Medicine, University of Illinois College of Medicine, Chicago, Ill.

Henk J. M. Dohmen, M.D., Department of Cardiology and Clinical Physiology, Wilhelmina Gasthuis, Amsterdam.

Eugene Downar, M.D., Department of Cardiology and Clinical Physiology, Wilhelmina Gasthuis, Amsterdam.

C. Dragodanne, M.D., Hôpital de la Salpêtrière, Paris.

Henry N. Dreifus, Cardiopulmonary Department, The Lankenau Hospital, Philadelphia, Pa.

Leonard S. Dreifus, M.D., Cardiopulmonary Department, The Lankenau Hospital, Philadelphia, Pa.

Marcelo V. Elizari, M.D., Service of Cardiology, Ramos Mejïa Hospital, Buenos Aires.

Nabil El-Sherif, M.D., Veterans Administration Hospital, Miami, Fla.

Daniel Flammang, M.D., Hôpital Lariboisière, Paris.

Guy Fontaine, M.D., Hôpital de la Salpêtrière, Paris.

R. Frank, M.D., Hôpital de la Salpêtrière, Paris.

John J. Gallagher, M.D., Clinical Electrophysiology Laboratory, Duke University Medical Center, Durham, N.C.

Henry Gelband, M.D., Department of Pediatrics and Pharmacology, University of Miami Hospitals and Clinics, Miami, Fla.

Robert Grolleau, M.D., Department of Cardiology, University of Montpellier.

Claude Guimond, M.D., Department of Cardiology, University of Montpellier.

G. Guiraudon, M.D., Hôpital de la Salpêtrière, Paris.

Ronald R. Hope, M.B., F.R.A.C.P., Veterans Administration Hospital, Miami. Fla.

Michiel J. Janse, M.D., Department of Cardiology and Clinical Physiology, Wilhelmina Gasthuis, Amsterdam.

Jackie Kasell, Clinical Electrophysiology Laboratory, Duke University Medical Center, Durham, N.C.

Henri E. Kulbertus, M.D., Hôpital Universitaire de Bavière, Liège.

Richard Langendorf, M.D., Michael Reese Medical Center, Chicago, Ill.

Sun H. Lau, M.D., Cardiovascular Program, U.S. Public Health Service Hospital, Staten Island, N.Y.

Ralph Lazzara, M.D., Veterans Administration Hospital, Miami, Fla.

Julio O. Lázzari, M.D., Service of Cardiology, Ramos Mejía Hospital, Buenos Aires.

Raúl J. Levi, M.D., Department of Electrocardiography, Ramos Mejía Hospital, Buenos Aires.

K. I. Lie, M.D., Department of Cardiology and Clinical Physiology, Wilhelmina Gasthuis, Amsterdam.

William J. Mandel, M.D., Department of Cardiology, Cedars of Lebanon Hospital Division, Los Angeles, Calif.

E. Neil Moore, D.V.M., Ph.D., F.A.C.C., School of Veterinary Medicine, University of Pennsylvania, Philadelphia, Pa.

Robert J. Myerburg, M.D., Division of Cardiology, University of Miami School of Medicine, Miami. Fla.

Onkar S. Narula, M.D., Division of Cardiology. The Chicago Medical School, Chicago, Ill.

Kristina Nilsson, Department of Pediatrics and Pharmacology, University of Miami Hospitals and Clinics, Miami, Fla.

Alejandro Navakosky, M.D., Department of Electrocardiography, Ramos Mejía Hospital, Buenos Aires.

Alfred Pick, M.D., F.A.C.P., F.A.C.C., Michael Reese Medical Center, Chicago, Ill.

Paul Puech, M.D., Department of Cardiology, University of Montpellier.

Ricardo A. Quinteiro, M.D., Department of Electrocardiography, Ramos Mejía Hospital, Buenos Aires.

Kenneth M. Rosen, M.D., Cardiology Section, The Abraham Lincoln School of Medicine, Chicago, Ill.

Mauricio B. Rosenbaum, M.D., Service of Cardiology, Ramos Mejía Hospital, Buenos Aires.

Manfred Runge, M.D., I. Medizinische Universitäts Klinik, Hamburg.

Jeremy Ruskin, M.D., Cardiovascular Program, U.S. Public Health Service Hospital, Staten Island, N.Y.

Benjamin J. Scherlag, Ph.D., Veterans Administration Hospital, Miami, Fla.

Francien J. G. Schopman, Department of Physiology, University of Amsterdam.

Reinier M. Schuilenburg, M.D., Department of Cardiology and Clinical Physiology, Wilhelmina Gasthuis, Amsterdam.

Will C. Sealy, M.D., Duke University Medical Center, Durham, N.C.

Joseph F. Spear, Ph.D., School of Veterinary Medicine, University of Pennsylvania, Philadelphia, Pa.

Harold C. Strauss, M.D., Duke University Medical Center, Department of Medicine, Cardiovascular Division, Durham, N.C.

Ruey J. Sung, M.D., Department of Pediatrics and Pharmacology, University of Miami Hospitals and Clinics, Miami, Fla.

A. C. Tans, M.D., Department of Cardiology and Clinical Physiology, Wilhelmina Gasthuis, Amsterdam.

Paul Touboul, M.D., Hôpital Cardiologique, Lyon.

Jørgen Tranum-Jensen, M.D., University of Copenhagen, Anatomy Department, Copenhagen.

Raymond C. Truex, Ph.D., Department of Anatomy, Temple University, Philadelphia, Pa.

Andrew G. Wallace, M.D., Division of Cardiology, Duke University Medical Center, Durham, N.C.

Yoshio Watanabe, M.D., Fujita Gakuen University School of Medicine. Toyoake, Aichi.

Menashe B. Waxman, M.D., Department of Medicine of the University of Toronto. Toronto.

Hein J. J. Wellens, M.D., Department of Cardiology and Clinical Physiology, Wilhelmina Gasthuis, Amsterdam.

Arnold C. G. Wenink, M.D., University of Leiden, Leiden.

Jay R. Wiggins, Ph.D., Department of Pharmacology, College of Physicians and Surgeons of Columbia University, New York, N.Y.

David O. Williams, M.B., M.R.C.P., Veterans Administration Hospital, Miami. Fla.

Andrew L. Wit, Ph.D., Department of Pharmacology, College of Physicians and Surgeons of Columbia University, New York, N.Y.

Delon Wu, M.D., Abraham Lincoln School of Medicine, University of Illinois College of Medicine, Chicago, Ill.

Iwao Yamaguchi, M.D., Department of Cardiology, Cedars of Lebanon Hospital Division, Los Angeles, Calif.

Douglas P. Zipes, M.D., Indiana University School of Medicine, Indianapolis, Ind.

ANATOMY AND ELECTROPHYSIOLOGY OF THE DEVELOPING CONDUCTING SYSTEM

1

THE DEVELOPMENT OF THE CARDIAC SPECIALIZED TISSUE

ROBERT H. ANDERSON, M.D., ANTON E. BECKER, M.D.,
ARNOLD C. G. WENINK, M.D., AND MICHIEL J. JANSE, M.D.

INTRODUCTION

It is a reasonable premise that knowledge of the development of any system provides a sound basis for the comprehension of both its normal and abnormal structure. It can also be argued that awareness of the morphogenetic nature of components of any system can provide some evidence relative to its function. In our opinion, all of these statements hold good for the cardiac specialized or conducting tissue. However, there is considerable divergence of opinion regarding the precise origin of certain parts of the conducting system, in particular the atrioventricular junctional area, while controversy continues to rage concerning the extent of specialized structures within the atrial tissues. Review of the relevant literature shows that in many cases these disagreements relate more to differences in interpretation than to variation in observations, while other arguments relate more to definitions and semantics. In this review we will present our own observations relative to the development of the cardiac specialized tissue. These have been based on histologic study of human embryos and specimens of congenitally malformed human hearts, together with combined morphologic and electrophysiologic studies of human fetal hearts. Where any topic is contentious we shall refer to the results of previous investigators. However, we shall not attempt to provide an exhaustive review of prior studies of development of the cardiac specialized tissue. Rather we will attempt to provide an outline of embryogenesis which we hope will facilitate interpretation and aid comprehension of the subsequent contributions to this book.

EARLY STAGES OF DEVELOPMENT

At the stage at which the heart is represented by a straight tube (approximately 2 mm CR length—3 weeks intrauterine development—Horizon X), various segments are recognizable. These can be designated, following the precedent of Keith (432), as sinus venosus, primitive atrium, primitive ventricle, bulbus and truncus. Each of the segments is separated by a constricted ring, and close examination of these rings reveals that they are histologically distinct from the walls of the intervening segments (fig. 1a) (62, 920). A close parallel to this situation is to be found in the hearts of lower vertebrates where some authorities hold the junctional tissues to be specialized (658). In contrast, others contend that conducting tissues are only observed in birds and mammals (179). Nonetheless, examination of the precise effect of cardiac looping and development on the disposition of

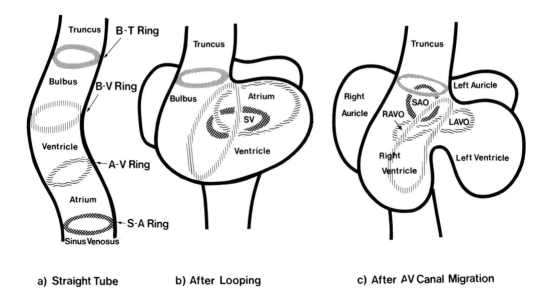

a) Straight Tube   b) After Looping   c) After AV Canal Migration

Early Stages - Distribution of Ring Specialized Tissues (Wenink,1975)

Fig. 1. Diagrams showing the effect of looping upon the rings of specialized tissue separating the components of the primitive heart tube, viz: sinus venosus, atrium, ventricle, bulbus and truncus. The four rings, the sinuatrial (SA), atrioventricular (AV), bulboventricular (BV) and bulbotruncal (BT) rings are indicated by differing varieties of cross-hatch or stipple, and these symbols will continue to be used throughout the subsequent diagrams. After looping (fig. 1b), the formation of the inner curvature brings the AV, BV and BT rings into close apposition. After canal migration, the SA ring is brought into contact with the AV ring posteriorly, while the BV ring is now juxtaposed to the AV ring in both medial and lateral parts of the right bulboventricular junction. These ring appositions are of considerable significance to subsequent development of AV junctional specialized tissues. Other abbreviations: SAO = sinuatrial orifice. RAVO = right atrioventricular orifice. LAVO = left atrioventricular orifice.

these junctional rings is of considerable significance to the subsequent formation of conducting structures (fig. 1).

Absorption of the sinus venosus into the right atrium places the sinuatrial ring in the posterior wall of the right atrial chamber. It impinges postero-inferiorly upon the atrioventricular ring, which following formation of the right ventricle is itself in apposition to the anteriorly situated bulboventricular ring in two sites, one septally and the other laterally (fig. 1c). Since the looping process produces an exceedingly short inner curvature of the heart, the cono-ventricular flange, it follows that atrioventricular, bulboventricular and bulbotruncal rings are all in close apposition at this point (fig. 2). This concept of disposition of the rings is dependent upon the premise that the definitive right ventricle is formed in part from the primitive ventricle and in part from the bulbus. Although some maintain that the right ventricle is an entirely bulbar structure (868), our own studies do not support this contention (34). Furthermore, if the primitive ventricle does contribute to both ventricles, as we believe, then the posterior ventricular septum is formed de novo from the primitive ventricle and is not a bulboventricular structure. As we shall show, conducting elements formed astride the posterior interventricular septum are of particular

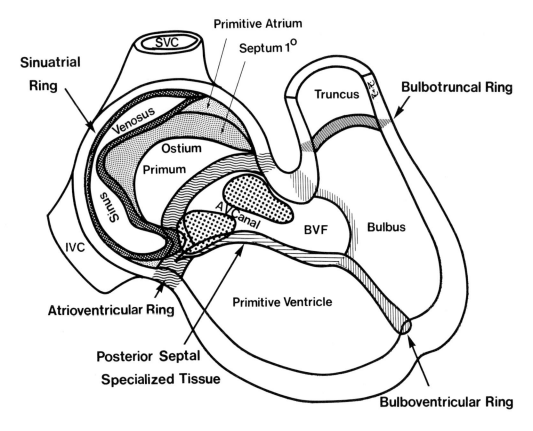

Horizon XV

Fig. 2. Diagram illustrating the disposition of specialized tissues following looping and canal migration, but prior to fusion of the endocardial cushions (bold stipple). The specialized rings are in the same symbols as for figure 1. The atrial septal primordia are depicted by various forms of hatching (primitive atrium, septum 1°). The heart is depicted as viewed from its right side looking through the as yet unseptated ostium atrioventriculare. The primitive ventricle is shown as though septated by the posterior septum. The primordium of the compact node is astride this septum (posterior septal specialized tissue). Although drawn in a differing cross-hatch, our results indicate that this tissue is derived from a posterior invagination of the atrioventricular ring. Note that the sinuatrial ring is in the posterior atrial wall. SVC = superior vena cava. IVC = inferior vena cava. BVF = bulboventricular foramen. 1° = primum.

significance to development of the junctional area. In the ensuing account, therefore, we will presume that the right ventricle is derived in part from the primitive ventricle and in part from the primitive bulbus.

CONDUCTING TISSUES PRIOR TO COMPLETION OF
ATRIOVENTRICULAR SEPTATION

Study of embryos in the stage at which fusion of the endocardial cushions is about to occur (Horizon XV) is of major significance to concepts of subsequent development of the conducting tissues. At this stage the septum primum is growing down to the cushions and is

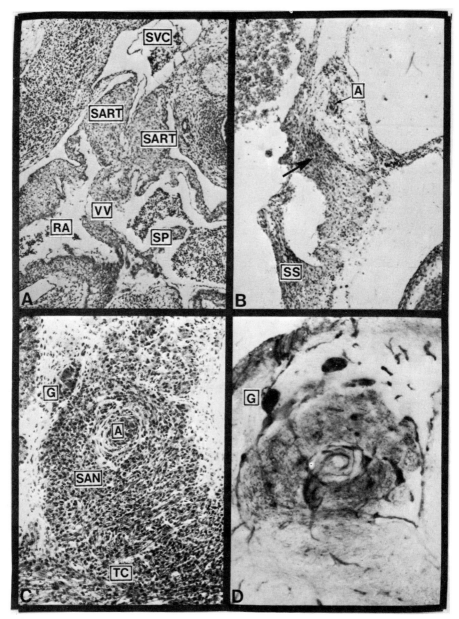

Fig. 3. Photomicrographs illustrating the development of the sinuatrial node. At approximately six weeks of development (fig. 3a) the sinuatrial ring tissue (SART) is thickened at the junction of the superior vena cava (SVC) with the right atrium (RA). Note the prominent venous valves (VV) depending from the sinuatrial junction and the perforated septum primum (SP) which is an outgrowth from the primitive atrial tissue. At approximately 8 weeks of development (fig. 3b) the sinuatrial ring thickening is confined to a small area of tightly packed cells (arrowed) above the septum spurium (SS). The cells do not surround the prominent artery seen at the cavo-atrial junction (A). By 10–12 weeks of development (fig. 3c and d) the cells have proliferated and now surround the nodal artery (A). The sinuatrial nodal cells (SAN) are minimally differentiated from those of the crista terminalis (TC) in histological terms (fig. 3c). However, an adjacent section processed for cholesterase activity (fig. 3d) shows that the nodal cells are ChE positive and are supplied by ChE containing nerves. Note the ganglion cell body which is also ChE positive (G).

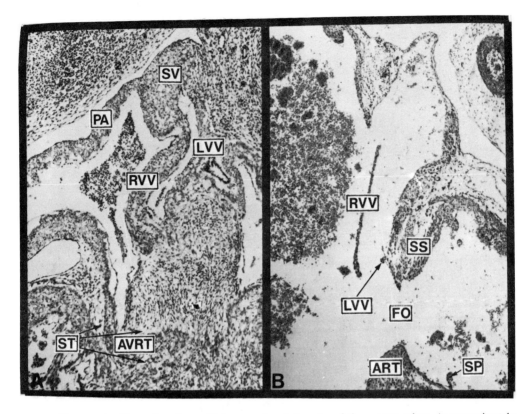

Fig. 4. Photographs illustrating the rapid decrease in relative size of the venous valves. At approximately 6 weeks of development (fig. 4a) the valves are bulky bilaminate structures. Note the extension of a layer of cells from both the primitive atrium (PA) and sinus venosus (SV) into the right venous valve (RVV) which inferiorly abuts against the endocardial cushion (EC). The left venous valve (LVV) is closely adposed to the posterior atrial wall. Note also the atrioventricular ring tissue (AVRT) encased in sulcus tissue (ST). By approximately 8 weeks of development (fig. 4b) the valves have decreased considerably in relative size. The right venous valve (RVV) is a thin sheet of cells while the left venous valve (LVV) is a small structure adherent to the septum secundum (SS). Note that the septum secundum is an invagination of tissue outside the sinus venosus. The inferior part of the foramen ovale (FO) is composed of the posterior invagination of the anterior ring tissue (ART) to which the septum primum (SP) is attached.

becoming perforate at its superior extent. The septum secundum has not yet become invaginated. The septating bulbotruncus is still situated above the proximal bulbus while the primary interventricular foramen is widely patent (fig. 2). The sinuatrial junction is clearly marked by the venous valves. The right venous valve is larger than the left, and superiorly both fuse to form the prominent septum spurium. The sinuatrial ring tissue is thickened at the junction with the superior vena cava, but this thickening is present round medial, lateral and anterior quadrants of the vein (fig. 3a). The venous valves are bilaminate structures, one layer derived from the primitive atrium, the other from the sinus venosus (fig. 4a). The junction with the atrium is confined to the posterior atrial wall, but inferiorly the sinuatrial ring tissue extends forwards around the left sinus horn and impinges upon the atrioventricular ring.

The atrioventricular ring tissue is well marked at this stage, particularly in the right

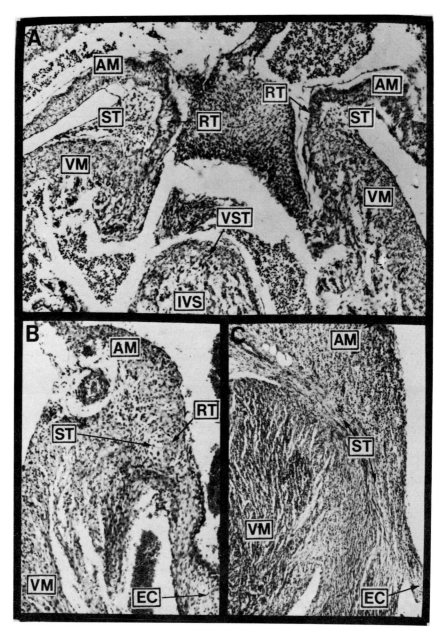

Fig. 5. Photomicrographs illustrating the development of the lateral atrioventricular junctions. At approximately 6 weeks (fig. 5a) atrial (AM) and ventricular (VM) tissues are continuous to both right and left, separated by segments of ring tissue (RT). Note that 'clear' sulcus tissue (ST) fills the epicardial space between atrium and ventricle. Note that the ventricular specialized tissue (VST) is also separated from the ventricular septum (IVS) by clear tissue. This tissue is continuous with the sulcus tissue. EC—endocardial cushions. By 8 weeks (fig. 5b) the sulcus tissue has started to migrate inwards and is sequestrating the ring tissue (RT) to the atrial side. Note that the cushion tissue (EC) is forming the valve cusp. By 16 weeks (fig. 5c) the sulcus tissue has thickened and fused with the valve cusp, derived from cushion tissue. Atrial and ventricular tissues are therefore separated. However, in many instances gaps can still be found in the anulus through which atrioventricular contiguities occur, often via segments of ring tissue. See also figure 19.

lateral segment of the right atrioventricular orifice where it is already differentiated into a circumferential bundle of cells (30). Elsewhere round the orifice the atrial and ventricular tissues are in free communication via the atrioventricular ring segment (fig. 5). The atrioventricular ring tissue is also in close communication with a discrete bundle of cells which sits astride the posterior interventricular septum. Study of our material indicates that this bundle astride the posterior septum is derived by invagination from the atrioventricular ring tissue and is continuous with this tissue (fig. 2). It forms the primordium of the compact atrioventricular node and is surrounded by a layer of 'clear' cells. These 'clear' cells are themselves continuous with the tissue occupying the atrioventricular sulcus, which can be termed 'sulcus tissue' (fig. 5a). Wenink (918,919) has previously emphasized the importance of this tissue, indicating that the nodal primordium is encased within tissue derived from the 'outside' of the heart. The sulcus tissue separates the nodal primordium from the underlying ventricular septum and the overlying endocardial cushion tissue. Since the primordium is derived from the AV ring, as would be expected it bifurcates posteriorly to continue as the right and left portions of the AV ring tissue (fig. 2). The sinuatrial ring tissue abuts against the AV ring derivatives posteriorly while the primitive atrial fibers impinge upon the lateral limbs of ring tissue (fig. 6,7). This arrangement was clearly described by Mall (518) as follows: 'There is a very marked (connection) from the sinus to the inferior septum below. This is composed of muscle fibers which arise as two horns to which the dorsal muscle fibers of the atria stream'.

Thus at this stage, prior to fusion of the endocardial cushions, the 'inputs' to the nodal primordium are via the sinus venosus and the posterior atrial wall. It is possible for anterior fibers to 'feed' the nodal primordium, but only via the circumferential segments of the atrioventricular ring tissue (fig. 6,7).

When the nodal primordium encased in its sulcus tissue is traced anteriorly, it passes into the postero-inferior rim of the primary interventricular foramen (fig. 2). It then becomes directly continuous with a sheet of cells draped across the bulboventricular part of the interventricular septum (fig. 2). Our studies suggest that this tissue is derived from the bulboventricular ring. It is the primordium of the bifurcating bundle and is also encased in 'sulcus' tissue. However, the studies of Wenink (918) indicate that this 'sulcus' tissue is continuous with and derived from the left bulbar ridge. The cells of the bulboventricular ring tissue astride the septum are in turn continuous with the subendocardial cell layers of the trabeculated pouches. As may be anticipated, this arrangement of conducting tissues prior to fusion of the endocardial cushions is reflected in that observed in endocardial cushion defects of the complete type (fig. 8; 484).

DEVELOPMENT OF THE SINUATRIAL NODE

At approximately six weeks of age most of the junction between the superior vena cava and the sinus venosus is thickened (fig. 3a). This is the region of the sinuatrial ring tissue. By approximately 9 weeks of age (40 mm CR fetus) the thickening is confined to the anteromedial quadrant of the cavo-atrial junction and the cells are small and densely packed. An artery is present around the junction, but the SA ring cells do not encase it (fig. 3b).

　　　　　　　R. H. ANDERSON ET AL.

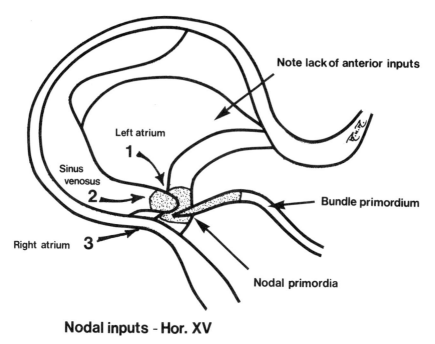

Nodal inputs - Hor. XV

Fig. 6. Diagram illustrating the 'contacts' with the compact nodal primordium prior to establishment of the atrial septum. The nodal 'inputs' are from the posterior atrial wall, occurring through the sinus venosus [2] tissue enclosed within the venous valves), left atrial wall [1] or right atrial wall [3]. There are no direct connections between the anterior atrial wall and the ventricular specialized tissue at this stage except through the circumferential atrioventricular ring specialized tissue.

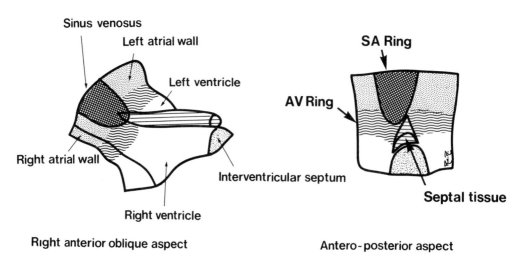

Right anterior oblique aspect　　　　　　　**Antero-posterior aspect**

Horizon XV

Fig. 7. Diagram illustrating the 'contacts' with the compact nodal primordium. This tissue, indicated by broad hatching, is itself derived by an invagination from the AV ring, and the right and left rings bifurcate posteriorly from the main primordium. The 'inputs' as indicated in figure 6 are from the right and left primitive atrial walls and the sinus venosus.

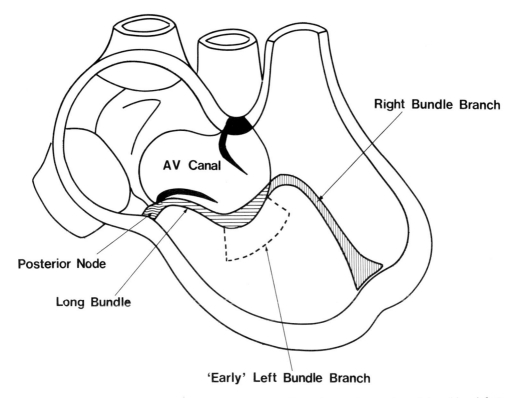

Fig. 8. Diagram illustrating the disposition of conducting tissues in complete endocardial cushion defects. Our own studies in this anomaly are in keeping with those of Lev (484). We believe that the 'long' AV bundle is the primordium of the compact node, which persists as a bundle owing to the deficiency of the atrial septum. The node is small, and makes contact only with the posterior atrial wall. The left bundle branch is related to the posterior septum. This arrangement is reminiscent of the embryonic conducting tissues prior to fusion of the endocardial cushions (see fig. 2).

In a single 28 mm fetus it was noted that cholinesterase containing nerves were also aggregated in this area, such fibers not being visible elsewhere in the heart. By 11 weeks of development (90 mm CR length) the antero-medial thickening is seen to have become aggregated around the prominent artery, and the area is recognizable as the sinuatrial node (fig. 4c). Histological differentiation is minimal but adjacent sections processed for cholinesterase show that the nodal cells are easily distinguished by their enzymic content and are supplied by cholinesterase containing nerve fibers (fig. 4d). The nodal cells are small and densely packed. The node is an antero-lateral structure and possesses a well formed tail or cauda which extends inferiorly and epicardially along the crista terminalis well below the opening of the inferior vena cava, as shown by reconstruction of one of our specimens (fig. 21). At the margins of the node the cells become less tightly packed and a zone of transitional cells, often elongated and attenuated, merges gradually with the atrial myocardium. The finding of relatively late differentiation of the sinuatrial node is in keeping with the results of Boyd (87). Tracts of specialized cells extending from the node into the atrial tissues were not identified.

DEVELOPMENT OF THE INTERNODAL MYOCARDIUM

The precise nature of development of the septum has a bearing upon both the nature of the internodal tissues and the formation of the atrioventricular junctional area. Study of our specimens indicates that the septum primum is an outgrowth of the primitive atrium, originating to the left of the sinuatrial ring. Similar prior observations were made by Los (505) and Van Praagh and Corsini (634). The septum secundum is an invagination of primitive atrial tissue, as also indicated by Los (505). This is well demonstrated by the finding of the remnant of the left venous valve adposed to the right fold of the invagination of the septum secundum (fig. 4b). The position of the left venous valve extends backwards along the superior limbus of the fossa ovalis, and then projects downwards behind the fossa overlying the septum primum (fig. 9). Thus the sinuatrial ring and the sinus venosus are positioned in the posterior atrial wall and are completely posterior to the foramen ovale. In our specimens larger than 40 mm the venous valves have become

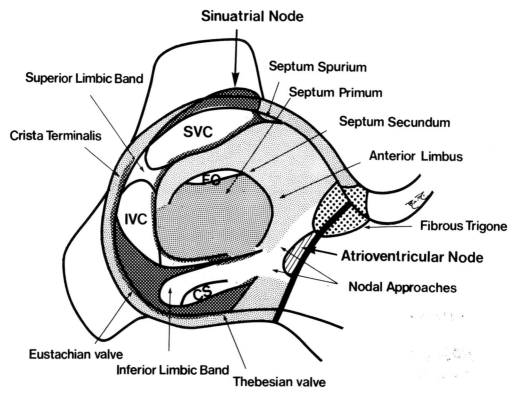

Fig. 9. Diagram illustrating the embryonic origins of the interatrial septum. The nodal appraoches are left blank, and these will be considered in detail in figure 12. The sinus venosus, enclosed by the right and left venous valves, is situated in the posterior atrial wall. The right venous valve persists as the Eustachian and Thebesian valves, while the inferior limbic band sweeps forwards into the nodal approaches as the sinus septum. The tissues above and in front of the foramen ovale (FO) are derived from the primitive atrial tissues. The septum primum is an ingrowth while the septum secundum is an invagination from the primitive atrial wall. Abbreviations as for other diagrams. CS = coronary sinus.

much reduced in size and their constituent cells are cytologically indistinguishable from atrial myocardium (fig. 4b). In contrast, the cells of the sinuatrial node and atrioventricular junctional area are becoming increasingly differentiated from atrial cells. Thus, although the sinuatrial ring tissue and sinus venosus musculature undoubtedly extend from the sinuatrial node to the atrioventricular junctional area (fig. 9) the constituent cells of this area do NOT constitute histologically specialized tracts. We are unable to find specialized tracts such as described by James (393) using either histological or histochemical criteria. We would also point out that two of these postulated tracts are to their largest extent outside the sinuatrial ring (fig. 10). This fact has previously been commented upon by Van Mierop (549). We have indicated elsewhere (410) that strict criteria regarding morphological specialization had been laid down early in this century regarding these tracts and would repeat that we do not yet consider that these criteria have been fulfilled. We there-

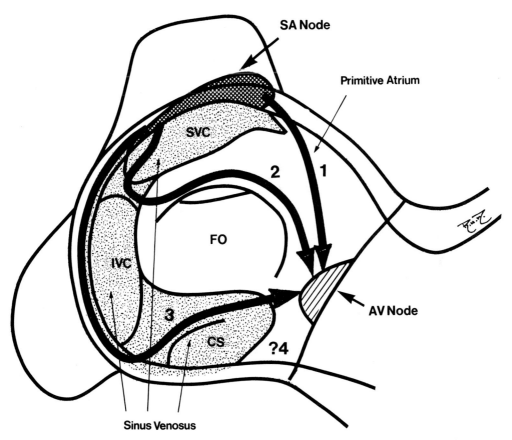

Fig. 10. Diagram illustrating the embryonic nature of the possible routes between the sinuatrial and atrioventricular nodes. (Compare with fig. 9.) The sinus venosus is the cross-hatched area. The postulated 'specialized pathways' reported by James (393) are indicated by arrows 1–3. We were unable to distinguish specialized tracts in these muscle bands, and it should be noted that the greater parts of routes 1 and 2 are without the sinus venosus. Note also that a fourth potential route (?4) exists beneath the coronary sinus. This pathway supplies a good proportion of nodal 'input' in our experience, but was not discussed by James (393). Abbreviations as for previous diagrams.

fore prefer on the basis of our histological investigations to describe the internodal tissues as the internodal atrial myocardium.

Subsequent studies using techniques other than light microscopy may well indicate that 'preferential' conduction is dependent upon a morphological property of a given cell. However, until such time as this is proven we prefer to stand by the criteria of Aschoff (39) and Mönckeberg (563) which were laid down for use by light microscopists.

DEVELOPMENT OF THE TRANSITIONAL ZONE OF THE JUNCTIONAL AREA

The precise nature of the tissues contributing to the nodal approaches is entirely dependent upon the mode of formation of the lower portion of the atrial septum. The potential contributors to this structure are shown in figure 11. The forward sweep of the venous

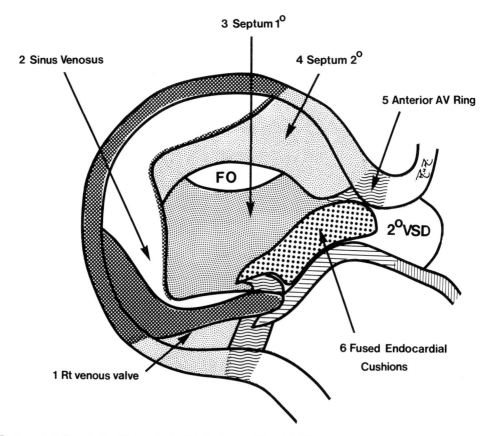

Potential Contributions to Inf. Limbus - Hor. XVII

Fig. 11. Knowledge of embryonic make-up of the inferior part of the atrial septum is essential in order to elucidate the nature of the nodal approaches. This diagram illustrates the potential contributors to this structure. Our findings indicate that the major contributors are 2) sinus venosus, 3) septum primum (1°) and 5) the anterior AV ring. Abbreviations as before. 2° = secondary. VSD = ventricular septal defect.

valves takes sinus venosus tissue on to the nodal primordium, and the sinus septum forms an important posterior contribution. The endocardial cushions, although prominent in early development, do not contribute markedly to the tissue of the septum. However, a backward invagination of the anterior AV ring tissue, together with its adjacent sulcus tissue, forms the important anterior component of the septum. This tissue, together with the lower edge of the septum primum, forms the main septum in front of and beneath the fossa ovalis. It is likely that the posterior invagination of the ring tissue forms the so-called 'inferior' limb of the septum secundum depicted by earlier investigations. However, our studies indicate that the ring tissue invagination is discrete from that forming the septum secundum at the superior margin of the foramen ovale.

DEVELOPMENT OF THE ATRIOVENTRICULAR NODE

It is evident that development of the definitive node is produced by a process of apposition of the inferior edge of the developing atrial septum with the nodal primordium

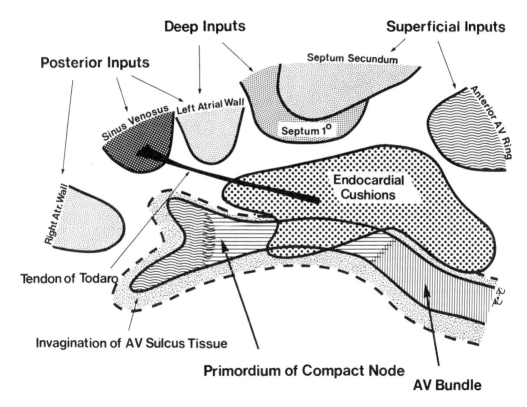

Fig. 12. Elaboration of figure 11 showing the possible origins of the atrioventricular junctional area. The AV bundle is a derivative of the bulboventricular ring. The primordium of the compact node is an invagination of the posterior AV ring tissue. Note that this primordium is separated by posterior AV sulcus tissue from the ventricular tissues, and that the endocardial cushions are situated superiorly to the compact node—AV bundle junction. The potential contributors to the transitional cell zone of the nodal approaches are shown in groups of posterior, deep and superficial inputs. The Tendon of Todaro is illustrated. This is probably derived from anterior and posterior sulcus tissue.

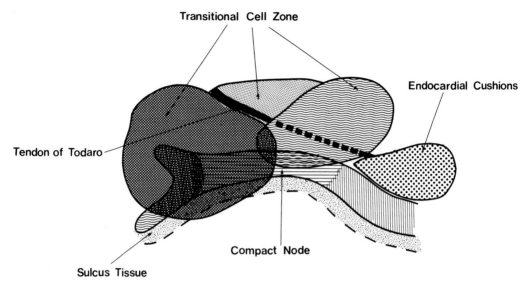

Fig. 13. Diagram illustrating the origin of the definitive atrioventricular junctional area. The compact nodal primordium is derived from the anterior invagination of the posterior AV ring tissue, and its two posterior extensions represent the right and left portions of the ring. It passes between the posterior sulcus tissue and endocardial cushion tissue to become the penetrating bundle, where it fuses with bulbo-ventricular ring tissue. The posterior transitional cell zone is derived from the anterior prolongation of the sinus venosus together with primitive atrial tissue. The deep transitional cells, beneath the Tendon of Todaro, are probably of septum primum origin while the superficial and anterior transitional cells are derived from the posterior invagination of the anterior AV ring tissue. The Tendon of Todaro is probably derived from sulcus tissue.

initially developed astride the posterior ventricular septum (fig. 2). In this way the anterior atrial myocardium is brought into direct contact with the nodal primordium. The invagination of the posterior AV ring tissue, together with its two posterior limbs, therefore forms the primordium of the compact node. The contributions from the sinus septum and posterior atrial wall become specialized to form the posterior transitional cell zone (fig. 12). Since the invagination of the anterior ring tissue forms the main part of the anterior septum, it follows that cells from this anlagen will form the main part of the anterior 'input' to the compact node, while cells from the septum primum and left atrial wall will form the deep 'inputs'. (Compare fig. 12 and 13.) As the endocardial cushions become less bulky structures, so more of these anterior transitional fibers overlay and make direct contact with the primordium of the compact node. It is important to appreciate that the endocardial cushions, together with anterior sulcus tissue, separate the compact nodal primordium from the atrial myocardial tissues. In contrast, the posterior sulcus tissues separate the compact node and its extensions from the ventricular myocardial tissues. It therefore follows that posterior sulcus tissue forms the anulus fibrosus and separates compact node from ventricles (fig. 14,15). It is by passage beneath the endocardial cushion and anterior sulcus tissue that the compact nodal primordium becomes isolated from the atrial myocardium, and by our definition becomes the penetrating bundle (fig. 14–16). The penetrating bundle is therefore sandwiched between posterior sulcus tissue inferiorly and endocardial cushion tissue superiorly (fig. 15,16). The formation of the anulus from the posterior sulcus tissue is a slow process.

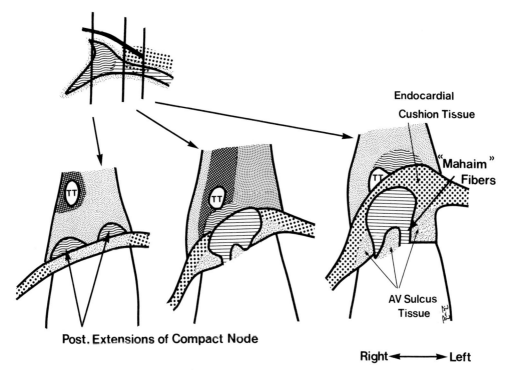

Endocardial Cushion Tissue

"Mahaim" Fibers

AV Sulcus Tissue

Post. Extensions of Compact Node

Right ◄───► Left

Fig. 14. Diagram illustrating the relationships between the compact nodal primordium, the posterior AV sulcus tissue and the endocardial cushion tissue. The anterior sulcus tissue and the upper reaches of the posterior sulcus tissue are not illustrated. The three diagrams are imaginary frontal sections through the junctional area in the planes shown in the inset (TT = Tendon of Todaro). Note that the sulcus tissue separates the compact node and its posterior extensions from the ventricular septum. The nodal primordium passes between the sulcus tissue and the endocardial cushion tissue to become the penetrating bundle (right hand diagram). Note also that until the fibrous anulus is formed from the sulcus tissue (a relatively late event) remnants of the compact nodal primordium continue to make contact with the ventricular septum. If these persisted into adult life they would constitute 'Mahaim' fibers. See also figure 15.

By twelve to fourteen weeks of development strands of conducting tissue are still present connecting the compact node to ventricular myocardium throughout the junctional area. In newborn specimens 'rests' of such strands are found scattered amongst the anulus and the central fibrous body, and in some cases nodo-ventricular connections are still present. We have identified these 'rests' in many adult specimens studied. We have never identified pathological changes in the 'rests', and we have not seen the so-called 'remoulding' of these fragments reported by James (400). Our findings are in keeping with those of Valdes-Dapena et al. (850) and we consider the 'rests' to be a consequence of normal nodal development. We have been unable to find evidence to implicate such changes in 'sudden death in infancy' syndrome (26).

COMMENT ON DEVELOPMENT OF THE ATRIOVENTRICULAR NODE

It is evident from the above description that our findings suggest that the atrioventricular junctional area is derived from multiple developmental sources. The 'compact' node is

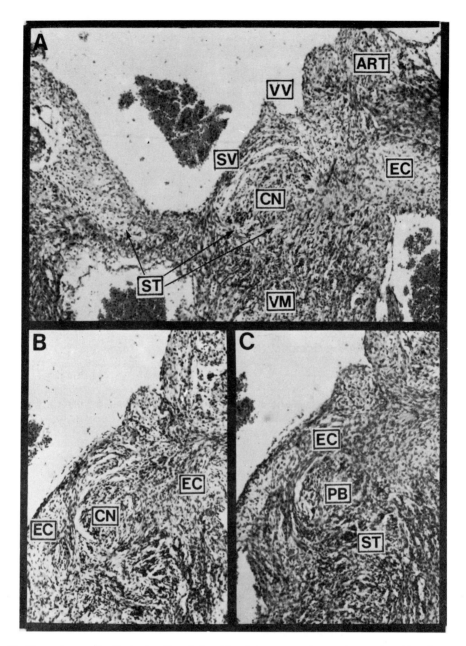

Fig. 15. Photomicrographs illustrating the relationship of compact node to sulcus and cushion tissue at approximately 8 weeks of development. Figure 15a shows a posterior section through the junctional area. The compact node (CN) is overlaid by the sinus venosus input (SV), note the remnant of the venous valve (VV), and the invagination of the anterior ring tissue is seen superiorly (ART). The cushion tissue is to the mitral side (EC), and elsewhere the nodal and atrial tissues are incompletely separated from ventricular myocardium (VM) by the developing anulus fibrosus, composed of sulcus tissue (ST). A more anterior section (fig. 15b) shows the nodal primordium (CN) sinking between the two extensions of the cushion tissue (EC). The sulcus tissue is separating the node from the septum, and the node is still in contact with the transitional cell zones superiorly. A section yet further anterior (fig. 15c) shows that the nodal primordium has passed beneath the cushions (EC) to become the penetrating bundle (PB). The sulcus tissue (ST) is still separating the bundle from the ventricular myocardium, while cushion tissue and anterior sulcus tissue separate it from the atrial septum.

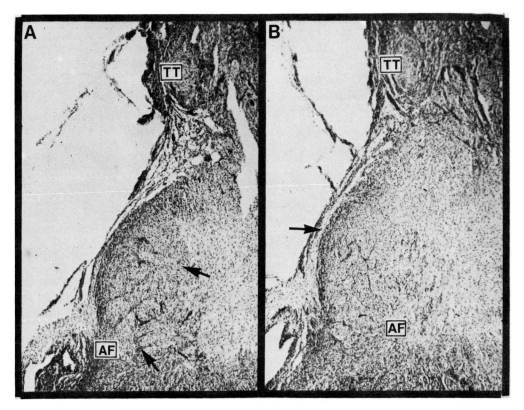

Fig. 16. Microphotographs of a later stage (about 16 weeks) showing development of the junctional area (compare with figure 15). Figure 16a is a section through the node which now approximates to its infantile appearance. Note, however, that 'rests' of compact node (arrowed) are interspersed amongst the developing anulus fibrosus (AF), derived from sulcus tissue. Note also the Tendon of Todaro (TT) separating superficial and deep inputs to the node. A section taken more anteriorly (fig. 16b) shows how an upward extension from the tricuspid valve (arrowed, cushion tissue) is beginning to separate the overlay cells from the nodal primordium. When this tissue is complete above the node, separating it from the atrial inputs, the node will become the penetrating bundle. Again note the extensions from the node into the fibrous anulus (FA). This is a natural consequence of development of the anulus from sulcus tissue.

developed from the atrioventricular ring tissue and its posterior invagination. The nodal approaches and their transitional cells are drived from a. the sinuatrial ring, b. the septum primum, c. the anterior part of the AV ring, and to a smaller extent from d. the primitive atrium (fig. 13). It follows therefore that in our opinion it is futile to argue as to whether the node develops from left sinus horn (129, 619, 651) or atrioventricular canal musculature (430, 518, 712) since we believe both structures contribute to the definitive node, together with other tissues. However, we would question theories which suggest that the junctional area develops by a process of 'active migration'. We question if it is possible to elucidate the nature of such dynamic events from microscopical study.

In summary, we consider the node to have multiple origins and we believe that this viewpoint is supported by both histochemical evidence (23) and by evidence adduced from cases exhibiting complete heart block (300).

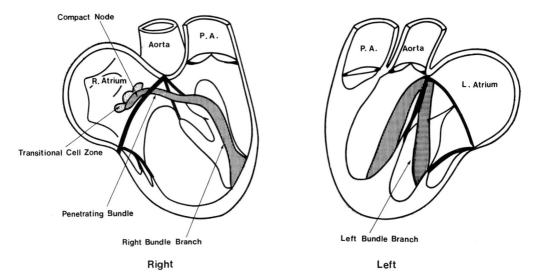

Fig. 17. Diagram illustrating the presumed origins of the definitive bundle branches. The right bundle branch is, we believe, the persisting bulboventricular ring, hence its position at the junction of primitive ventricular and bulbar portions of the interventricular septum. In contrast, we believe the left bundle branch to be formed in part from the bulboventricular specialized tissue and in part from the atrioventricular specialized tissue. This would account for its wider distribution and the fact that distally in the ventricles it forms two divisions.

DEVELOPMENT OF THE VENTRICULAR SPECIALIZED TISSUE

It is our belief that the ventricular conducting tissues are developed by expansion of the bulboventricular ring. This origin provides a good explanation for the position of the thin right bundle branch beneath the trabecula septomarginalis, which marks the point of bulboventricular junction (fig. 17). It also explains why the conducting fibers are related to the trabecular portion of the right ventricle but not the inflow portion. However, it is possible that the left bundle branch is derived in part from the posterior nodal primordium. In favour of this origin is the more widespread distribution of the left bundle branch and the fact that in atrioventricular canal deformities the left bundle fibers are undoubtedly related to the posterior ventricular septum. The finding that distally in the ventricle the left bundle tends to divide into two radiations with a thinly dispersed septal radiation would also support a dual origin for the left bundle branch.

DEVELOPMENT OF THE LATERAL ATRIOVENTRICULAR JUNCTIONS

The atrioventricular ring tissue becomes particularly well developed in the right atrioventricular orifice by the 20 mm stage, and at this stage morphological atrioventricular connections are still present throughout the AV orifices (30). An expansion of the AV ring tissue is almost always present at the right anterior quadrant of the tricuspid orifice in the position in which Kent (434) described his 'node' (fig. 18). It may well be significant that this anterior node is formed above the lateral bulboventricular junction. When traced

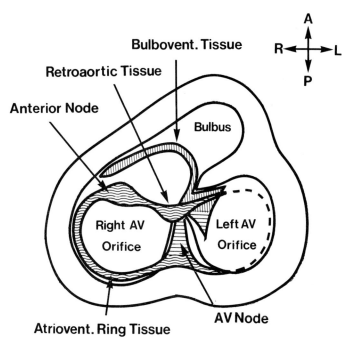

Fig. 18. Plan view illustrating the disposition of the ring tissues in an embryo up to mid-term. The AV node is itself an invagination of the AV ring tissue, and its right posterior extension is continuous with a ring encircling the tricuspid (right AV) orifice. The ring is expanded anterio-laterally at the bulboventricular junction, and here in earlier embryos is in close contact with the bulboventricular ring tissue. This is the situation of the anterior node described by Kent (434). The ring tissue continues medially and expands into a second node like structure in the retro-aortic tissue. The bulbotruncal ring probably contributes to the formation of this structure. Orientation is indicated by the compass: A = anterior. P = posterior. R = right. L = left.

medially the ring tissue again expands into a second node-like structure in the retroaortic position, and it is from this tissue that conducting fibers can be traced into the anterior nodal inputs. The ring tissue, and the atrial tissues in general become separated from the ventricular myocardium by an ingrowth of atrioventricular sulcus tissue (fig. 5,19). As with the septal region, it is the sulcus tissue which forms the anulus fibrosus, and also as in the septum complete division of atrial and ventricular tissues is a relatively late event (fig. 5). Careful examination of most full term specimens reveals the presence of defects in the anulus through which atrial and ventricular musculatures are contiguous, frequently via persisting segments of ring tissue. However, well formed bundles of myocardium crossing or perforating the anulus fibrosus have yet to be identified in our 'normal' material.

The anterior 'node' is of considerable significance in malformed specimens. In situations when the posterior septum is misplaced or absent we have found that the normal node is not properly formed, but its place is taken by the anterior 'node'. Such situations are primitive ventricular hearts (27) and classically corrected transposition (28). It is tempting to speculate that in these situations the anterior bundle is derived from the right lateral part of the bulboventricular ring tissue (fig. 20) in this way coming into direct contact with the ventricular specialized tissue, also part of the bulboventricular ring. This concept is further supported by situations in which both anterior and the normally

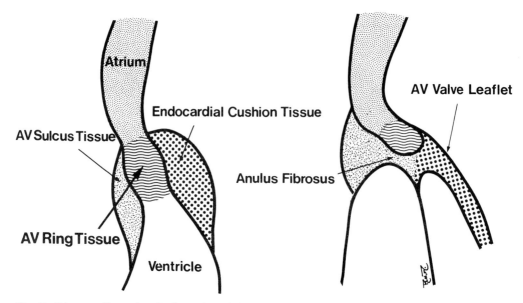

Fig. 19. Diagrams illustrating the formation of the anulus fibrosus. The left hand diagram is an early stage
when atrioventricular connection is effected through a segment of ring tissue. AV sulcus tissue is seen
epicardially and cushion tissue endocardially. The anulus is formed (right hand diagram) by inward migration
of the sulcus tissue. This sequestrates the ring tissue in the atrial myocardium. The endocardial cushion tissue
forms the valve cusp. See also figure 5.

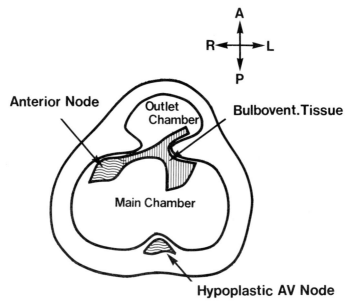

Fig. 20. Diagram illustrating how the anterior node can form the atrioventricular connection when absence
of the posterior septum prevents formation of the normal node. Primitive ventricle with outlet chamber is illustrated as an example of this disposition (27) but a similar disposition is encountered in classically corrected
transposition (28). Orientation as for figure 18.

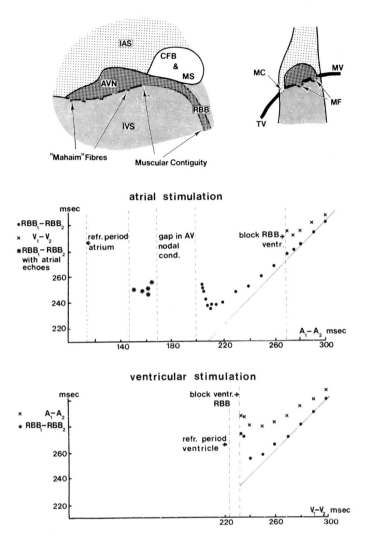

Fig. 21. Upper panel: diagrammatic representation of the atrioventricular junctional area from a twelve week fetal heart on which electro-physiological experiments had been conducted, demonstrating that atrioventricular conduction was comparable to that of an adult heart. However, on sectioning the heart, the anulus fibrosis was found to be incompletely formed, permitting widespread atrioventricular continuity through 'Mahaim fibers' (MF) and direct muscular contiguities (MC). IAS = interatrial septum. IVS = interventricular septum. TV = tricuspid valve. MV = mitral valve, AUN = atrioventricularnode. CFB = central fibrous body. MS = membranous septum. RBB = right bundle branch. *Middle panel:* the right atrium was stimulated close to the sinus node at a cycle length of 350 msec. After every 10th beat, a premature stimulus was given. Recordings were made at the right bundle branch, about halfway between the tricuspid valve base and the conal papillary muscle, and at the apex of the right ventricle. Note 'gap' in AV conduction at A1A2 intervals between 170 and 200 msec. At shorter intervals, atrial premature beats were conducted to the right bundle branch accompanied by atrial echo's. The ventricular myocardium was protected by the AV conducting system, since the shortest interval between conducted impulses at the level of the right bundle branch was 235 msec, which is 10 msec longer than the refractory period of the ventricular myocardium. *Lower panel:* the right ventricle was stimulated at the apex. Block occurred at the junction of ventricular myocardium and the right bundle branch at an interval of 230 msec. In antegrade direction, block occurred at an interval of 268 msec (middle panel), indicating that retrograde conduction had a larger margin of safety than antegrade conduction across the RBB-myocardial junction.

positioned posterior nodes are connected to ventricular conducting tissues by anterior and posterior bundles. Such cases were described by Mönckeberg and Anderson (24, 28, 562). We find it difficult to account for the presence of two bundles using any other concept of development.

PHYSIOLOGICAL DEVELOPMENT OF CONDUCTING TISSUE

An important consideration in development is the stage at which the conducting system functions in an 'adult' fashion. We have recently studied developing hearts using both electrophysiological and anatomical techniques in an attempt to elucidate this problem (411). In these human fetal specimens, ranging in age from 11 to 16 weeks, it was significant that the conduction pathways were to all intents and purposes functionally 'normal'. However, anatomical studies demonstrated that the anulus fibrosus was improperly formed throughout the junctional area, and that multiple connections were present between the compact node and its overlay fibers and the ventricular myocardium (fig. 21). This finding demonstrates the dangers inherent in implying functional characteristics from morphological observations. It also illustrates that the human conducting tissue is functionally mature from an early age, unlike the situation reported in other mammals by Preston et al. (636). It further suggests that immaturity of the conducting system is unlikely to be a factor in producing 'sudden death in infancy', as proposed by Dawes (184). We also studied the atrial tissues of these specimens, and were only able to record 'specialized' action potentials from the areas subsequently shown to be nodal by three-dimensional reconstruction (fig. 22). 'Plateau' action potentials in contrast were widely distributed through the atrial myocardial tissues. Our maps of the spread of activation supported the contention of Spach and his colleagues (775, 776) that the sinus impulse was conducted to the atrioventricular node through the atrial myocardial bands delineated by the holes in the interatrial septum (fig. 23).

POSTNATAL DEVELOPMENT OF THE CONDUCTING TISSUES

It is our experience that the conducting tissues in the full term fetus have reached their complete state of development. We would consider that from birth onwards there is a gradual reduction in the overall size of both the sinuatrial and atrioventricular nodes relative to the rest of the heart. Certainly in the adult the atrioventricular junctional area is much less well differentiated than in the infant, and this point will be elaborated in a subsequent chapter. Whether such changes should be considered as 'development' of conducting tissue is questionable. James (403) has described considerable 'moulding' of the tissue occurring postnatally. We have already alluded to the presence of 'rests' of the compact node in the central fibrous body and septal anulus fibrosus. We consider these an inevitable consequence of normal development, and as will be demonstrated subsequently (page 268), such 'rests' are found in the majority of normal adult hearts. In our experience they have not been the seat of pathological change and we would hesitate before implicat-

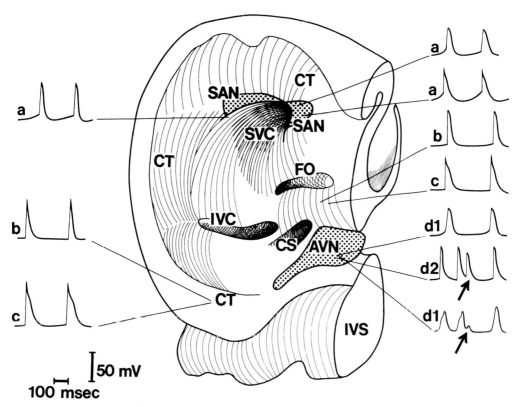

Fig. 22. Reconstruction of another twelve week human fetal heart showing action potentials recorded from the approximate site indicated by the pointers. Potentials with diastolic depolarization (a) were confined to the region of the sinuatrial node (SAN). Cells which exhibited a typical Wenckebach phenomenon (d1, d2) were recorded only from the atrioventricular node (AVN). Cells with a 'plateau' action potential (c) were scattered through the atrial musculature, and non-plateau cells (b) with similar activation times were always recorded in adjacent positions. In the specimen the reconstruction also showed that the tail of the sinus node extended caudally along the crista terminalis (CT) outside the ostium of the inferior vena cava (IVC). Other abbreviations as before. Reproduced from Janse et al., (411), by permission of the *Amer. Heart J.*

ing them as a possible source for circus movement (406). We would certainly agree that formation of the anulus fibrosus continues after birth, and disruption of septal atrioventricular connections such as described by Truex et al. (834) may well be an explanation of the benign nature of some forms of infantile paroxysmal tachycardias (510). However, examination of 'normal' adult lateral and septal junctions again reveals presence of multiple potential atrioventricular contiguities, and emphasises the dangers of extrapolating from structure to function without careful electrophysiological control.

DEVELOPMENT OF INNERVATION OF CONDUCTING TISSUE

We have studied the innervation of conducting tissues up to the midterm stage using both cholinesterase and fluorescence techniques (23). In our experience, cholinesterase-

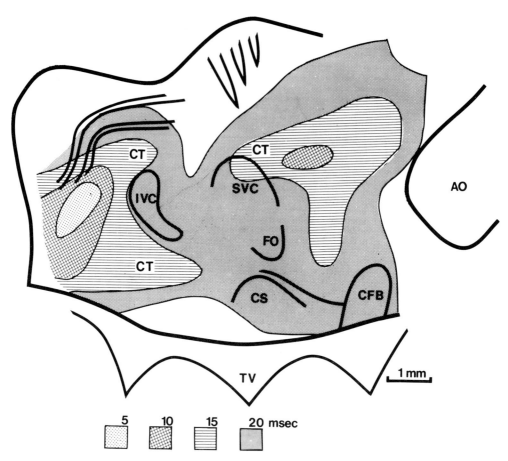

Fig. 23. Diagram of the spread of activation in the atrial tissues of the fetal heart reconstruction shown in figure 22. The cross-hatched and stippled areas represent the areas enclosed within 5 msec isochrones as shown in the key. The two earliest areas correspond to the two cristal 'insertions' of the sinus node to the posterior crista terminalis and the anterior limbus respectively. Note that spread is almost uniform and is governed by the geometry of the atrial septum. Narrow tracts conducting in advance of the remaining atrial tissues are not observed. Abbreviations as before. Reproduced from Janse et al. (411) by permission of the *Amer. Heart J.*

containing nerves appear early during development, being observed adjacent to the sinus venosus in a 28 mm embryo. By 12 weeks of development, a rich cholinesterase containing nerve plexus is distributed throughout the atria and around the coronary arteries, being particularly abundant in relation to the sinuatrial node (fig. 4) and the transitional cells of the atrioventricular junctional area (fig. 24a). The compact node itself is not well innervated, but is conspicuous by its cholinesterase content, as is the ventricular specialized tissue (fig. 24). We did not find cholinesterase positive nerves related to the ventricular conducting tissues in the human fetus, unlike Kent et al. (435) who reported such nerves in adult tissues. However, we have grave doubts as to whether the so-called 'nerves' are indeed nerve fibers. We ourselves observed similar activity in canine preparations to that reported by these investigators, but we attributed it to surface activity (fig. 24). We hesitate to consider the human or canine ventricular specialized tissue as being innervated by

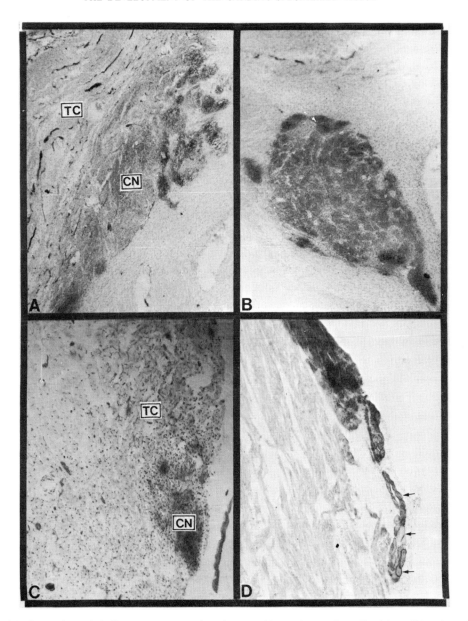

Fig. 24. Comparison of cholinesterase preparations from a mid-term human fetus (fig. 24a and b) and an adult dog (fig. 24c and d). Figure 24a is from the atrioventricular node. Note that its transitional cell (TC) and compact zones (CN) can be distinguished by their innervation pattern and enzymic contact. The transitional cell zone is innervated; the compact node is devoid of nerves but is itself ChE positive. Figure 24b is from the atrio-ventricular bundle. Note that the cells are ChE positive, but that nerves are not seen. Figure 24c is from the dog node and is counterstained with haematoxylin. As in the human fetus, the transitional cells are well in-nervated (TC), and the compact part of the node (CN) is richly ChE positive. In contrast, the cells of the canine left bundle branch (fig. 24d, section not counterstained) are themselves ChE positive but do not contain nerves. The circumferential activity around individual cells (arrowed) is in our opinion sarcolemmal activity, and not neural as claimed by Kent et al. (435). Compare this activity with the nerves seen in relation to transitional cells in figure 24c. All sections are processed using Gomori's technique as described in Anderson and Taylor (23).

cholinergic fibers until proven by ultrastructural studies. We were unable to detect adrenergic fibers related to the conducting tissues by the midterm stage, and as James (403) suggested, this probably suggests late development of sympathetic control as opposed to parasympathetic control. Nonetheless, failure of demonstration of fluorescence is not proof of lack of adrenergic activity, and again it is likely that ultrastructural studies are necessary to elucidate fully the development of the innervation pattern of the conducting tissues.

CONCLUSIONS

We believe that the definitive conducting tissues are remnants or expansions of discrete junctional rings of specialized tissue identifiable in the young embryo. The sinuatrial node represents the antero-lateral part of the sinuatrial ring at its junction with the superior vena cava. Histological differentiation of this node is a relatively late event. Although the sinuatrial ring remnants extend between the differentiated sinuatrial node and the atrio-ventricular junctional area, we are unable to detect evidence of histologically or histochemically discrete specialized tracts connecting the nodes. The definitive atrio-ventricular junctional area is not formed until septation is complete. However, the primordium of the compact node is clearly identified at the stage of development of the posterior interventricular septum. It is transformed into the definitive junctional area only with the establishment of deep and superficial inputs from the atrial septum. It is of great significance that the anulus fibrosus is formed from the sulcus tissue which originally surrounds the nodal primordium and separates it from the ventricular septum, whereas the endocardial cushion remnants, together with the sulcus tissue, separate the compact node from the anterior atrial myocardium at the site of formation of the penetrating bundle. We consider the definitive junctional area to be derived from multiple developmental sources and therefore believe arguments relative to a single origin for the node to be non-productive.

We have emphasized the importance of other remnants of the atrioventricular ring tissue, both to unusual atrioventricular connections in malformed hearts and to possible accessory atrioventricular connections in normal hearts. It is our experience that the specialized tissues are fully developed at term and we question if subsequent changes should be considered as 'development'. Finally, we have presented evidence from combined functional and anatomic studies which highlight the possible dangers of extrapolating from morphologic investigations without electrophysiological controls.

ACKNOWLEDGEMENTS

We are grateful to our colleagues who collaborated with us in previous investigations, and whose co-operation was instrumental in formulating some of the concepts here presented. We are particularly indebted to Mrs. Audrey Smith, Mr. R. Stuckey and Miss Mary Huntington for their assistance in the preparation of both material and the final manuscript.

2

ELECTROPHYSIOLOGY OF THE INTACT NEONATAL CANINE ATRIOVENTRICULAR CONDUCTING SYSTEM[1]

HENRY GELBAND, M.D., KRISTINA NILSSON, RUEY J. SUNG, M.D.,
ARTHUR L. BASSETT, Ph.D., AND ROBERT J. MYERBURG, M.D.

INTRODUCTION

Over the past few years, there have been several clinical investigations concerning the electrophysiology of the cardiac conducting system in the neonate and pediatric patient (1,57,89,213,450,660–662). These studies using His bundle electrograms, have indicated that there are a number of significant differences between the clinical electrophysiological parameters measured in pediatric patients and adults. For example, it is well known that heart rates are faster, intracardiac conduction times are shorter (57,89,660–662), and atrial and atrioventricular (AV) nodal refractory periods are shorter in children (213). Additionally, there are reports which suggest antiarrhythmic and cardiotonic drugs have cardiac electrophysiological effects which are different from those noted in adult animals (299,665,680). However, there is a paucity of experimental data on the basic electrophysiological properties of the neonatal atrioventricular conducting system. Preston et al. (636) in 1959 described AV transmission in young experimental puppies and observed that premature atrial responses were able to propagate to the ventricle during the vulnerable period of the ventricle and induce ventricular fibrillation. This apparently was possible because the refractory period of the AV node was less than that of the ventricle. More recently, the sequence of excitation of an impulse from sinoatrial node through atrial septum and AV node was described for the puppy heart (770). Rosen (683), as well as Roberts (663) have used microelectrode techniques to define the effects of age on trans-membrane action potential characteristics of Purkinje and ventricular muscle fibers.

None of the clinical or basic electrophysiological studies in the neonate have dealt with the sequence of ventricular endocardial excitation; although this topic has been extensively evaluated in the adult animal (2,96,97,219,224,257,451,476,496,575,577,637,727,728, 769,832,848). Most of the studies on the sequence of ventricular endocardial excitation has been derived from experiments either on intact dog hearts utilizing intramyocardial plunge electrodes or epicardial or endocardial surface electrodes, during cardiopulmonary bypass, on explanted perfused hearts or on models consisting of large areas of isolated

1. Supported in part by grants from the National Foundation March of Dimes, the Heart Association of Greater Miami, the Broward County Heart Associaion and Institutional Research Funds of the Miami Veterans Administration Hospital.

segments of ventricular endocardium which were studied in the tissue bath by micro-electrode or surface electrode recording techniques.

Because of the problems inherent in evaluating partial segments of endocardium, we have developed a system whereby it is possible to simultaneously determine the pattern of endocardial excitation of the total right and left ventricular endocardial surface by micro-electrode and surface electrogram mapping techniques. The model has made possible the study of the mechanism and sequence of endocardial excitation during atrial stimulation with an intact A-V node and His-Purkinje network. We used the 1–2 week puppy heart for this model since information regarding the mechanism and sequence of His-Purkinje and ventricular endocardial activation is not available in the puppy heart, and as indicated above, significant differences may be present between the puppy and its adult counterpart.

PREPARATION OF THE MODEL

Hearts from 1–2 week old puppies were rapidly excised after the animals were anesthetized with ether. The hearts were dissected in oxygenated cooled Tyrode's solution. Initially the right atrial free wall was removed leaving all of the atrial septum and appendage intact. A cut was then made from the anterior junction of the right atrioventricular groove along the superior aspect of the right ventricle to the pulmonary artery and anterior junction of the right ventricular free wall and septum. This cut was extended along the anterior junction of the free wall and septum to the right ventricular apex. The ventricular cavity was carefully opened and the leaflets of the tricuspid valve were removed as well as the chordae tendineae which were severed close to the papillary muscles.

The heart was then turned over and the entire left atrium removed. The left ventricle was opened by an incision through the free wall, midway between the two papillary muscles. This incision extended to the apex of the left ventricle. The anterior leaflet of the mitral valve was cut vertically in its midportion and the cut extended through the aortic root. The chordae tendineae were cut close to the papillary muscles and the mitral valve removed. This procedure exposed the main left bundle branch, its major divisions, the left ventricular septum, papillary muscles and free wall endocardium.

Finally, by careful blunt dissection, the central plane of the ventricular septum was split from the apex of the heart to the base. This dissection was made using the anterior descending branch of the left coronary artery as a landmark for the interventricular septum. It was then possible to lay the myocardium with its two 'flaps' flat in a tissue bath with the right atrium separating right and left ventricles, thus exposing the entire cardiac endocardium and specialized conducting system in one plane (fig. 1).

GENERAL CONSIDERATIONS

Surface stimulation of the right atrium resulted in propagation of an impulse to both ventricles following a delay of 82 to 108 msec depending upon the rate of atrial stimulation.

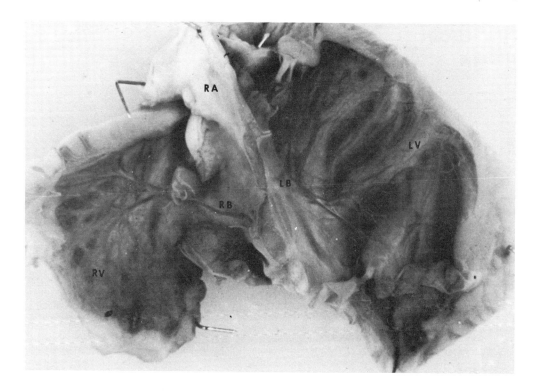

Fig. 1. Pertinent anatomic features of the model. The preparation has been stained with Lugol's solution to demonstrate the glycogen rich ventricular conducting system. The right atrial free wall and left atrium have been removed. Incisions were made to expose the entire right endocardial surface by an incision from the tricuspid valve to the pulmonary outflow tract where it joins the septum, and then down to the apex of the right ventricle along the junction of the right ventricular free wall and septum. An incision along the free wall of the left ventricle from the mitral valve to the apex makes it possible to expose the entire left endo-cardial surface. A final incision then is made through the central plane of the interventricular septum from its apex to its base. Thus, it is possible to lay the preparation flat in a tissue bath and pin it down so the entire right atrium, right ventricle and left ventricular endocardium are in one plane. Note that the right atrium (RA) separates the two ventricular cavities. The right bundle branch (RB) courses down the septum to the base of the anterior papillary muscle, after which it becomes a free running false tendon which then branches profusely on the free wall of the right ventricle (RV) as a dense network of subendocardial Purkinje fibers. The left bundle branch (LB) enters the left ventricle (LV) under the aortic ring. The main LB bifurcates into an anterior and posterior division which course toward the apical regions of their respective papillary muscles. A network of septal subendocardial Purkinje fibers is present between the two divisions. Endocardial ventricular muscle is visible between the conducting tissue.

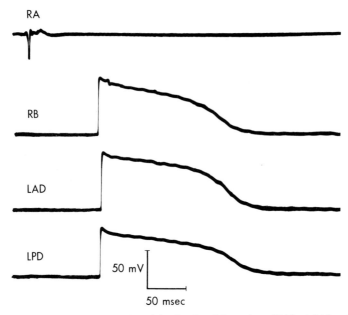

RA

RB

LAD

LPD

50 mV

50 msec

Fig. 2. Simultaneous recording of electrical activity in the right atrium (RA), right bundle branch (RB), left anterior division (LAD), and left posterior division (LPD). In this preparation, the right atrium was generating automatic impulses. A bipolar surface electrogram records RA activity (upper trace). Following transmission of the impulse through the intact atrioventricular junction, transmembrane action potentials are recorded (in the lower three traces) from the RB, LAD and LPD at their junctions with their respective papillary muscles. The transmembrane action potential is recorded in the RB 94 msec after RA activation, Following RB depolarization there is rapid activation of the LPD and then the LAD. Horizontal calibration = 50 msec; vertical calibration = 50 mV.

The right bundle branch (RBB) was usually activated before the left bundle branch (LBB) (fig. 2). In 20 to 23 experiments, activation of the proximal RBB occurred 2 to 9 msec before the main LBB. These measurements were made at the most proximal portion of each bundle as it penetrated the membraneous portion of the ventricular septum. This pattern continued through the Purkinje network at comparable levels of excitation, right ventricular Purkinje fibers being activated before left ventricular Purkinje fibers (fig. 3). The sites of impulse input into ventricular muscle (described in detail below) occurred 4 to 12 msec earlier in right ventricular muscle than in left ventricular muscle. This differs from observations in the adult canine heart, in which left ventricular septal activation precedes right ventricular septal activation (97,728). However, clinical observations substantiate our finding, since newborns frequently lack the small initial q wave in the left precordial leads which is normally interpreted to indicate left to right activation of the septum. Nonetheless, activation of the base of the right and left ventricular endocardial surface occurred almost simultaneously. Thus, it appears that most of the Purkinje fiber and ventricular muscle of the right ventricle is activated prior to their counterparts in the left ventricle except at their respective bases. In order for an excitatory wave front to occur simultaneously at the base of the right and left ventricle, either: 1. conduction has to be faster through ventricular muscle in the left ventricle; 2. right ventricular conduction

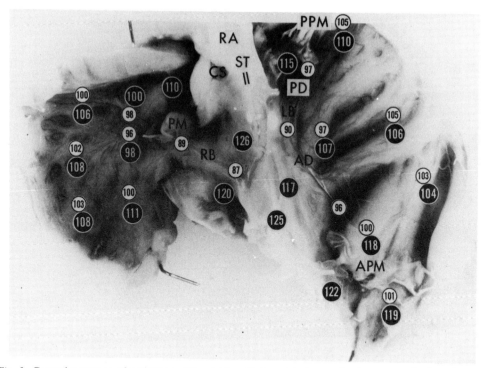

Fig. 3. General sequence of activation of the right and left ventricular conducting system. Surface electrodes (ST) stimulate the right atrium (RA) close to threshold at a cycle length of 800 msec. Black numbers on white backgrounds represent time intervals from stimulus to Purkinje fiber (PF) depolarization. White numbers on black backgrounds are the time intervals from stimulus to ventricular muscle (VM) depolarization, recorded immediately adjacent to PF. The earliest area of ventricular excitation occurs at the penetrating portion of the right bundle (RB). The excitation wave then precedes rapidly down the proximal RB to the anterior papillary muscle (PM), across to the false tendons to the network of conducting tissue on the free wall. VM is initially activated on the apical free wall. The wave of excitation then spreads to the remaining right ventricular free wall and to the base of the septum. The left bundle branch (LB) in this preparation was activated 3 msec after the RB. The sequence of activation then spreads along the anterior (AD) and posterior division (PD) as well as down into the septal interconnecting fibers between the two divisions. Earliest muscle to be activated is the lower third of the septum. This is followed by a divergent wavefront of VM depolarization. One is to the base of the left ventricular septum and the other is to the left ventricular apex. It is obvious that throughout PF and VM depolarization the right ventricle was excited before its counterparts in the left ventricle, except at the basal regions, where right and left ventricle were almost simultaneous. CS = coronary sinus, PPM = posterior papillary muscle, APM = anterior papillary muscle.

delay occurs; or 3, there is a greater mass of right ventricle to be depolarized. We favor the last hypothesis since it is well appreciated that newborns have a relative preponderance of right ventricular mass secondary to a sustained increase in pulmonary arteriolar resistence in utero (581).

In this model, if the RBB, LBB, or free wall of either ventricle was stimulated, propagation of the impulse to the contralateral ventricle occurred; as well as retrograde conduction to the right atrium. There was a delay of 8–14 msec in conduction between bundle branches (fig. 4). However, following this delay, the sequence of excitation was normal for that ventricle. Retrograde conduction to the right atrium occurred following an 80–95 msec delay in the Bundle of His and AV node.

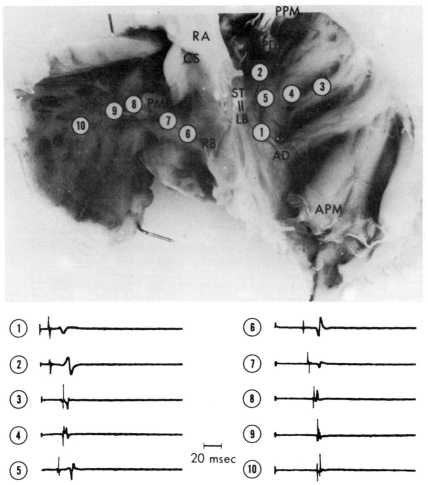

Fig. 4. Patterns of ventricular excitation with bundle branch stimulation. In this preparation, the left bundle branch (LB) was stimulated by surface electrodes (ST) and bipolar surface electrograms were recorded from the numbered sites indicated. The first deflection of each trace represents Purkinje fiber (PF) activation followed by a second deflection which indicates ventricular muscle activation. The numbered electrogram tracings correspond with the numbered sites. The shortest PF-VM interval is located at site 3 in the left ventricular endocardium. This site is the junction of the middle and lower third of the septum. On the right ventricular endocardium the shortest PF-VM interval is located at site 9 which is the right ventricular apical free wall. The sequence of endocardial excitation is similar to that described in figure 3. Similar patterns of endocardial excitation were obtained with RB stimulation. Horizontal calibration 20 msec, CS = coronary sinus, PM = papillary muscle. APM = anterior papillary muscle. PPM = posterior papillary muscle, AD = anterior division, PD = posterior division.

SEQUENCE OF EXCITATION OF THE RIGHT VENTRICULAR ENDOCARDIUM

The RBB is an isolated structure, both anatomically as well as physiologically throughout its course. The RBB descends the septum to the base of the anterior papillary muscle, crosses it, then separates into many free running false tendons which terminate on the

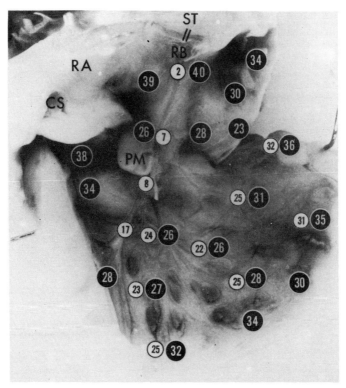

Fig. 5. General sequence of activation of the right ventricular (RV) conducting system and muscle. Preparation consists of RV septum, apex, and free wall. The proximal right bundle branch (RB) was stimulated (ST) with surface electrodes where it penetrated the uppermost area of the ventricular septum. The sequence of excitation was from proximal to distal in specialized conducting tissue along the RB. Conduction proceeds across the base of the papillary muscle (PM) and then to the false tendons and finally to diffuse ramifications on the RV free wall. Initial muscle activation was the apical and free wall endocardium where the Purkinje fiber-ventricular muscle (PF-VM) interval was 2 msec. Black numbers on white backgrounds represent time intervals from stimuli to PF depolarization. White numbers on black backgrounds are times from stimulus to VM depolarization. Note that after initial depolarization of the apical wall two divergent wavefront occurs. One is through the septum (from apex to base). The PF-VM interval progressively increases as the impulse travels closer to the base of the RV septum. The second wave of excitation procedes to the remaining free wall of the RV where the PF-VM interval again increases. The base of the septum and free wall are depolarized almost simultaneously.

free wall of the RV as a profuse subendocardial Purkinje network. Because of the physio-logical isolation, impulse input from the RBB directly into septal muscle fibers does not occur. As shown in figure 5, the propagating impulse spreads along the RBB toward the apex of the heart, across the false tendons to the subendocardial Purkinje network on the free wall of the right ventricle.

The earliest muscle to be activated is the apical free wall which is followed by almost simultaneous depolarization of the remaining lower portions of the ventricular free wall. The spread of excitation then proceeds through ordinary muscle to the basal portions of the free wall and septum. Thus septal and free wall muscle is activated from distal (apical) to proximal (basal) portions. During septal depolarization the papillary muscles are also activated (base to apex orientation). It is of interest to note that the time of activation of the basal portion of the septum always occurred after activation of the basal areas of the free wall (fig. 5).

SEQUENCE OF EXCITATION OF THE LEFT VENTRICULAR ENDOCARDIUM

The sequence of excitation of the left ventricular endocardium is more complex than that of the right because of the anatomy of the specialized conducting fibers of the left ventricle (fig. 6). The LBB immediately divides into the left anterior division (LAD) and left

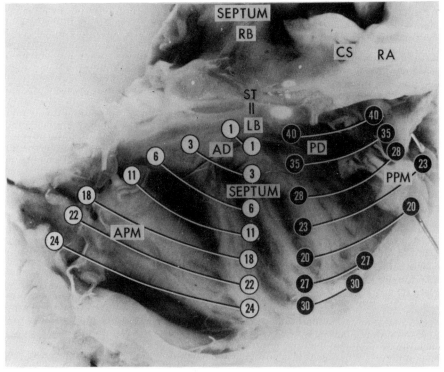

Fig. 6. Sequence of activation of the left ventricular septum and free wall. The left bundle branch (LB) was stimulated close to threshold by surface electrodes at a cycle length of 800 msec. Isochronic lines on the left connecting the black numbers on white backgrounds represent the sequence of excitation of the conducting system tissue. Isochronic line on the right, connecting white numbers on black backgrounds represent the sequence of activation of ventricular muscle. The same sequence applies to conducting tissue or muscle on either side of the septum. The numbers represent time in milliseconds from the onset of stimulus to activation at each site. The pattern of activation on the upper two thirds of the ventricular septum is from the bundle branch to the major divisions and subendocardial Purkinje fibers. At the junction of the middle and lower thirds of the septum muscle activation is initiated. Septal muscle is then depolarized from apex to base. Impulses traversing through the lower septal conducting fibers to the base of each papillary muscle (APM, PPM) arrived about the same time as impulses traveling down the longitudinal axis of the PM from the anterior (AD) or posterior division (PD). Ventricular muscle in the septum and free wall are activated from apex to base, while ordinary muscle in the PM is activated from its base to apex. RA = right atrium. CS = coronary sinus. RB = right bundle.

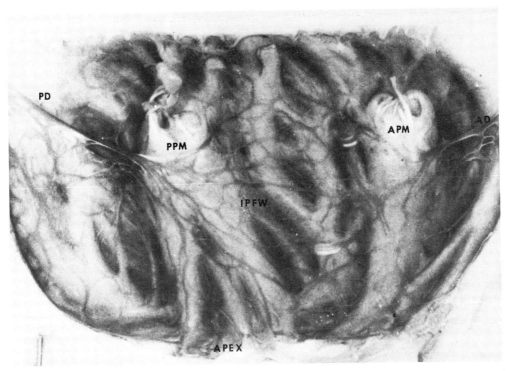

Fig. 7. Pertinent anatomic features of the intact left ventricular free wall. The left ventricle (LV) was opened by an incision through the ventricular septum, bisecting the left bundle branch. The incision extended to the apex of the LV. The anterior division (AD) and posterior division (PD) are indicated. Note that these two divisions course to their respective anterior papillary (APM) or posterior papillary muscle (PPM). Fibers course down the longitudinal axis to the base of each papillary muscle. Note the profuse merging network of conducting fibers in the interpapillary free wall (IPFW). This network extends throughout most of the free wall. The preparation is stained with Lugol's solution to identify the specialized conducting system.

posterior division (LPD). These divisions course to their respective papillary muscles but are connected by a very profuse endocardial network of specialized conducting fibers. As the LAD and LPD cross the apex of the papillary muscles some fibers descend each papillary muscle to their bases (fig. 7). However the major portion of these divisions continue across to the superior aspect of the interpapillary free wall. The ramifications of each division merge with each other to complete a circumferential ring of specialized conduction tissue similar to that observed in the adult animal (575).

Additionally, the specialized conducting fibers in the septal endocardial network in the lower half of the septum provide input to the base of each papillary muscle as well as the apex of the left ventricle. These fibers then continue to the mid and lower interpapillary free wall where they provide a second network of interconnecting conducting fibers. The abundant subendocardial Purkinje fibers which emerge from the lower half of each papillary muscle merge with the fibers from the apex of the left ventricle on the interpapillary free wall (fig. 7). Thus it appears that both the septum and free wall have 'protective' mechanisms whereby each has numerous interconnections of specialized conducting fibers.

A propagating impulse traverses the major divisions of the LBB toward the papillary muscles as well as down the septal subendocardial Purkinje network simultaneously. However, septal muscle activation does not occur until the impulse arrives at the lower septum. This area on the lower septum is the earliest site of left ventricular muscle excitation. After

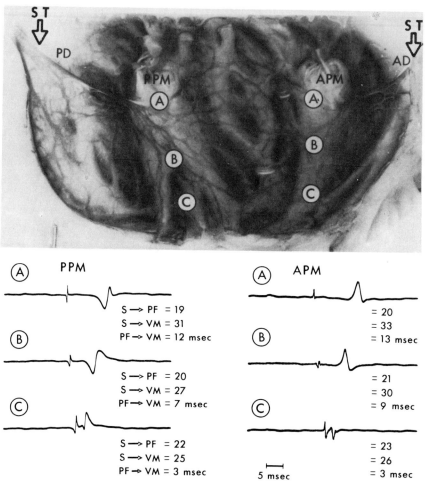

Fig. 8. Sequence of excitation of the anterior and posterior papillary muscle of the left ventricle. A preparation similar to that shown in figure 7 was utilized. The anterior division (AD) and posterior division (PD) are seen coursing to their respective papillary muscles (APM, PPM). Upon reaching the papillary muscles conducting fibers course down toward the base. Additionally, specialized conducting fibers on the septum cross to the base of each papillary muscle. The AD and PD were simultaneously stimulated by close bipolar surface electrodes (ST). Surface electrograms were recorded on each papillary muscle at sites labeled A, B, and C. Each tracing labeled A, B, and C, correspond to the site on each papillary muscle. Electrograms recorded at each site demonstrate two deflections. The first is a Purkinje fiber (PF) spike which is followed by a second deflection indicating ventricular muscle (VM). PF were initially activated on the apex of each papillary muscle. PF at the base were activated 3 msec later. However, VM cells were depolarized at the bases 6 and 7 msec respectively before VM cells were activated at the apex. The PF-VM interval at the base was 3 msec, while this interval increased to 12 and 13 msec at the respective bases. Thus, impulse input into VM is essentially simultaneous at the base of each papillary muscle. Horizontal calibration = 5 msec.

entering muscle at this site, the wave front propagates in a divergent manner. One wave front is towards the base of the septum through ordinary muscle and the second continues towards the left ventricular septo-apical area (fig. 6).

Shortly after the ventricular apex depolarizes, the anterior and posterior papillary muscles are activated beginning at their bases. They receive input from two sources; one being fibers which originate from reflections down the papillary muscles from the major divisions of the LBB, and the second source is from fibers from the subendocardial septal network of conducting fibers which have an input into the base of each papillary muscle. Similar to that found in the adult, muscle activation occurs initially at the base of each papillary muscle then proceeds towards the apex of each respective papillary muscle (fig. 8).

After traversing the apical regions of the papillary muscles, the continuation of the LAD and LPD merge with each other on the superior portion of the interpapillary free wall. Specialized subendocardial fibers which spread along the septum to the left ventricular apex and also to the base of each papillary muscles also continue to the interpapillary free wall and apical free wall. Thus impulse input to the free wall is made up of numerous sources, all of which merge and interconnect.

Experiments designed to study free wall activation were done on preparations shown in figure 7. The right and left atria and right ventricle were removed. An incision was then made through the left ventricular septum, bisecting the LBB, from base to apex. Thus, excitation of the entire left ventricular endocardium with an intact free wall could be evaluated with the LAD and LPD remaining on respective ends of the preparation. The preparations were stimulated either from the proximal LAD or LPD and maps of the pattern of endocardial excitation were made. Additional experiments included simultaneous stimulation of the LAD and LPD in an attempt to simulate the physiologic state. These experiments revealed that impulse input into ordinary muscle occurred initially in the apical portion of the free wall (fig. 9). The propagating wave front spreads through muscle towards the base of the free wall between the papillary muscles.

It is apparent that the entire apical region of the left ventricle (septum and free wall) is the first to be electrically excited. After the apex of the heart is depolarized there is an orderly spread of electrical activity to the base of the heart (septum and free wall). This is consistent with the contraction pattern of the left ventricle which is also from apex to base.

It appears that there is no significant difference in the sequence of excitation between the neonate and adult dog when considered individually. The right interventricular system is primarily a single branch which terminates in numerous ramifications on the apical area of the free wall, right ventricular muscle depolarization proceeds from apex towards base through the free wall and the septum. The left bundle branch, though there are two major divisions, has profuse subendocardial Purkinje fiber interconnections on the septal and interpapillary free wall. The left conducting system supplies input into muscle at the lower portions of the septum and free wall and then there follows an orderly spread of excitation through muscle from apex to base. On the other hand, when considered together, there is one significant normal physiologic variation between the neonatal and adult dog. This concerns the observation that the right ventricular septum is activated just prior to

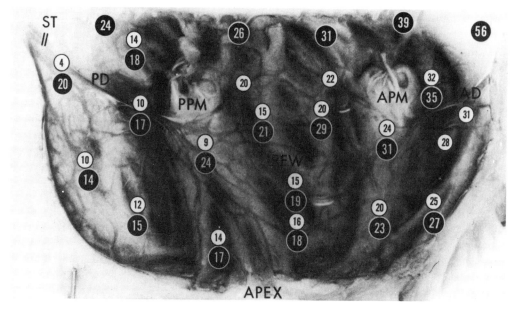

Fig. 9. Excitation of the left interpapillary free wall. Preparation is similar to that shown in figure 8. The posterior division (PD) was stimulated (ST) with surface electrodes at a basic cycle length of 800 msec. Note that the two major divisions of the left bundle branch (PD, AD) course towards the apex of their respective papillary muscles (PPM, APM). Additionally septal conducting fibers course to the base of the papillary muscles and to the apex of the left ventricle. The entire free wall surface between the papillary muscles has multiple impulse inputs. The continuation of the major divisions merge in the superior aspect of the inter-papillary free wall (IPFW). Note that the fibers from the base of each papillary muscle continue and merge with each other in the lower portion of the IPFW. Thus, there is profuse interconnecting of specialized conducting fibers on the IPFW from the apex to the base. Depolarization times of specialized conducting fibers are shown in black numbers on white backgrounds and for muscle cells in white numbers on black backgrounds. The numbers represent time in milliseconds from the onset of stimulus to activation at each site. The impulse originating in the PD courses down to the PPM. At the same time it descends the septal conducting fibers. The impulse crosses the PPM to have input into the IPFW. Additional input into this area is from the base of the PPM. The sequence of activation then proceeds to the interconnecting conducting fibers on the IPFW towards the anterior papillary muscle (APM) and finally to the AD. Muscle activation is initiated in the lower third of the septum which then depolarized the septum from apex to base. Papillary muscles are depolarized as described in the previous figure. Muscle of the IPFW is also depolarized in an apex to base orientation as well as the septal endocardial surface medial to the APM. The most basal areas of each longitudinal section of the left ventricle (area above PD, IPFW, and AD) are last to be depolarized in each section.

left ventricular septal activation, and that the excitatory wave front reaches the most basal portions of the right and left ventricles almost simultaneously. As suggested above, this may be due to the relative preponderance of the muscle mass of the right ventricle and septum which is found in the neonatal mammal.

ACTIVATION PATTERNS DUE TO LESIONS IN THE SPECIALIZED CONDUCTING SYSTEM

The left bundle branch has been described as a bifascicular structure (321,638,690) or as a diverging network of interconnected fibers (819). Recent physiologic evidence (476,575) strongly suggests that the LBB of the canine heart can be best described as the latter. We used the 1–2 week puppy heart to evaluate these divergent concepts.

For these experiments, activation patterns of the endocardium were studied after discrete lesions were made in the LAD, LPD or left ventricular septum. Control activation maps were obtained prior to any incision. All lesions were made as close to the bifurcation of the main left bundle branch as possible. A discrete lesion in either the LAD or LPD had little or no influence on the sequence of endocardial activation of either the specialized conducting system or ventricular muscle. As can be observed in figure 10, panel B, there is a slight delay in conduction distal to the incision in the posterior division, but the overall pattern of right and left ventricular excitation remained essentially normal. Following this lesion in the posterior division, interruption of the LAD was completed. With these combined discrete lesions, there is a slight delay (~10–15 msec) of the impulse to a site on the LAD or LPD distal to the transection. However, the impulse rapidly entered the upper septum and traversed the dense interwoven network of septal subendocardial fibers and reentered the anterior or posterior division distal to the transection. From this point the sequence of activation was entirely normal (fig. 10, panel C). Any lesion or combination of such lesions did not influence right ventricular endocardial excitation.

When a third lesion was made in the preparation in the proximal RBB, there was a significant alteration in the sequence of activation; but not surprisingly it was limited to the right ventricle. As shown in panel D of figure 10, there are no further changes in

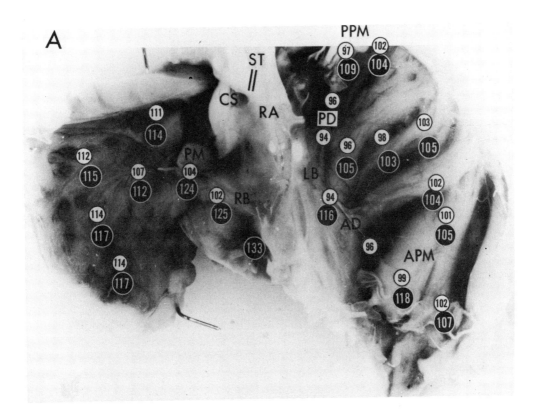

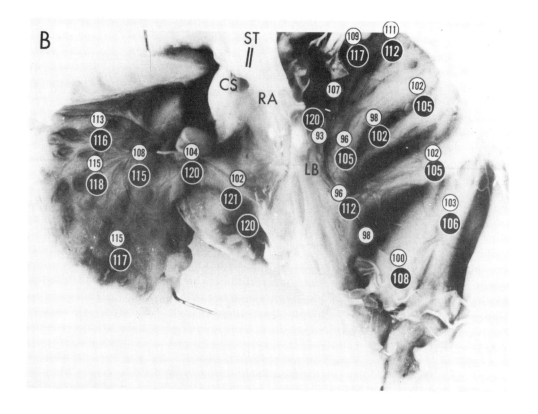

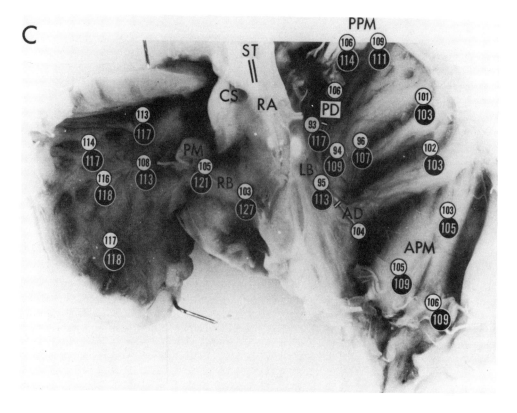

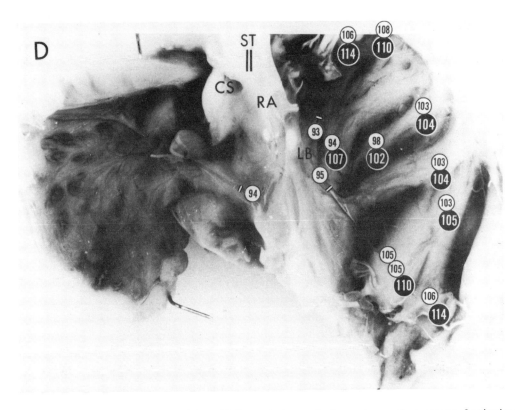

Fig. 10. The effect of lesions in the right and left ventricular conducting system on the sequence of activation of the endocardium. The right atrium (RA) was stimulated (ST) by bipolar surface electrodes at a basic cycle length of 800 msec. Conduction to the left ventricle (LV) preceeded right ventricular conduction in this experiment. Numbers represent intervals from stimulus to response at each site. Black numbers of a white backgrounds represent Purkinje fiber (PF) activation, while white numbers on black backgrounds indicate ventricular muscle (VM) activation. Panel A is control. Panel B shows activation after a discrete lesion was made across the posterior division (PD). Note that there is a 14 msec delay in propagation to a site on the PD distal to the incision. However, the sequence of excitation of the right and left ventricle was essentially unchanged. In panel C, an additional lesion was made across the anterior division (AD). No significant change in the sequence of excitation occurred since the impulse preceded down the septal interconnecting PF and reentered the major divisions distal to the sites of transection. From this point on the sequence of excitation was essentially normal. In panel D, a discrete lesion transected the right bundle branch (RB). Note that there was no change in the sequence of excitation of the left ventricular endocardium. Electrical activity could not be elicited distal to the transection of the RB. This obviously would not occur in a clinical situation since conduction may proceed through the interventricular septum which was severed in this preparation. CS = coronary sinus. PM = papillary muscle. APM = anterior papillary muscle. PPM = posterior papillary muscle. LB = left bundle branch.

the sequence of activation of the left ventricular endocardium. However, the impulse propagated down the RBB to the site of the lesion where it was completely blocked. No electrical activity could be recorded in either Purkinje or muscle cells distal to the transection of the proximal RBB. From this experiment a number of points become evident. First, a discrete lesion of the proximal right bundle can result in complete right bundle branch block in this model. Secondly, this is not true for the left ventricle. Lesions in both the LAD and LPD do not significantly alter the sequence of activation because of the profuse Purkinje interconnections between the two divisions of the LBB. Third, since complete block occurred at the site of the transverse incision of the RBB (no electrical activity in muscle or Purkinje fibers occurred distal to the incision), a limitation of this model is evident. We assume that all specialized conducting fibers and ventricular muscle between the right and left ventricle within the ventricular septum were severed in the preparation of the model. This obiously does not occur in the clinical situation since there is conduction through the ventricular septum from left to right (97, 728). Thus, in the clinical situation an impulse could traverse the septum distal to the lesion in the proximal RBB. This would then result in depolarization of the right ventricle.

Other experiments were carried out to further elucidate the effect of endocardial lesions on the patterns of endocardial excitation. Figure 11, panel B shows that once a transverse lesion is made across all of the anterior division of the LBB the spread of excitation by-passes the site of block by way of the interconnecting specialized pathways on the upper septum. When a second lesion is made across the posterior division the main access for the wave of excitation is still via the specialized fibers in the upper septum. At a point distal to the block the impulse reenters the LAD and LPD with a delay of ~ 20 msec (fig. 1, panel C). However, if these two lesions are connected in a manner shown in panel D of figure 11, there is a significant change in the sequence of excitation so that the wave front of excitation spreads initially antegrade to the site of the incision in the anterior and posterior division. Excitation then proceeded superior to the incision in myocardial tissue. The impulse reentered the posterior division at a site distal to the incision but prior to the LPD joining the posterior papillary muscle (conduction through this area was delayed ~ 10 msec). The sequence of endocardial activation then proceeded to the base of the

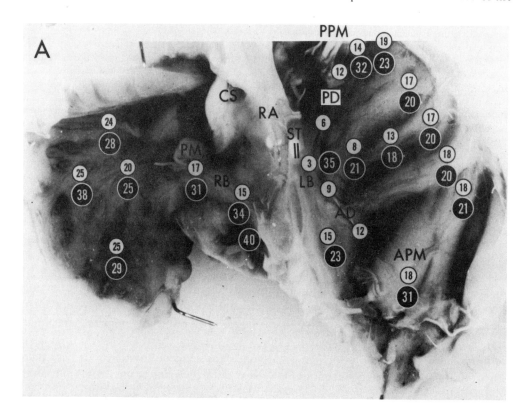

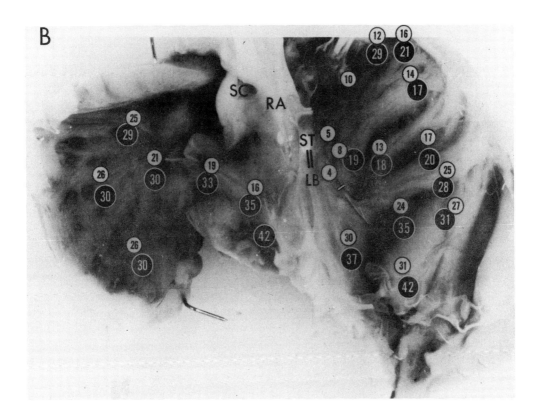

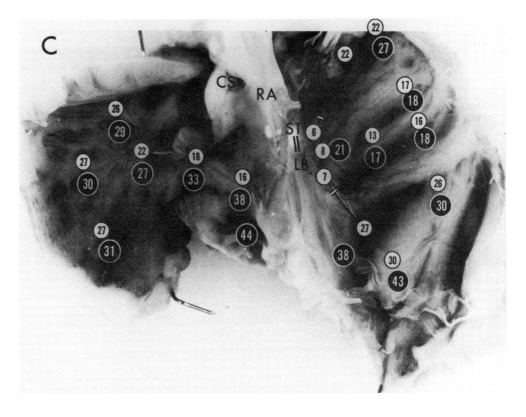

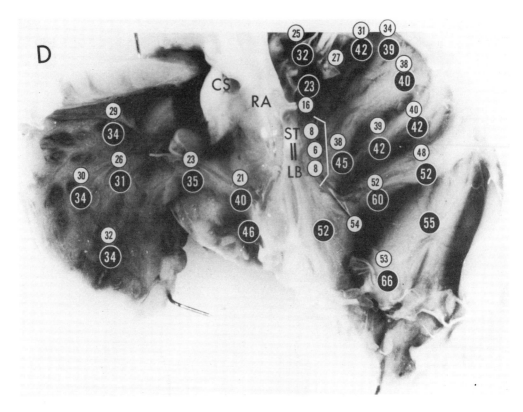

Fig. 11. Activation of the distal left ventricular conducting system after sequential incisions of its major divisions (AD, PD) and septum. The left bundle branch (LB) was stimulated (ST) by surface electrodes at a cycle length of 800 msec. Activation of conducting tissue (black numbers on white background) and neighboring ventricular muscle (white numbers on black background) is indicated at each recording site. The numbers represent intervals from stimulus to response at each site. Panel A represents control recordings. In panel B, after a discrete lesion was made across the AD; except for a 13 msec delay around the site of transection of the AD, there was no change in the sequence of activation of the endocardium. After an additional lesion was made across the PD (panel C) there was a delay of 15–20 msec of the impulse around the lesions, the impulse reentered the major divisions distal to the site of transection, thus there is no significant change in the sequence of endocardial excitation. In panel D the two lesions in the AD and PD were joined by a third lesion as indicated. This resulted in a significant change in the sequence of left ventricular endocardial excitation. Note that the impulse was blocked septally, so it traversed the lesion in the PD, superiorly to the transection. It then reentered the PD distal to the site of transection but prior to the PD joining the posterior papillary muscle (PPM). The sequence of endocardial excitation then proceeded down to the PPM and then back to the septal interconnecting conducting fibers. Finally the impulse reentered the AD. The diffuse interconnections on the septum in the apical area between papillary muscles also had an impulse input into the base of the anterior papillary muscle (APM). Ventricular muscle of the septum, free wall and papillary muscles were activated in the usual manner. No change in right ventricular activation occurred throughout the experiment. RA = right atrium. CS = coronary sinus. PM = papillary muscle.

posterior papillary muscle which was depolarized in the usual manner. Subsequently, the wave front spread from the base of the posterior papillary muscle medially towards the septum with simultaneous depolarization of the upper septum (presumably through the septal Purkinje network distal to the lesion). Excitation then spread down toward the apex of the heart followed by a pattern of normal septal muscle depolarization (from apex to base). The portion of the left ventricle normally excited by the LAD was depolarized from a propagating impulse from the apical area of the septum. It spread to the base of the anterior papillary muscle, then to the apex of the papillary muscle and subsequently depolarized the remaining myocardium after considerable delay (20–30 msec greater than control).

This delay would undoubtedly produce a significant axis shift on the surface electro-cardiogram. This supports some of the published observations, but conflicts with others. Lazzara et al. (476) demonstrated that transection of the major divisions of the LBB did not produce complete block of the left conducting system. However, complete transection from one division through the septal endocardium to include the second division did result in complete block. We assume on the basis of our experimental observations (fig. 11), that there may be cases where such an extensive lesion may not result in complete

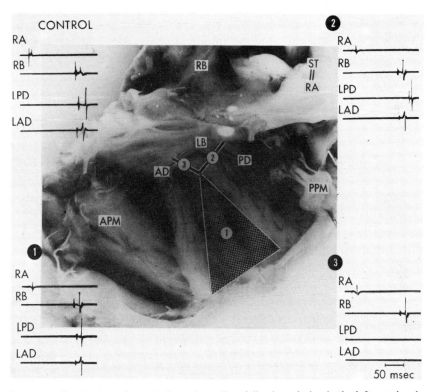

Fig. 12. Sequence of activation of ventricular endocardium following a lesion in the left septal endocardium. Bipolar surface electrograms were recorded following surface stimulation (at threshold) of the right atrium (RA) at a basic cycle length of 800 msec. The electrograms were recorded from the RA, at the junction of the right bundle branch (RB), left anterior and posterior divisions (LAD, LPD) with their respective papillary muscles. Each electrogram tracing has two deflections. The first represents Purkinje fiber (PF) activation, and the second, ventricular muscle (VM) activation. Following RA stimulation, the RB is activated first, followed by activation of the LAD and then the LPD. Following a triangular incision in the endocardium of the left septum (shaded area labeled 1) there was no change in the sequence of activation (panel 1). When the incision was extended from the apex of the triangle across the LPD (incision 2), there was a transient delay to the LPD recording site but the sequence of depolarization at the recording sites did not change (panel 2). The last incision (labeled 3) was made across the LAD. This resulted in activation of the RB only. Complete block of the left conducting system occurred (panel 3). Horizontal calibration = 50 msec.

block of the left ventricular conducting system. It seems evident that in order to have complete block of the left conducting system distal ot the LBB, at least a lesion which is extensive enough to involve the LAD, LPD and interconnecting septal conducting fibers (and perhaps more) has to occur.

Under certain limited experimental conditions propagation did not always bypass discrete areas of block in the major divisions of the LBB. Figure 12 demonstrates such a condition. Initially a triangular incision of endocardium was completed in the lower two thirds of the septum. Simultaneous surface electrograms were recorded at the junctions of the LAD and the LPD with their respective papillary muscles, as well as the RBB and right atrium. There was no change, nor did we expect any, in the sequence of activation to the recording sites with this large septal "lesion". When an extension of this incision was made across the posterior division (fig. 12, panel 2) there was a delay of 24 msec to the recording site on the posterior papillary muscle; conduction to the other recording sites were normal. When a third incision was made from the apex of the wedge across the anterior division, conduction to both the anterior and posterior papillary muscles failed. Conduction from right atrium to the RBB was intact (fig. 12, panel 3).

GENESIS OF CARDIAC ARRHYTHMIAS AND CONDUCTION DISTURBANCES

An abnormality in the electrical activity of a cardiac cell which results in a change in the rate, regularity, or site of origin of the cardiac impulse may result in an arrhythmia. We have shown that a disturbance in the normal sequence of activation of an impulse (block) will result in a conduction disturbance. Additionally, combinations of the above (163), the concept of reentry (935), and slow conduction (162) have all been elucidated as determinants of cardiac arrhythmias. Many of the studies defining the mechanisms for cardiac arrhythmias have been evaluated in isolated segments of specialized conducting system or ventricular myocardium. Although there is strong evidence that the mechanisms defined in utilizing isolated segments of myocardium in the tissue bath may pertain to the cardiac system in situ, we feel that this relatively intact model may be more appropriate for the study of the mechanism and perpetuation of cardiac arrhythmias.

The most common arrhythmia encountered and most easily produced was one related to conduction. An increase in the rate of atrial stimulation (200/min) usually resulted in 2:1 block across the AV node. With higher rates of stimulation (240–300/min) we were able to induce 3:1 or higher degrees of block. The sequence of excitation of both ventricles were normal for those impulses conducted to the Bundle of His. This supports the clinical observations of Krongrad et al. (450) who demonstrated that 2:1 AV block occurred secondary to rapid atrial stimulation in infants and children undergoing cardiac catheter ization. Rates which achieved this degree of block were in the range of 200–300 stimuli/min. However, our demonstration that newborn puppies will have varying degrees of block at atrial rates as low as 200/min is not consistent with the clinical observation that infants with paroxysmal atrial tachycardia (rates up to 300/min) have the ability to conduct 1:1 to the ventricles (albeit with aberrency). Additionally the observations of Preston et al. (636)

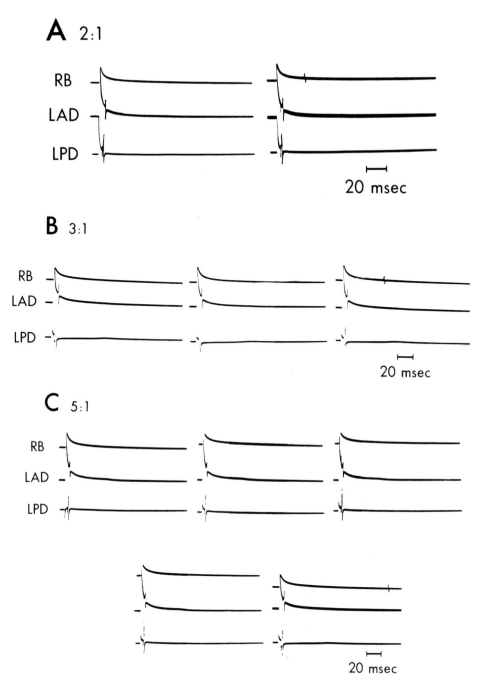

Fig. 13. Conduction block between the right bundle branch (RB) and left bundle branch (LB). The LB of the preparation was stimulated by surface electrodes during this experiment. Bipolar surface electrograms were recorded at sites on the RB, left anterior (LAD) and left posterior division (LPD), at their junction with their respective papillary muscles. After superfusion with Tyrode's solution for 3 hours, the impulse was blocked in a 2:1 fashion proximal to the RB recording site (panel A). The degree of block increased to 3:1 (panel B) and then finally 5:1 (panel C). Note that as the degree of block increased, the time to activation of conducted impulses to the RB also markedly increased; from 28 msec when 2:1 conduction was present, to 140 msec (panel C). Thus as the degree of block increased, conduction time slowed on those impulses which were conducted to the RB.

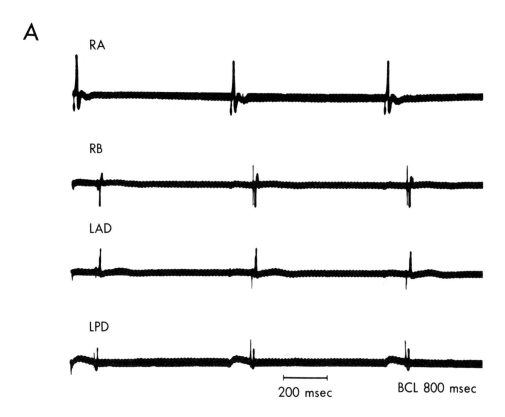

A

RA

RB

LAD

LPD

200 msec   BCL 800 msec

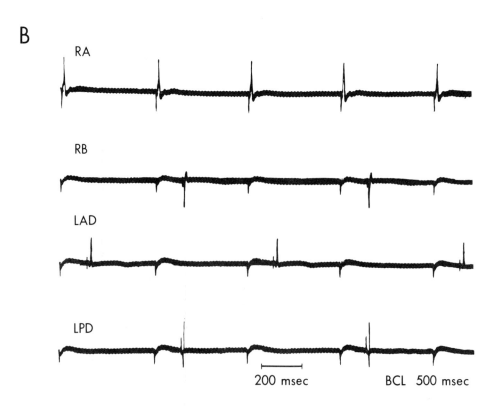

B

RA

RB

LAD

LPD

200 msec   BCL 500 msec

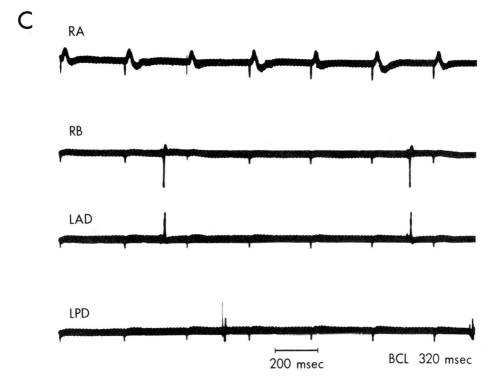

Fig. 14. Alternating conduction block in the ventricular conducting system. Following right atrial (RA) surface stimulation, simultaneous bipolar electrograms were recorded from the RA, the right bundle branch (RB), left anterior and posterior divisions (LAD, LPD) of the left bundle branch. In panel A, RA stimulation at a basic cycle length of 800 msec, resulted in 1:1 conduction to the RB, LAD, and LPD. Conduction across the atrio-ventricular junction to the recording site was ~102 msec. In panel B the rate of stimulation of the RA was increased to 120/min (BCL = 500 msec). This resulted in 2:1 conduction from the RA to RB and the LPD. RA to RB or LPD interval was 148 msec. During these conducted beats, the impulse was blocked proximal to the LAD recording site. However, the impulses which were not conducted to the RB or LPD, conducted to the LAD, also in a 2:1 fashion. Note that RA to LAD interval (150 msec) is approximately equal to the RA to RB and LPD interval when an impulse to these sites is conducted. A further increase in the rate of atrial stimulation (BCL = 320 msec) resulted in an increase in the degree of conduction block (panel C). Note that there is 4:1 conduction from RA to RB and LAD. For those impulses which are conducted to the RB and LAD, conduction is blocked in the LPD. The RA to RB and LAD interval equals 180 msec. When conduction of an impulse from the RA to the LPD (4:1) is present, the impulse is blocked in the RA and LAD. The interval from RA to LPD for conducted beats is equal to the RA to RB or LAD interval. See text for further discussion.

that the refractory period of the A-V node did not exceed the refractory period of the 'ventricles' in newborn mammals indicate that the refractory period of the 'ventricles' is the prime determinant for the maximum frequency at which the neonatal heart may follow atrial stimulation. Further experiments using this model are mandatory to clarify these conflicting reports as to whether the A-V node, the proximal ventricular conducting system, or the gate (572), serves most effectively as the filter for excessive rates between the atria and ventricle in the neonatal animal.

Some preparations which had impulses originating in the LBB would on occasion fail to conduct to the contralateral bundle branch system or would do so with varying degrees of block. This abnormality in conduction began in preparations after they were in the tissue bath for 3 hours. Initially block between the bundle branch systems would be either 2:1 or 3:1. However with time (4 hours) higher degrees of bundle branch block occurred (fig. 13).

Other preparations revealed rather bizarre conduction defects. We observed, in one of our preparations, alternating LAD and LPD block as well as varying degrees of block between the right atrium and right ventricle (fig. 14). In panel A of this figure the right atrium was stimulated at a basic cycle length of 800 msec. Simultaneous bipolar surface electrograms were recorded from the right atrium, RBB at its junction with the papillary muscle, and the LAD and the LPD at the junctions with their respective papillary muscles. There is 1:1 conduction from the right atrium to the recording sites within the right or left ventricle after the normal delay across the A-V node. When the frequency of atrial stimulation was increased to 500 msec (panel B), 2:1 conduction occurred between the right atrium and the RBB and LPD. Those impulses which conducted to the RBB and LPD were blocked in the distribution of the LAD proximal to the site where the surface electrogram was recorded. On alternate beats, impulses from the atria propagated to the LAD (2:1) but were not conducted to the RBB and LPD. Thus, there appears to be RBB and LPD block alternating with LAD block. When the rate of atrial stimulation was further increased to a basic cycle length of 320 msec, the pattern of block changed (panel C). Now there was 4:1 block between the right atrium and the RBB and LAD with complete block in the LPD. On each impulse following the conducted beat to the RBB and LAD, the right atrial impulse propagated only to the LPD, also in a 4:1 fashion.

Thus in a single preparation we were able to observe alternating rate dependent block in the major fascicles of the ventricular conducting system. Though we were not able to determine the exact mechanism of this electrophysiologic phenomenon in this experiment, we assume that there had to be rate dependent changes in the refractory periods or an imbalance of the temporal-spatial relationships of the major fascicles of the ventricular conducting system.

SUMMARY

A model utilizing 1–2 week old puppies has been developed whereby the electrophysiological properties of the intact specialized conduction system can be evaluated in the tissue bath using microelectrode or surface recording techniques. The unique feature of this model is that the preparation consists of right atrium, an intact atrioventricular junction and the entire endocardium of the right and left ventricle. Using this model it has been shown that there are normal physiologic differences in the sequence of endocardial excitation in the puppy when compared to the adult dog. These differences are: 1. right ventricular septal activation preceeding left ventricular septal activation; and 2. simultaneous right ventricular and left ventricular basal activation. Both of these differences are probably secondary to the increase in right ventricular mass which is a physiological response in the newborn to pulmonary artery hemodynamics.

Additionally it has been demonstrated that the model is excellent to study the effects of discrete lesions in the specialized conducting system on the sequence of ventricular endocardial excitation. It may also be used to determine the mechanism and perpetuation of arrhythmias; be they due to conduction abnormalities, enhanced automaticity or combinations of the two.

ELECTRONMICROSCOPY OF THE CONDUCTING SYSTEM

3

THE FINE STRUCTURE OF THE ATRIAL AND ATRIO-VENTRICULAR (AV) JUNCTIONAL SPECIALIZED TISSUES OF THE RABBIT HEART[1]

J. TRANUM-JENSEN, M.D.

The widest range of morphological and physiological specializations of the conducting system (CS) are found in the atrial and especially in the AV junctional components. The study of these very heterogeneous tissues encounters a number of difficulties which are of importance for the interpretation of fine structural observations and which may account for some of the divergencies found between different studies.

a. In both light (LM)- and electron microscopic (EM) studies of the CS the characterization and distinction between cells and tissues in many regions rest upon rather minute differences in cellular and histological structure.[2] The criteria used for distinction are generally of a quantitative nature which do not allow a sharp definition, particularly difficult at the LM level, and in the nodal regions gradual transitions between different tissues are observed. These conditions, together with a small but marked individual variation in the topographical location and the mutual relations of the CS elements (835), complicate the precise definition and the reproducible sampling of representative areas for EM. Consequently comprehensive systematic EM studies of particular regions of the CS have hitherto been few in number.

b. Many of the criteria used for characterization of the various cell types in the CS and their distinction from the working cardiocytes (e.g. diameter and 'paleness' of cells, nuclear and mitochondrial morphology, glycogen content and myofibrillar organization) are sensitive to preparative procedures, notably fixation, and particularly to the conditions of the tissues prior to fixation.

c. A considerable species variation recognized in the structure of the CS (835, 837) makes experiences from one animal difficult to apply in the study of others.

d. Only few morphological studies are made directly on samples preceeded by electrophysiological identification (31, 262, 830) and at the cellular level such studies are still absent, primarily due to lack of appropriate techniques. This together with the nearly complete lack of systematic quantitated EM studies on the atrial and AV junctional

---

1. All sectioned material presented derives from the hearts of young rabbits fixed *in vivo* during Nembutal-N_2O anaesthesia, while artificially ventilated, by perfusion retrogradely through the aorta of phosphate or cacodylate buffered glutaraldehyde-formaldehyde mixtures. Tonicity of fixative vehicles kept at 280–300 mOsm, of total fixatives 700–750 mOsm, pH 7.3. The intraaortic pressure was monitored during perfusion and kept by regulating the fixative flow to within 120–160 mm Hg. Postfixation in OsO_4, epon embedding. Sections for light microscopy stained with toluidine blue, for EM with uranyl and lead stains.
2. The visibility of glycogen granules in EM thin sections appear among a number of other preparatory steps to depend on the thickness of the sections. In sections cut about 30 nm,—as used for most illustrations in this paper—, most of the glycogen granules will be exposed to the surfaces of the section and are likely to be eluated in the water-bath during sectioning and in the subsequent staining of the sections at high pH. The section of figure 6a is approx. 60 nm.

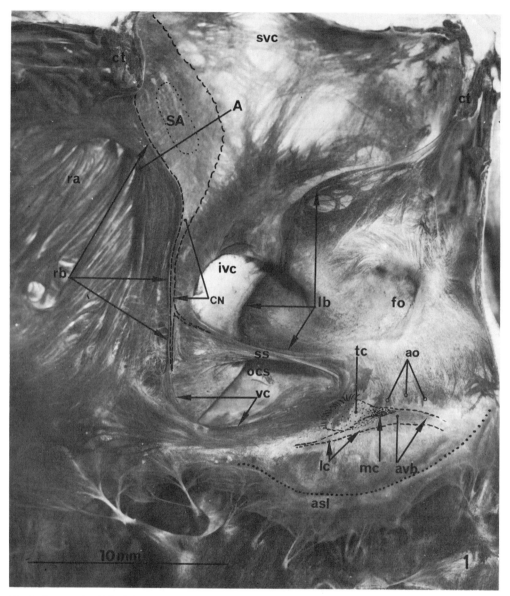

Fig. 1. Survey of rabbit right atrium demonstrating macroscopical structures referred to in the text and the approximate localization and organization of the nodal structures. The contrast of the specimen has been enhanced by supravital staining with methylene blue which stains superficially located muscle cells.

ct: cut ends of crista terminalis; ra: right auricle; fo: fossa ovalis; svc: superior vena cava; ivc: inferior vena cava; ocs: ostium of the coronary sinus; vc: valve of the coronary sinus; ss: sinus septum; asl: attachment of septal tricuspid leaflet marked by dotted line; SA: sino-atrial (SA) node. Letters inside approximate area termed central portion; cn: location of the cauda of the SA node; rb: right branch of the sino-atrial ring bundle (SARB); lb: left (septal) branch of the SARB; tc: transitional-; lc: lower nodal-, and; mc: compact midnodal zone of the atrio-ventricular (AV) node; The 'open node' corresponds to that part of the tc zone which receives atrial inputs (fanned) avb: AV bundle; ao: atrial overlay fibres. (Magn.: 5.7:1).

specialized tissues limits the possibilities for the precise identification of the morphological substrates for the physiological specializations observed.

In a search for a heart combining extensive study by both physiologists and morphologists, the rabbit would be among the favourites, and important past and recent advances on the correlation of structure and function in the CS has been achieved in this animal. In this paper it is intended to present briefly the ultrastructural characteristics of the rabbit atrial and AV junctional specialized tissues, with special attention being given to structures of possible physiological interest, in order to provide some morphological details for the discussions to come. With the existence of a large number of often cited papers and recent comprehensive reviews (122,845,866) on these subjects it is inevitable that some well known facts will be restated but it is beyond the scope of this chapter to do an extensive review of the available literature.

THE SINUATRIAL (SA) NODE AND ITS RELATED STRUCTURES

Topographic and LM identification
The bulk of the SA node of the rabbit heart is located above the crista terminalis (CT) in the wall of the superior vena cava (SVC) and extends backwards in the thin wall of the atrium formed by the root of this vessel (84,399) (fig. 1,2). In the central portion of the node the tissue appears in the LM as an interweaving aggregate of very irregular cells, the boundaries of which are difficult to resolve with the LM. The cells contain sparse and thin, branching myofibrils, which anastomose irregularly with fibrils in other cells (fig. 3,4). Towards the peripheral portions of the node an increasing number of cells with more numerous and regularly ordered myofibrils occur, identified as the transitional cells. The degree of myofibrillar organization is the only criterium for distinction between these cell types in the LM.

Besides these cells a third cell type may be observed which is characterized by being larger and paler than the surrounding cells and typically occurs singly (fig. 3). These 'intercalated clear cells' (863) are not unique to the SA node and have been found in several species in many other locations in the atrium (839) as well as in the AV node (864) and will be dealt with separately. Apart from a relatively sparce amount of interspersed connective tissue, the LM appearance of the rabbit SA nodal cells seems similar to that of other mammalian species (835,837 and chapter of Truex in this book).

The node is in contact with the medial aspect of the CT (fig. 1,2), and thin nodal extensions may encircle the root of the SVC (84). From the posterior end of the node a strand of nodal tissue, the cauda, consistently departs and passes down, medial to and parallel with the CT, to the posterior border of the ostium of the coronary sinus (OCS) from where fine strands may be followed into the sinus septum and the valve (Thebesian) of the coronary sinus (84,247). During the course along the CT the cauda comes in close relation to the right branch of the sinuatrial ring bundle (SARB). This is a thin bundle of slender and regularly cross striated muscle cells which take up a position corresponding to or within the rudiments of the right and left venous valves (84,247,611) (fig. 1). In its cranial course the SARB crosses the CT from the lateral to the medial side and marks approximately the most lateral border for the extension of the SA node over the medial aspect of the CT (fig. 2).

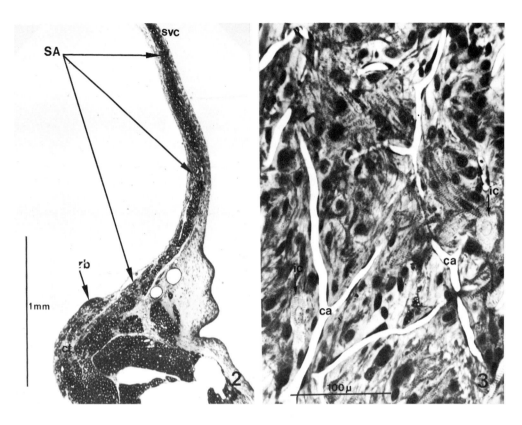

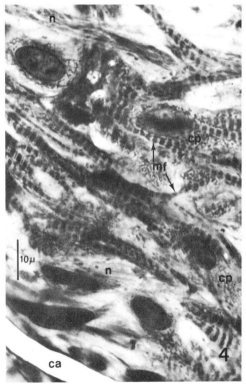

Fig. 2. Cross section of rabbit SA node from a position corresponding to line A of figure 1. The nodal tissue (SA) extends from the wall of the superior vena cava (svc) onto the medial aspect of the crista terminalis (ct). rb: right branch of the SARB (Magn.: 42:1).

Fig. 3. Section of the central portion of the SA node cut tangentially to the epicardium. Note the structural heterogeneity of the tissue. In center of the picture the thin myofibrils of nodal cells form an anastomosing network, typically found in the central nodal portion. ic: intercalated clear cells; ca: capillaries (Magn.: 290:1).

Fig. 4. High power light micrograph of section similar to that of figure 3 showing typical cells from the central nodal portion. The boundaries of the very irregular single cells cannot be resolved. The cells contain poorly aligned myofibrils (mf), which connect with myofibrils in neighbouring cells. Large areas of the cytoplasm (cp) is not occupied by myofibrils and contain granulate and thread-like structures mainly representing mitochondria. n: nerves coursing between the nodal cells. (Magn.: 1100:1).

THE SA NODE

Fine structure
Ultrastructural studies on the SA node of several mammalian species (rat: (124,862), rabbit: (121,822,830), dog: (350,396,428), cow: (349), monkey: (139,863) and man: (396)) seem to indicate that the principal cellular structure do not differ between the species. Most divergencies in descriptions of the cellular structure are of a nature which may be ascribed to the different possibilities for ultrastructural preservation available for the particular studies.

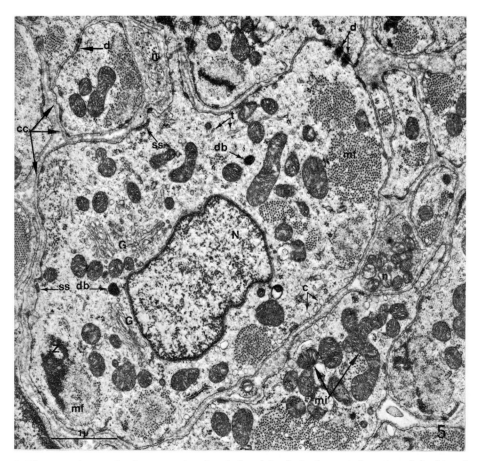

Fig. 5. Electron micrograph of cross sectioned typical nodal cells in the central portion of the SA node. A nodal cell sectioned at level with the nucleus (N) is surrounded by several irregularly contoured extensions of neighbouring cells. The cells contain few small myofibrils (mf) sectioned at various levels, at lower left including part of a Z disc (Z). Golgi complexes (G) are located around the nucleus, and irregularly shaped mitochondria (mi) are randomly distributed in the cells. Two dense bodies (db) which might correspond to the specific granules of working atrial cardiocytes are seen. Subsarcolemmal cisterns (ss) and small caveolae and vesicular profiles (c) are located along the cell membrane. The cell coat (cc) is seen as a faint staining layer lining the cells. Large areas of adjacent cell membranes are in close apposition separated by an approx. 20 nm gap along which a few small desmosome structures (d) are located. t: tubular profiles of sarcoplasmic reticulum Nerves and single axons (n) are seen in the intercellular space. (Magn.: 20,700:1).

There is no direct evidence at the cellular level to indicate which cells function as the normal pacemaker. In the following account a description is given of the cell type which pre-dominates in the central portion of the node. In the adult rabbit these cells are located in the wall of the SVC 1–2 mm above the CT, corresponding to the region where the pacemaker is normally located (613). It also corresponds to the cell type reported to be the exclusive type found in tiny biopsies taken at the site of the electrophysiologically identified pacemaker in the rabbit heart (830). This is considered the *typical nodal cell.* The combined cross- (fig. 5) and longitudinally sectioned profiles of these cells suggests an irregular, roughly spindleshaped, sometimes branching cell with thin tapering ends (428). The more precise shape, the average length of the cells, whether they normally branch and their precise three dimensional relations, are not known. They typically possess one nucleus and have a diameter of 3 to 9 μ in the nuclear region.

The most conspicuous feature of the internal structure of these cells is the poorly developed contractile apparatus. Organized myofibrils occupy less than half the cell volume. The single fibrils are loosely organized, they often branch and split up, and are less axially aligned in the cells compared to the working cardiocytes. The Z discs are irregular and show interruptions and thickenings. M lines are very indistinct or cannot be recognized and the H bands are slurred, which may be ascribed to improper transverse alignment of the filaments within sarcomeres (fig. 6,6a). Unorganized thin filaments are widely distributed in the cytoplasm in addition to a few thick myosin-like filaments (fig. 6, 7).

Mitochondria of very variable shape and size are distributed at random in the cells (fig. 5). Their closely applied foliate cristae have no marked preferential orientation, and the mitochondrial matrix has a density equal to the mitochondria of working cardiocytes. Small Golgi complexes are regularly located in the nuclear region (fig. 5). The specific atrial dense granules (58,63), which are characteristic regular structures in the atrial working cardiocytes, often located in the vicinity of Golgi complexes, have been found in nodal cells also (139). However, they are not mentioned in most studies on the SA node, and do not occur with the frequency observed in atrial working cells (fig. 5).

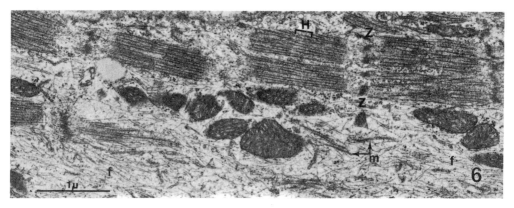

Fig. 6. Longitudinal section of typical SA nodal cell. The poorly developed myofibrils exhibit interrupted Z discs (Z) and slurrish H bands (H). Numerous thin actin-like filaments (f) and a few thick myosin-like filaments (m) are randomly distributed in the cytoplasm. (Magn.: 20,700:1)

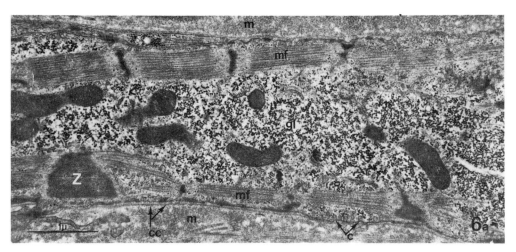

Fig. 6a. Longitudinal section of a SA nodal cell exhibiting a large number of distinct stained glycogen particles (gl). The thin, poorly developed myofibrils (mf) possess very irregular Z-discs some of which show extensive thickenings (Z). The cell coat (cc) is seen as a faint staining layer along the cell membrane, and material (m) with similar staining properties almost fills the adjacent intercellular space. c: cluster of small caveolae. (Magn.: 20,000:1).

Particulate material in the size range of 15–30 nm is widely distributed in the cytoplasm. The distinction between these particles is not straightforward, and is dependent on the preparative methods involved. Large 25–30 nm particles which stain densely with routine uranyl and lead stains are identified as glycogen β-particles (fig. 6a). Such particles are not particularly numerous in most SA nodal cells compared to the working cardiocytes, although they occasionally occur in striking numbers in a few cells, eventually forming large aggregate α-particles (863). Among the particles ranging between 15–25 nm some are associated with membranes and are identified as ribosomes. Due to the overlap in size of small glycogen particles and ribosomes in the vicinity of 20 nm a precise distinction cannot be made for free particles of this size (261) unless special measures are taken. In comprehensive studies on ventricular Purkinje fibres of the cow evidence has been presented by specific stainings and enzyme digestions, that a notable number of the small cytoplasmic particles in these cells are ribosomes (816), which have also been identified as a prominent constituent of working cardiocytes (815). Ribosomes were often found associated with thick filaments in arrangements similar to those found in developing (123,865) or cultured (480) cardiocytes and it has been hypothezised, that the poor organization of myofibrils in the Purkinje fibres reflect an imbalance in degradation and synthesis of myofibrillar proteins (814). The myofibrillar organization observed in nodal cells has evidently many similarities to developing and cultured cardiocytes. Specific studies have not been made on nodal cells, but it seems very probable that a proportion of the small particles observed in these cells are ribosomes (fig. 8).

The sarcoplasmic reticulum (SR) does not have the degree of development seen in working cardiocytes (261, 534) and its smooth tubular profiles course for long distances without relation to myofibrils (fig. 5,9).

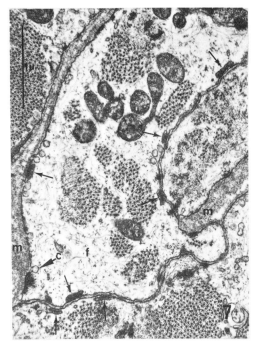

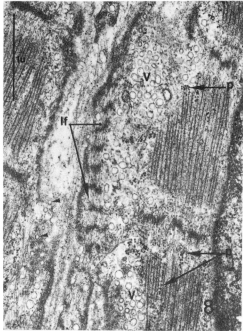

Fig. 7. Cross section of extensions of typical nodal cells with a number of densely stained subsarcolemmal cisterns (small arrows) distributed along the cell membranes which are in close apposition over long stretches. c: caveola; f: unorganized thin filamentous material; m: cell coat like material accumulated in larger intercellular spaces. (Magn.: 23,400:1).

Fig. 8. Section cut tangentially to SA nodal cells revealing accumulations of subsarcolemmal vesicular profiles (V). A number of the small pores (arrowheads) seen in areas of tangentially sectioned cell membrane are likely to be the narrow necks of caveolae. A leptomere fibril (lf) showing 220 nm banding on bundles of thin filaments is located in the subsarcolemma. These fibrils of unknown significance—preferentially located in the subsarcolemma—may be found in all cardiocytes but seems particularly numerous in cells of the CS. (Virágh & Challice, *J. Ultra-Struct. Res.*, 28: 321, (1969). p: small ribosome-like particles in rows and clusters among myofibrils. (Magn.: 23,400:1).

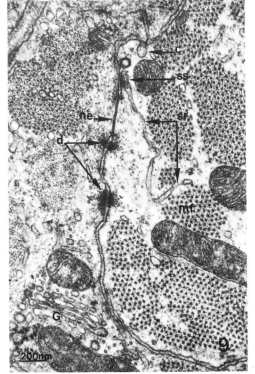

Fig. 9. Cross section of nodal cells showing one of the rare cases of nexus formation (ne) between cells in the central nodal portion. Two small desmosome structures (d) are seen in addition along the apposed cell membranes. sr: tubule of SR forming lateral coupling by a subsarcolemmal cistern (ss) and weaving among myofibrils (mf); G: Golgi complex; c: caveola. (Magn.: 35,300:1).

Structures related to the cell membrane

Subsarcolemmal cisterns (lateral couplings) of the SR are found as small densely staining sacs irregularly scattered along the cell periphery (fig. 5,7,9). They exhibit the same basic structure as seen in other cardiocytes (261,534,773) being separated from the cell membrane by a gap of 15–20 nm containing particulate dense material and sometimes exhibiting a faint line of particulate densities in the middle of their lumen. In the dog heart (350) it has been noted that the cisterns of the nodal cells are smaller and more homogeneously dense than those of the Purkinje fibres. By cytochemical methods the subsarcolemmal cisterns have been identified as accumulation sites for calcium ions in working cardiocytes (479,711), and they are generally believed to play the important role in the exitation-contraction coupling by release of calcium ions triggered by the action potential. Calcium diffuses in the cytoplasm and binds to the thin filaments of the I band and is removed by a Ca pump in the tubules of the SR for restorage in the subsarcolemmal cisterns.[3] The presence of energy consuming transport processes at the subsarcolemmal cisterns is evidenced by the localization of ATP-ase activity at these sites (701). The frequency of subsarcolemmal cisterns in nodal cells compared to other cardiocytes and whether they have preferential locations has never been quantitated. They may seem conspicuous in some nodal cells (fig. 7) and not in others. Some investigators have noted localizations where cell membranes are in close apposition and opposite to nerve varicosities. The nodal cells are obviously not specialized for a contractile function. The presence of SR couplings in nodal cells may be a consequence of the development of the rudimentary contractile apparatus, or they may have significance for other functions as well. It might be suggested that the relative amount of subsarcolemmal cisterns, Ca-binding filaments, and SR, in proportion to the cell volume, ceteris paribus, will influence the magnitude and rate of intracellular Ca-concentration variations.

It is generally agreed that the specialized system for inward spread of excitation, the T-tubule system, is not developed in any part of the CS, and the subsarcolemmal (lateral) cisterns are therefore the only type of SR coupling found. T-tubules are not observed regularly in atrial working cardiocytes (63,357,534,758), and the proposed consistent definition of Purkinje-fibres in the ventricles (in this sense termed P-fibres), being cells lacking T-tubules (771) cannot be readily applied to atrial specialized tissues.

Small caveolae are frequently observed along the cell membrane of nodal cells, and several may be found clustered side by side (fig. 5,6a). In sections cut tangential to the cell membrane large areas of the subsarcolemma may be found occupied by vesicular profiles, many of which will be caveolae (fig. 8). These caveolae are observed in all cardiocytes and their number seems to vary from cell to cell (758). Their number may seem quite conspicuous in some nodal cells, but their frequency has not been quantitated. Whether they just serve in a transport process as micropinocytotic structures or may have other functions is not known. Their presence might have an electrophysiological significance by increasing the membrane capacitance per unit area of cell surface as proposed for ventricular working cardiocytes by the presence of T-tubules in these cells (771).

The nodal cells are, as are other cardiocytes (381) and a variety of other cell types (647),

---

3. For recent review on the model for excitation-contraction coupling see e.g. Bassingthwaighte (51).

lined by a cell coat (external lamina), the main components of which are believed to be glycoproteins and acidic mucopolysaccarides (647). The coat appears as a moderately dense staining layer of 20–40 nm thickness lining the cell membrane and often most densely stained at its outer surface (fig. 5,6a). Accumulations of similar material often are also located in clefts between the cells (fig. 6a,7). Very little is known about the significance of surface coats on muscle cells. They stain intensely with cationic dyes (55,381,647), and might play an important role by influencing the local ionic environment of the cell membrane and eventually act as a selective barrier for certain substances (61,539). Part of the explanation for the low sensitivity of pacemaker cells and other cardiac specialized tissues to the action of enzymes which disturb the integrity of working cardiac cell membranes, might be sought in specialized properties of the cell coat (539). Glycoproteins of the cell coat have been demonstrated to be continously synthesized in the Golgi apparatus of the cell to which the coat belongs (60), and should probably be considered an important, integrated, perhaps cell specific, component of the sarcolemma.

'One of the very characteristic features of the typical SA nodal cells is their paucity in specialized intercellular contacts.[4] The cells are in close apposition over large areas of their surface, separated by a rather uniformly spaced gap of about 20 nm. The only specialized zones of contact regularly encountered along this gap are fascia adherentes type junctions into which myofibrils insert, and irregularly scattered small desmosomes (fig. 5,7, 9). Nexuses (gap junctions) are exceedingly rare compared to working cardiocytes, and when observed are always small (fig. 9). The only function normally ascribed to the fasciae adherentes and the desmosome type junctions is to serve the mechanical adhesion of the cells. There is substantial evidence that the nexus is the principal low resistance junction between cardiocytes.[5] The very low conduction velocity within the central nodal region (613) and the low margin of safety may find its explanation in the exceptional sparsity of nexuses in this region, as suggested by many authors.

The transitional cells in the peripheral portions of the node, e.g. adjacent to the CT, differ from the typical nodal cells by containing more and better organized and aligned myofibrils. The most significant difference recognized is probably the more frequent engagement of these cells in nexus junctions, a frequency which among the transitional cells close to the CT approximates that of the working atrial myocardium.

The cauda of the sinus node over its full length onto the posterior circumference of the OCS is composed of cells with essentially the same characteristics as the typical nodal cells (828).

The SARB, in its right as well as its left (septal) branch is formed of regular cylindrical muscle cells which differ from the working atrial cardiocytes virtually only by their very small diameter. They are like those connected at their ends by well developed intercalated discs, and along their lateral surface by occasional nexuses (828).

---

4. The distribution of intercellular contacts in various cardiac tissues has recently been reviewed by Kawamura and James (429).
5. For recent review see e.g. Berger (64).
6. The rabbit received 5-OH-dopamine (80 mg/kg i.v. $\frac{1}{2}$ hour prior to fixation) producing a stable precipitate in the small vesicles of adrenergic axons (Tranzer, J. P. & Thoenen, H., *Experientia*, 23: 743 (1967); Chiba, T., *Anat. Rec.* 176: 35 (1973).

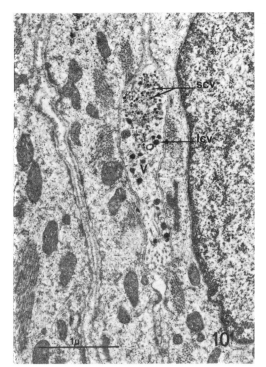

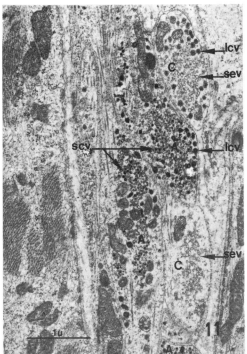

Fig. 10[6]. Axon varicosity (V) in close contact with SA nodal cells, the membranes of the nerve and muscle cells being separated by a 15 nm gap. No signs of subsynaptic specialization is seen in the muscle cells. The varicosity is identified as adrenergic by the presence of small dense cored vesicles (scv) in addition to large dense cored vesicles (lcv). (Magn.: 23,400:1).

Fig. 11. Bundle of axons between SA nodal cells. Adrenergic varicosities (A) containing large (lcv) and small (scv) dense core vesicles are in close apposition to cholinergic varicosities (C) containing small empty vesicles (sev) in addition to lcv. (Magn.: 18,300:1).

Innervation of the SA node[7]

In fluorescence microscopy for catecholamines (36,233), and staining for cholinesterase (84,233), the node, including the transitional portions, is outlined by its ample supply with adrenergic and cholinergic nerve fibres compared to the working myocardium. Most axon profiles and varicosities seen in electron micrographs are separated from the nodal cells by distances of 100 nm or more, completely or partly covered by Schwann cell extensions and are preferentially located in the larger interstices between the nodal cells. Naked varicose axons are mostly found in the narrower clefts between the cells, and some of these engage in close contacts. At these sites the membranes of the axon swelling and the muscle cell are separated by a 15–20 nm gap (fig. 10), and the same axon swelling may often be seen in close contact with both of the apposed muscle cells. Close contacts are fairly common in the rabbit SA node, and they have been observed in studies on the SA node of several species (58,63,428,613,830).

7. The innervation of mammalian cardiac tissues has recently been comprehensively reviewed by Yamauchi (954).

There are no conspicuous signs of postsynaptic specialization in the muscle cells. The location of subsarcolemmal cisterns of the SR at the site of the contact has been noted in several studies, and may often seem striking. However, they are not always seen, and whether the location is preferential lacks quantitation.

It may be noteworthy that cholinergic and adrenergic axons regularly course together in the same bundles with no Schwann cell extensions between the opposing axolemmas (fig. 12). Thickenings of the axon membranes have been observed at these sites, suggestive of an interaction between the different axons (599).

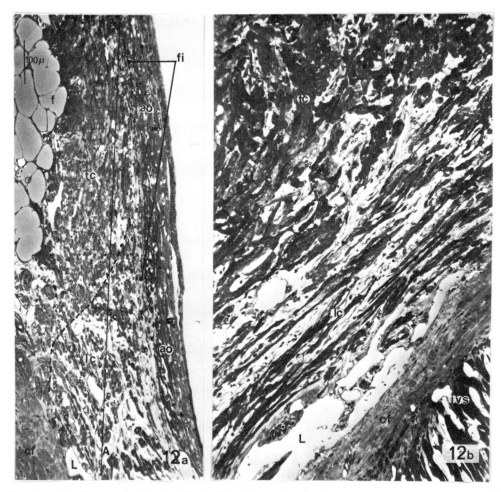

Fig. 12 a and b. Cross section (to the left) of rabbit AV node shortly after the entrance into the enclosed nodal compartment. The zone of transitional cells (tc) is located above and beneath the zone of lower nodal cells (lc). The zones are not readily distinguished in transverse sections (approximate border marked by stippled line) and the two tissues blend along the border. In the corresponding longitudinal section (obtained by 90° re-orientation of the block, the left margin of fig. 12b corresponding to line A of fig. 12a) the subdivision is clearly demonstrated. The lc form longitudinally oriented bundles of slender cells and the tc appear as irregular trabeculae. A layer of atrial muscle (ao) covers the nodal tissues with a layer of fibrous tissue (fi) intervening. ivs: Interventricular septum inserting into the central fibrous body (cf); f: fat cells; L: lymphatic space. Direction of AV bundle towards the right. (Magn.: 120:1) The rather considerable individual variation in the microtopographical relations of the tissues in this region is illustrated by comparison with figures 25a and 26a.

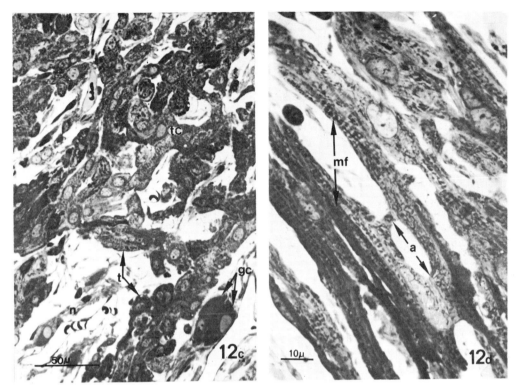

Fig. 12c. (Detail of fig. 12b) The rounded and irregular transitional cells (tc) are joined in trabeculate strands (t) with little predominant orientation. gc: ganglion cells which are frequently found inside and around the AV nodal tissues of the rabbit. n: nerve fibre containing a small ganglion cell. (Magn.: 370:1)

Fig. 12d. (Detail of fig. 12b). The long slender lower nodal cells contain comparatively regularly aligned myofibrils (mf) and the cells are joined together in longitudinally oriented, branching and anastomosing (a) bundles. (Magn.: 950:1)

THE AV JUNCTIONAL SPECIALIZED TISSUES

The AV junctional tissues, defined as the AV node, its atrial connecting fibres, and the non-branching part of the AV bundle (353), comprise very heterogeneous tissues, the structural and cellular complexity of which are still very incompletely clarified. Considerable individual and species variations in the shape and histological structure have been observed in these tissues (835,837), and marked regional differences in the structure and cellular composition of the AV nodal tissues have recently been demonstrated in systematic ultrastructural studies in some species (mouse: (810), rabbit: (262) and monkey: (864)).

Topographical and LM identification
The AV junctional tissues of the rabbit (fig. 1) are located in the triangular region bound distally by the attachment of the septal tricuspid leaflet, posteriorly by the OCS, anteriorly by the membraneous septum and superiorly by the anterior extension of the sinus septum from where a strand of fibrous tissue, the tendon of Todaro, takes a straight course to the central fibrous body, and when visible may serve as a useful landmark for the cranial

extension of the nodal tissues ((31) and chapter 15 by Becker and Anderson). The variations in the position of the landmarks of this region are generally too great to allow a precise
macroscopical location of the different compartments of the junctional tissues. Recent
studies (20) have demonstrated the presence of histologically and histochemically distinct
cellular zones within the rabbit AV nodal tissue, which subsequently have been correlated
with characteristic electrophysiological (EP) specializations in a combined EP and
morphological study (31 and chapter 17 by Janse et al.).

Based on these studies, the rabbit AV node can be histologically divided (fig. 1) into
two compartments: a posterior *open node* which receive the atrial inputs along its upper
and posterior margins, and an anterior *enclosed node* surrounded by and isolated from the
atrial myocardium by a sheath of fibrous tissue formed by the fibrous annulus of the
tricuspid orifice and extensions from the central fibrous body. The upper portion of the
open node is occupied by the *transitional cell (TC) zone*, which receives the atrial inputs.
Anteriorly this zone proceeds into a *zone of compact- or mid-nodal cells (MC)* located in
the enclosed nodal compartment. The *zone of lower nodal cells (LC)* is a longitudinally
oriented bundle extending the full length of the nodal area, proceeding posteriorly along
the fibrous annulus, and anteriorly into the AV bundle.

The TC zone of the open node which receives the atrial inputs is composed of small
flattened cells, sparse in myofibrils. In longitudinal sections they form a network with a
predominant orientation corresponding to the longitudinal axis of the node. Proceeding
anteriorly the appearance of the TC tissue progressively changes. At about the entrance
into the enclosed node (fig. 12a and b) the TC are made up of small rounded cells forming a
complicated network of anastomosing trabecula with little predominant orientation (fig.
12c). Proceeding into the enclosed node the size of the TC zone decreases and the cells
become more closely applied. The MC zone (fig. 13) is recognized as a relatively small
mass of very closely applied intertweening muscle cells, the boundaries of which can not
be resolved by the LM (fig. 14), and located well inside the enclosed nodal compartment.

The bundle of LC is not very characteristic in transverse sections but in the corresponding longitudinal sections (fig. 12a and b) the bundle is clearly recognized. It is formed by
small, slender and mostly regularly cross striated muscle cells joined together in longitudinally oriented anastomosing fascicles (fig. 12d). Posteriorly the bundle is very thin
and is located below, and sometimes a little medial to the zone of TC. Proceeding anteriorly
the bundle widens and extends often an appreciable distance onto the medial side of the
TC zone (fig. 12a, 25a). During the course in the open node, contacts between the TC and
LC are not apparent. From about the point of entrance into the enclosed node, bundles
of muscle cells derived from the TC zone blend with the LC (fig. 12a and b) and more
anteriorly connections become more frequent. The anteriorly located connecting fibres
(fig. 13, 15) form discrete bundles which blend with the LC and proceed with these into
the AV bundle. It is not clear whether these fibres should be considered as being derived
from the TC, MC, LC or constitute a fourth fibre type. This zone of transition from the
AV node into the AV bundle is further complicated since superiorly located TC seem
to by-pass the compact nodal portion and proceed anteriorly. The transition from the AV
node to the AV bundle is for these reasons ill defined in the rabbit, and in agreement
with the findings in the monkey heart (864), the transition exhibit marked individual
variations.

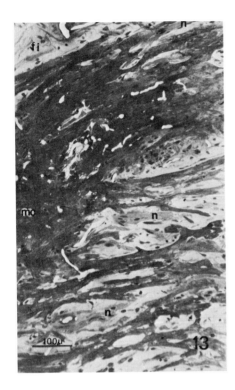

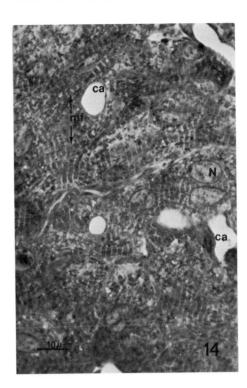

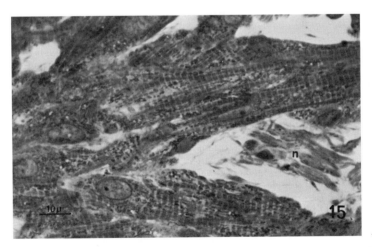

Fig. 13. Zone of transition from AV node into AV bundle seen in longitudinal section. Longitudinally oriented bundles of muscle cells depart from the compact midnodal tissue (mc) and proceed into the AV bundle towards the right. More longitudinally oriented strands of nodal cells resembling transitional cells proceed over the mc towards the AV bundle. n: nerves; fi: fibrous sheath of enclosed nodal compartment. (Magn.: 120:1)

Fig. 14. High power light micrograph of compact midnodal tissue. The cells form a compact mass with no recognizable cell borders. Myofibrils (mf) course in nearly random directions leaving large cytoplasmic areas free. N: nuclei; ca: capillaries. (Magn.: 960:1)

Fig. 15. High power light micrograph of muscle cells departing from the compact midnodal tissue. The individual cells contain longitudinally oriented myofibrils and are joined in bundles. n: nerve fasicle. (Magn.: 960:1).

The *AV bundle* of the rabbit comprises throughout its length a very heterogeneous tissue with cells of very varying diameters collected in bundles as described in several other species (835,837,864). A compartmentalization of the fibres is usually pronounced in the rabbit, and small diameter cells seems predominant in the lower right portion of the bundle (fig. 16).

Fine structure
The AV nodal tissue shows many similarities with the SA nodal cells with respect to their organization of myofibrils, SR, mitochondria and other cell organelles and shall not be gone over in detail again. The most marked differences are concerned with the cellular

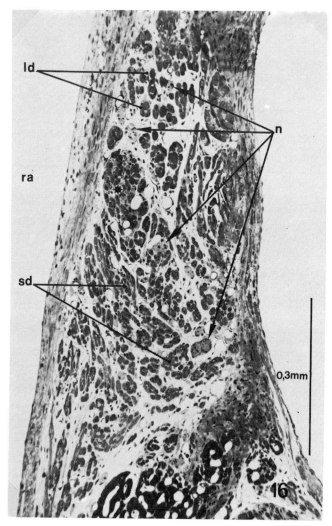

Fig. 16. Cross section of penetrating portion of the AV bundle. The bundle is composed of cells of very varying diameters. Small diameter cells (sd) are predominant in the lower right part of the bundle, and large diameter cells (1d) at the top and towards the left of the bundle. The individual cells are joined in fibres which are collected in groups. Numerous nerve fasicles (n) are located between the muscle cells and dense aggregates of nerves and muscle fibres are formed (asterix). ra: right atrium. (Magn.: 140:1)

shapes and distribution of intercellular contacts. Although obvious differences in cellular shapes exist in the various zones of the AV node, the differences are difficult to define more precisely in single sections in the EM than when observed by the LM and measurement of their size does not mean very much due to their irregularity. Careful EM serial section work on the AV node of the mouse (810) has clearly revealed great individual variations in the shape of adjacent cells, but with a tendency for zonal differences. Regional differences in the distribution of nexus junctions were clearly demonstrated. Such regional

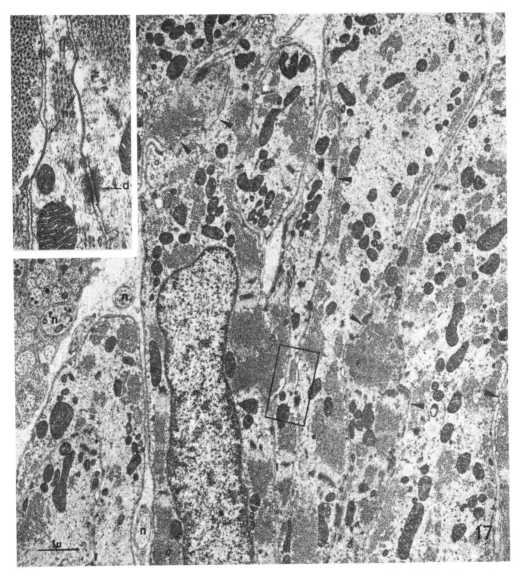

Fig. 17. Cross section from the lower posterior region of the transitional cell zone. Interlacing cell extensions come into close apposition over long stretches. Nexus junctions are frequently observed in this tissue. (Position of nexuses marked by arrowheads and inset.) ne: nexuses; d: desmosome; n: nerve and single axons. (Magn.: 11,500:1)

differences have also been observed in the rabbit (262), and an overall low frequency of these junctions compared to the working myocardium has been a consistent finding in EM studies on the AV node of several species (349, 350, 428, 439, 810, 822, 864).

In the posteriorly located TC zone in the open node of the rabbit, the cells are typically flattened in the plane of the endocardium, and the cells are closely applied over large areas of their surface (fig. 17). In this region nexuses are fairly common and several can be observed in nearly all low power micrographs. Anteriorly in the TC zone, where the cells are more rounded (fig. 18), and form trabeculae, the nexuses are more scarce.

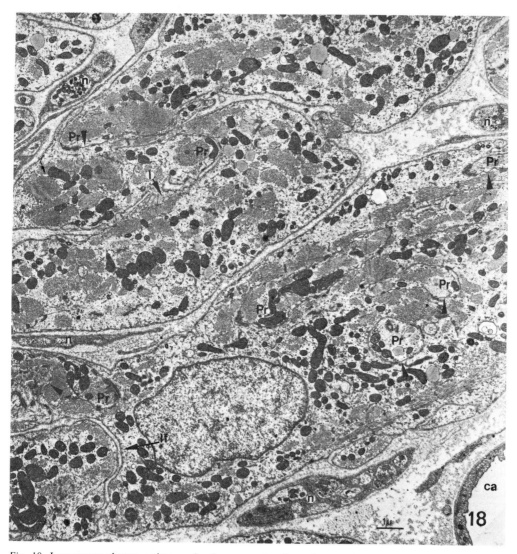

Fig. 18. Low power electron micrograph of cross section from the anterior region of the transitional cell zone. The irregularly contoured cells are collected in groups and send processes (Pr) into each other. Complex interdigitations (I) are formed between apposed cell membranes. Position of nexuses marked by arrowheads. lf: subsarcolemmal leptomere fibril; n: nerves; ca: capillary. (Magn.: 7580:1)

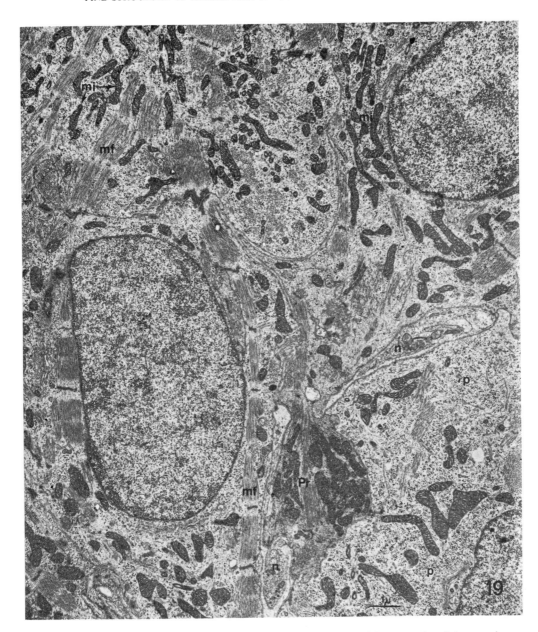

Fig. 19. Compact midnodal tissue. The cells are closely packed together with long stretches of close membrane apposition leaving little intercellular space between the cells. Large quantities of particulate material (p) are seen in the cytoplasm between the poorly developed and irregular coursing myofibrils (mf) together with irregularly shaped mostly slender mitochondria (mi). Nexus junctions are rarely found among these cells. Pr: cell process bulging into the body of another cell; n: nerves located in the sparse intercellular spaces. (Magn.: 8550:1)

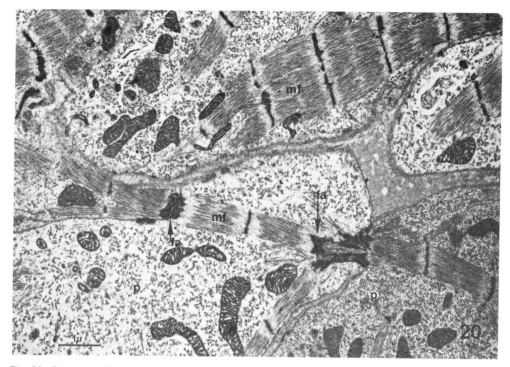

Fig. 20. Compact midnodal tissue. The myofibrils (mf) are coursing in various directions in the cells and connect by fasciae adherentes (fa) with myofibrils in other cells to form an anastomosing network in the tissue. Many of the small particles (p) seen in these cells form short rows and are likely to be ribosomes. (Magn.: 12,000:1)

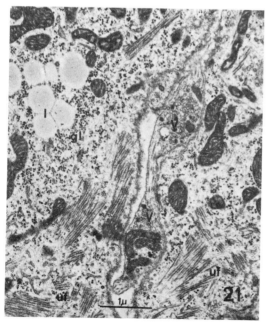

Fig. 21. Compact midnodal tissue. An example on the very frequent neuromuscular contacts encountered in the AV nodal tissues of the rabbit. The same axon is seen in close contact by two varicosities (V) with the muscle cells to the right with no signs of subsynaptic specialization. Distinct glycogen granules (gl) are seen among lipid droplets (l) in the cell to the left. uf: very poorly organized sarcomere structures. (Magn.: 14,700:1)

The MC tissue has a highly characteristic appearance (fig. 19). The irregularly contoured cells are closely applied over almost their entire periphery. Their poorly developed myofibrils have very varying orientations and connect by frequent fasciae adherentes with myofibrils in other cells forming an irregular network of connected myofibrils throughout the tissue (fig. 20). These cells contain very large amounts of small particles many of which are probably ribosomes owing to their small size and their tendency to occur in rows while others are distinct glycogen granules (fig. 21). This tissue is further characterised among the

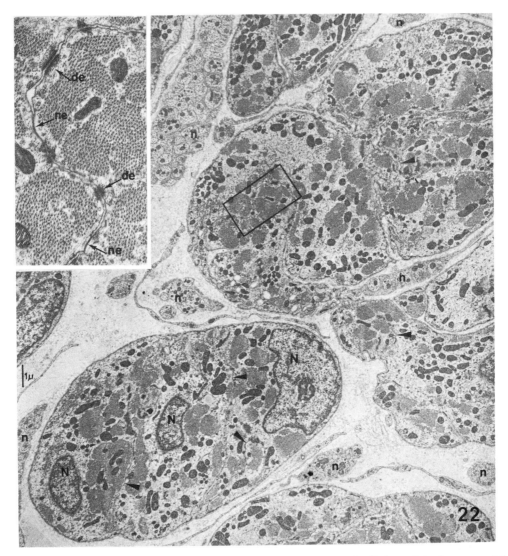

Fig. 22. Low power electron micrograph of cross sectioned lower nodal cells located in the open nodal compartment. The cells are joined together in discrete bundles with extensive areas of close membrane apposition along which nexus junctions are frequent (arrowheads and inset). Three muscle cells are cut at level with the nuclei (N) at lower left. Several nerves (n) are located in the intercellular space. ne: nexuses; d: desmosomes. (Magn.: 6,300:1, inset 22,000:1)

AV nodal tissues by a very low frequency of nexuses, particularly in proportion to the large areas of close membrane apposition. Usually only a few nexuses can be found in each section.

The LC (fig. 22) as seen in the LM form discrete bundles of closely applied long slender cells. Their internal structure show, as in the other AV nodal tissues, many similarities to the SA nodal cells except for a more regular myofibrillar organization. Nexuses are frequently observed along the areas of close membrane apposition as in the posterior TC region.

The cells of the *AV bundle* as seen in the LM are very heterogeneous with respect to cell diameter, a feature they share with Purkinje fibres of the ventricles of several species (771,864). No attempts have so far been made to classify them in the rabbit. They are like the ventricular Purkinje fibres connected by frequent and large areas of nexus formation (fig. 23).

THE INNERVATION OF THE AV JUNCTIONAL TISSUES

The AV node receives an abundant supply of adrenergic and cholinesterase-containing nerve fibres (84,233). Regional differences both in the density and type of nerve fibres has been evidenced histochemically in the rabbit (20). Close contacts between nerves

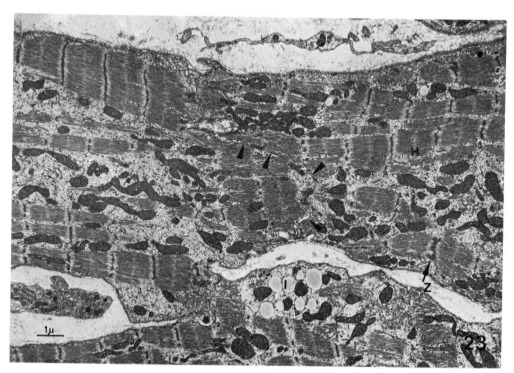

Fig. 23. Low power electron micrograph of longitudinally sectioned cells in the upper portion of penetrating AV bundle. The cells are largely cylindrical and connect at their ends by frequent and long stretches of nexus formation (arrowheads). The myofibrils are also here relatively poorly developed with interrupted and often thickened Z discs (Z) and slurrish H bands (H). l: lipid droplets. (Magn.: 7550:1)

and muscle cells have been observed in several species, and careful EM serial sectioning studies on the mouse AV node (809,810) have revealed the presence of extensive neuro-muscular contacts, which however show regional differences in frequency.

Neuromuscular contacts may regularly be found in all of the AV nodal tissues of the

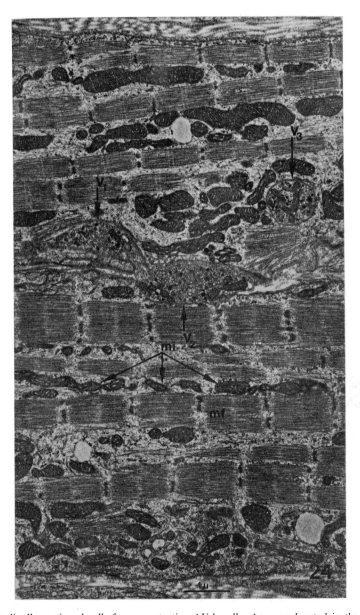

Fig. 24. Longitudinally sectioned cells from penetrating AV bundle. An axon located in the space between two cells form two varicosities (V_1 & V_2) which make close contacts engrooved in the muscle cells. A third varicosity profile (V_3) is seen in the upper muscle cell. Rows of slender mitochondria (mi) are located among parallel aligned myofibrils (mf). (Magn.: 12,000:1)

rabbit (fig. 21) and may appear particularly numerous among the TC. The areas of contact show the same features as seen in the SA node.

The AV bundle of many species has been shown to contain a large number of nerve fibres, but the density and relative proportion of cholinergic and adrenergic fibres may not be equal in all species (954). In the rabbit, nerves occupy a considerable percentage of the cross sectioned area of the bundle (fig. 16) (84). Axons are seen in close relation to nearly all of the muscle cells, and close contacts are frequently observed, sometimes very large (fig. 24).

THE 'INTERCALATED CLEAR CELLS'

The occurrence of a cell type, whose main characteristics are, that in contrast to the surrounding cells they are large, pale and contain few and poor myofibrils in proportion to the cell volume, has been described in many cardiac tissues in a variety of species. Such cells

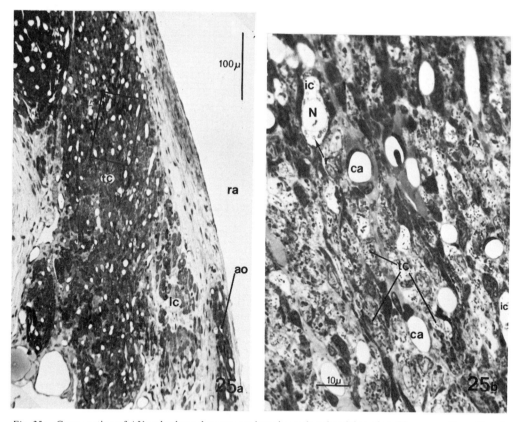

Fig. 25a. Cross section of AV node about the entrance into the enclosed nodal portion. The zones of transitional (tc) and lower nodal (lc) cells are clearly distinguished. Myocardium of interatrial septum is seen at upper left. A few strands of atrial overlay fibres (ao) is seen at lower right. (Magn.: 185:1)

Fig. 25b. (Detail of fig. 25a (frame)). A few intercalated clear cells (ic) are found among the normal appearing transitional cells (tc). The nucleus (N) of the intercalated clear cell is large and waterclear, and in the cytoplasm ring shaped structures (r) are seen. ca: capillaries. (Magn.: 960:1)

have particularly been noted in the nodal regions, in the valvular structures around the coronary sinus, and in the interatrial septum (396, 399, 828, 839, 862–864). The nature and significance of these cells remain uncertain. For a morphological consideration of their nature the following features may be taken into account.

They often occur singly, intercalated among cells which exhibit the normal morphological characteristics of the particular tissue in which they are located, and they possess the same types of intercellular connections which are characteristic for the particular tissues (828, 863).

Their number within the same tissue may vary considerably. In the TC zone of the rabbit AV node they may be found in greatly varying numbers in different hearts (fig. 25, 26), and within the same heart very varying degrees of 'clearnes' are observed, ranging from cells which differ little from the surrounding cells to very large, nearly waterclear cells (fig. 26b).

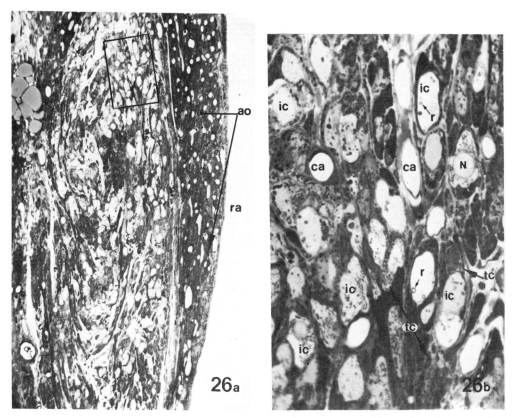

Fig. 26a. Cross section of another AV node than that of figure 25 in the same position at about the entrance into the enclosed nodal portion, (identified by the cessation of atrial connections along the upper nodal margin when serially sectioned from behind). The heart is fixed and processed as in that of figure 25 and illustrates the puzzling phenomenon of the varying amounts of intercalated clear cells. The atrial overlay (ao) is in this heart very pronounced. An excessive amount of clear cells occupy the entire nodal tissue and the lower nodal cells can hardly be distinguished. (Magn.: 185:1)

Fig. 26b. (Detail of figure 26a (frame).) Large numbers of intercalated clear cells (ic) with round pale nuclei (N) are intercalated among normal appearing transitional cells (tc). The varying degree of "clearness" is very conspicuous. Ring shaped structures (r) are found in the cytoplasm of the most clear cells. (Magn.: 960:1)

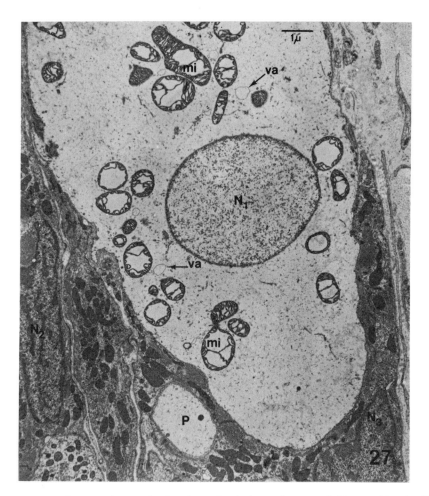

Fig. 27. Low power electron micrograph of an intercalated clear cell surrounded by transitional cells of the AV node. The nucleus (N) of the clear cell is cut outside the equatorial plane, and exhibits a homogeneous finely granular distribution of chromatin compared with the nuclei of surrounding cells (N_2 & N_3), which on the other hand appear somewhat condensed. The mitochondria (mi)—corresponding to the ring shaped structures seen in the LM—exhibit large empty spaces and the cristae are distorted. Empty vacuoles (va) are seen in the cytoplasm which does not contain other recognizable structures. A process likely to belong to a clear cell is seen surrounded by normal appearing cells below. (Magn.: 7400:1)

Ultrastructurally they are characterized by their poor content of myofibrils, which exhibit a low degree of order, and in the most waterclear cells (fig. 27) organized myofibrils are virtually absent. The nuclei are large and rounded compared to the surrounding cells, and exhibit a finely granular, homogeneous distribution of chromatin, most pronounced in the most waterclear cells. Their mitochondria are also large, the inter-cristal spaces being widened, often considerably, while the cristae are thinned and distorted, changes which are again most pronounced in the most clear cells. Empty vacuoles are often present in the cytoplasm. The cells may or may not contain glycogen granules, and it seems that the most clear cells are devoid of these.

It may appear that the morphology of these cells could be formally explained by osmotic swelling together with internal disorganization of cell organelles of the cells characteristic for the particular tissues. Changes of this kind may be observed in many other tissues where they are recognized as products of the preparative procedures, notably the circumstances of fixation, and the changes are often not uniform in the tissues. It is the author's opinion that these large clear cells observed in cardiac tissues may have an artefactual origin, caused by unphysiological conditions prior to the fixation, and it is felt that the nature of these cells, to which so many important functions have been ascribed is in need for further investigation.

IMPULSE FORMATION AND CONDUCTION

4
RECENT OBSERVATIONS SUPPORTING THE ROLE OF SLOW CURRENT IN CARDIAC ELECTROPHYSIOLOGY[1]

DOUGLAS P. ZIPES, M.D.

INTRODUCTION

Within the past ten years, the concept has emerged that the ionic currents underlying the cardiac action potential involve calcium as well as sodium and potassium. The purpose of this communication is to review the development of this concept and attempt to relate it to our understanding of clinical electrophysiology and of the pathogenesis of some arrhythmias.

BASIC ELECTROPIIYSIOLOGIC CONCEPTS

Twenty-six years ago, Hodgkin and Katz (359) demonstrated that a large and relatively specific increase in the membrane permeability to sodium ions accounted for the amplitude and rate of voltage change of the depolarization phase of squid nerve action potentials. Using the voltage-clamp technique, Hodgkin and Huxley (360) dissected the currents underlying the nerve action potential into two constituents, an inward sodium flow followed by an outward potassium flow, and formulated equations to describe how these currents vary with transmembrane voltage potential and time. Over the ensuing years, cardiac electrophysiologists, assuming that exclusively sodium and potassium movements were involved, applied the Hodgkin-Huxley analysis of transmembrane current flow to explain the markedly more complex waveforms of cardiac action potentials (600). However, as early as 1956, Coraboeuf and Otsuka (143) noted that the overshoot of the action potential in the guinea pig ventricle was rather insensitive to the extracellular sodium concentration and in the early 1960s, many investigators working independently, for reviews, see Weidmann (900), Trautwein (831), Reuter (653)], showed that the kinetics of the inward ionic flow in cardiac fibers could not be satisfactorily described in terms of sodium ion movement alone. Neidergerke and Orkand (596) soon demonstrated a sodium-calcium competition for entry into myocardial cells, and indicated that the upstroke of the frog heart action potential, but not its peak overshoot potential, were altered by variations in the sodium concentration. Hagiwara and Nakajima (333) developed a very important pharmacologic tool by demonstrating that cardiac fibers possessed one current (fast current) sensitive to tetrodotoxin (TTX) and another current (slow current) sensitive

1. Supported in part by the Herman C. Krannert Fund; by Grants HL-06308, HL-05363 and HL-05749 from the National Heart and Lung Institute of the National Institutes of Health; and by the Indiana Heart Association.

to manganese (Mn). In the late 1960s, Reuter (652) presented evidence for a slow component of depolarization which is not very sensitive to variations in the extracellular concentration of sodium ions, but is uniquely sensitive to the extracellular concentration of
calcium ions, and is sluggish in its kinetics of activation and, especially, inactivation.
Subsequent work established that the fast sodium inward current, responsible for the
rapid upstroke of the cardiac action potential, triggers this second slower current, which is
carried by calcium ions or by sodium ions (or possibly by both) and which is responsible
primarily for the plateau phase of the cardiac action potential. These two inward currents,
the fast and the slow current, are probably interdependent; depolarization is undoubtedly
more complex than simply a rapid component followed by a slow component. Both
currents are present in specialized conducting tissues and in atrial and ventricular muscle
cells. In cardiac muscle cells, the slow inward calcium current is essential for coupling
excitation of the cell membrane to activation of the contractile proteins (653,831,900).
Although some species differences among characteristics of the slow current may
eventually be found, it is now clear that this current is a fundamental physiological
property of all myocardial tissue (653,831,900).

MANIPULATION OF INWARD CURRENTS

Both the fast and slow currents are voltage and time dependent, but have sufficiently
different characteristics to allow their independent study. For example, the fast inward
channel may be inactivated under conditions which do not interrupt the function of the
slow channels. Partial loss of resting membrane potential in ventricular fibers, which
ordinarily exhibit a large fast component, may allow emergence of action potentials that
are dependent on the slow component during depolarization. The fast channels may be
inactivated by depolarizing fibers using either voltage-clamp techniques or by increasing
extra-cellular potassium concentration (108,250,900). Also, TTX which has been shown
to specifically block the fast sodium conductance in nerve tissue (587), pharmacologically
inactivates the rapid current in cardiac fibers without altering resting potential (108,333).
Under these conditions the tissue becomes inexcitable. Factors which augment transmembrane calcium flux restore regenerative, propagated action potentials to the tissue.
For example, agents such as catecholamines, histamine, xanthines, and dibutyryl cyclic
adenosine monophosphate, which all increase intracellular cyclic adenosine monophosphate (cAMP) levels, directly augment the slow inward current (617,817,892). Recent
evidence suggests that the increase in slow inward current caused by elevated cAMP levels
is responsible for the positive inotropic effects of these agents (892).. These restored
responses do not occur in a calcium free medium unless calcium is replaced by certain
other divalent cations such as strontium or barium (333,617). The restored action potentials are characterized by a slow upstroke velocity, delayed recovery of excitability and
their propagation through the tissue is slow and exhibits unidirectional block, summation,
inhibition and re-entry (161,162).
    The slow current can be selectively blocked by the cations manganese, cobalt, nickel,
and lanthanum as well as by the synthetic organic compounds verapamil and D600 (a

Table 1.

Electrophysiologic Property	Rapid Current	Slow Current
Activation and inactivation kinetics	Rapid	Slow
Dependent on extracellular ion concentration of:	Sodium	Calcium
Abolished by:	Tetrodotoxin	Manganese, cobalt, nickel, lanthanum, verapamil, D600
Threshold of activation	−60 to −70 mV	−30 to −40 mV
Resting membrane potential	−80 to −95 mV	−40 to −70 mV
Conduction velocity	0.5 − 3.0 M/Sec	0.01–0.1 M/Sec
Overshoot	+20 to +35 mV	0 to +15 mV
Rate of rise (dV/dt) of action potential upstroke	200–1000 V/Sec	1–10 V/Sec
Action potential amplitude	100–130 mV	35–75 mV
Response to stimulus	All-or-none	Affected by characteristics of stimulus
Safety factor for conduction	High	Low
Recovery of excitability	Prompt, ends with repolarization	Delayed, outlasts full repolarization

methoxy derivative of verapamil) (273). Verapamil appears to block slow calcium current at a site distal to the beta adrenergic receptor, and therefore allows catecholamine-induced elevation of cAMP levels without permitting an increase in calcium influx (891). The characteristics of the rapid and slow currents are compared in table 1.

AUTOMATICITY

Automaticity, the property of a cell to spontaneously depolarize, has been thought to be due to a decrease in potassium conductance during a steady inward sodium movement, which results in a net intracellular accumulation of positive changes. Such automaticity is a normal characteristic of specialized fibers in the atria and ventricles (653,831,900). Recent observations suggest that slow inward currents may underlie automaticity which occurs during conditions facilitating slow-channel mechanisms. For example, oscillatory after-potentials capable of reaching threshold have been recorded in bovine cardiac Purkinje fibers in which only slow responses were present (108). Repetitive firing of canine Purkinje fibers has recently been demonstrated in a sodium-free, calcium-rich bathing medium where the slow-current rather than both currents is probably operative (38). Furthermore, toxic digitalis concentrations may induce a loss of resting potential in Purkinje fibers to a range in which they demonstrate oscillatory afterpotentials resembling those seen in sodium-free, calcium-rich solutions (167,677), (fig. 1). Repetitive firing has been shown in such digitalis intoxicated Purkinje fibers (265). The exact nature of the ionic fluxes responsible for diastolic depolarization in these preparations is presently

D. P. ZIPES

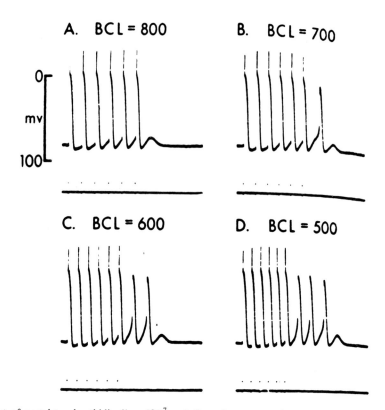

A. BCL = 800   B. BCL = 700

C. BCL = 600   D. BCL = 500

Fig. 1. Effect of acetylstrophanthidin (1×10^{-7} gm/ml) on the transmembrane potentials of canine Purkinje fibers driven for 6 cycles at different cycle lengths. Top tracing recorded from isolated false tendon; bottom tracing, stimulus artifacts. A, basic cycle length (BCL) 800 msec; driven train followed by a subthreshold transient depolarization (TD). B, BCL 700 msec; TD reached threshold and was followed by a subthreshold TD. C, BCL 600 msec; two consecutive TDs reached threshold, followed by a subthreshold TD. D, BCL 500 msec; three consecutive TDs reached threshold, followed by a subthreshold TD. Reproduced from Ferrier, G. R., Saunders, J. H., and Mendez, C., A cellular mechanism for the generation of ventricular arrhythmias by acetylstrophanthidin, *Circulat. Res.* 32:600, 1973, by permission of the American Heart Association, Inc.

unknown. The response of such automaticity to calcium-stimulating and slow-channel blocking agents suggests that the slow inward current is probably involved (267,279,679).

CLINICAL RELEVANCE OF THESE CONCEPTS

These data, borne originally of electrophysiological studies on isolated preparations, have important clinical relevance. For example, it would appear that normal sinus rhythm, (481,509,752,953,959), and normal A-V nodal conduction (614,705,958,959) are maintained by operation of slow-channel mechanisms. In addition to having most of the properties of slow-current responses (table 1), sinus and A-V nodal action potentials have contours similar in many ways to contours of slow-current dependent action potentials. In the sinus node and in the N region of the A-V node (fig. 2,3), it is possible that only the second slow-current may be present and propagation through these areas may normally

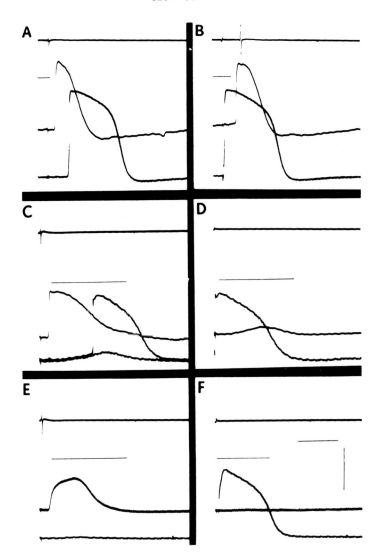

Fig. 2. Action of manganous chloride (MnCl$_2$) on AN and His bundle fibers during anterograde (left) and retrograde (right) propagation in the rabbit A-V nodal preparation. A and B: Control records obtained from the same cells; C and D: Results obtained from similar regions in the presence of 2 mM MnCl$_2$. E and F: Results obtained after 4 mM MnCl$_2$. Top tracing, atrial electrogram recorded with external electrode; middle tracing, transmembrane potential of an AN cell; bottom tracing, transmembrane potential of a His bundle fiber. Two sweeps illustrated in panel C. Horizontal lines preceding or above action potentials indicate 0 potential for the AN cells. MnCl$_2$ resulted in block at the level of the A-V node, by selectively suppressing activity in nodal cells without suppressing activity in the atrium or His bundle. Retrograde block generally preceded anterograde block at a concentration of 2 mM MnCl$_2$. Calibrations: 100 msec and 50 mV. Reproduced from *Circulat. Res* 32: 447, 1973, by permission of American Heart Association, Inc.

occur without engaging the fast component. Transitional cells on either side of the A-V node may demonstrate a continuum of relatively less dependence on slow-current contribution to depolarization, as a function of the distance from the N region (59). Summation, the ability of spatially separated wavefronts to exert, at a common site, an excitatory

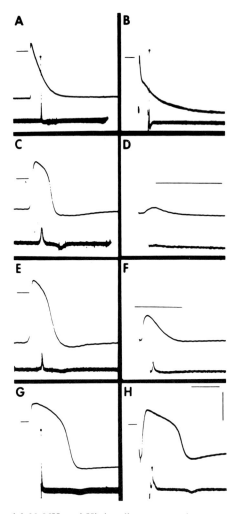

Fig. 3. Effects of MnCl$_2$ on atrial, N, NH, and His bundle trans-membrane potentials in the rabbit A-V nodal preparation. Left: Control observations. Right: After administration of MnCl$_2$ (3 mM). Top tracing, trans-membrane potentials; bottom tracing, dV/dt. A and B: Atrial cells; C and D: N cells; E and F: NH cells; G and H: His bundle cells. Atrial stimulation, A, B, C, D; His bundle stimulation, E, F, G and H. Horizontal lines preceding or above action potentials indicate 0 potential for each impaled cell. MnCl$_2$ selectively suppressed activity in the N region of the A-V node. Calibrations: 100 msec and 50 mV for all panels. Vertical calibration: 40 V/sec in A, B, E, G and H and 20 V/sec in C, D and F. Reproduced as in fig. 2, by permission of the American Heart Assn., Inc.

event which exceeds the effect produced by either wavefront alone, has been demonstrated in the A-V node (fig. 4) (366, 957) and may be present in the S-A node as well. Cells in the A-V node also exhibit recovery of excitability which is delayed beyond the time required for restoration of the membrane potential to its full diastolic level (548). Summation and delayed recovery of excitability are both features of slow-channel responses (161, 162). Maximum membrane potential is less negative in sinus and A-V nodal cells than in other cardiac fibers. It is probable that this lower membrane potential influences the nature of

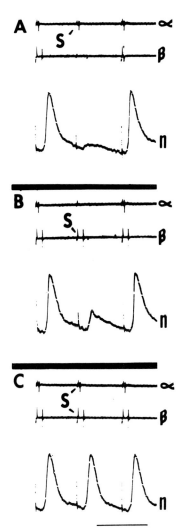

Fig. 4. Site of summation in the rabbit A-V node. This example was obtained by dividing the rabbit atrium into two sections to provide separate atrial inputs (arbitrarily called alpha and beta) into the A-V node. Top tracing, atrial electrogram recorded from the alpha side of the preparation; middle tracing, atrial electrogram recorded from the beta side of the preparation; bottom tracing, transmembrane action potential recorded from the cell impaled in the N region of the A-V node. Test stimulus (S) was delivered to either alpha (A) or beta (B) side of the atrium alone or to both sides together (C). Premature stimulation of either side alone resulted in block at the level of the A-V node. Stimulation of both sides together at the same intervals which previously failed to conduct resulted in summation and conduction. Time calibration in C, 300 msec. Reproduced from *Circulat. Res.* 32: 170, 1973, by permission of the American Heart Assn., Inc.

the currents and that hyperpolarization of sinus or A-V nodal cells might unmask an inherent rapid sodium current (756).

Slow-channel blockers may be used to detect which arrhythmias, or cell types, might be suppressed by such selective drug action. Because of the similarity noted above between nodal cells and slow-channel dependent cells, we have used slow-channel blockers to inhibit sinus and A-V nodal activity. Manganese suppresses (fig. 2, 3), while TTX fails to

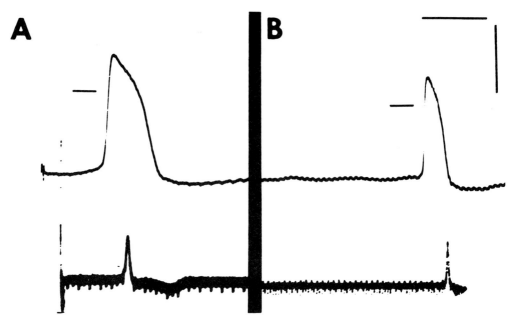

Fig. 5. Effect of tetrodotoxin (TTX) on transmembrane action potentials of N cells and the corresponding dV/dt in the rabbit A-V node. A: Control. B: After administration of tetrodotoxin, (5×10^{-6} gm/ml Tyrode's solution). TTX did not affect transmembrane action potentials obtained from the N region of the A-V node, while rendering atrium and His bundle inexcitable (not shown). Horizontal lines preceding action potentials indicate 0 potential. Horizonal calibration: 100 msec for A and 200 msec for B. Vertical calibration, 50 mV and 20 V/sec. Reproduced as in fig. 2, by permission of the American Heart Assn., Inc.

affect (fig. 5), sinus and A-V nodal potentials in isolated preparations (481, 509, 953, 958, 959). Slow-channel blockers infused into the sinus nodal and A-V nodal arteries (959) (or verapamil given IV) reduce sinus node discharge rate, depress A-V nodal conduction and lengthen the effective and functional A-V nodal refractory periods (fig. 6, 7). His-Purkinje conduction remains normal. In the whole dog, isoproterenol and epinephrine overcome the electrophysiologic effects of the slow-channel inhibiting agents, and this effect of the catecholamines is prevented by propranolol (959). Some of these observations have been recently confirmed in isolated preparations (937). It would appear that the generation of *normal* action potentials in the sinus and A-V nodes depends upon the slow ionic current, and therefore the slow current appears to be involved in both impulse formation (sinus node) and impulse conduction (A-V node). The physiologic role of the slow current may be different at these two nodal sites since the sinus node demonstrates automaticity while the N region of the A-V node normally does not. These findings have important clinical relevance because they suggest an entirely new pharmacologic approach, such as with verapamil, in treating tachyarrhythmias which involve the sinus and A-V nodes.

Calcium currents may play a part in the genesis of other cardiac arrhythmias and, if this is so, antiarrhythmic agents with a specific mechanism of action can be used to treat arrhythmias according to their specific ionic pathogenesis. The fact that automaticity may be due to different ionic mechanisms may explain why some drugs, e.g. lidocaine, suppress automaticity in normal Purkinje fibers but not in the sinus node.

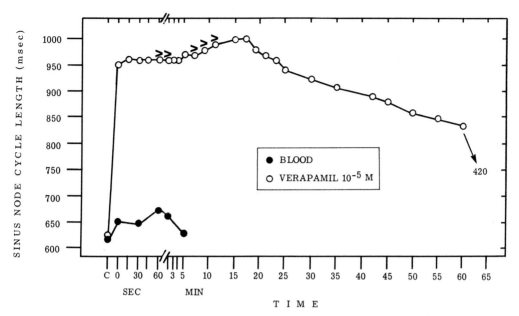

Fig. 6. Effects on the spontaneous sinus node cycle length of a single infusion of 1×10^{-5} M verapamil into the canine sinus node artery. Control, after infusing blood alone. At 60 minutes, isoproterenol (2 ml, 1.0 μg/ml) was infused into the sinus nodal artery. The symbol >, placed over a value indicates that the value was greater than that which could be recorded due to a junctional rhythm. C, spontaneous control cycle length prior to infusion; 0, first measurement of cycle length recorded 30 seconds after completion of a 2 ml flush injection which followed the verapamil infusion. Verapamil markedly slowed spontaneous sinus node discharge, which returned toward control values with time. Isoproterenol overcame the effects of verapamil and shortened the spontaneous sinus node cycle length to 420 msec, as indicated by the arrow. Reproduced from *Circulat. Res.* 34: 184, 1974, by permission of the American Heart Assn., Inc.

Such concepts may be important in patients with myocardial infarction. The infarct, because of the milieu of elevated potassium which has been released from dead or dying cells, plus local endogenously released catecholamines would seem quite conducive to slow-current mechanisms (162, 163, 892). It is well-known that experimental acute coronary artery ligation is associated with clearly defined stages of peak arrhythmic activity (342). These stages may relate to totally different electrophysiologic mechanisms which become operative at different times during the evolutionary changes following myocardial infarction. Not only may arrhythmias due to re-entry or automaticity occur at different times but whether they involve predominantly slow-current or fast-current mechanisms may vary in a temporal sequence. Conceivably, different parts of the myocardium may be at different evolutionary stages at the same time, and different pathogenic mechanisms may operate simultaneously. Although these thoughts are largely speculative, they are supported by some recent experimental data and could help explain why certain anti-arrhythmic agents may be more effective at different times during the evolution of the myocardial infarction (286, 474). The protective effects of sympathectomy (157) may relate, in part, to eliminating its stimulating role for slow-current dependent arrhythmias.

Other conditions which result in a reduction of the level of resting membrane potential also may be responsible for the production of slow-current arrhythmias and may be more

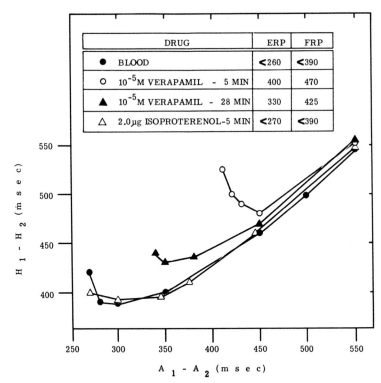

DRUG		ERP	FRP
●	BLOOD	<260	<390
○	10^{-5}M VERAPAMIL　-　5 MIN	400	470
▲	10^{-5}M VERAPAMIL　-　28 MIN	330	425
△	2.0 µg ISOPROTERENOL-5 MIN	<270	<390

Fig. 7. Effects on A-V nodal conduction of a single infusion into the canine posterior septal artery of 1×10^{-5} M verapamil, followed by a single infusion of isoproterenol (2 ml, 1.0 µg/ml). The values obtained after infusion of blood alone served as the control. Effective refractory period (ERP) and functional refractory period (FRP) of the A-V node at various times are indicated. Verapamil markedly prolonged the ERP and FRP, which gradually improved with time. Isoproterenol returned the values to the control state. Reproduced as in fig. 6, by permission of the American Heart Assn., Inc.

effectively treated with slow-channel blockers than with conventional anti-arrhythmic agents. One such area of interest involves the recent *in vivo* and *in vitro* demonstration of rather specific digitalis-induced arrhythmias, which exhibit overdrive acceleration rather than overdrive suppression, in response to rapid stimulation (fig. 1,8) (167, 265, 332, 677, 941, 961). The mechanism responsible for this overdrive acceleration is unknown, but clearly sets these arrhythmias apart from normal automaticity which exhibits overdrive suppression. Recently, similar ventricular arrhythmias exhibiting overdrive acceleration have been created with barium and strontium (280).

Although the evidence is far from overwhelming, some data suggest that these digitalis-induced arrhythmias may be caused by slow-channel dependent automaticity. In favor of such a conclusion is the observation that the arrhythmias *in vivo* and *in vitro* are enhanced by calcium administration and suppressed by slow-channel blockers (267, 279, 679). In the intact dog, these ouabain-induced arrhythmias resist suppression with routine doses of most antiarrhythmic agents, responding best to aprindine (279), a new antiarrhythmic agent which appears to suppress both the fast and the slow channels (650), (fig. 9). Calcium or isoproterenol administration reverses this suppression. It would be interesting to

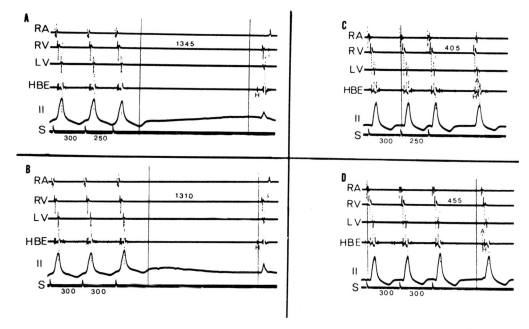

Fig. 8. Ouabain-induced repetitive ventricular response (RVR) and accelerated ventricular escape (AVE) in the dog. Panels A and B, control; panels C and D, after ouabain administration; panel C, RVR; panel D, AVE. Stimuli delivered simultaneously to right atrium and ventricle for ten cycles (300 msec). Following the last basic stimulus, either a premature stimulus was introduced (RVR, panel C) at an interval of 250–275 msec or pacing was abruptly terminated (AVE, panel D). Last three stimuli for each period of pacing are depicted. In the control state, a supraventricular escape beat initiated by discharge in or near the His bundle followed cessation of pacing (H-V interval, 35 msec). After ouabain administration, a ventricular escape followed termination of pacing (H activation begins after onset of ventricular activation). RA, right atrial electrogram; RV, right ventricular electrogram; LV, left ventricular electrogram; HBE, His bundle electrogram; II, Scalar lead II; S, stimulus. Time lines 1 second; paper speed, 100 mm/sec. Escape intervals in msec. Reproduced from *Circulation*, in press (Feb. 1976), by permission of the American Heart Assn., Inc.

establish overdrive acceleration as a feature of slow-current automaticity and apply that concept clinically. For example, the increased incidence of arrhythmias in ischemic hearts discharging at more rapid rates may reflect not just the effects of heightened ischemia, but also the rate-accelerating effects on slow-current dependent automaticity.

In this regard are some recent observations from our laboratory (280). We have recently been able to induce rate-accelerated ventricular escapes following calcium administration *in vivo*, (Foster, P. R., Elharrar, V., Zipes, D. P., unpublished). Because barium and strontium have been successfully substituted for calcium in preparations apparently dependent on slow-channel mechanisms (109, 260, 333, 617, 858, 859) we attempted to produce ventricular arrhythmias which exhibited overdrive acceleration by infusing barium or strontium intravenously. In these *in vivo* canine studies, barium administered IV, or strontium administered IV while concomitantly reducing serum potassium with glucose and insulin, resulted in ventricular escapes which shortened their escape interval following faster basic pacing rates (fig. 10) (280). Preliminary studies in isolated canine Purkinje fibers have confirmed the *in vivo* observations and revealed a rate-accelerated increase in automaticity in Purkinje fibers superfused with barium (fig. 11).

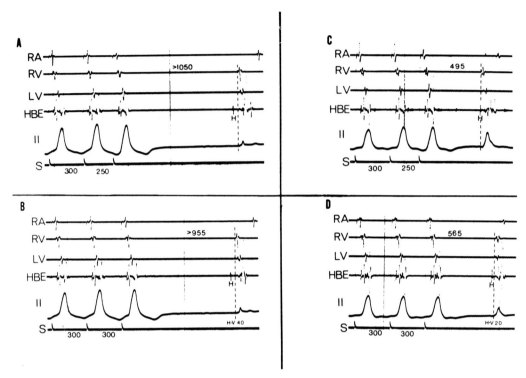

Fig. 9. Suppression of ouabain-induced RVR and AVE with aprindine, and return of RVR and AVE follow-ing calcium administration in the dog. Same experiment as in figure 8. After initiation of ouabain-induced RVR and AVE (fig. 8), aprindine administration (panels A and B) suppressed the ventricular escapes. In this example, a supraventricular escape beat initiated by discharge in or near the His bundle followed cessation of pacing or premature stimulation (H-V interval prolonged to 40 msec following aprindine). Thus, an RVR or AVE escape interval would exceed the supraventricular escape interval. After calcium administration (panels C and D), a ventricular escape beat followed termination of pacing (H-V interval shortened to 5 msec in panel C and 20 msec in panel D, indicating ventricular initiation of a probable fusion beat). Aprindine suppressed, while calcium reinitiated, the RVR and AVE. Interrupted line indicates earliest recorded onset of ventricular activation. Reproduced as in fig. 8, by permission of the American Heart Assn., Inc.

When comparing data obtained on the digitalis-induced arrhythmias and the normal sinus and A-V nodes, the observations do not all fit a cohesive picture. For example, these specific digitalis-induced arrhythmias have been shown to occur *in vitro* before digitalis has produced significant resting membrane depolarization, at voltage levels which should initiate the fast, not the slow current (265). Also, the response to pacing and calcium administration differ. As mentioned, digitalis, barium and strontium-induced arrhythmias exhibit overdrive *acceleration*, rather than overdrive *suppression*. Yet, the sinus node, thought perhaps to be a prototype of slow-current automaticity, exhibits overdrive suppression (508). Calcium administration reverses the suppressive effect which vera-pamil exerts on the digitalis-induced arrhythmias (279), but does not reverse the sup-pressive effect of slow-channel blockers on the sinus and A-V nodes in the whole dog (959). In addition, in vivo sensitivity to verapamil of the digitalis-induced arrhythmias and both nodes differ markedly. Generally, about 200 μg/Kg verapamil intravenously sup-

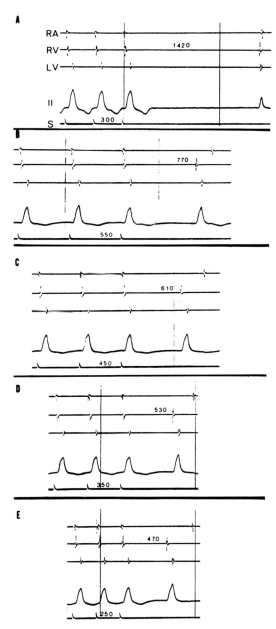

Fig. 10. Barium-induced overdrive acceleration in the intact dog. Recordings and method of testing as in figure 8, B and D. Panel A, control; panels B through E following intravenous barium infusion (10.9 *m*M/Kg) and pacing at progressively shorter basic cycle lengths. A supraventricular escape followed cessation of pacing in panel A, while accelerated ventricular escapes followed cessation of pacing in panels B through E. The interval between the last paced beat and the ventricular escape beat progressively shortened as the basic cycle length shortened.

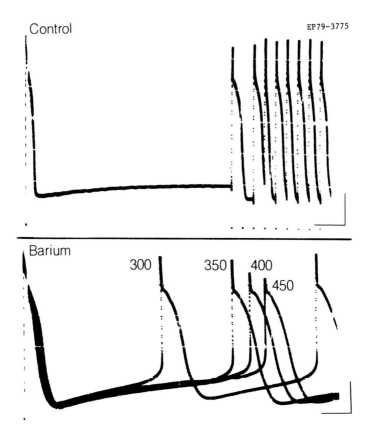

Fig. 11. Barium-induced overdrive acceleration in isolated canine Purkinje fiber ventricular muscle preparation. Tracings are transmembrane action potentials recorded from a Purkinje fiber. In the control state, (top), no spontaneous discharge followed a train of 10 stimuli delivered at a basic cycle length of 350 msec. After infusing barium chloride (0.1 mM in Tyrode's solution), automatic activity occurred in the Purkinje fiber and exhibited overdrive acceleration. The first action potential is the last of each train of ten driven action potentials that preceded cessation of pacing. After a pause, the first escaping action potential following cessation of pacing at different cycle lengths is depicted in superimposed sweeps. The numbers identify the basic cycle length which gave rise to each action potential. Calibration: Vertical calibration, 25 mV; horizontal calibration, 1, second top; 20 msec, bottom.

presses sinus and A-V nodal activity (unpublished observations), while more than 10 times that amount is needed to suppress the rate-dependent digitalis-induced arrhythmias. Aprindine was far more effective than was verapamil (fig. 9), (279).

Although manganese suppresses slow inward current of both catecholamine-evoked slow responses and those normally occurring in sinus nodal cells, not all slow currents appear sensitive to manganese. For example, ouabain directly accelerates sinus rate in isolated sinus nodal preparations, and this acceleration is blocked by manganese. On the other hand, the acceleration of sinus rates induced in the same preparation by catecholamines is *not* blocked by manganese given in concentrations which completely suppress ouabain-induced sinus node acceleration (346). Furthermore, ouabain is unable to *directly* augment the slow inward current evoked by catecholamines in potassium depolarized atrial and ventricular muscle cells even in concentrations which do produce positive inotropic effects (532,617,892). Perhaps the digitalis-induced arrhythmias, and sinus and A-V nodal cells are not both slow-current dependent; or maybe more than one calcium-dependent slow channel exists, with different electro-physiologic features.

It is obvious that much work needs to be done to place the roles of slow inward current in proper clinical perspective. However, it is exciting to consider the possible electro-physiologic and therapeutic implications of this concept, which, in its present form, is less than 10 years old. One must not forget that the slow current is important in both the electrical and mechanical properties of the heart and therefore, agents which block the slow channel also depress contractility. The therapeutic goal will be to use slow-channel blockers which exert a clinically beneficial antiarrhythmic effect at doses which do not significantly reduce cardiac output. It may even be possible to develop drugs which selectively affect slow-channel dependent arrhythmias while leaving contractility relatively unimpaired.

ACKNOWLEDGEMENT

Parts of this manuscript appeared as an Editorial in *Circulation*, June 1975, to which H. R. Besch, Jr. Ph.D. and August M. Watanabe, M.D. contributed enormously. The studies on ouabain, aprindine, barium and strontium were done in collaboration with a number of associates: Peter R. Foster, M.D., Victor Elharrar, Ph.D., J. Christopher Bailey, M.D., and David A. Lathrop, Ph.D.

5

EFFECT OF AUTONOMIC ACTIVITY ON PACEMAKER FUNCTION AND CONDUCTION[1]

E. NEIL MOORE, D.V.M., Ph.D., AND JOSEPH F. SPEAR, Ph.D.

The effect of the autonomic nervous system on impulse formation and conduction within the heart is well known. The time course of the effect of a brief vagal volley on sinus node cycle length was first measured by Brown and Eccles in 1934 (93). Subsequent workers described the discrete effect of phasic changes in vagal tone on spontaneous sinus rhythm in both animals and man during complete atrioventricular conduction block (40, 443, 448, 490, 685). Several laboratories have defined the time course of autonomic stimulation on atrioventricular conduction (186, 542, 778, 872), however there have been few studies concerning the role of phasic variations in autonomic tone on arrhythmia production. The present studies describe effects of phasic stimulation of the sympathetic and parasympa-

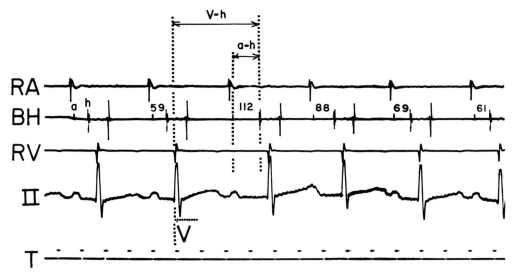

Fig. 1. The influence of brief vagal stimulation on AV nodal conduction time. Bipolar electrograms were recorded from the right atrium (RA), the bundle of His (BH), and the right ventricle (RV), simultaneously with a lead II electrocardiogram (II). In the His bundle electrogram, a and h indicate septal and His bundle activation respectively. The a-h intervals are indicated in msec for the subsequent beats. V indicates the timing of a 100 msec train of stimuli delivered to the left vagus. Timing signal t denotes 100 msec intervals. V-h indicates the interval between the beginning of the vagal stimulation and the His bundle activation of the subsequent beat. a-h indicates the atrial to bundle of His conduction time for the first beat following vagal stimulation.

1. This study was supported by U.S. Public Health Service Grants HL-16076 and HE-4885 and by grants from the American Heart Association.

thetic nervous system upon atrioventricular conduction in the anesthetized open-chest dog.

Figure 1 presents analog data describing the basic techniques used in these experiments. Close bipolar electrograms were recorded from the right atrium, the bundle of His, and the right ventricle, together with a simultaneously recorded lead II ECG. In order to eliminate complications due to variations in cycle length induced by autonomic stimulation, the hearts were paced from the right atrial appendage at constant basic cycle lengths. The conduction time through the AV node is approximated by the time interval between the low atrial septal component (a) and the His spike (h) as registered by the bundle of His electrogram (BH). At the time indicated by V a 100 Hz 100 msec duration train of 4 msec square wave pulses was delivered to the decentralized right vago-sympathetic trunk. The a-h interval preceding vagal stimulation was 59 msec. The a-h conduction times for the subsequent beats were 112, 88, 69 and 61 msec. In the upper graph of figure 2, the time of occurrence of vagal stimulation was varied relative to the cardiac cycle. The atria were paced at a constant basic cycle length and the a-h conduction intervals were plotted versus the time following vagal stimulation. The times after vagal stimulation are plotted on the abscissa. The time after vagal stimulation as plotted in figure 2 is represented

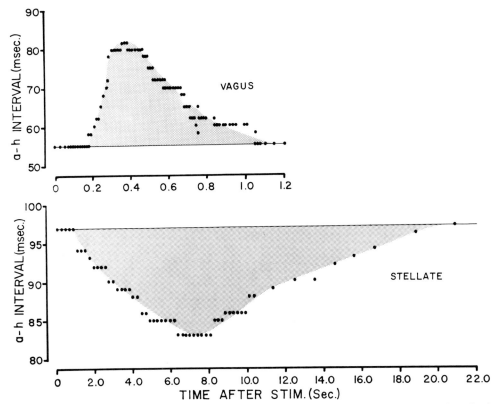

Fig. 2. A comparison of the effects of vagal and stellate stimulation on AV nodal conduction time. On the ordinates are plotted the intervals from the atrial septal activation to the His bundle activation (the a-h interval in the His bundle electrogram). On the abscissa are plotted the times after stimulation of either the left vagus (top) or right stellate ganglion (bottom). There is a ten-fold difference in the scaling factor of the abscissa between the vagal and stellate plots. (Reproduced by permission, Spear & Moore, *Circulat. Res. 32*: 33, 1973.)

in figure 1 as the v-h interval; i.e. the interval between the beginning of vagal stimulation and the His spike of the subsequent conducted beat. The resulting a-h intervals at varying v-h intervals were plotted on the ordinate of figure 2. Figure 2 thus presents the time course of the effect of a brief period of vagal stimulation upon AV nodal conduction (a-h interval). In a similar manner, the effect of a 100 msec, 100 Hz stimulation of the decentralized right stellate ganglion was determined. The time course of the effects of this brief stellate ganglion stimulation is presented in the bottom graph of figure 2. It can be noted in figure 2 that following a period of brief vagal stimulation there is a latency of about 200 msec before AV conduction time increases. Following this latency, conduction time rapidly prolongs with peak delays in AV conduction being reached at about 400 msec following the beginning of vagal stimulation. The AV conduction time rapidly returns to its pre-stimulation values within about 1 to $1\frac{1}{2}$ seconds following the vagal stimulation. In contrast, the lower graph of figure 2 shows that following a similar brief period of stimulation of the stellate ganglion that there is a latency for acceleration of conduction through the AV node of about 1000 msec. In addition, it takes about $7\frac{1}{2}$ seconds before the peak effect of stellate

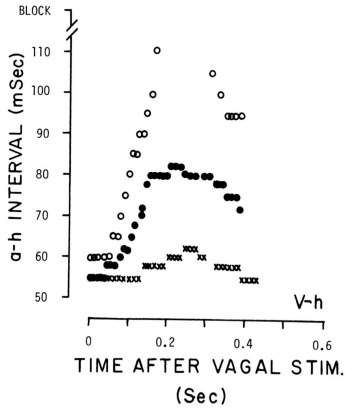

Fig. 3. The effect of increasing the intensity of vagal stimulation on AV nodal conduction. On the ordinate are plotted the a-h times as in the previous figure; the times after vagal stimulation are plotted on the abscissa. The x's indicate the responses with the lowest intensity of vagal stimulation. The filled circles are the responses following a higher intensity vagal stimulation and the open circles are the responses following an intensity of vagal stimulation that produced block in the AV node.

stimulation is seen. The decreased AV conduction time following stellate stimulation dissipates over approximately 20 to 25 seconds. The relatively brief influence of a vagal volley on AV conduction as indicated in the upper graph of figure 2 suggests that vagal effect on AV conduction can be very discrete and may even influence single beats while increases in sympathetic tone result in more prolonged and less discrete effects on AV conduction.

Experiments also were performed to determine the variability of the vagal time course from animal to animal and to determine the effect of changes in the intensity of vagal stimulation upon the time course of the changes in AV conduction. Figure 3 presents data from a single animal in which three different intensities of vagal stimulation were used to scan the cardiac cycle. The data are plotted in the same manner as in figure 2. With increasing intensities of vagal stimulation, the peaks of the curves were shifted to longer a-h times due to increased AV nodal conduction time. The curve indicated by the open circles shows that atrioventricular block occurred between 200 and 300 msec following the highest intensity vagal stimulation. The maximum conduction time through the AV node preceding the blocked beats was 110 msec. The latency to the first slowing of AV conduction for the lowest intensity of stimulation was difficult to determine because of the small increment in a-h conduction time but appeared to be at about 130 msec following the vagal stimulation. Higher intensities of vagal stimulation (filled dots and open circles) resulted in the latency for onset of AV nodal slowing being definitely shortened, and were

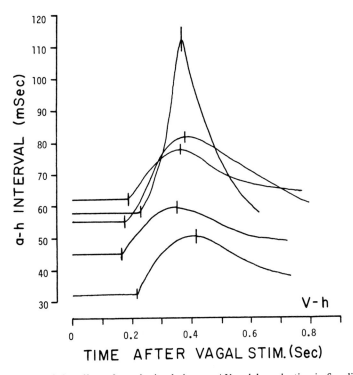

Fig. 4. The time course of the effect of vagal stimulation on AV nodal conduction in five different animals. The ordinate and abscissa are the same as in figure 3. Vertical lines are placed on each curve to indicate the time at which AV conduction delays were first seen and the time at which peak effects on AV conduction were exhibited.

approximately 80 msec in figure 3. However, the time to peak effect for all three intensities of vagal stimulation appeared to be similar and occurred between 280 and 300 msec following vagal stimulation.

Figure 4 presents superimposed records indicating the time course of vagal influences upon AV nodal conduction in five different animals. It is impossible to be assured of equal degrees of vagal stimulation among these different animals. However, in each of these cases, the intensity of vagal stimulation was below that necessary to induce AV nodal block. For these five different animals the latency from the beginning of the vagal stimulation to the first slowing of AV conduction time varied from 170 to 230 msec. The times to peak effect for the five animals ranged between 350 and 410 msec following vagal stimulation. Therefore, figures 3 and 4 indicate that there is relative consistency with regard to time to peak effect of vagal influences on AV nodal conduction time from animal to animal and with variations in intensity of vagal stimulation. This observation allows us to study the effects of phasic changes in vagal stimulation and to be reasonably confident about the time course of vagal influence from animal to animal.

Figure 5 presents analog data showing the effects of a single vagal volley having sufficient intensity to induce complete block within the AV node. The electrograms are labeled as in figure 1. In addition to the recorded cardiac electrical potentials the idealized time course for the effect of vagal stimulation is represented below (VT). This curve was generated from the normalized data of figures 3 and 4. In this figure, a brief period of vagal stimulation (V) was applied to the right vagus 280 msec preceding the third atrial stimulus. As can be seen in the VT record below, the timing of this vagal stimulation was such that the

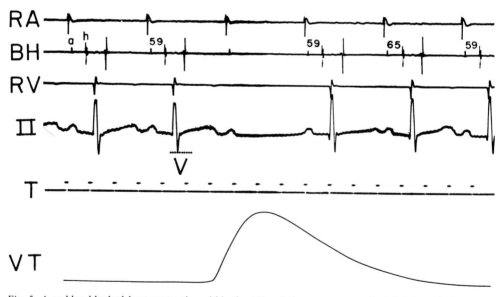

Fig. 5. A sudden blocked beat occcurring within the AV node in response to a single brief vagal stimulation. Bipolar electrograms were recorded from the right atrium (RA), bundle of His (BH), and the right ventricle (RV) simultaneously with the lead II electrocardiogram (II). In the His bundle electrogram a and h indicated atrial septal and His bundle activation respectively. The a-h intervals are indicated in msec for the following beats. V indicates the onset and duration of vagal stimulation; the timing signal t denotes 100 msec. VT indicates the idealized time course of the vagal influence.

third beat in the series was attempting to transit the AV node at the time when the vagal influence was from 60 to 80 percent of maximal. This intensity of vagal tone resulted in the atrial response being concealed within the AV node as indicated by the absence of a His spike (h) in the BH electrogram. In this experiment the atrium was paced at a basic cycle length of 320 msec so that vagal influences on sinus rhythm were prevented. However, a cycle length influence on AV conduction was seen since the atrioventricular block of the third beat provided an increased recovery time for the AV node, permitting the fourth beat of the series to be conducted at a faster rate than normally would have been expected at this time following vagal stimulation. In fact, this atrial beat was conducted through the AV node with a normal control a-h conduction time when vagal influence (VT) was still from 50 to 70 percent of maximal. The fifth atrial beat of the series (the second atrial beat following the blocked beat), conducted with a slightly prolonged conduction time of 65 msec since at this time the influence of the preceding brief period of vagal stimulation had not completed receded and this beat did not have the advantage of the increased long cycle length afforded by a blocked beat. This figure demonstrates the complex inter-relationships that cycle length and autonomic tone have upon AV nodal conduction. Brief vagal stimulation can determine conduction of a single beat even though the vagal influence extends over three to four beats, i.e. the interaction of the increased cycle length provided by the blocked beat and the level of residual vagal influence following the blocked beat can cause a beat to be conducted fortuitously with a normal appearing con-duction time. It should be pointed out that this pattern of a sudden blocked beat with AV conduction times preceding and following the blocked beat being unchanged mimic Mobitz type II heart block. However, second degree AV block occurred within the AV node rather than within the His-Purkinje system as usually reported.

The observation that Mobitz type II second degree AV block could result from brief vagal stimulation suggested that other complex patterns of AV conduction might be generated by appropriate cyclic vagal stimulation at precise times during the cardiac cycle.

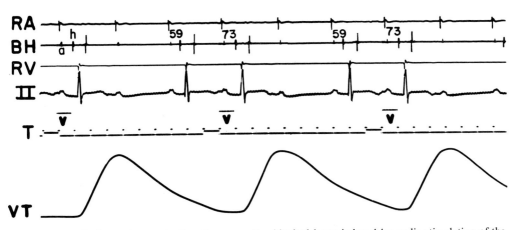

Fig. 6. Gradually increasing conduction time preceding blocked beats induced by cyclic stimulation of the right vagus. Electrograms were recorded simultaneously from the right atrium (RA), bundle of His (BH), right ventricle, and a lead II electrocardiogram. VT indicates the idealized time course of vagal effect fol-lowing the three periods of brief vagal stimuli indicated by V.

Figure 6 presents the data from an experiment in which vagal stimulation was repeated every three beats at a consistent time of the cardiac cycle. Vagal stimulation occurred 50 msec preceding every third atrial stimulus. In this experiment the heart was paced from the right atrium at a basic cycle length of 320 msec to eliminate vagal effects on sinus rhythm. The relative intensity and vagal time course (VT) is shown below the analog records. In these records, the beat following the blocked beat conducted with an a-h time of 59 msec. The second conducted beat following the blocked beat had an a-h time of 73 msec; this pattern repeated itself as long as phasic vagal pulsing continued. As indicated in the VT record below, a vagal pulse 50 msec preceding the atrial driving stimulus is timed such that the subsequent atrial beat would have been conducting through the AV node at a time when the vagal influence upon AV nodal conduction was between 80 and 90% maximal. This high level of vagal influence caused the second atrial beat to be blocked in figure 6. The subsequent atrial response was conducted with a control AV nodal conduction time of 59 msec as a result of the interaction of the increased coupling interval provided by the blocked beat and the residual vagal influence following vagal stimulation. In this case the vagal influence would have fallen to about 30% of maximum. The second atrial beat following the dropped beat (fourth RA electrogram) had a longer a-h interval of 73 msec. This resulted from the small residual vagal influence still present at this time and more importantly, this beat was conducted without the advantage of a long preceding cycle length which would permit total recovery of the AV node. Figure 6 demonstrates that this pattern of pacing and vagal stimulation produced a progressively increasing atrial

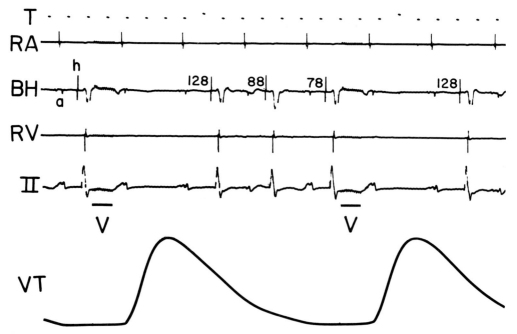

Fig. 7. Gradually decreasing AV nodal conduction time preceding blocked beats induced by brief vagal stimulation. The electrograms were recorded as in the previous figures. In this case only two brief periods of vagal stimulation are shown.

to His conduction time preceding a blocked beat. This pattern mimics a 3 to 2 second degree heart block of the Mobitz type I or Wenckebach type. Other types of repetitive block could be simulated with this technique of phasic vagal stimulation and the patterns were critically dependent upon the relationship between the basic cycle length of the atrial drive and the time in the cardiac cycle at which vagal stimulation occurred.

Figure 7 presents still a different pattern of second degree heart block induced by another slight variation in the time of occurrence of the vagal stimulation. In this figure the analog electrical cardiac records are similar to those described in the previous two figures. However, in this case, the atrial driving rate was 310 msec. The vagal stimulation was delivered every fourth beat and preceded the atrial stimulus by 130 msec. Conduction of the second atrial response through the AV node failed because it arrived in the AV node when the vagal influences were 50 to 70% of maximal. This degree of vagal influence was sufficient to cause the beat to be completely blocked within the AV node in this animal. The beat following the blocked beat was conducted with an a-h interval of 128 msec. Although this beat was conducted with the advantage of the increased coupling interval provided by the preceding blocked beat, the vagal influence had only fallen to 70 to 80% of maximal, and this beat was conducted with a long a-h interval because of this high degree of residual vagal influence. The second beat following the blocked beat was conducted with an a-h interval of 88 msec. In this case, the beat did not have the advantage of following an increased preceding cycle length provided by the dropped beat. Since vagal influence was still about 20% of maximal at this time a delay in AV nodal conduction resulted. The third beat following the dropped beat was conducted at an a-h interval of 78 msec; at this time the effect of vagal stimulation upon the AV node had probably been fully dissipated. The pattern of 4 to 3 AV conduction produced by this cyclic variation in vagal stimulation was one of a gradually decreasing AV conduction time preceding a blocked beat. Of course

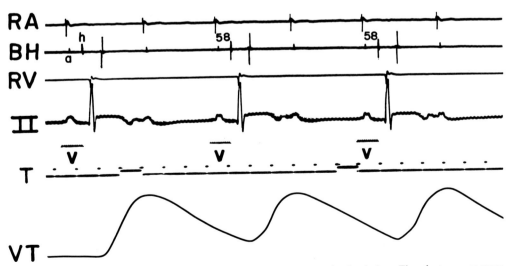

Fig. 8. Alternate block and conduction induced by repetitive vagal stimulation. The electrograms were recorded as in the previous figures. In this case a brief period of vagal stimulation was associated with every other beat producing 2:1 block within the AV node.

most examples of 4 to 3 second degree AV block exhibit gradually increasing a-h intervals. This might be called an inverse Wenckebach block with supernormal acceleration in conduction before the blocked beat.

Figure 8 presents findings in another animal in which phasic variations in vagal stimulation were timed to occur 50 msec before every other atrial pacing stimulation. The lead II electrocardiogram (II) shows a 2 to 1 conduction pattern with every other beat being blocked within the AV node. This figure further demonstrates the discrete effect that brief vagal stimulation can have on conduction.

The time course of brief stellate stimulation upon AV nodal conduction is about 20 times longer than that of similar vagal stimulation (fig. 2). It is therefore much more difficult to

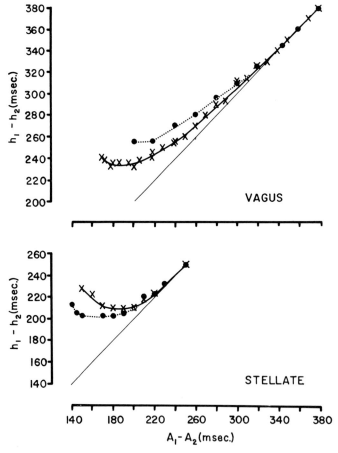

Fig. 9. A comparison of the effects of vagal and stellate stimulation on AV nodal conduction during premature atrial beats. The A_1-A_2 intervals (the intervals between the last of a series of 12 basic atrial beats and a premature atrial beat introduced at progressively more premature times) are on the abscissa. The ordinates are the h_1-h_2 intervals (the intervals between the His bundle activation of a premature atrial beat). The crosses connected by the solid lines are the control points determined without background nerve stimulation and the circles connected by the broken lines are the experimental points determined during autonomic nerve stimulation. The experimental points of the top graph were determined during continuous 100 Hz stimulation of the right vagus. The experimental points of the bottom graph were determined during continuous 100 Hz stimulation of the right stellate ganglion. (Reproduced by permission, Spear & Moore, *Circulat. Res.* 32: 38, 1973).

demonstrate discrete effects of stellate stimulation on AV conduction. Figure 9 presents data in two different animals demonstrating the effects of vagal and stellate stimulation on AV nodal conduction of premature atrial beat. In both graphs the abscissae are the A_1–A_2 intervals (the intervals between the last of a series of 12 basic atrial beats to premature atrial beats introduced at progressively earlier time intervals). The ordinates are the corresponding h_1–h_2 intervals; i.e. the intervals between the basic His bundle response (h_1) resulting from conduction of the A_1 atrial response and the premature His bundle activation (h_2) resulting from conduction of the premature atrial beat (A_2). In the upper graph the crosses connected by the solid line are the control points determined without vagal stimulation. The filled circles connected by the broken lines are the experimental points determined during continuous vagal stimulation at 100 Hz delivered to the right vagus. The intensity of vagal stimulation was sufficiently low so that AV nodal conduction time (h_1-h_2 intervals) was identical to the AV nodal conduction time of beats at the basic cycle length without vagal stimulation. Note in the upper graph of figure 9 that while the effect of a continous subliminal stimulation of the vagus did not cause a prolongation in AV nodal conduction time of the normal basic beats, that nevertheless the AV nodal conduction time of premature atrial beats evoked earlier than 300 msec underwent an AV nodal delay. Thus premature atrial beats brought out the subliminal vagal influence upon AV nodal conduction. In the lower graph of figure 9, a similar experiment was performed in which continuous stimulation of the right stellate ganglion was carried out to evaluate the subliminal sympathetic effect on AV conduction of premature atrial beats. The x's connected by the solid line are the control AV conduction time of premature atrial beats evoked without stellate ganglion stimulation. The solid circles connected by the dotted line are premature atrial beats conducted during continuous 100 Hz stimulation of the right stellate ganglion. The degree of stellate stimulation was not sufficient to cause acceleration of conduction times for normal atrial beats at the basic cycle length; however, at intervals below a coupling interval of 200 msec the premature atrial beats during background stellate stimulation were conducted through the AV node with a faster AV conduction time (shorter h_1–h_2 intervals) than during AV nodal conduction of control beats. Therefore, it can be seen that the influence of sympathetic stimulation on AV conduction was manifest only for those premature atrial beats with coupling intervals of less than 200 msec. Thus, autonomic influence on AV nodal conduction can be very subtle.

Figure 10 presents an example of a discrete effect of stellate ganglion stimulation on AV nodal conduction of a single supraventricularly conducted beat. The records of figure 10A and B were obtained from an animal in which second degree heart block was experimentally induced by damage of the AV node. Note that the right ventricular electrogram in the third trace (RV) and the right atrial electrogram (RA) appear just below the RV electrogram. This preparation exhibited stable 4 to 3 Wenckebach cycles at a relatively slow basic cycle length of 450 msec as shown in A of figure 10. In figure 10B, a record was obtained during stimulation of the right stellate ganglion during the period of time indicated by ST. The record in B of figure 10 demonstrates that the severity of second degree heart block was reduced by the stellate stimulation. The ventricular beat indicated by the arrow, was conducted from the atrial only following stellate stimulation. The delay time between the beginning of stellate stimulation and the effect on AV nodal conduction of the conducted beat at the arrow is characteristic of the slow onset of sympathetic effects

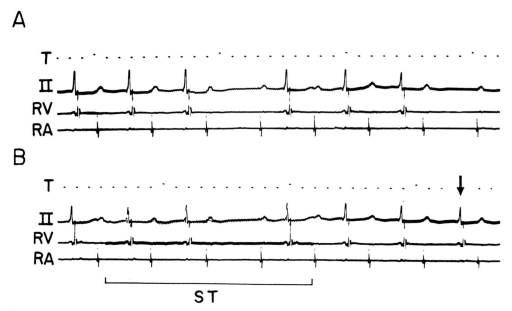

Fig. 10. An example of a reduction in the severity of second degree heart block following stellate ganglion stimulation. Bipolar electrograms were recorded from the right ventricle (RV) and the right atrium (RA) simultaneously with a lead II electrocardiogram (II). ST indicates the timing of a 1.6 second train of 100 Hz stimuli delivered to the right stellate ganglion. The time signal (T) denotes 100 msec intervals. The arrow indicates the beat that was conducted due to the stellate stimulation. (Reproduced by permission, Spear & Moore, *Circulat. Res.* 32: 39, 1973.)

upon AV nodal conduction. In contrast, the degree of heart block in this preparation was increased by vagal stimulation (not shown). Figure 10 therefore shows that stellate stimulation had a discrete effect on the conduction of a single beat. In fact, conduction of the atrial response might be considered 'supernormal conduction'.

In summary, these experiments describe ways in which phasic variations in autonomic tone can have discrete influences upon AV conduction. The experiments demonstrate that appropriately timed phasic vagal or stellate stimulation can produce patterns of first or second degree AV heart block including Wenckebach periods and Mobitz type II heart block. In addition, the concealed effects of both vagal and stellate stimulation can be brought out during AV conduction of premature atrial beats. As pointed out in previous publications (561), changes in autonomic tone can be the mechanism(s) responsible for many types of pseudo-supernormal conduction. Pseudo-supernormal conduction was demonstrated for vagal influence in figure 7 and for stellate stimulation in figure 10. The precise way that phasic changes in vagal and stellate stimulation influence AV nodal conduction depends on many factors including: 1. the intrinsic time course for the onset and duration of vagal or stellate effects; 2. the intensity of the increase or decrease in autonomic tone; 3. the immediate sensitivity of the AV node to autonomic influence; 4. the time during the cardiac cycle in which the change in autonomic tone occurs; and 5. the basic underlying rhythm of the heart during the change in autonomic tone.

6

SUPERNORMAL EXCITABILITY AND CONDUCTION[1]

JOSEPH F. SPEAR, Ph.D., AND E. NEIL MOORE, D.V.M., Ph.D., F.A.C.C.

Supernormal conduction, that is, conduction which is better than anticipated or conduction that occurs when block is expected, can theoretically be caused by a variety of mechanisms including the presence of a period of supernormal excitability (127,561). The term supernormal excitability refers to a reduced current requirement to excite a tissue at a specific period of its activity cycle. Periods of supernormal excitability were first described for nerve in 1912 by Adrian and Lucas (4) and for heart muscle in 1938 by Hoff and Nahum (158). In these early experiments the tissues were excited by electrodes placed on the surface. Recent studies have emphasized the complexity of surface stimulation in testing myocardial excitability (158,170,380). Because a conducted beat relies on depolarizing currents for its propagation, in situations where one is interested in correlating changes in membrane excitability with characteristics of conduction, a pure depolarizing current is more appropriate for evaluating excitability. A pure depolarizing current can be delivered to a cell through an intracellular microelectrode. Using this technique Weidmann (898) first demonstrated a period of supernormal excitability in sheep Purkinje fibers and Childers et al. (125) showed that specialized atrial fibers within Bachmann's bundle in dogs possessed a period of supernormal excitability. The present studies will describe attempts to correlate supernormal excitability in the Purkinje system of the dog with associated conduction phenomena in this tissue.

THE TECHNIQUE OF INTRACELLULAR STIMULATION

Figure 1 demonstrates the technique for measuring excitability utilizing depolarizing current passed to the cell by way of an intracellular microelectrode. False tendons were removed from right and left ventricles of anesthetized dogs and equilibrated in Tyrode's solution with 95% oxygen and 5% carbon dioxide. The tissues were maintained at 37°C. In figure 1, PF_1 is a recording from a Purkinje fiber with a microelectrode capable of both stimulation and recording. PF_2 is a differential recording from an impalement within a space constant of the PF_1 fiber. The second pair of action potentials in the PF_1 and PF_2 records were evoked by applying a depolarizing current through the PF_1 electrode at just threshold intensity. The record labelled (PF_2) is the PF_2 action potential evoked by intracellular stimulation displayed on an expanded time scale. The intensity of the current utilized to evoke the response is shown on the same expanded time scale below the

1. This study was supported by U.S. Public Health Service Grants HE-4885 and HL-16076.

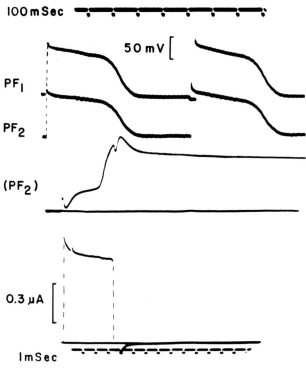

Fig. 1. Analog data demonstrating the technique used to measure excitability and threshold potential. All traces were recorded simultaneously. The 100 msec time pulses apply to traces PF$_1$, PF$_2$. The 1 msec time pulses apply to traces (PF$_2$) and the current record. PF$_1$ indicates transmembrane action potentials recorded with a microelectrode capable of both passing current and recording potentials. The PF$_2$ transmembrane action potential were recorded within a space constant of the PF$_1$ recording site using a difference amplifier. The second action potentials in the PF$_1$ and PF$_2$ records were evoked by a threshold depolarizing current delivered through the PF$_1$ electrode. The PF$_2$ action potential evoked as a result of this current is shown on the expanded time scale below as (PF$_2$).

(PF$_2$) record. By scanning the conducted beat with threshold depolarizing pulses, the excitability of the tissue could be obtained throughout the time course of an action potential. In the (PF$_2$) record the threshold potential was determined as the potential at which the rapid upstroke of the action potential was initiated. Because of the complications of cable properties that play a role in cardiac excitation when current is injected at a single point in the tissue, the threshold potential indicated in (PF$_2$) of figure 1 is not the true membrane threshold potential. During intracellular injection of a depolarizing current a certain minimum amount of surrounding membrane (liminal length of membrane) must be raised above the membrane threshold potential to counter the repolarizing effect of local currents from adjacent inactive membrane (709). Changes in excitability as measured by intracellular stimulation can be due at least in part to changes in cable properties of the membrane. However, since a conducted wave of activity relies on local depolarizing current to excite fibers downstream, the factors that modify excitability as measured by intracellular stimulation in these experiments would be expected to similarly modify excitability in the case of a conducted beat.

SUPERNORMAL EXCITABILITY

Figure 2 presents a typical excitability curve measured in a Purkinje fiber using intracellular depolarizing current. The abscissa is the time following the upstroke of a normally
conducted action potential evoked at a basic cycle length of 800 msec. The ordinate is

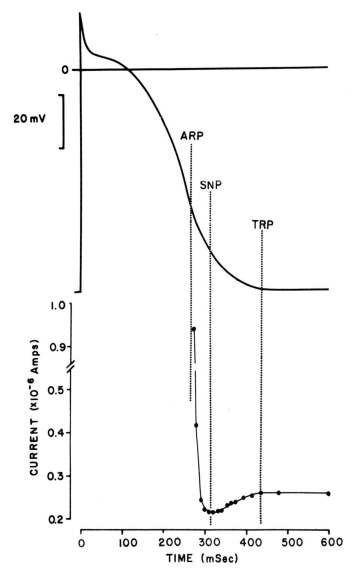

Fig. 2. A representative excitability determination in a canine Purkinje fiber. The action potential voltage
time course is displayed at the top and the excitability curve is displayed at the bottom. The abscissa indicates
the time after the upstroke of the action potential. The ordinate is the minimum depolarizing current necessary to evoke a response at the times indicated on the abscissa. TRP indicates the total refractory period
or the time in which the membrane potential and the excitability returned to their resting values. ARP
indicates the time of the absolute refractory period and SNP indicates the minimum current requirements to excite the fiber during the supernormal period.

the minimum current required to excite the impaled fiber at the various times indicated on the abscissa. The voltage time course of the normally conducted action potential is displayed above the graph using the same time axis. The vertical dotted lines correlate specific times on the action potential time course and the excitability curve. For a period of 260 msec following the upstroke of the action potential, the tissue could not be excited by the highest current which the intracellular microelectrode was capable of passing. This period is the absolute refractory period and its boundary is indicated by the vertical dotted line labelled ARP. When the action potential has repolarized beyond about −55 mV the fiber can be re-excited as can be seen in the excitability curve. During this period of time, the current necessary to excite the fiber falls to a minimum value and then as the fiber repolarizes to full resting potential, the current increases gradually to a steady level which is maintained during the steady resting potential (diastole). The minimum current required to excite the fiber occured at 315 msec following the upstroke of the action potential and this time is indicated by the vertical dashed line labeled SNP. Excitability returns to a constant value when the membrane potential returns to its steady resting value. This period of time is indicated by the vertical dashed line labeled TRP. In 24 excitability curves measured in left and right Purkinje tissues (779) it required an average of $17.0 \pm 4.6\%$ less current to evoke an action potential during the period of supernormal excitability than required during diastole. In these experiments the period of supernormal excitability lasted 88.2 ± 23.6 msec in fibers driven at a basic cycle length of 800 msec. Weidmann (898) originally showed that the period of supernormal excitability results partly because during the later phase of repolarization as compared to the resting state the threshold potential has recovered more completely than has the membrane potential. The membrane potential therefore has to undergo a smaller degree of additional de-polarization to reach threshold potential and thus excitation can be brought about by a weaker depolarizing current.

Intracellular stimulation methods have demonstrated that not all of the tissues of the mammalian heart exhibit a period of supernormal excitability. Supernormal excita-bility has been verified in the bundle branch-Purkinje system (779,898) and in the specialized atrial fibers of Bachmann's bundle (125). Supernormal excitability was not present in the AV node (548), in the bundle of His (779) and in atrial and ventricular working muscle (125,779).

SUPERNORMAL CONDITION

The presence of a period of supernormal excitability in atrial specialized fibers and in Purkinje tissue implies that conduction of the cardiac impulse may be facilitated during this period. According to the local circuit theory of conduction a reduced current re-quirement for excitation during late repolarization would mean that cells could be brought to threshold potential faster downstream and therefore, an increment in conduc-tion velocity would be realized. In addition, under conditions in which marginal con-duction exists, a beat could be conducted or blocked, depending on whether or not it engaged the tissue during its supernormal period of excitability. This possibility has special implications when one considers conduction in a potential reentrant pathway. In experiments in which the voltage time course of the action potential was modified by changing the pacing rate and rhythm it was shown that the characteristics of the period of supernormal excitability remained relatively unchanged in the presence of large

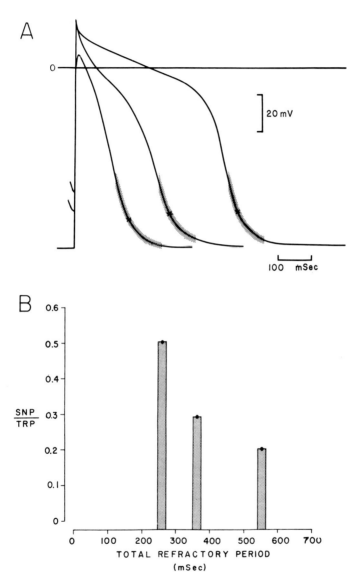

Fig. 3. The relationship between the supernormal period and the total refractory period. Above are shown superimposed action potentials. The longest duration action potential was evoked at a basic cycle length of 800 msec. The shorter action potentials were successively evoked premature beats at cycle lengths of 460 msec and 251 msec. The shaded areas delineate the boundaries of the period of supernormal excitability. The x's within the shaded area indicate the point of minimum current requirements. The histograms on the common time scale are the ratios of the supernormal period to the total refractory period (SNP/TRP) plotted vs. the total refractory period for each of the action potentials shown above. (Reproduced with permission, Spear and Moore, *Circulation*, 50: 1974.)

changes in action potential duration; i.e. supernormal excitability was membrane potential dependent rather than action potential configuration dependent (780).

Figure 3 summarizes the data from one of these experiments. Above are shown three
superimposed action potentials. The longest duration action potential was at a basic
cycle length of 800 msec. The next shorter action potential was due to a single premature
beat evoked at a cycle length of 460 msec. The shortest action potential was obtained
during a second premature beat following the first at a cycle length of 251 msec. The
shaded areas on each action potential delineate a period of supernormal excitability.
The x's within the shaded area indicate the points of minimum current requirements for
eliciting a propagated response. In the lower graph the ratio of the duration of the
supernormal period to the duration of the total refractory period is plotted on the ordinate
and the total refractory period corresponding to each of the action potentials is plotted
on the abscissa. In figure 3, the total refractory period was shortened in associated with
successively evoked premature beats. Although the supernormal periods occurred earlier
in time with abbreviation of the refractory period, their duration, minimum current and
configuration remained relatively unaffected. Since the duration of the period of supernormal excitability is independent of the total duration of the action potential, cycle
length reductions in action potential duration will result in the supernormal period comprising a greater percentage of the total duration of the action potential. At the shortest
action potential duration, the supernormal period comprised half of the total action
potential duration. The experiments of Sasyniuk and Mendez (719) demonstrated that
proximal to a site of conduction block in Purkinje fibers, the action potential duration is
greatly abbreviated. The early recovery of the tissue at the site of block allows the possibility of early re-excitation of this tissue and therefore may provide a local reentrant
pathway. The experiment of figure 3 demonstrates that since the duration of the period
of supernormal excitability is not proportionately abbreviated for short duration action
potentials, in these cases not only does the tissue recover more rapidly, but it recovers
with a proportionately longer period of supernormal excitability. Thus a period of
supernormal excitability may play a role in facilitating reentry by allowing reactivation
of the tissue in situations where a potential reentrant beat had a slow rate of depolarization and low amplitude (low safety factor for conduction) and would only continue to
be conducted if it entered a region of supernormal excitability.

Figure 4 is a simulation to suggest how a subthreshold excitation could be facilitated
by a premature beat. In figure 4, MP indicates a transmembrane potential recorded with
a microelectrode also capable of stimulation. The intensity of the current pulse displayed on an expanded time scale is indicated by I. In A of figure 4, the action potential
was evoked in a Purkinje fiber by pacing upstream through extra-cellular electrodes at
a basic cycle length of 800 msec. At the time indicated by the arrow, a subthreshold
current was passed through the recording microelectrode. In the present hypothetical
simulation, such a subthreshold current, could represent a potential reentrant beat which
is unable to excite the final common pathway as indicated by the small non-propagated
stimulus artifact in the MP record. In B a premature beat was interposed between the
conducted beat and the subthreshold intracellular stimulus. The premature action potential exhibited a brief duration and occurred with the appropriate timing so that its super-

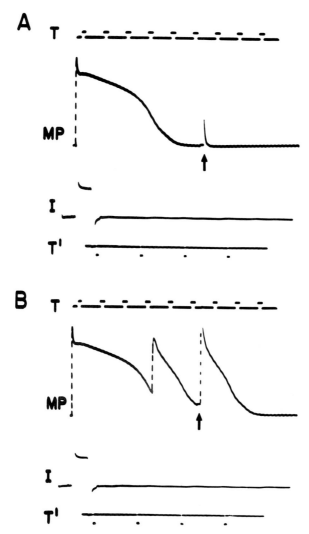

Fig. 4. A demonstration of the interaction between a subthreshold current pulse and a premature action potential. In the records of A and B, MP indicates a transmembrane potential recorded with an electrode capable of both passing current and recording. I is a record indicating the intensity of current delivered through the microelectrode at the time indicated by the arrow in A. T indicates 100 msec time pulses for the MP action potential. T′ indicates 10 msec intervals and this signal is associated with the current record. In B a premature beat was evoked between the action potential and the previously subthreshold stimulus. The interval between the upstroke of the action potential and the intracellular stimulating current was the same in both A and B.

normal period was engaged by the previously subthreshold stimulus. Thus in the presence of the premature beat, the intracellular current evoked an action potential.

Recent studies have correlated a period of supernormal conduction with the period of supernormal excitability in atrial specialized tissues and in the Purkinje system (125, 779). In order to be confident that the period of supernormal excitability is in fact the cause of acceleration in conduction, one must first of all show a temporal coincidence

of the two phenomena. To correlate supernormal excitability with a period of supernormal conduction, Purkinje fibers were isolated and superfused with Tyrode's solution
as described in figure 1. A third microelectrode was inserted in the preparation at some
distance from the current passing and voltage recording electrodes. Figure 5 demonstrates
records obtained from this type of experiment. Two superimposed action potentials from
proximal (P) and distal (D) cells are shown at the top of the figure. By passing current
through the microelectrode located near the P recording electrode, intracellular excitability during repolarization was determined as previously described. In addition the
conduction times of the evoked responses could be determined as the time difference

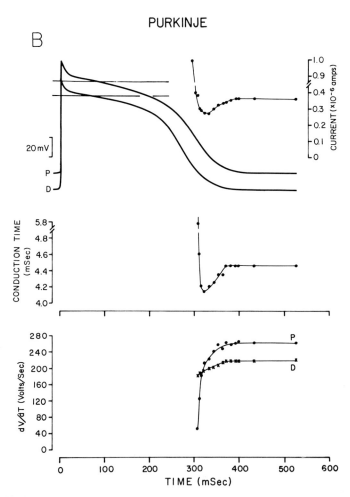

Fig. 5. Relationship between supernormal excitability and supernormal conduction in the isolated Purkinje
fiber. The time courses of transmembrane action potentials are displayed above. P represents an action
potential recorded near the stimulating intracellular microelectrode and D indicates a distal action potential
4 mm downstream. All data are plotted on the common time axis below. The graph at the top indicates
threshold currents necessary to evoke conducted responses. The middle graph plotted on the same time
course as the action potential indicates the conduction times between proximal and distal recording sites.
The corresponding rates of rise (dV/dT) of the evoked action potential for both proximal and distal cells
are shown in the bottom graph. (Reproduced with permission, Spear and Moor, *Circulat. Res.* 35: 1974.)

between activation of the proximal and distal recording sites. Conduction time is plotted in the middle graph. The rates of maximal depolarization (dV/dT) for the evoked responses for both proximal and distal recording sites were electronically determined and are plotted in the graphs at the bottom of figure 5. All data are on a common time axis with 0 time being the upstroke of the action potential. The excitability curve plotted at the upper right of the action potentials shows the typically observed decrease in current requirement associated with repolarization of the Purkinje system. It can be seen from the middle graph that a decrease in the conduction time corresponds to the period of supernormal excitability. Premature beats evoked during the time when the proximal cell was supernormally excitable are conducted to the distal cell with a shorter conduction time than those beats evoked during diastole; the very early premature beats, evoked before the period of supernormal excitability, exhibited conduction times that were longer than during diastole.

In other experiments, however, the conduction times of these early premature beats could be decreased as well as increased. This very early phase of the relative refractory period was associated with depressed rates of rise of action potentials as indicated in the bottom graph of figure 5. In addition, the current required to excite the Purkinje fibers was increased above diastolic current requirements during this time until the fiber was no longer excitable (absolute refractory period).

Figure 6 presents normalized data for five Purkinje fiber experiments. Zero on the normalized time axis is the upstroke of the action potential. The time of full repolarization is noted by 1.0. Plotted on the ordinate above is the normalized conduction time between proximal and distal electrodes. Diastolic conduction time is indicated by 1.0. The lower ordinate is the normalized dV/dT for the proximal Purkinje cells in each experiment, while 1.0 indicates the diastolic maximum rate of depolarization of the action potentials. Both graphs are plotted on the normalized time scale seen on the abscissa. The shaded areas in both graphs delineate the boundaries of the period of supernormal excitability. The boundary at normalized time 1.0 (full recovery) can be precisely defined. However, the left hand border occurring at about 0.82 is less discretely defined on this graph because it varied somewhat among the experiments. During the supernormal period of excitability as delineated by the shaded areas, there was an average of 9.8% decrease in conduction velocity in all preparations. The dV/dT during the supernormal period of excitability only averaged a decrease to about 60% of maximum. Interestingly, very premature beats evoked prior to the start of the period of supernormal excitability exhibited conduction times that could be either increased or decreased. It is probable that the slow rate of rise of the action potentials coupled with the increased current requirements caused a slowing of conduction. In those cases in which the apparent conduction times between proximal and distal cells were decreased, the conduction time for the very early premature beats appeared to approach zero. That is, proximal and distal activation appeared to be very nearly simultaneous. This phenomenon was described previously by Van Dam et al. (171) and is probably due to dissociated conduction.

Figure 6 demonstrates that there was a consistent decrease in the conduction time between proximal and distal cells associated with the period of supernormal excitability. However to be confident that dissociated conduction during this time was not responsible

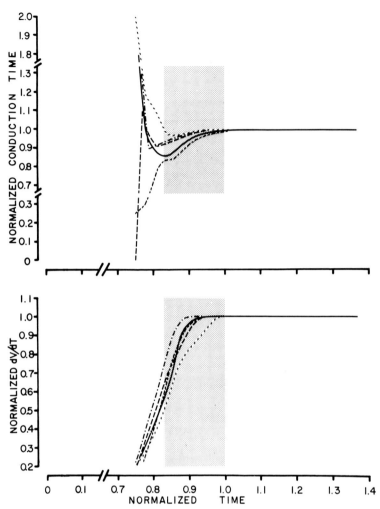

Fig. 6. Normalized data from 5 experiments on isolated canine Purkinje fibers comparing conduction times and maximum rates of rise of action potentials evoked during the period of supernormal excitability. Common abscissa is the normalized time after the upstroke of the action potential. The shaded area delineates the boundaries of the period of supernormal excitability. Full repolarization is indicated by 1.0 and the upper ordinate is the normalized conduction time. Diastolic conduction time is noted by 1.0 and the ordinate below is the normalized maximum rate of depolarization of the proximal cells. The maximum rate of depolarization during diastole is also indicated by 1.0.

for an apparent supernormal conduction, microelectrode recordings near the site of current injection were used to investigate the characteristics of the conduction of very early premature beats. Figure 7 presents records similar to those seen previously in figure 1. The upper traces and lower traces were recorded simultaneously but at different sweep velocities, (see the legend for details). In this case the premature beat was very early as shown by the second action potentials in all three of the upper traces and was evoked near the absolute refractory period. Because of the high current being passed through the stimulating electrode at this time, the stimulus artifacts, particularly in the

(PF$_3$) record are large. The parts of the (PF$_3$) record obscured by the stimulus artifact, are connected by a dotted line. Notice that the (PF$_2$) cell near the current passing electrode (first trace on the expanded time scale) is activated very late after the beginning of the stimulus and that there appears to be a slow wave preceding a more rapid phase of depolarization. A distal cell (PF$_3$) appears to be activated coincidently with the proximal cell's rapid phase of depolarization. The arrows indicate what we consider to be the beginning of the rapid phase of depolarization in each case. In these cases even with the highest current intensities that we could deliver, the latency between the beginning of

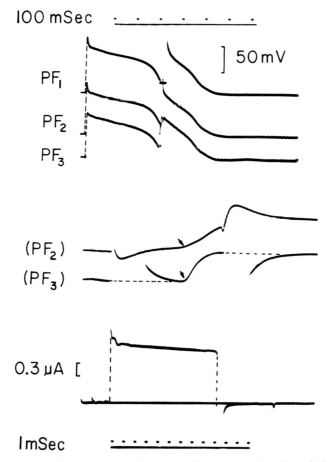

Fig. 7. Analog data demonstrating conduction of a very early premature beat in an isolated Purkinje fiber. PF$_1$ indicates transmembrane action potentials recorded with a microelectrode capable of both passing current and recording potentials. The PF$_2$ transmembrane action potentials were recorded within 0.02 mm of the PF$_1$ recording using a difference amplifier. Transmembrane action potentials in PF$_3$ were recorded downstream from the PF$_1$ electrode. (PF$_2$) and (PF$_3$) are the PF$_2$ and PF$_3$ recordings on an expanded time scale. Below on the same expanded time scale is shown the current record. The 100 msec time pulses above are time references for the upper three action potentials, while the bottom 1 msec pulses are for the lower time expanded traces. The second triad of action potentials in the upper three records were evoked by prematurely exciting the Purkinje fiber through the PF$_1$ electrode. The records (PF$_2$) and (PF$_3$) on the expanded time scale show the conduction characteristics of the evoked premature beat. The small arrows note the initiation of the rapid phase of depolarization in each case.

the current pulse and the rapid phase of activation of the (PF$_2$) fiber could not be reduced significantly. This phenomenon was characteristic of very early premature beats when the rates of the action potentials were considerably reduced and the current required to excite the fiber was relatively large. In contrast the latency between the beginning of the stimulus and the upstroke of the action potential during the period of supernormal excitability or during diastole could be reduced to virtually zero. It can be seen from figure 7 that the coincident activation of proximal and distal recording sites is only apparent. Slow conduction away from the stimulation site must have occurred. However the real site of all-or-none activation was most probably at some distance from the

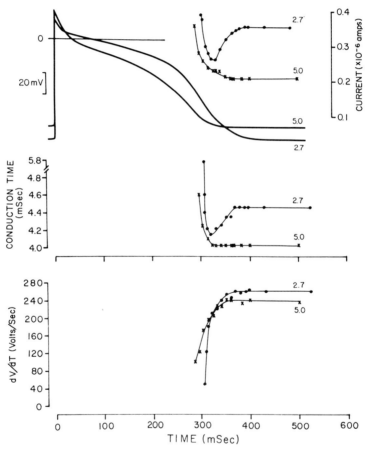

Fig. 8. The effect on supernormal excitability and supernormal conduction of elevating the potassium in the Tyrode's solution from a concentration of 2.7 to 5.0 mM. The data in the two potassium concentrations are superimposed and plotted on the same time axis. The time courses of the action potentials recorded during the same impalement in two potassium solutions are superimposed at the top of the figure. The graphs at the upper right present threshold currents necessary to evoke responses at the two potassium concentrations. The middle graphs show the conduction times of the evoked responses between proximal and distal electrode sites separated by 4 mm for 2.7 and 5.0 mM potassium. The maximum rates of rise of the action potentials recorded at the proximal electrode site in the two potassium solutions are shown in the graph at the bottom. (Reproduced with permission, Spear and Moore, *Circulat. Res.* 35: 1974.)

stimulation site with retrograde reflection to the proximal site and antegrade conduction to the distal recording site. This type of conduction is not true accelerated conduction since actual conduction time is from the beginning of the slow wave (not definable in our records) to the activation of the distal cell. The rapid phase of depolarization in proximal and distal cells does not indicate conduction time in this circumstance.

Besides a temporal coincidence of the period of supernormal excitability and super-normal conduction, there are additional data which indicate that supernormal excit-ability is the cause of supernormal conduction. If the period of supernormal excitability is eliminated by elevating the level of potassium in the external medium, then the period of supernormal conduction is also eliminated. This is demonstrated in figure 8. The figure shows superimposed data from a single cell impalement in 2.7 mM and 5.0 mM potassium.

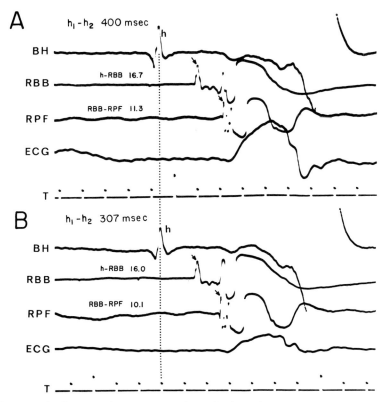

Fig. 9. Analog records demonstrating supernormal conduction of a premature beat in the open chest anesthetized dog. Bipolar plunge electrodes were used to record electrograms from the bundle of His (BH), the right bundle branch near the anterior papillary muscle (RBB) and a right Purkinje fiber in the free wall of the right ventricle (RPF). A lead II electrocardiogram was simultaneously recorded (ECG). The records displayed in A were obtained during constant pacing at a basic cycle length of 400 msec. The interval between successive His depolarizations in this case was 400 msec. The records displayed in B were obtained during AV conduction of a premature atrial beat evoked at an interval of 240 msec. The interval between the His spike of the last basic beat (h_1) and the His bundle spike of the premature beat (h_2) was 307 msec. The records are arranged so that the His bundle spikes in A and B are time aligned. The interval between the His bundle spike and right bundle branch spike (h-RBB) and the interval between the right bundle branch spike and the Purkinje fiber spike (RBB-RPF) are designated in both A and B. Due to respiratory movements of the heart in the open chest dog the ECG record in B was distorted.

The change from 2.7 mM to 5.0 mM potassium caused a 12 mv depolarization in the cell and reduced the action potential duration. In addition there was a 41% decrease in the current required to excite the fiber during diastole and a decrease in the conduction time between proximal and distal recording electrodes during this time. The supernormal period of excitability was eliminated in the 5.0 mM potassium solution as indicated in the excitability curves at the right of the action potential. The supernormal period of conduction was also eliminated.

Because the normal plasma potassium concentration in the dog is from 2.9 to 5.5 mM, it is possible to demonstrate supernormal conduction in the canine Purkinje system *in vivo*. Previous investigators have described such a phenomenon in the dog (37, 266). Figure 9 presents analog records from an open-chest anesthetized dog. The plasma potassium concentration was 3.9 mM. Using close bipolar plunge electrodes, records were obtained from the bundle of His, the right bundle branch near the base of the right anterior papillary muscle and from a right Purkinje fiber in the free wall of the right ventricle. A lead II electrogram was simultaneously recorded. The records in A of figure 1 show a normally conducted beat occurring during right atrial pacing at a basic cycle length of 400 msec. The h_1-h_2 interval in this case was 400 msec. As indicated, the His spike to right bundle branch spike time was 16.7 msec. The right bundle branch spike to right Purkinje fiber spike time was 11.3 msec. The records in B of this figure were obtained during a premature atrial beat occurring at a coupling interval of 240 msec. Due to delay in conduction through the AV node, this atrial coupling interval resulted in an h_1-h_2 coupling interval of 307 msec. In this case, the His bundle spike to right bundle

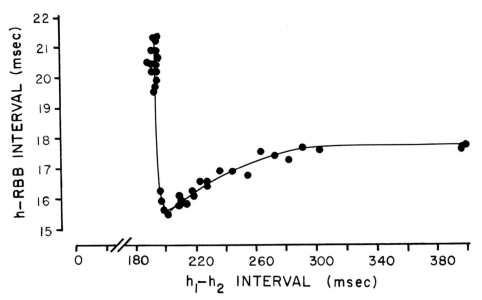

Fig. 10. The conduction time between the His bundle spike and the right bundle branch spike in the open chest anesthetized dog during premature supraventricular beats. On the abscissa are plotted the times from the His bundle spike of the last of a series of 12 basic beats and the His bundle spike of a premature atrial beat (h_1-h_2). On the ordinate are plotted the conduction times from the His bundle spike to the right bundle branch spike for the premature beats indicated on the abscissa.

spike was reduced to 16.0 msec and the right bundle spike to Purkinje fiber spike time was reduced to 10.1 msec. The total increment in conduction time in B as compared to A was therefore 1.9 msec. This represents a 6.9% increase in the conduction time between the His bundle to peripheral Purkinje fiber during the premature atrial beat. The data of figure 10 present the results of a full scan of premature beats in a second animal whose plasma potassium concentration was 3.5 mM. On the abscissa are plotted the h_1-h_2 coupling times for the various premature beats. On the ordinate are plotted the corresponding His bundle spike to right bundle spike conduction times for the different premature beats. Notice that at h_1-h_2 intervals between 195 and 290 msec there was an acceleration in the conduction time between the His bundle and right bundle branch spikes. The maximum increment in conduction time was about 2.2 msec and this represents about a 12.4% increase in conduction time as compared to normal diastole conduction times. At h_1-h_2 coupling interval earlier than about 195 msec, the conduction time between His and right bundle branch increased. The data of figures 9 and 10 indicate that the phenomenon of supernormal conduction described in the isolated Purkinje system also occurs in the whole animal preparation. It is also of interest that the magnitude of the increment in conduction time as well as the configuration and duration of the period of supernormal conduction are comparable to those observed in the isolated tissue experiments.

A decrease in conduction time of 12% was observed for beats traversing the normal bundle branch-Purkinje system. This small increment in conduction time of only a few milliseconds which is directly attributable to supernormal excitability, can only be detected by high resolution recording and measuring techniques and therefore normally goes unrecognized. The role of supernormal excitability under conditions of marginal conduction remains to be defined. However, it is possible that in circumstances of first and second degree heart block within the bundle branch-Purkinje system the period of supernormal excitability may be responsible for larger increments in conduction velocity. In addition a beat may be conducted or blocked depending on whether or not it engages the period of supernormal excitability.

7
THE ROLE OF PHASE 3 AND PHASE 4 BLOCK IN CLINICAL ELECTROCARDIOGRAPHY[1]

MAURICIO B. ROSENBAUM, M.D., JULIO O. LÁZZARI, M.D., AND
MARCELO V. ELIZARI, M.D.

In the past, automaticity and conduction were thought to be independent and totally unrelated physiologic properties of the specific tissues of the heart. It was then only natural that, abnormalities of conduction and alterations of automaticity (the latter still poorly known and almost unexplored) were discussed in separate and disconnected chapters in books of arrhythmias and electrocardiography. However, in the last few years, the development of the concept of phase 4 block (144, 237, 240, 241, 691–694, 696) brought into focus the existence of a relationship between automaticity and conduction, which may prove to have significant physiologic as well as clinical and electrocardiographic and even therapeutic consequences. This relationship may perhaps open a new chapter in contemporary electrocardiography; and although this statement may at first glance appear as too provocative or overhasty, it is greatly supported by Alfred Pick (632), teacher, friend and deep thinker of the electrocardiography of all times, when he says that 'hemiblocks and phase 4 block are the two most important advances of electrocardiography in the last ten years'. However, whether or not a new chapter will open its way, this is less important than the fact that the concept of phase 4 block (together with its closely associated phase 3 block) may be dealt with as a multipurpose concept which may serve to explain a series of old and still puzzling problems of clinical electrocardiography. Among these, I have selected for this chapter the following five: intermittent bundle branch block (BBB), paroxysmal AV block, parasystole, Wolff-Parkinson-White syndrome and the effects of certain drugs upon conduction. Essentially, I will try to show how these five problems, apparently so dissimilar and heterogeneous, can be aligned together on behalf of the newly established relationship between automaticity and conduction.

A. INTERMITTENT BUNDLE BRANCH BLOCK

Intermittent BBB was the original model from which all the other relationships between automaticity and conduction were derived, and its mechanism should be thoroughly understood for a full comprehension of phase 3 and phase 4 block (237, 240, 692, 694). Figure 1 shows a typical example, in which left (L) BBB beats alternate with normally conducted beats. The first two beats, after pauses shorter than 1.00 sec show tachycardia-dependent or phase 3 LBBB; the two following beats, after pauses of 1.00 to 1.22 sec

1. This work was supported in part by the Comision Para el Estudio Integral de la Enfermedad de Chagas. School of Medicine, Buenos Aires University and by the Fundacion de Investigaciones Cardiologicas Einthoven, Buenos Aires, Argentina.

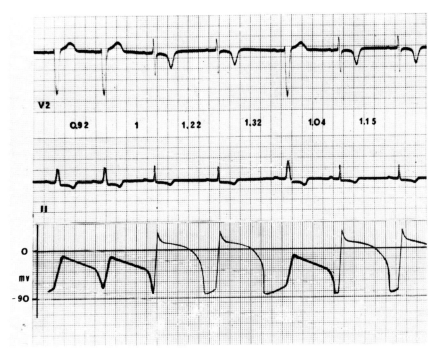

Fig. 1. Typical example of intermittent BBB. Leads V2 and II simultaneously recorded during carotid sinus massage. R-R intervals, in seconds. The first two beats show phase 3 LBBB, closing relatively short R-R intervals; the fifth beat, ending a relatively longer R-R interval, reveals phase 4 LBBB; and the third, fourth, sixth and seventh beats, ending R-R intervals of intermediate length, show normal conduction. Bottom: schematic representation of the underlying electrophysiologic mechanisms.

show normal conduction; and the fifth beat, after a pause of 1.32 sec shows bradycardia-dependent or phase 4 LBBB. As illustrated schematically at the bottom of figure 1, phase 3 block occurs when an impulse falls (or arrives at the injured region of the LBB) during electrical systole of the preceding beat, whereas phase 4 block occurs when an impulse falls relatively late in diastole. Therefore, phase 3 and phase 4 block can also be called 'systolic' and 'diastolic' block, respectively. Figure 2, B and C, illustrates again that phase 3 BBB is related to a prolongation of the electrical systole and is, hence, systolic, whereas phase 4 BBB is related to slight hypopolarization and a probably enhanced spontaneous diastolic depolarization (SDD) and is, thus, diastolic. Figure 2A shows that the aberrant ventricular conduction of premature supraventricular beats may simply be considered as a functional or physiologic variety of systolic or phase 3 block. Figure 3 displays the results of a study of 14 cases of intermittent BBB, and illustrates the occurrence, in all of them, of an early range of systolic or phase 3 BBB, followed by a normal conduction range during the initial part of electrical diastole, after which comes a late range of phase 4 or diastolic BBB. Figure 3 also shows what we have termed 'accordion effect' (692) meaning that the two block ranges seem to compress more or less the intermediate normal conduction range. In Argentina, the accordion effect is often referred to as the 'bellows-like effect' or the 'Troilo effect'.

When patients with intermittent BBB are explored, it is rather easy to demonstrate

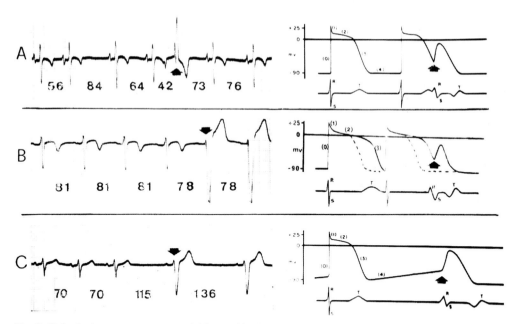

Fig. 2. Strip A shows a premature atrial beat with aberrant ventricular conduction of the RBBB type. Strip B shows phase 3 LBBB. Strip C shows phase 4 LBBB. The three strips (lead V1) belong to three different patients. Intervals, in hundredths of a second. To the right of each strip, the underlying physiologic mechanisms are shown schematically, in conventional symbols.

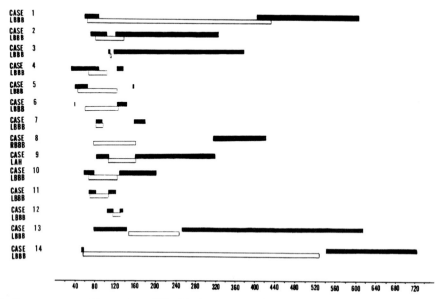

Fig. 3. Fourteen cases of intermittent BBB. Black bars to the left = phase 3 block; black bars to the right = phase 4 block; white bars = normal conduction. The extension of the normal conduction range varies from case to case (accordion effect). Scale indicates cycle length in hundredths of a second.

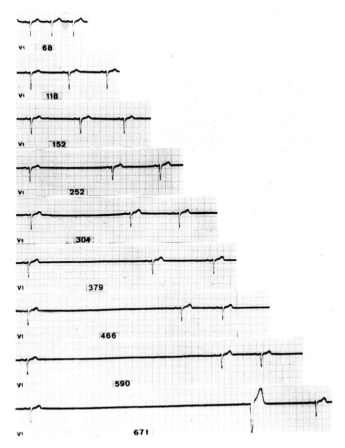

Fig. 4. Several strips from a long tracing (1220 sinoatrial beats), arranged according to progressive increase in cycle length. R-R intervals in hundredths of a second. Conduction is normal at R-R intervals of 0.68 sec up to 5.90 sec, and a pause of 6.71 sec is needed to uncover the existence of phase 4 LBBB.

the existence of phase 3 BBB, but it may be extremely difficult to uncover the presence of phase 4 BBB, as shown in figure 4. In this particular instance, a pause of 6.71 sec had to be provoked to bring out the presence of phase 4 BBB, and this was possible only because the patient was extremely sensitive to carotid sinus massage. Obviously, the demonstration of phase 4 BBB depends on the possibility of provoking long enough diastolic intervals, which in many patients may not be feasible or safe; and this explains why, in the past, this variety of BBB was considered to be exceptional, or only a 'paradoxical' manifestation of intermittent BBB. However, through the careful use of vagal stimulation during the study of many patients with intermittent BBB, our group in Buenos Aires was able to demonstrate that phase 4 BBB is rather frequent. Moreover, and as supported by recent experimental studies on the intact canine heart (241, 696) as well as on the isolated conduction system (242), it appears now that both phase 4 and phase 3 BBB represent a common type of response to injury of the ventricular conducting fascicles. However, not every kind of fascicular injury will cause the simultaneous occurrence of phase 3 and phase 4 block. It is only when the conducting fascicles are *slightly or moderately injured* that they will respond physiologically with an accordion, more or less open or closed according to the degree of injury (695). A reasonable extrapolation is that an accordion may be a manifestation of slightly or moderately injured Purkinje fibers anywhere in the heart. To support this view, accordions of the same type will now be shown to exist in such a wide variety of conditions as paroxysmal AV block, parasystole, the WPW syndrome, and during the effect of certain antiarrhythmic drugs. However, for a better understanding of the relationships between automaticity and conduction which underly the mechanism of phase 4 block, a few words must be said before about escapes of the injured fascicle (EIF).

EIF are more readily studied experimentally than in clinical cases. When one of the main ventricular conducting fascicles is moderately injured, the sequence is as illustrated

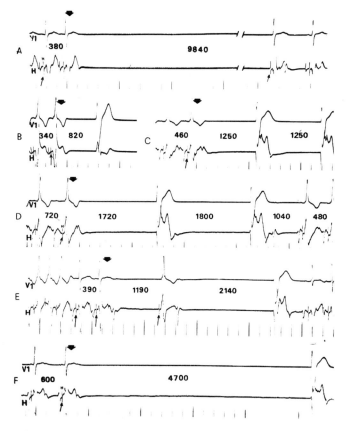

Fig. 5. Experiment during which the RBB was mechanically injured in a dog. In all strips, VI was simultaneously recorded with a His bundle potential. The large arrows indicate vagal stimulation. In the control (A), a His bundle escape (small arrow) occurs after a pause of 9840 msec. Immediately after injuring the RBB (B), RBBB occurs, and an EIF showing a LBBB pattern appears after a pause of 820 msec. C and D were recorded during the next three minutes and show that the coupling of the EIF lengthens progressively, while RBBB is still present for any diastolic interval. E was recorded a few minutes later. The first three beats show phase 3 RBBB, the next two beats show normal conduction, and the sixth beat, after a pause of 1190 msec is a His bundle escape showing phase 4 RBBB. The seventh beat is an EIF, with a coupling of 2140 msec. Note the progressive lengthening of the coupling interval of the EIF, as injury declines and the conduction disturbance improves.

in figure 5. In the control and during vagal stimulation, there is a His bundle escape after a pause of 9,840 msec (A). After injuring the RBB (B to F), EIF showing a LBBB pattern occur with an initial short coupling (of only 820 msec in B), and this coupling increases progressively as the injury diminishes or subsides. Figure 5 also shows that the EIF display a pattern of LBBB when the RBB is injured, and that the coupling of the EIF is much shorter than the coupling of the His bundle escapes in the control. This clearly indicates that the EIF are specifically related to a great increase of automaticity in the Purkinje fibers of the injured fascicle. Figure 6 shows the average sequence of 40 similar experiments on the intact canine heart (241). In this sequence, the normal conduction range was extremely narrow at the beginning and widened progressively in a few minutes at the expense of both the phase 3 and phase 4 block ranges (mostly the latter) in such a way that the phase 4 BBB shifted progressively to the right, always accompanied by a shift of the EIF in the same direction. Thus, as the accordion opens, the phase 4 BBB and the EIF tend to go always together, and this documents the existence of a close relationship between depressed conduction and increased automaticity. During the opening of the accordion, the coupling of the EIF was usually slightly longer than the critical diastolic interval for phase 4 block, and this should be kept in mind when discussing later the mechanism of parasystole.

Figure 7 shows that EIF, as well as their relationship with phase 4 BBB, can also be documented in clinical cases of intermittent BBB. This association of EIF and phase 4

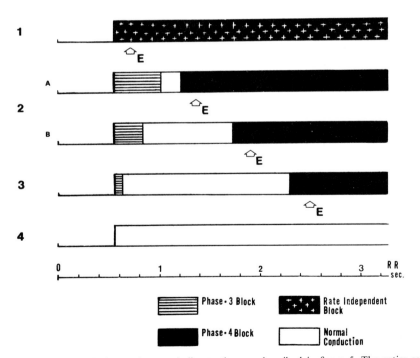

Fig. 6. Average sequence of 40 experiments similar to the one described in figure 5. The entire sequence, from 1 to 4, lasts 10 to 20 minutes, according to the initial degree of fascicular injury. E = escape from injured fascicle.

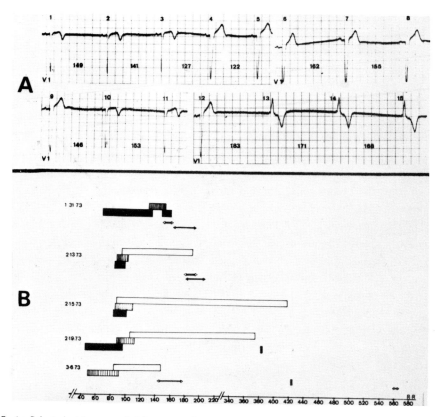

Fig. 7. A: Selected strips recorded from a patient with intermittent LBB and anteroseptal ischemia. Beats 1, 2, 3 and 10 show a small degree of incomplete LBBB; beats 4 and 5 show phase 3 LBBB; beats 6, 7 and 8 show phase 4 LBBB; and beat 11 is a junctional escape with incomplete LBBB. Beats 13 to 15 are EIF, showing a RBBB pattern. B: Sequence of conduction changes, from the same patient. Black bars to the left = phase 3 LBBB; black bars to the right = phase 4 LBBB; striped bars = incomplete LBBB; white bars = normal conduction; white arrows = junctional escapes; black arrows = EIF. R-R intervals, in hundredths of a second.

BBB will be used later to construct a model for studying the effects of drugs on injured Purkinje fibers of the human heart (695).

B. PAROXYSMAL ATRIOVENTRICULAR BLOCK

Figure 8A shows a typical example of paroxysmal AV block. As the sinoatrial rate slows spontaneously, AV conduction changes from 1:1 into complete AV block, and 1:1 conduction is restablished only after a ventricular escape, provided a sinus impulse falls at a proper time after the escape. Figure 8, B to D, illustrates other examples in which paroxysmal AV block was triggered by atrial or ventricular extrasystoles (144,693). Obviously, paroxysmal AV block is an extremely serious condition, which at first sight does not seem to keep any relationship with the much less dangerous and much more common intermittent BBB. They look indeed so dissimilar, both clinically and electro-cardiographically, that it is no wonder that in the past, they were assumed to belong

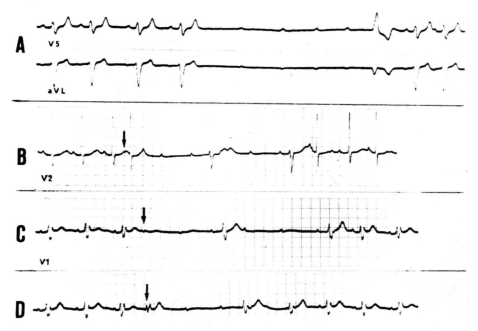

Fig. 8. Paroxysmal AV block precipitated by sinoatrial showing in A, by a conducted atrial extrasystole in B, by a blocked atrial extrasystole in C, and by a ventricular extrasystole in D. In the four examples, AV conduction changes suddenly from 1:1 into complete heart block, and back to 1:1, whenever a P wave falls at a proper time after a ventricular escape.

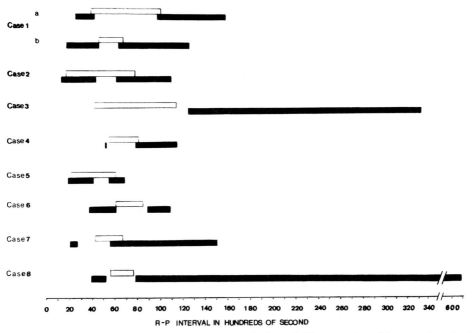

Fig. 9. Eight cases of paroxysmal AV block. Symbols, as in figure 3. The extension of the normal conduction range varies from case to case (accordion effect), or even in the same patient from day to day (a and b in Case 1).

into different parts of electrocardiography. However, figure 9 shows that, in physiological terms, paroxysmal AV block expresses itself by the same kind of accordion which so well characterizes the much simpler intermittent BBB. In the last analysis, paroxysmal AV block is also a simple form of intermittent BBB, but occuring in patients in whom the other fascicles are totally interrupted by previous lesions (693).

C. PARASYSTOLE

In our view, parasystole is physiologically related to the occurrence of a 'microaccordion', in which phase 3 and phase 4 block are limited to a small group of moderately injured Purkinje fibers, or perhaps even a single fiber. Figure 10A shows an example of parasystole, in which sinus impulses falling within certain limited range of the inter-parasystolic interval were able to discharge the parasystolic focus and reset the parasystolic mechanism. Careful measurements showed that, in addition to the automatic beats, the parasystolic

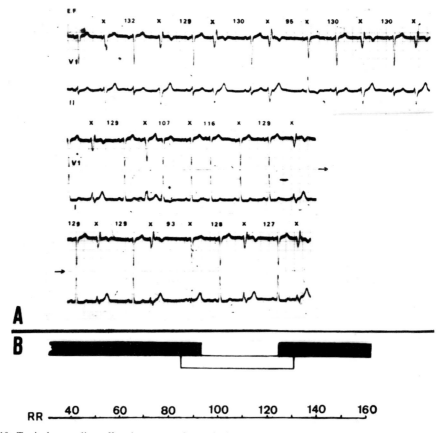

Fig. 10. Typical accordion effect in a case of ventricular parasystole. The X indicate the parasystolic beats (sometimes as fusion beats), or the sinoatrial impulses which penetrate and discharge the parasystolic focus. Intervals, in hundredths of a second. The black bar to the left corresponds to phase 3 block in the parasystolic focus, and the black bar to the right, to phase 4 block in the same focus.

focus gave rise to a typical accordion (fig. 10B). Note that the inter-parasystolic interval (equivalent to the coupling of an EIF) is only slightly longer than the critical diastolic interval for phase 4 block (compare with fig. 6).

On the basis of similar observations, several years ago we developed a still unpublished and most amusing model of parasystole. Any one can imagine accordions of variable opening (different duration of the normal conduction range), more or less shifted to the right or left, and this is of course the principal and rather complex variable. The other two variables are the heart rate and the rate of discharge of the parasystolic focus. With these three variables, an infinite number of examples of 'artificial' parasystole can be constructed, several of which closely resemble known varieties and features of clinical parasystole. Figures 11 and 12 illustrate two examples. Most of the features of clinical parasystole can thus be explained in a very simple way. 1. The protection or entrance block can be considered as the result of phase 3 and phase 4 block with an extremely narrow or sometimes absent intermediate normal conduction range, within the small group of slightly to moderately injured Purkinje fibers forming the parasystolic focus. 2. The parasystolic beats are equivalent to the EIF, which as shown in the first section of this paper, are so commonly associated with the existence of phase 4 block. 3. The rate of discharge of the parasystolic focus depends on how much SDD is enhanced within it. In most clinical cases of parasystole the rate of discharge is such that it suggests that SDD is not greatly enhanced, and this matches the observation that in most cases of

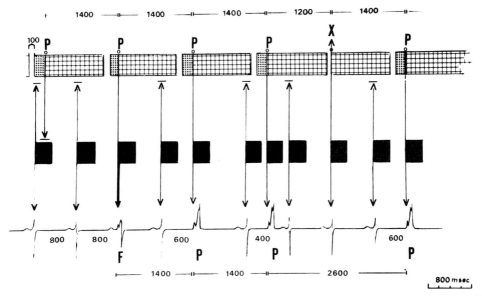

Fig. 11. 'Artificial' ventricular parasystole, according to theoretical model described in text. The bars with squares represent the phase 3 block range of the parasystolic focus; the bars with dots represent the phase 4 block, which is always interrupted by discharge of the parasystolic focus. The interval between the phase 3 and phase 4 block ranges represents the opening of the parasystolic accordion. The black bars represent the normal duration of refractoriness in the ventricular tissues around the parasystolic focus. P = parasystolic impulses or beats. F = fusion beat. A sinoatrial impulse may penetrate, discharge, and reset the parasystolic focus, only when it falls during the intermediate normal conduction range, as in beat X.

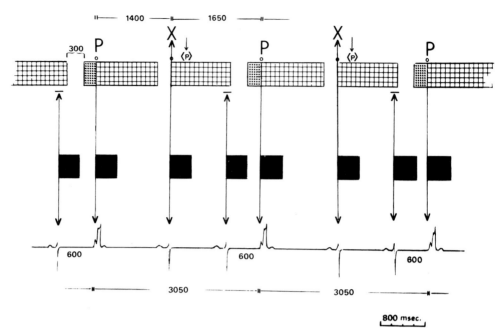

Fig. 12. Demonstration of how parasystole can give rise to a fixed coupling, if the variables of the model are properly adjusted. Description and symbols as in figure 11.

intermittent BBB, SDD need not be greatly enhanced for phase 4 BBB to occur, provided a slight degree of hypopolarization and a shift of the threshold potential toward zero are present (237,693–694). In the case of parasystole, the possibility should be considered that a shift of the threshold potential toward zero may lower the original rate of discharge or that which would result from the slope of SDD alone. 4. Entrance block without exit block, which is most common in typical parasystole, requires the existence of unidirectional block, which is also common and nearly constant in most cases of phase 3 and phase 4 block (693). Exit block, when present, is perhaps equivalent to what we have called 'concealed escapes' (692).

The most important factor determining the characteristics of parasystole and even more, whether parasystole may exist or not, or be transient or intermittent, is the width of the normal conduction range, that is, the opening of the accordion. Thus, if the parasystolic accordion is widely open, it will be penetrated continuously by sinus impulses, protection of the focus will be limited to short initial and terminal segments of the interparasystolic cycle, and no parasystole as classicaly described will exist at all. At the most, some automatic or 'parasystolic' beats will emerge here and there, probably with a variable coupling, but a parasystolic cycle will be extremely difficult or impossible to document. The possibility that isolated ventricular extrasystoles with variable coupling but without manifest evidence of parasystole may actually be caused by a widely open parasystolic focus becomes, in the light of this concept, extremely appealing. Moreover, the notion of absolute or total protection of the parasystolic focus should perhaps be changed into the more elastic concept of varying or mutable degrees of protection, which can be expressed both qualitatively and quantitatively by the opening of the accordion or the parasystolic focus itself. On the other end of the spectrum, if the opening of the parasystolic accordion is extremely narrow, the degree of protection will be great, penetration of the focus by sinoatrial impulses will occur rarely and, even then, the resetting of the parasystolic cycle will cause only minor changes in the inter-parasystolic interval. Small variations of this kind which are often attributed to changes in the parasystolic rate of discharge, may thus be caused by a narrow parasystolic accordion. A totally closed accordion means that block occurs during any part of the cycle, and phase 3 and phase 4 block cannot longer be claimed to be present, at least in the entire injured region. However, even then, automatic beats can be shown to emerge from the injured region (241,696), probably due to unidirectional block. Since under such conditions protection of the focus will be total or absolute, such a situation may perhaps give rise to a 'perfect' parasystole. However, although this is probably true, it is remarkable that perfect parasystole will be closer to spontaneous extinction than imperfect parasystole, because a totally closed accordion indicates a greater degree of injury, which only will require the unidirectional block to change into bidirectional block for the parasystole to disappear. Thus, like in the case of intermittent BBB and paroxysmal AV block or for any kind of accordion, parasystole can occur only if the Purkinje fibers of the parasystolic focus are slightly to moderately injured.

The analysis of a series of cases of parasystole published by Cohen et al. (134) greatly support our view that parasystole may be related to the existence of a microaccordion.

D. WOLFF-PARKINSON-WHITE

Figure 13 illustrates the occurrence of phase 3 and phase 4 block and a typical accordion, uncovered or caused by the administration of Ajmaline in a patient with the WPW syndrome. It can be seen that, beats following either relatively short or long diastolic intervals show a normal QRS, which indicates block in the anomalous bundle; whereas beats terminating diastolic intervals of intermediate duration show the WPW configuration, which means normal conduction in the Kent bundle. Similar results were observed in 4 to 17 patients with the WPW syndrome (639), when similarly studied. Thus, the same accordions that we have described in intermittent BBB, paroxysmal AV block and parasystole, can also occur, and not uncommonly, in the WPW syndrome. The similarity in physiological behavior of all these four apparently different conditions is strikingly impressive, and extrapolation is again unavoidable. Thus, two significant ideas were imposed on our mind by these observations. First, the anomalous bundle, like the main intraventricular conducting fascicles or like a parasystolic focus, may be composed of Purkinje or Purkinje-like fibers, or at least of fibers normally or abnormally endowed with the property of automaticity. In the light of our present knowledge, there is no other apparent way to account for the occurrence of phase 4 block (which necessarily implies the existence of enhanced or normal SDD) in the Kent bundle. Obviously, this notion may constitute an essential step in the final determination of the disputed anatomical nature of the anomalous bundle. Secondly, if accordions are related to a slight to moderate degree of injury in the affected fascicle or group of Purkinje fibers, this brings into focus the possibility that the

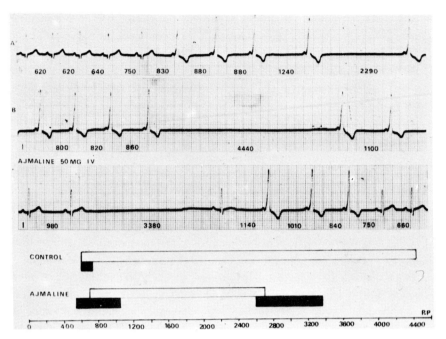

Fig. 13. Phase 3 and phase 4 block, and accordion effect in the Kent bundle of a patient with the WPW syndrome, after administration of Ajmaline. The black bars to the left indicate the phase 3 block range in the Kent bundle (causing normalization of the QRS), the black bars to the right correspond to the phase 4 block range (causing also normalization of the QRS), and the white bars indicate the range for normal conduction (causing persistence of the WPW pattern). All intervals, in miliseconds. See text for further description.

Kent bundle may be either normal or diseased, and that such a distinction can eventually be established clinically and electrocardiographically. Observations from our laboratory (639) suggested that the Kent bundle was healthy in a group of patients in whom there was no maneuver or drug able to cause either phase 3 or phase 4 block (in the same way that there is no drug or maneuver that will cause phase 3 or phase 4 block in a normal right or left bundle branch). On the other hand, it seems quite obvious that, Kent bundles in which phase 3 and/or phase 4 block occur either spontaneously or under the effect of drugs, must be at least moderately injured or diseased. This discrimination between a healthy and a diseased Kent bundle may prove to be of far reaching consequences regarding the prognosis and treatment of patients with the WPW. In this regard, it should be mentioned that, drugs which tend to close the accordion in cases of intermittent BBB (695,696), tend also to close the accordion in patients with the WPW syndrome (693). In the latter case, a totally closed accordion implies that the anomalous bundle will no longer be functionally available for the occurrence of reentrant arrhythmias characteristic of the WPW syndrome.

E. DRUGS AND ACCORDIONS

Figure 14 illustrates the effects of therapeutic doses of lidocaine (a bolus i.v. injection of 1 to 2 mg per kg) on automaticity and conduction, in two clinical cases of intermittent BBB (A and B) and in one example of intermittent BBB provoked experimentally in a dog.

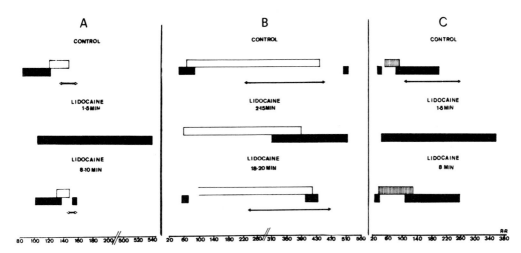

Fig. 14. Panels A and B show the effects of a bolus injection of lidocaine (1 mg/kg) on two different patients with intermittent LBBB. Panel C shows the effects of an i.v. bolus injection of 20 mg (2 mg/kg) during a canine experiment in which phase 3 and phase 4 BBB were present, with a narrow intermediate conduction range, and frequent EIF. Symbols, as in figure 3 and 7. See text for further description.

During the peak effect of the drug all escape beats were suppressed and the accordion tended to close partially or totally. In the latter case, conduction was totally interrupted in the affected fascicle (A and C). This result was unexpected. Since it is well known that lidocaine depresses SDD in normal and abnormal Purkinje fibers, as indeed documented in the present study by the suppression of the escape beats, it was thought that this would be accompanied by a shift of the phase 4 BBB range to the right with widening of the normal conduction range, particularly because lidocaine may also shorten action potential duration and refractoriness. A possible way of accounting for this unpredictable result in which automaticity and conduction were simultaneously depressed is by postulating that lidocaine caused a significant depression of membrane responsiveness. Since it has been shown that at therapeutic doses lidocaine has little effect on membrane responsiveness or that it may even improve it in normal Purkinje fibers (69–70), our results suggest that the opposite effect may occur in abnormal or critically injured Purkinje fibers, and furnish and explanation for the reported development of severe intraventricular or atrioventricular block during the administration of therapeutic doses of lidocaine (303, 499, 668).

Figure 15 shows another example of how lidocaine can be used fruitfully to explore the physiological behavior of intermittent BBB. In a patient with phase 3 LBBB, the ocurrence of EIF made it impossible to determine whether or not phase 4 LBBB was also present. After a single injection of lidocaine, the EIF were suppressed and the phase 4 BBB was readily documented.

These studies with lidocaine serve to illustrate how the concept of phase 3 and phase 4 block and the idea of an accordion can be used as a model for testing the effects of various antiarrhythmic drugs (695). For instance, drugs which depress SDD are expected to shift the phase 4 BBB range and the EIF to the right (if this is the only or predominant effect), whereas drugs which enhance SDD will be expected to cause the opposite effect. Drugs

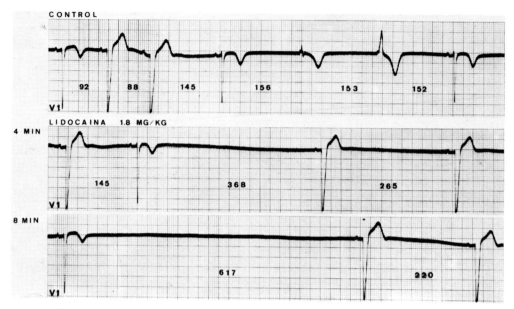

Fig. 15. Effects of lidocaine on a patient with intermittent LBBB and EIF. The control tracing shows phase 3 LBBB (second and third beats), normalization of conduction after relatively longer diastolic intervals (fourth and seventh beats), and EIF after slightly longer pauses (fifth and sixth beats). The EIF preclude visualization of the phase 4 block. However, after injection of an i.v. bolus of lidocaine, the EIF are suppressed, and the much longer diastolic intervals are terminated by sinoatrial beats revealing the phase 4 LBBB.

which prolong action potential duration and/or refractoriness are anticipated to prolong the phase 3 BBB range. Drugs which cause hyperpolarization or tend to restaure membrane potential toward more normal values, will be expected to widen the normal conduction range. Of course, most of the drugs can share several effects, in such a way that the net end result may eventually be difficult to interpret. However, the main advantage of the present model is that it may reflect better the true effect of the drugs upon injured Purkinje fibers in the intact human heart. Figure 16 shows preliminary results obtained with four different drugs. Indeed, the fact that phase 3 and phase 4 block and EIF can be identified in patients or provoked in the intact canine heart, and that under such conditions conduction and automaticity can be simultaneously changed with certain drugs, provides a model of great potential value for studying the effects of antiarrhythmic drugs.

CONCLUSIONS

Intermittent BBB, paroxysmal AV block, parasystole, and the WPW syndrome are well known clinical-electrocardiographic conditions. Apparently, nothing brings them together, and everything seems to keep them apart. However, the present study shows that, at least under certain conditions, all of them can share a similar physiological behavior, showing the occurrence of phase 3 and phase 4 block and the development of a typical accordion. Thus, no matter how dissimilar and heterogeneous they may appear

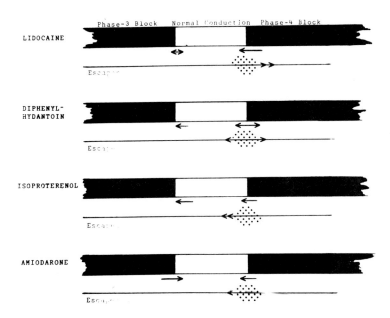

Fig. 16. Effects of drugs upon automaticity and conduction. The arrows indicate the direction in which the phase 3 block range, the phase 4 block range and the escape beats shift after administration of each drug.

or look, they can be assembled together, thanks to the concept of phase 3 and phase 4 block. This common physiological behavior suggests that they can also share a similar anatomical basis. It is postulated that this is the occurrence of slightly to moderately injured Purkinje or Purkinje-like fibers, in the diseased bundle branch, diseased fascicle constituting the only remaining AV connection, parasystolic focus, and anomalous bundle, respectively.

The fact that intermittent BBB, paroxysmal AV block, parasystole and the WPW syndrome can be aligned together because of sharing certain physiological properties, may by itself provide a lot of new information. By simple extrapolation, known features or mechanisms of any of these conditions can be applied to a better understanding of the other conditions, from a totally new angle. For example, the information previously gathered from the study of intermittent BBB helped to explain most of the features of parasystole, including the mechanism of entrance and exit block, the concept of partial versus total protection of the parasystolic focus, the mechanism of ventricular extra-systoles with variable coupling and no apparent parasystole, the reason for some variations in the rate of discharge of the parasystolic focus, and the very reason why parasystole may exist or not, be stable or transient. By the same token, physiological evidence is first presented suggesting that the anomalous bundle responsible for the WPW syndrome is or may be composed of Purkinje or Purkinje-like fibers, and that it is possible to determine whether the Kent bundle is healthy or diseased. The latter may have essential importance for determining the prognosis and treatment of patients with the WPW syndrome and disabling arrhythmias. Moreover, all these conditions can be used as a clinical model for studying the effects of antiarrhythmic drugs on diseased Purkinje fibers in the human. If science can be defined as 'the search for unity in hidden likenesses

(90), the results presented in this article can be considered as a modest scientific contribution within the field of clinical cardiology. And although some of the concepts and ideas are speculative and still unproven, they can be at least used as working hypothesis which may provide a new approach to the understanding of several still obscure problems of clinical electrocardiography.

These conclusions invite to a final comment on the significance of facts and ideas. There is a definite tendency in scientific research to overestimate the value of facts as compared to ideas. It is thus not uncommon for important cardiological journals to publish papers plagued with facts and void of ideas, and to reject papers with excellent ideas but few 'hard facts'. Of course, such a stand is highly respectable when it fulfills the healthy approach to force young investigators to explore thoroughly and correctly whatever they explore. However, the scale has shifted too much in this direction, to the point that the omnipresence of hard facts has become the paradigm of too many dull and unpromising studies. In my view, 'the special intelectual satisfaction of connecting facts to each other constitutes the real fascination of knowledge' and the true mother of ideas and hypothesis. This comment is meant as a plea for research men in the field of cardiology and for editors of journals, to bring the lever of the scale that weighs facts and ideas to a more proficient equilibrium.

8

THE ELECTROPHYSIOLOGIC BASIS OF PARASYSTOLE
AND ITS VARIANTS[1]

ALFRED PICK, M.D., F.A.C.P., F.A.C.C.

INTRODUCTION

Development of new electrophysiologic techniques in recent years has led to the experimental reproduction in the animal laboratory, as well as at the bedside, of various cardiac arrhythmias. Hypothetic mechanisms deduced from the analysis of clinical electrocardiograms could thus be verified, and new concepts emerged for the understanding of previously obscure causes of certain disorders of the cardiac rhythm (630). One such example is parasystole.

Electrocardiographic features of a typical parasystolic rhythm are well known. Not all its classical criteria (729,856), however, need to be fulfilled. Thus: 1. the coupling intervals may become constant transiently or over a protracted period of time; 2. the two simultaneously acting rhythms may become linked temporarily or permanently to each other; 3. the parasystolic beats may not be manifest when expected; or 4. the manifest or calculated ectopic cycles may not maintain the expected regularity. Examples of such deviations from the classical postulates, their various causes, and the relation of parasystole to bundle branch block are the topic of this communication.

MECHANISMS OF FIXED AND REVERSED COUPLING

In figure 1, the upper record of panel A shows four ventricular premature beats during a sinus tachycardia of 115. Their distance ('coupling') to a preceding sinus beat varies from 0.32 to 0.50 sec and the latter permits fusion of an ectopic with a sinus impulse. Longer (3.75 sec) and shorter (1.50 sec) interectopic intervals have a common denominator of 0.75 sec, revealing the presence of a ventricular parasystole discharging at a rate of 80. In the lower record of panel A the same interectopic intervals of 1.50 sec are measured, but now at a constant coupling of 0.36 sec, recurring after every second sinus beat. This change of varying to fixed coupling of the parasystolic beats is the consequence of a slight acceleration of the sinus rate to 120, so that two parasystolic cycles (2 × 0.75 sec) equal precisely three sinus cycles (3 × 0.5 sec). Thus, fixed coupling and repetitive group beating (trigeminy) have developed by chance as, temporarily, two totally independent pacemakers became synchronized.

Panel B shows, in a case of artificial parasystole produced by fixed rate ventricular

1. Supported in part by funds contributed by the Marion G. & S. Max Becker Fund and the Michael Reese Medical Research Institute Council.

A

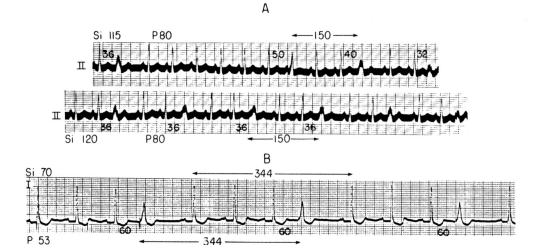

Fig. 1. Fixed coupling due to a simple numerical relation between parasystolic and basic rate (A) in spontaneous parasystole, (B) in artificial parasystole. Si = sinus rate/min. P = parasystolic rate/min. Numbers between horizontal arrows are multiples of cycle lengths; numbers within records are coupling intervals (in sec/100, as in all subsequent figures except fig. 15B). From Langendorf and Pick, *Circulation* 35, 304 (1967). Reproduced by permission.

pacing (without retrograde conduction to the atria), how constant coupling was achieved when the pacing rate was adjusted so that the sum of three artificial cycles measuring 3.44 sec equalled precisely the sum of four regular sinus cycles.

A more complex variant of parasystolic group beating with fixed coupling, observed during asynchronous ventricular pacing, is shown in figure 2. A series of four sinus beats alternates with four paced beats. The transition from artificial to natural complexes takes place via a ventricular fusion beat, whereas the change back to artificial rhythm occurs at a constant coupling interval of 0.40 sec. Again the explanation of this unusual behavior of a parasystole is found in comparative measurements, as indicated in lead III. The sum of eight sinus cycles (5.60 sec) equals the sum of seven paced ones. Since both rhythms are regular this must result of necessity in periodic appearance and disappearance of the two

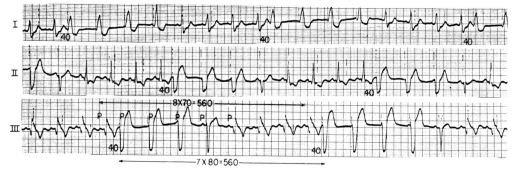

Fig. 2. Repetitive group beating with fixed coupling as a result of a simple numerical relation between sinus and pacing rates. P = consecutive sinus impulses. Numbers as in figure 1. From Langendorf and Pick, *Circulation* 35, 304 (1967). Reproduced by permission.

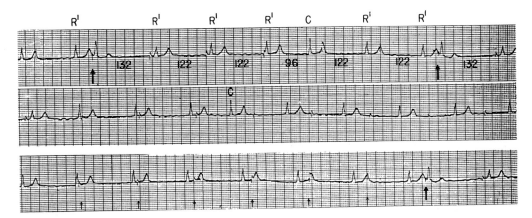

Fig. 3. Artificial ventricular parasystole with fixed coupling due to supernormal phase of excitability and reversed coupling of junctional escapes (R′). Other symbols explained in text. From Langendorf and Pick, *Circulation* 35, 304 (1967). Reproduced by permission.

independent rhythms, and in a fixed coupling of the first beat of each group of paced (parasystolic) beats. On the other hand, fusion beats occur when the least common multiple of the two different cycles is reached representing a new 'starting point' of the repetitive interplay of the two rhythms.

A different cause of constant coupling in an artificial parasystole is shown in figure 3, a case of atrial fibrillation in whom an advanced A-V block produced by digitalis permitted only occasional capture of the ventricles by atrial impulses (labelled C). Otherwise consecutive regular A-V junctional escapes (R′) caused A-V dissociation. Subthreshold fixed rate pacing of the right ventricle (arrows) elicited only rare responses; they occurred invariably and predictably when the pacer impulse fell 0.36 sec after a spontaneous beat (heavy arrows). Such responses to sub-threshold stimulation limited to an early point in the ventricular cycle, at the end of repolarization, are characteristic of a supernormal phase of excitability (770, 780, 898). In this instance the artificial parasystole manifested itself merely in the form of occasional fixed coupled ventricular premature beats. This record shows, moreover, that after these premature beats the first junctional cycle is lengthened from 1.22 to 1.32 sec. Thus, during the supernormal phase not only the ventricles were depolarized but the effective pacer impulses also propagated back to the site of the junctional pacemaker and postponed its spontaneous discharge (concealed retrograde conduction). Protection of the two ectopic pacemakers was here not mutual but only unidirectional (see fig. 4 and 5).

In figure 4 is illustrated, in a patient with left bundle branch block with normal A-V conduction, competition between a regular sinus rhythm and fixed rate atrial pacing (atrial parasystole with unidirectional protection). Effective pacing impulses produce small, diphasic atrial deflection (P′) in contrast to normally shaped sinus P waves, some of which are labelled P. Ventricular complexes, all conducted at the same P-R interval of 0.20 sec, occur in repetitive groups separated by longer R-R intervals. The latter are induced by block within the A-V junction of atrial responses to pacer stimuli that fall early after a ventricular complex. Within these ventricular groups, four different atrial cycle

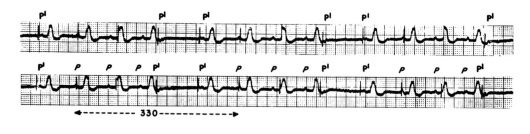

| P-P | 64 | P'-P' | 84 |
| P-P' | 38 | P'-P | 80 |

Fig. 4. Artificial atrial parasystole causing repetitive group beating with fixed coupling. P' stands for paced atrial beats. P indicates sinus P waves. The two strips are a contiguous portion of a long lead I. Measurements indicated below the record are explained in the text.

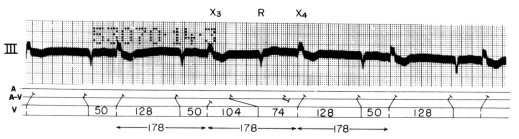

Fig. 5. Atrial fibrillation with complete A-V dissociation. Spontaneous ventricular parasystole causing bigeminy. 'Reversed' coupling causing fixed coupling. In the diagram the horizontal line at level A-V indicates the site of a junctional pacemaker. Explained in text. From Langendorf and Pick, *Circulation* 35, 304 (1967). Reproduced by permission.

lengths recur, always in the same sequence: two sinus cycles (*P-P*), each measuring 0.64 sec, are followed by the short 'coupling' (0.38 sec) of a blocked paced impulse (*P-P'*); this in turn is succeeded by a pacing cycle (*P'-P'*) of 0.84 sec and a 'return cycle' (*P'-P*) of 0.80 sec. Thus, the sum total of these five successive atrial cycles, indicated by the horizontal arrows, remains 0.30 sec.

The constancy of these various atrial cycles (notably the identical length of the two sinus cycles after the return cycle) permits the following conclusions: a. the natural (sinus) and the artificial (pacing) impulses are discharged and propagated through the atria in a regular manner; b. a significant transient depression or acceleration (445) of spontaneous sinus impulse formation by its extraneous (artificial) depolarization can be ruled out; and, therefore, c. an estimation becomes possible of conduction times between the sinus pacemaker and the site of the pacing electrode, by subtracting the length of the sinus cycle (0.64 sec) from that of the return cycle (0.80 sec) (466, 793). This difference of 0.16 sec represents the sum of the antegrade and retrograde conduction times between the two atrial pacemakers. Although the two conduction times may not be equal, both can be considered to be well within normal limits.

Figure 5 shows atrial fibrillation with complete A-V dissociation and bigeminy caused by ventricular premature beats alternating with A-V junctional beats. The spacing of the junctional beats is regular (1.28 sec) except for one (R), and the coupling of premature beats is constant (0.50 sec) except in the middle of the record. Here one junctional cycle (X_3-R) is shortened to 1.04 sec, and the coupling of the premature beat lengthened by the same amount to 0.74 sec. However, the distance between the premature beats remains constant (1.78 sec), revealing their parasystolic nature. The interpretation of this disturbance in the otherwise orderly arrangement of the bigeminy is indicated in the diagram.

With the exception of X_3 all parasystolic beats are conducted back to the site of the junctional pacemaker (concealed retrograde conduction), discharge it and postpone its spontaneous firing. The retrograde impulse of X_3, however, is stopped in the lower part of the junction. Consequently: a. the junctional center can release a spontaneous impulse on time; but b. this impulse is delayed in reaching the ventricles because it encounters partial refractoriness in the lower junction; and c. the next junctional impulse is completely blocked. The fixed coupling (0.50 sec) of the other parasystolic beats is the consequence of 'reversed' coupling of junctional escapes to premature ventricular beats. Without this transient change from unidirectional to mutual protection of the two pacemakers, the parasystolic origin of the bigeminy could not be recognized.

Figure 6, obtained in a digitalized patient, shows atrial fibrillation with incomplete A-V dissociation, an occasional ventricular capture (labelled C) occurring in lead II. Elsewhere similar beats with a QRS of 0.10 sec occur in regular sequence (R-R 0.86 sec) before starting to alternate with earlier QRS complexes widened to 0.14 sec. During the resulting bigeminy, the cycle of the wider beats progressively shortens from 0.62 to 0.52 sec, whereas the narrow beats occur at intervals progressively lengthening from 0.94 to 1.06 sec. However, distances between the wider beats maintain a constant length of 1.54 sec. The interpretation of this ventricular irregularity is presented in diagrammatic form. The A-V dissociation is the result of a combination of high degree A-V block with acceleration of A-V junctional impulse formation to 70/min and a ventricular parasystole with a manifest discharge rate of 38/min. The parasystole emerges whenever the ventricular myocardium is in a nonrefractory state, and is protected from all junctional impulses, but each parasystolic impulse penetrates backwards to reset the junctional center (reversed coupling cf. fig. 3 and 5). However, this link between the two ectopic rhythms is not constant. Retrograde (concealed) conduction becomes slower as the distance of para-

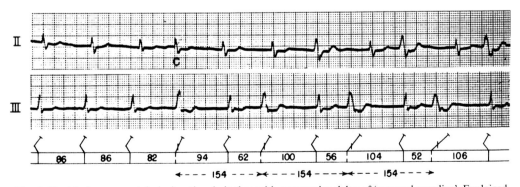

Fig. 6. Ventricular parasystole in junctional rhythm with progressive delay of 'reversed coupling'. Explained in text.

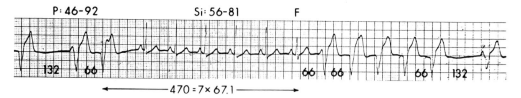

P: 46-92   Si: 56-81   F

132   66   66   66   66   132

←————————470 = 7 × 67.1 ————————→

Fig. 7. Accelerated parasystolic ventricular rhythm with intermittent 2:1 (type II) exit block in recent inferior wall infarction (monitored chest lead).

systolic to junctional beats lengthens and with it the coupling shortens. Therefore, spontaneous junctional discharges, although coupled to the parasystole, are postponed to an increasing extent, giving rise to the unusual phenomenon of reversed coupling that is *not* fixed (cf. fig. 3 and 5).

TYPES OF EXIT BLOCK OF PARASYSTOLIC IMPULSES

In figure 7, P waves can be identified at rates varying between 56 and 81/min (sinus arrhythmia). Ventricular complexes are of three types: a. five consecutive ones with normal QRS duration are sinus beats conducted with a normal P-R of 0.16 sec; b. the second type at the beginning and the end of the record with QRS prolonged to 0.14 sec occurs independent from P waves and represents idioventricular discharges with A-V dissociation. Their ventricular origin is supported by the occurrence of a ventricular fusion beat, labelled F, at the transition of sinus to the ectopic rhythm. The cycle of the ectopic beats is either 0.66 sec or precisely twice as long, corresponding to a rate of 46 or 92. The long interval of 4.70 sec between the third ectopic and the fusion beat corresponds to about 7 short ectopic cycles. Thus, an accelerated ventricular parasystolic rhythm with a 2:1 exit block competes with a sinus arrhythmia for ventricular depolarization. It emerges whenever the ventricles are no longer, or not yet, completely refractory from responses to sinus impulses. The sinus rhythm, on the other hand, takes over when the ectopic cycle happens to be prolonged by the intermittent exit block and no parasystolic impulse is ready at that time to collide with the sinus impulse in the A-V junction. Since the long and short successive parasystolic cycles maintain a precise numerical (2:1) relation, the exit block may be considered to be of Mobitz Type II.

In figure 8, two or three instances of ventricular bigeminy alternate with two consecutive sinus beats. During this bigeminy the 'coupling' of the premature beats (vertical bars in the diagram) progressively shortens from 0.64 to 0.46 sec. The first 'coupling' of each series is almost as long as the sinus cycle resulting in ventricular fusion beats (interrupted

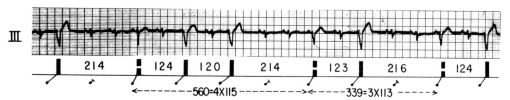

III

214   124   120   214   123   216   124

←- - - - - - -560 = 4 × 115 - - - - - - - - →←- - - -339 = 3 × 113 - - - - - →

Fig. 8. Intermittent bigeminy due to Type I second-degree exit block of a ventricular parasystole. Explained in text.

vertical bars). Long intervals between consecutive ectopic beats (2.14 or 2.16 sec) measure less than the sum of two short ones (1.24 and 1.20 sec). However, distances between fusion beats have a common denominator of about 1.14 sec. Using this value as cycle length of a regular ectopic ventricular rhythm (the dots in the diagram), the various manifest inter-ectopic intervals can be fitted to correspond to the structure of Wenckebach periods. Thus, a Mobitz Type I exit block of a protected ventricular parasystole, at propagation ratios of 4:3 or 3:2 can be postulated as a cause of the intermittent bigeminy.

In figure 9, lead III in the upper record shows a sinus bradycardia at a rate of 58 (beats #1, 4, 5 and 8) in competition with a slower A-V junctional rhythm (rate 46) for ventricular and atrial activation. QRS of both sinus and junctional beats measures 0.10 sec. Junctional discharges are manifested: a. by three premature retrograde P waves (resetting the otherwise regular sinus cycle), one with a ventricular response (beat #2); or b. by escape beats which coincide with a sinus P wave (beats #3 and 6) or are preceded by it at a short distance (beat #7). The true junctional cycle length can be established by the distance between two successive escapes (beats #6 and 7) which measures 1.30 sec (rate 46/min). When two sinus beats (#4 and 5) intervene between junctional impulses, the interval between the latter of 3.88 sec corresponds to three simple junctional cycles. Based on these measurements, the diagram was constructed representing an A-V junctional parasystole with varying antegrade and retrograde conduction.

Junctional discharges (indicated by dots) occur in a regular sequence regardless of whether they precede, follow or coincide with a sinus impulse. Thus, the junctional pace-

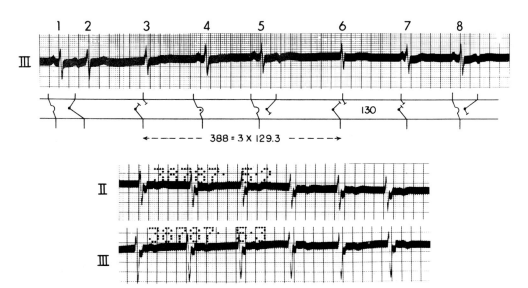

Fig. 9. Slow A-V junctional parasystole in sinus bradycardia (upper lead III) changing after several days to junctional rhythm with persistent retrograde conduction to the atria (lower leads II and III). In the diagram, small semicircles indicate protection of regular junctional discharges (dots) from sinus impulses that traverse the A-V junction. The different inclination of diagonal lines connecting dots with the symbols of atrial and ventricular activity indicate differences in conduction speed (not absolute values) of antegrade or retrograde propagation of junctional impulses. The numbers above the record correspond to consecutive ventricular complexes of different supraventricular origin (explained in text).

maker is protected from invasion by sinus impulses, either by the latter's collision with a junctional impulse traveling backwards (beats #3, 6 and 7) or by refractoriness of junctional tissues surrounding the ectopic focus. In beats #3 and 6 this may be attributable to phase 3 depolarization; in beats #1, 4, 5 and 8 to late diastolic (phase 4) depolarization of the area of the junctional pacemaker, probably in the His bundle (747) (see Discussion). However, this protective (entrance) block is only unidirectional since both antegrade and retrograde propagation of junctional impulses to atria and/or ventricles, without or with delay, is possible unless prevented by physiologic refractoriness of tissues proximal or distal to the site of the junctional pacemaker. The degree of this refractoriness and the speed of completed conduction in either direction depends on the time that has elapsed since the last traversal of the junction by a sinus impulse. Thus, antegrade conduction is delayed in beat #2 and retrograde conduction after beat #8.

In the two leads of the bottom record, regular junctional discharges have become faster (61/min) and each propagates at constant and equal speed to atria and ventricles. Sinus activity appears to be completely suppressed so that the parasystolic nature of the junctional rhythm can no longer be recognized.

MECHANISMS AND VARIANTS OF PROTECTION OF PARASYSTOLIC CENTERS

In figure 10A the upper lead II, obtained in a 68-year-old woman on admission to the hospital for dehydration and anemia, shows atrial fibrillation with a fast completely irregular ventricular response (average rate 170/min). Three ventricular complexes with QRS slightly prolonged to 0.10 sec, indicated by dots in the diagram, are ventricular ectopic beats. Their coupling intervals are 0.36, 0.44 and 0.48 sec but intervals between them are equal, 2.50 sec. This indicates a parasystolic rhythm, the rate of which appears to be very slow (24/min).

In three limb leads obtained the following day after commencement of digitalis medication, the irregular ventricular response is reduced to an average rate of 104/min. Ventricular ectopic beats of the same configuration (except one in lead II discussed in figure 10B) are more frequent and alternate at times with conducted beats (bigeminy) but at widely varying coupling intervals, from 0.28 to 0.62 sec. However, the interectopic intervals are again 2.50 or exactly one-half of it (1.25). This indicates that: a. the actual parasystolic discharge rate is 48/min and physiologic ventricular unresponsiveness reduced at times their manifest rate to one-half; and b. digitalis has slowed A-V conduction (and modified the ST-T configuration) but has not altered the protected ectopic impulse formation in the ventricles. Therefore, the intermittent bigeminy is not a manifestation of impending digitalis toxicity. The marked right axis deviation of the ectopic beats and their only moderate QRS widening suggest origin of the parasystole in the anterior fascicle of the left bundle branch.

Figure 10B is a reproduction of lead II of figure 10A. In the diagram solid arrows indicate responses of the ventricles to regular parasystolic impulses (dots) discharged at a rate of 48/min. The broken-line arrow in front of the second dot stands for discharge of,

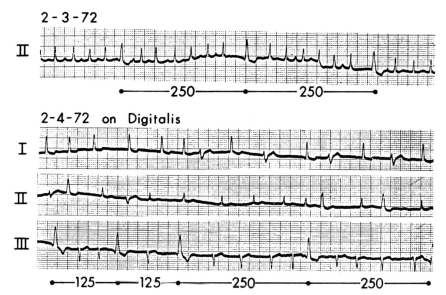

Fig. 10A. Ventricular parasystole in atrial fibrillation not influenced by digitalis.

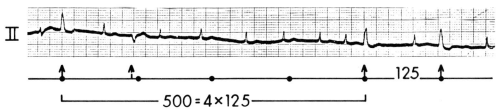

Fig. 10B. Diagrammatic demonstration in lead II of figure 10A of total (bidirectional) protection of the parasystolic center and dependence of exit of its impulses on physiologic ventricular refractoriness (see text).

and response to, another (non-parasystolic) ventricular focus. It thus becomes evident that the parasystolic discharge is shielded from both supraventricular and the idioventricular impulses (bidirectional protection, cf. fig. 3 and 5). Furthermore, comparison of 'coupling' intervals of effective and latent parasystolic intervals reveals that the shortest response interval is 0.32 sec, the approximate duration of ventricular refractoriness after a conducted supraventricular impulse. At an average ventricular rate of 104/min this is a normal value, though somewhat longer than the average Q-T interval of 0.30 sec determined in figure 10A (168,627).

In figure 11 regular sinus P waves at a rate of 75 (cycle length 0.80 sec) can be spaced throughout tracing. There are four types of ventricular complexes. Two of bizarre shape, with a QRS duration of 0.12 sec and a short coupling interval of 0.36 sec, are ventricular premature beats. The other three types are similar in shape and in direction of QRS and T but differ in the size of the two deflections. The smallest ones with a QRS of 0.08 sec are sinus beats conducted at a constant P-R of 0.18 sec. The largest ones, with a QRS of 0.10 sec, occur in a regular sequence (except after the premature beat) with a cycle of 0.78 sec (rate 77), which is somewhat shorter than the sinus cycle, and are independent from sinus impulses (intermittent A-V dissociation). The transition from one into the other rhythm takes place over one or two ventricular fusion beats labelled F. The similar-

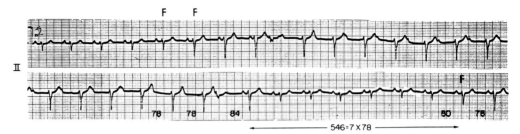

F   F

II

78   78   84   80   78

546≡7 X 78

Fig. 11. Accelerated ventricular, probably posterior, fascicular parasystole, unidirectionally protected, causing intermittent A-V dissociation. Continuous monitored lead II. The last beat of the upper strip is reproduced as the first of the lower strip.

ity of the ectopic and sinus beats as well as their minor QRS prolongation suggest their origin in the posterior fascicle of the left bundle branch (133) (a non-paroxysmal fascicular tachycardia).

In the lower strip is indicated that the long distance of 5.46 sec separating an ectopic from a fusion beat corresponds precisely to the sum of seven regular ectopic cycles. Here the ectopic rhythm is protected from the six intervening sinus beats and is, therefore, parasystolic in nature. However, the pause of 0.84 sec after the ventricular beats occurring prematurely during the parasystole is less than compensatory but 0.06 sec longer than the parasystolic cycle. This indicates that ventricular ectopic beats from a different focus penetrate to the side of the parasystole and reset its cycle. Or, in short, the protection of the parasystole is only unidirectional. Assuming equal conduction times to and from parasystolic focus, both would be short (0.03 sec, cf. fig. 4).

The two records illustrated in figure 12 were obtained in a patient with recent inferior wall infarction in the morning and afternoon of the same day. They have *in common*: a. runs of a rapid ventricular rhythm, probably originating in the posterior fascicle of the left bundle branch, with A-V dissociation (atrial rate 100, ventricular rate 158/min); b. capture of the ventricles by two consecutive sinus impulses when the fast ventricular rhythm spontaneously and abruptly stops; c. resumption of the ectopic tachycardia after the second capture at a 'coupling' interval of 0.38 sec, which equals the ectopic cycle. The

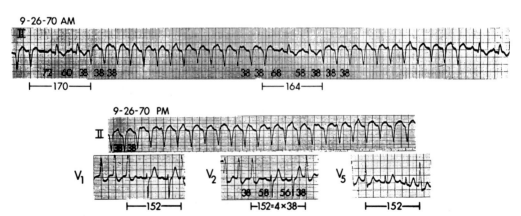

9-26-70 AM

II

72 60 38 38 38   38 38 68   58 38 38 38

├──170──┤   ├──164──┤

9-26-70 PM

II

38 38

V₁   V₂   38 38 56 38   V₅

├──152──┤   ├─152≡4×38─┤   ├──152──┤

Fig. 12. Repetitive, changing to a parasystolic ventricular tachycardia with intermittent exit block. The numbers are explained in the text.

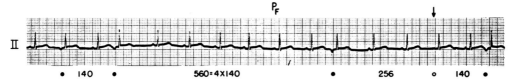

Fig. 13. Intermittent supraventricular parasystole. Symbols and numbers explained in text.

records *differ* in that interectopic interval containing the two captures is a precise multiple of the ectopic cycle in the afternoon (1.52 = 4 × 0.38 sec) but not in the morning (1.70 and 1.64 sec). Thus, in the afternoon the ectopic rhythm has developed the characteristic feature (protection) of a rapid parasystole.

In both records this sudden intermission may be caused by a temporary exit block of the ectopic impulses. In the afternoon, a complete entrance block appears to have developed of the area from which the rapid impulses are released. In the morning record, this area was either unprotected, or protected only from the first of the pair of captures (cf. fig. 14). Such a variable dynamic state of conductivity is not unusual nor unexpected in or around a freshly infarcted area (939), located here in a vicinity of the posterior fascicle of the left bundle branch.

In figure 13 the regular sequence of upright sinus P waves (P-R 0.16 sec) is on six occasions disturbed by P waves of different shape. Four inverted P waves (P-R 0.14 sec), labelled by solid circles, appear more or less prematurely. They originate either low in the atria or in the A-V junction, and their retrograde impulses reset the sinus nodal discharge as indicated by the less than compensatory pause following them. Two smaller, broader and notched P waves are not (P_f) or only slightly premature (↓). These are ectopic atrial impulses from a different area which do not reach the sinus node; the first (P_f), an atrial fusion beat, collides with the sinus impulse, and after the other (↓) the returning sinus cycle is fully compensatory.

Intervals between the first three retrograde P waves measure 1.40 sec and a precise multiple thereof (5.60 sec) revealing their parasystolic nature. However, the interval between the last two retrograde P waves (2.56 + 1.4 sec) is 0.22 sec shorter than the sum of three parasystolic cycles; the latter is resumed only after the second non-parasystolic P wave (↓). Therefore, the parasystolic focus is protected from sinus impulses but not from another ectopic atrial impulse which can penetrate to its site and reset its cycle (open circle). Thus, due to the selective protection, the parasystole is not continuous but intermittent (cf. fig. 14–16).

In figure 14 are reproduced three selected representative portions of a long lead II in which ventricular premature beats (X) or ventricular fusion beats (XF) are separated by one or two sinus beats (bigeminy and trigeminy). During the bigeminy the coupling of X progressively shortens from 0.56 to 0.38 sec, but the X-X intervals remain constant (1.12 sec). When two successive sinus beats intervene, the X-X interval bridging them is 0.20 sec shorter than the sum of two short X-X intervals. However, the distance of the first of the pair of sinus beats to the next ectopic beat following it is again 1.12 sec. Thus a parasystolic rhythm can be diagnosed that is not continuous but at times reset by, and linked to, a sinus impulse that penetrates past the barrier of parasystolic protection.

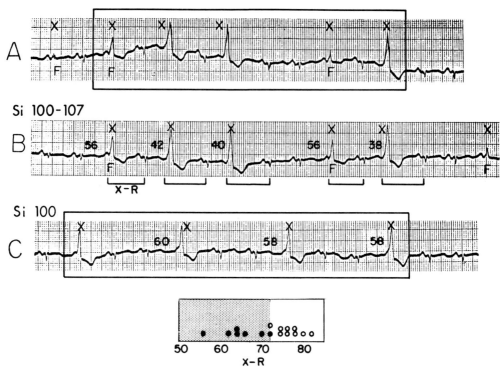

Fig. 14. Intermittent ventricular parasystole causing bigeminy and trigeminy. Symbols and diagram explained in text. This and Figures 15A–D and 16 are from Cohen, Langendorf and Pick, *Circulation* 48, 761 (1973). Reproduced by permission.

Further measurements reveal that the intermittence of the parasystole depends on the time interval (X-R) at which a sinus impulse reaches the ventricles following a parasystolic ventricular depolarization. The diagram below shows that the protection of the parasystole (shaded area) ceases after 0.70 sec, which is somewhat longer than half of the parasystolic cycle of 1.12 sec. Thus this record demonstrates the mechanism causing fixed coupling of the first of a series of parasystolic beats, which is characteristic of an intermittent type of parasystole (see Discussion).

Figures 15A–D are from another, similar case of an intermittent parasystole which could be analyzed in greater detail. Figure 15A shows in three limb and precordial leads a sinus beat paired with a premature ectopic one. Both have the earmarks of old anteroseptal infarction with a QRS axis of $-60°$ in a right bundle branch block, the latter more distinct in the premature complex of lead V_1. The origin of the ectopic beats could be located to the posterior fascicle of the left bundle branch in a His bundle record (fig. 15B). It showed abnormal shortening of both A-H and H-Q intervals in the ectopic beats when compared with corresponding intervals of the sinus beats and this revealed the retrograde His bundle depolarization by the ectopic impulses, with one fusion His deflection (133).

The parasystolic nature of these fascicular beats was documented in long records, two representative portions of which are shown in figures 15C and D. The upper record A in figure 15C shows a series of premature (fascicular) beats (X) 'coupled' in a bigeminal

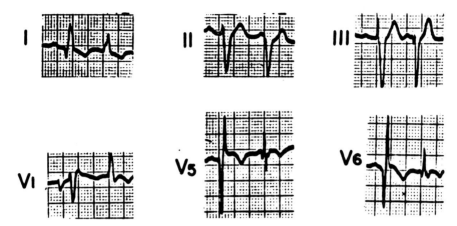

Fig. 15A. In each of six standard leads a parasystolic beat follows a sinus beat (see text).

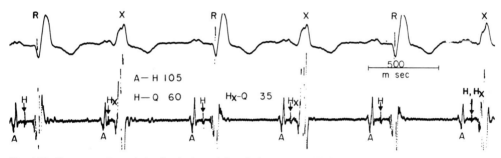

Fig. 15B. Demonstration of the fascicular origin of the parasystolic beats. Above standard lead I; below His bundle recording. R = sinus beats. X = parasystolic beats. H = antegrade His potential of sinus impulse. H_x = retrograde His potential of parasystolic beat. The last His deflection labelled H, H_x represents fusion within the His bundle of antegrade and retrograde impulses. Paper speed, 100 mm/sec. Measurements in millisecond. (See text.)

mode to each sinus beat at intervals progressively lengthening from 0.44 to 0.60 sec, after which the bigeminy ceases. The interectopic intervals are constant (1.44 to 1.48 sec) corresponding to a parasystolic rate of 42. In B, where the sinus rate has slowed from 86 to 78/min, most of the parasystolic discharges occur so early during physiologic ventricular refractoriness after a sinus beat that they remain ineffective, cause a compensatory pause and a 2:1 pseudo A-V block (456, 669). The diagram below derived from the entire material shows within the ventricular cycle a period (X-R intervals) of early and late protection (shaded areas with solid circles) equivalent to a phase 3 and phase 4 depolarization of a ventricular action potential. In between is a gap of about 0.20 sec, during which sinus impulses can penetrate into the parasystolic center and reset its cycle. These mechanisms of intermission of the parasystole and of the pseudo A-V block are depicted diagrammatically in figure 15D, which represents the framed portions of figure 15C. The explanation is given in the legend of this illustration.

In figure 16 are shown diagrammatically ten cases of intermittent ventricular parasystole analyzed as outlined in figures 14 and 15. Only in one, No. 3, both an early (phase 3) and a late (phase 4) zone of protection could be demonstrated; in the others, one or the other was found. Its length and occurrence had no relation to the parasystolic rate.

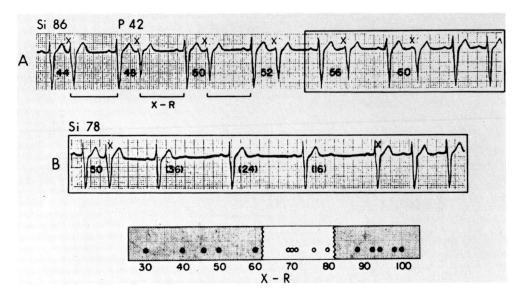

Fig. 15C. Demonstration of the parasystolic nature of the ectopic beats and of zones of their 'early' and 'late' protection. Si = sinus rate/min. P = parasystolic rate/min. Numbers within the records are manifest and latent coupling intervals, the latter in brackets. Other symbols as in figure 14. The framed portions are reproduced with a diagram of interpretation in figure 15D.

THE RELATION OF PARASYSTOLE TO BUNDLE BRANCH BLOCK

Figure 17 is a representative portion of a long lead III in a patient with left bundle branch and first-degree A-V block (P-R 0.24, QRS 0.16 sec). Three ventricular beats with less QRS prolongation (0.12 sec) correspond to complete or partial ventricular responses to a co-existent parasystolic rhythm, the regular cycle of which (1.50 sec) is indicated in the diagram by successively numbered dots. Impulses #1 and 6, having the contour of a right bundle branch block, suggest that the parasystolic focus is located in the left bundle branch distal to its blocked area. In the fusion complex #5, the parasystolic impulse depolarizes all or part of the blocked area in the left ventricle. Impulses #2, 3 and 4, falling earlier in the sinus cycle, cannot propagate at all, or not far, within the left bundle branch, refractory after its retrograde transseptal penetration by the preceding sinus impulse.

In figure 18 is shown a right bundle branch block in combination with a second-degree 2:1 A-V block. During the ensuing ventricular pauses, a subsidiary pacemaker escapes with the contour of a left bundle branch block suggesting origin in the blocked right ventricle (cf. fig. 17). It continues to discharge with a cycle length of 1.30 to 1.32 sec (corresponding to a rate of about 45), undisturbed by intervening sinus impulses (right ventricular parasystole). However, some of the effective parasystolic impulses collide with faster, slightly irregular sinus impulses either in the A-V junction (causing transient A-V dissociation) or within the ventricles causing fusion beats of variable contour illustrated in the bottom row. Depending on the varying time relation of the two activation fronts, sinus (A) or parasystolic (H-I) impulses can gain control of both ventricles; or

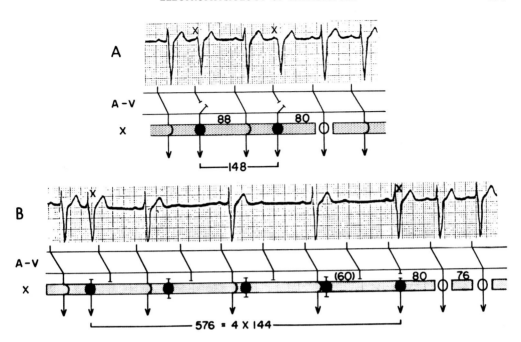

Fig. 15D. The framed portions of figure 15C with a diagram of the mechanism of intermittence of the parasystole and of the pseudo A-V block. The symbols are as follows: A-V indicates the atrioventricular junction where some of the sinus impulses collide with a retrograde parasystolic impulse (second and fourth beat in A); the horizontal stippled bars at the level of X represent protection of the parasystolic focus within the ventricles (posterior fascicle); the blank spaces in between indicate temporary loss of the portective entrance block. Solid circles represent spontaneous firing of the parasystolic focus circumvented by passing sinus impulses (vertical arrows with a semicircle in region X). The vertical arrows transecting open circles within the blank spaces indicate sinus impulses that enter, depolarize and reset the parasystolic center. The numbers above the stippled bars indicate (in sec/100) X-R intervals at which the parasystolic center is protected (in brackets) or reset (cf. diagram in figure 15C). Numbers below the stippled bars are the parasystolic cycle (in A) and a multiple thereof in B. The second to fourth parasystolic impulses are latent but prevent passing of the next sinus impulse (compensatory pauses manifested as transient 2:1 pseudo A-V block).

one or the other gains predominant control of ventricular depolarization, (B-C) and (F-G) respectively; or they share in the ventricular activation process to about the same extent (D-E).

In figure 19, during a regular sinus rhythm (rate 81, P-R 0.14 sec), QRS is prolonged to 0.12 sec due to the combination of a right with an anterior fascicular bundle branch system block (frontal QRS axis about $-50°$). Ventricular premature beats of similar shape but with a more prolonged QRS (0.16 sec) and more left axis deviation to about $-60°$ (labelled by solid circles) occur at widely varying coupling intervals (0.40 to 0.64 sec). The intervals between them are either 2.0 or 4.0 sec, corresponding to a regularly discharging ventricular parasystole at a rate of 30. Calculated coupling intervals shorter than 0.40 sec are ineffective (open circles), all falling within the normal ventricular refractory phase. A coupling interval slightly shorter than a sinus cycle produces a ventricular fusion beat (labelled F).

Contrary to the usual finding (cf. fig. 17, 18), the parasystolic center appears to be located in the only conducting (posterior) fascicle of the left bundle branch. This suggests

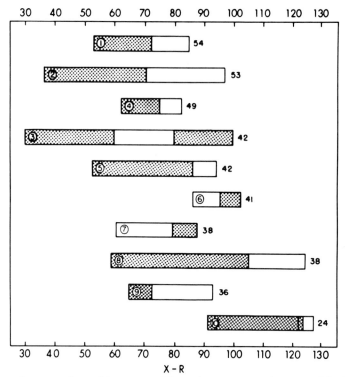

Fig. 16. Diagrammatic comparison of ten cases of intermittent parasystole arranged in descending order according to the parasystolic rate (numbers at the right, in beats/min). Each case is represented by a horizontal bar and successively numbered (numbers at the left). Cases #1 and 3 are described in this report. Hatched areas indicate (in sec/100) the range of X-R intervals protecting the parasystolic center. The zone of its depolarization by extraneous impulses is indicated by the clear portion of the bar. Only the last case shows overlap between the two areas.

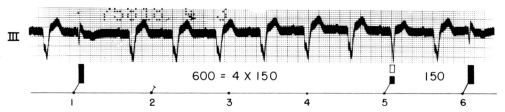

Fig. 17. Left ventricular parasystole in left bundle branch block. Explained in text.

that the intraventricular conduction defect is actually trifascicular, but different in degree. It is bidirectional in the right and left anterior fascicle, but only circumscribed and unidirectional in the posterior fascicle of the left bundle branch, maintaining undisturbed regular parasystolic discharges as well as their propagation whenever the myocardium is responsive.

DISCUSSION

The electrophysiologic basis of parasystole

The most significant contribution to the understanding of mechanisms operating in parasystole is the recognition by Hoffman in 1966 (371) and by Singer, Lazzara and Hoffman in

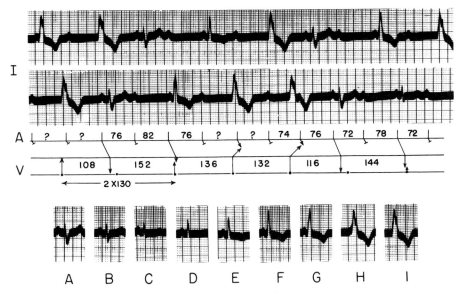

Fig. 18. Right-sided ventricular parasystole in the presence of a right bundle branch and second-degree (2:1) A-V block. The two strips above are respresentative continuous (overlapping) portions of a long lead I. In the diagram, numbers under A are measurable P-P intervals and those under V are intervals between consecutive ventricular complexes. Downward directed arrows indicate propagation of sinus impulses towards and into the left ventricle. Upward directed arrows originating in dots represent discharges and propagation of a regular parasystolic pacemaker in the right ventricle. Varying points of collision of the two impulses, some of which result in ventricular fusion beats, are indicated by the length of the opposit arrows. The single P-QRST complexes below (A to I) are examples of the various ventricular configurations encountered in lead I of the entire material arranged to illustrate the gradual transition of a pure right bundle branch block pattern (A) to that of a pure left bundle branch block pattern (H and I), with different types of fusion beats (B-G) in between. Discussed in text.

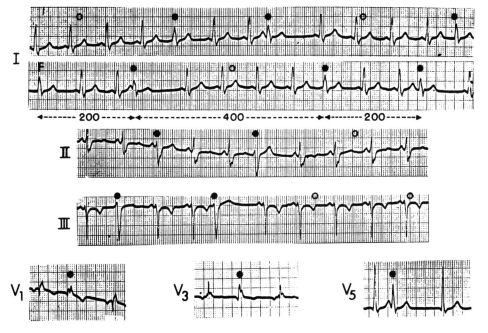

Fig. 19. Posterior fascicular parasystole in bilateral (right and left anterior fascicular) bundle branch system block. The two strips of lead I are continuous with overlap of one beat. The symbols are explained in the text.

1967 (760) that in myocardial cells having the property of automaticity, spontaneous diastolic (phase 4) depolarization not only initiates release of impulses but impairs propagation into and out of these cells. Thus, protection of a parasystolic rhythm from other impulses as well as all varieties of exit block are no longer hypothetical postulates but have gained a firm experimental background. This unifying concept has been applied by Watanabe in his reassessment of clinical cases of parasystole (887) and by Rosenbaum and co-workers in their explanation of intermittence of bundle branch and A-V block (696). The potential for development of a parasystolic rhythm by summation or inhibition of impulses in depressed Purkinje fibers has been pointed out by Cranefield and associates (163), and of slow response activity in other diseased regions of the heart by Wit and associates (934).

A hypothesis has been advanced that the mere presence of bundle branch block may provide conditions necessary to the emergence of a parasystole (627). For instance, a complete left bundle branch block can preserve undisturbed impulse generation in an automatic center distal to the blocking lesion. Expressed in electrophysiologic terms, a small circumscribed area within the specific conduction system can be visualized which contains cells injured to a different degree (696). Some of these cells cause unindirectional block due to hypopolarization, while in other neighboring ones the slope of phase 4 depolarization and/or the threshold for automatic firing is altered (761). In clinical electrocardiograms such a condition can be assumed when in the presence of a bundle branch block parasystolic beats have a shape characteristic for block of the contralateral ventricle (887). Examples are illustrated in figures 17 and 18.

The site of parasystolic impulse formation

As mentioned above, a relationship seems to exist between bundle branch block and parasystole, and this may account for the predominant origin of parasystolic rhythms in the ventricles as well as for their common association with organic heart disease. In contrast, A-V junctional parasystoles are known to occur in young persons with clinically normal hearts. A-V junctional parasystole may, in standard electrocardiograms, be indistinguishable from atrial parasystole (fig. 13). However, an unquestionable case of His bundle parasystole has been observed by Grolleau and associates (326) in a patient with unidirectional A-V block. Premature 'H' depolarizations, with or without conduction to the atria, revealed the concealed site of the parasystolic pacemaker and this finding lends credence to our interpretation of figure 9. Concealed conduction of junctional parasystolic impulses giving rise to pseudo A-V block has been described (504, 724), and the first case of fascicular intermittent parasystole with intermittent pseudo A-V block was reported from our laboratory (134).

Atrial parasystole seems to be rare. Most cases published as such may actually be junctional in origin, but atrial parasystole can be produced without doubt artificially by asynchronous atrial pacing (fig. 4). An unusual case of intermittent, probably atrial, parasystole was reported by Fisch and Chevalier (271). Double ventricular and the combination of atrial with ventricular parasystole have been illustrated by Chung and associates (130, 131).

Coupling in parasystole

One of the cardinal features of a parasystole is the widely varying 'coupling' interval of premature beats of uniform shape. It is present if basic and parasystolic rates differ and are totally independent. It will be absent, permanently or in a recurrent fashion, if and when some simple numerical relationship exists between the two rates. For instance, there may be a 1:1, 2:1, or other simple ratio of the different cycle lengths, or they may have a common multiple (131,458). Under such circumstances, persistent or recurrent fixed coupling may produce repetitive groups with each consisting of the same number of basic and parasystolic beats, as was pointed out by Kaufmann and Rothberger in 1917 (426) (fig. 1,2). Levy and co-workers (491) have shown in animal experiments that an artificially produced ventricular parasystole at about half the rate of the sinus rhythm initiates, via baroreceptors, a feedback mechanism that maintains the synchronization and that produces fixed coupling of the parasystole in the form of continued bigeminy. This will persist as long as the rate and propagation time of either of the two pacemakers remains constant and can be readily reproduced by using a well-functioning asynchronous artificial pacemaker (fig. 1B). However, a pacemaker releasing only sub-threshold stimuli may also give rise to fixed coupling although by a different mechanism, a supernormal phase of excitability (770,780,898) (fig. 3). Singer and co-workers (762) recently reported an unusual case in which fixed coupled premature beats suggested a re-entry mechanism in or near the point of origin of a ventricular parasystole.

When the two rhythms are not mutually protected from each other, a fixed permanent or recurrent link can be established between them, and this in two ways (462). Parasystolic impulses that can reach, discharge and reset the dominant pacemarker will produce a condition called 'reversed coupling' (462) (fig. 3–5). On the other hand, a temporary loss of protection of the parasystolic center results in 'intermittent parasystole' which is discussed below. Under both circumstances, constant rates and propagation times of the two types of impulses can give rise to a variety of repetitive group beating (462) (fig. 1,2). Thus, reversed coupling of the basic (sinus or ectopic) rhythm may enforce fixed coupling of parasystolic beats (fig. 3–5). Rarely sinus impulses may in this manner become coupled to unprotected ectopic atrial impulses imitating a sinus parasystole (721). Figure 6 shows that occasionally reversed coupling may be associated with a varying coupling interval of the parasystolic beat.

Intermittent parasystole (fig. 13–16) is characterized by 1. recurrence between successive regular parasystolic beats of long intervals that are not multiples of the measurable parasystolic cycle, and 2. fixed coupling of the first beat of a parasystolic series to a sinus beat. The mechanism of this variant appears to be transient loss of protection of the parasystolic focus from other impulses (134,785). In ten cases of intermittent ventricular parasystole during sinus rhythm, it was found that sinus impulses could break through the protective entrance block during a limited period within the parasystolic cycle (134) (fig. 16). Complete entrance block appeared to be present only early and late in the ectopic cycle, with a short period of no protection in between. In electrophysiologic terms, this loss of protection could be attributed to a short interval between incomplete repolarization (phase 3) and subthreshold diastolic repolarization (phase 4) of automatic cells discharging slowly ectopic impulses. Since under such circumstances the penetrating sinus impulse resets the start of an automatic cycle, a link is established between the two rhythms in that the first of a sequence of parasystolic beats becomes coupled to one of the preceding sinus impulses (134,785). This coupling will be constant when the intermittent entrance block is of a Mobitz Type II or it may vary, in which case the presence of a Wenckebach (Type I) entrance block may be stipulated (441).

Exit block in parasystole
Exit block, which reduces the number of responses to a regularly firing ectopic pacemaker or makes them irregular, has been postulated in the interpretation of a variety of atrial, A-V junctional and ventricular arrhythmias (631). In the specific case of a parasystole, the exit block may be viewed as a manifestation of unidirectional block of particular type (627). It prevents entrance of all extraneous impulses into, but only reduces the rate of impulse propagation out of a cell or group of cells having the property of automaticity. There is ample experimental proof for this interrelation of automaticity and conduction (168,371,696,934).

In analogy to A-V block, two types (17,322) and various degrees of exit block may exit. First-degree (simple delay) and third-degree (complete failure) of parasystolic impulse propagation cannot be proved, at least not in clinical electrocardiography. However, second-degree block (intermittent propagation failure beyond the limits of physiologic refractoriness) is easy to recognize, especially when the parasystolic cycle can be directly measured and the block is of Mobitz Type II (cf. fig. 7). Rarely, progressive impairment of parasystolic impulse spread can be surmised from a Wenckebach-like arrangement of irregular parasystolic intervals, as in figure 8, or from gradual lengthening of A-V junctional escape intervals in a ventricular parasystole that is due to concealed retrograde conduction with progressive delay, as in figure 6. Occasional random development of second-degree exit block may provide a clue to the establishment of an otherwise unrecognized parasystole (cf. fig. 5,12).

SUMMARY

Various mechanisms that cause deviations from the classical manifestations of a parasystolic rhythm are reviewed and illustrated by selected clinical electrocardiograms. They consist of:
1. Transient or continued fixed coupling of the ectopic beats due to a. synchronization of basic and parasystolic rhythms; b. reversed coupling of the basic to the ectopic rhythm (unidirectional protection); c. the operation of a supernormal phase of excitability; and d. intermittent parasystole due to a gap in the protection of the parasystolic center.
2. Irregularities in response to a regular parasystolic discharge may be caused by a second-degree exit block, usually of Mobitz Type II, rarely of Type I.
An electrophysiological basis for the emergence and maintenance of parasystolic rhythms appears to be abnormal states of spontaneous diastolic (phase 4) depolarization in otherwise latent subsidiary cardiac pacemakers.

9

SOME EFFECTS OF ELECTRICAL STIMULATION ON IMPULSE INITIATION IN CARDIAC FIBERS; ITS RELEVANCE FOR THE DETERMINATION OF THE MECHANISMS OF CLINICAL CARDIAC ARRHYTHMIAS[1]

ANDREW L. WIT, Ph.D., JAY R. WIGGINS, Ph.D.,
and PAUL F. CRANEFIELD, M.D., Ph.D.

I. INTRODUCTION

Circus movement of excitation, spontaneous diastolic depolarization and other causes of rhythmic activity have been the subject of intensive investigation for many years, and studies utilizing microelectrode techniques have defined many important mechanisms (163, 168). These studies have suggested physiological and pharmacological interventions which can terminate such ectopic impulse initiation. Some interventions are specific for arrhythmias that depend on automaticity and others for arrhythmias that result from reentry (374). An ideal goal for therapy of any human cardiac arrhythmia would require determining the mechanism underlying its origin and the use of a therapeutic intervention specific for that mechanism to terminate the arrhythmia. Although attaining this goal is still in the future many basic electrophysiological discoveries have been applied to determine the mechanisms for human arrhythmias.

Electrical stimulation of the heart in the cardiac catheterization laboratory has become a widely used and valuable investigative procedure in the study of ectopic tachycardias in humans. The effects of electrical stimulation on impulse initiation due to reentrant and automatic mechanisms have been carefully documented by cellular electrophysiologic studies and these studies demonstrate a difference in the response of the two mechanisms. It seems logical to apply these results to the clinic and attempts therefore have been made to differentiate reentrant rhythms from automatic ones.

It is our purpose here to first briefly review a few of the ways by which electrical stimulation can initiate and terminate tachycardias by reentrant mechanisms and then to discuss the effects of stimulation on diastolic depolarization. In light of more recent findings concerning the effects of electrical stimulation on impulse initiation by this latter means, we suggest that the criteria utilized to distinguish reentrant from automatic human arrhythmias must be reevaluated.

II. REENTRY

Basic requirements
Under physiological conditions the conducting impulse dies out after sequential activation of the atria and ventricles because it is surrounded by recently excited and thus refractory tissue. After the refractory period the heart must await a new impulse, normally arising

1. Certain studies reported here were supported by U.S. Public Health Service Grants HL 12738 and HL 14899 from the National Heart and Lung Institute and by a grant-in-aid from the American Heart Assoc.

in the sinus node for subsequent activation. The concept of reentry implies that the propagating impulse does not die out after complete activation of the heart but persists to reexcite the heart after the end of the refractory period. For this to happen the impulse must remain somewhere in the heart while the cardiac fibers it has excited, regain excitability so that the impulse can reenter and reexcite them (163). The importance of slowed conduction and unidirectional conduction block in establishing the conditions necessary for reentry was originally stressed in the studies of Schmitt and Erlanger and we have recently discussed them in detail (163, 168, 930, 931). Slowed conduction allows the cardiac impulse to conduct over a reasonably short functional pathway during the refractory period of the rest of the heart and unidirectional block provides an excitable route through which the reentering impulse can return to reexcite the heart. We have recently emphasized that 'slow response' action potentials exhibit both these properties of slow conduction and unidirectional conduction and can result in reentry (163, 168).

Reentry may well occur in diseased areas of myocardium where cardiac fibers are partially depolarized and where slowed conduction and unidirectional block are consistently present. Conditions favorable to reentry may also exist in the heart but conduction of the basic rhythmic impulse may be slowed insufficiently to permit reentry, or a strategically located site of potential unidirectional conduction block may show two-way conduction during the basic cardiac rhythm. Under these conditions reentry may be induced by changes in the rate or rhythm of the heart, and electrical stimulation can be used to change this rate or rhythm, bringing out the necessary slow or one-way conduction.

Some mechanisms by which electrical stimulation may induce and terminate reentrant tachycardias

Increasing the heart rate by rapid electrical stimulation may slow conduction in depressed cardiac fibers, and conduction of a premature impulse may also be slowed (163). The same alterations in rhythm can also result in unidirectional block, by causing an impulse to invade a previously excited region before it completely recovers excitability. Alterations in rate or rhythm can take advantage of natural dispersions in refractoriness, or induce dispersions in refractoriness, to set up functional reentrant pathways.

Reentry due to these mechanisms has been studied in detail using microelectrode techniques, and although it is always difficult to exactly document reentry no matter what the technique employed, the ability to induce reentry in isolated tissues and to record the electrical activity of individual cells in the reentrant pathway has numerous advantages. Using microelectrode techniques Mendez and Moe demonstrated a mechanism for reentry in the AV node (544) which had previously been postulated by electrocardiographic studies (730). They emphasize the ability of premature or rapid electrical stimulation to produce non-uniform conduction of impulses through the AV node bringing about unidirectional conduction block in some, but not all, nodal fibers and thus setting the stage for reentry. The premature impulse must be properly timed to take advantage of the dispersions in refractoriness and to conduct slowly enough to result in reentry. The mechanisms described for single reentry of atrial impulses in the AV node can also result in continuous reentry as shown in microelectrode studies on isolated tissues by Mendez and Moe (544), Janse et al. (409) and Wit et al. (929).

Microelectrode studies on isolated tissues have indicated that electrical stimulation can initiate and terminate reentry in other cardiac tissues by similar mechanisms. Myerburg et al. have suggested that reentry can occur in the peripheral ventricular conducting system after premature stimulation due to abnormalities in the gating mechanism (572). Sasyniuk and Mendez have demonstrated reentry resulting from premature stimulation due to unidirectional conduction block at the Purkinje fiber muscle junctions (719). Wit, Hoffman and Cranefield have shown premature stimuli to induce reentry in loops of Purkinje fibers with depressed action potentials (931), and Friedman et al have shown premature stimulation to cause reentry in subendocardial Purkinje fibers surviving in areas of myocardial infarction (285). In all instances, the premature impulse conducts slowly and takes advantage of dispersions in refractoriness within its pathway of propagation so that it blocks in some regions but continues to conduct slowly through others, allowing recovery of excitability and return conduction through the region of initial block. The area of conduction block becomes the area of unidirectional conduction which is necessary for reentry. The premature impulse must be properly timed to take advantage of the dispersions in refractoriness and to conduct slowly enough to result in reentry as in the AV node and continuous reentry may occur and result in sustained impulse initiation.

When continuous reentry occurs, either in the AV node or in other cardiac fiber types, the continuation of reentry is dependent on the impulse being able to find excitable tissue as it conducts throughout the reentrant pathway. Any intervention which makes the pathway refractory to the circulating impulse will cause it to block and terminates reentry. If the heart is excited by a properly timed electrical stimulus either during premature or rapid stimulation the induced impulse may penetrate the reentrant pathway, causing it to become refractory and thus terminate reentry. This has been demonstrated both in the *in situ* heart, in experimental animals and in microelectrode studies (929).

Clinical implications
Certain criteria derived from the experimental studies have been applied to clinical arrhythmias and have been used to indicate that a tachycardia is due to reentry. Reentry in the AV node as a cause of supraventricular tachycardia is suggested when: 1. tachycardias can be induced by premature atrial stimulation or rapid atrial stimulation, and the stimulated impulse which initiates tachycardia is conducted slowly through the AV node, i.e., a well defined echo zone is present; 2. the rate of atrial tachycardia is a linear function of AV nodal conduction time during tachycardia—the slower the AV nodal conduction, the longer the cycle length of tachycardia; 3. premature atrial impulses or rapid atrial stimulation can terminate tachycardia; and 4. atrial activation during tachycardia is in a retrograde sequence (68,154,309,310). Other criteria are also used (68). However, the criterion most strongly suggesting AV nodal reentry is the well defined relationship between AV nodal conduction delay and tachycardia, and the conduction delay necessary to produce tachycardia can be induced by electrical stimulation.

Electrical stimulation has also been used to define the mechanism of the supraventricular tachycardias in patients with Wolff-Parkinson-White Syndrome (589,902). Although in this case the relationship between onset of tachycardia and the conduction delay cannot be precisely demonstrated, the induction of unidirectional conduction block in

the accessory pathway which results in reentry can often be deduced from electrocardiographic observation.

Similar criteria have been used to decide whether ventricular tachycardias are re-
entrant (903,904,906,956). Tachycardias can be initiated by electrical stimulation and
may result from any of the mechanisms for reentry described above or other mechanisms
(904,906). These tachycardias can also be terminated by electrical stimulation, presumably because the stimulated impulse(s) enters the reentrant pathway, rendering it
refractory to the reentering impulse. Correlations between the onset of ventricular
tachycardia and conduction delays or conduction block cannot easily be made since the
delays or blocks which may cause ventricular reentry are not readily apparent on surface
electrograms or electrocardiograms.

III. SUSTAINED RHYTHMIC ACTIVITY CAUSED BY
DIASTOLIC DEPOLARIZATION

The effects of electrical stimulation on sustained rhythmic activity resulting from spontaneous diastolic depolarization are different in many ways from its effects on sustained
rhythmic activity caused by reentry, and this strengthens the assertion that the response of
the heart to stimulation can be used to indicate the mechanism of origin of an arrhythmia. However, more recent studies on the slow response strongly suggest that there is
more than one mechanism for impulse initiation by diastolic depolarization (168) and
certain forms of rhythmic activity in fibers with slow response action potentials may be
initiated and terminated by electrical stimulation in a way that is very similar to the response of reentrant arrhythmias.

Spontaneous diastolic depolarization occurring at high levels of membrane potential
Spontaneous diastolic depolarization leading to impulse initiation in cardiac fibers with
high levels of membrane potential is best exemplified by phase 4 depolarization in normal
Purkinje fibers. The behavior of normal phase 4 activity in Purkinje fibers has been fully
analyzed by voltage-clamp techniques. Phase 4 depolarization results from a time dependent fall in potassium permeability that shifts the transmembrane potential away from
E_k towards E_{Na} (852). The extent and time course of phase 4 depolarization is further
determined by inward going rectification (601). The slow potassium current which underlies the pacemaker current has been designated as i_{K_2} and its time and voltage dependence
can be described by a Hodgkin-Huxley variable, s, which changes from near zero to
unity between -90 and -60 mV (601). This is the range of potentials over which this
type of pacemaker activity occurs. Spontaneous diastolic depolarization of this kind may
also occur in other pacemaker fibers which have high levels of membrane potentials such
as the atrial fibers in the crista terminalis (375).

*Effects of electrical stimulation on spontaneous diastolic depolarization occurring at high
levels of membrane potentials*
The effects of electrical stimulation on spontaneous diastolic depolarization which occurs
between membrane potentials of -90 and -60 mV has been carefully studied in Purkinje

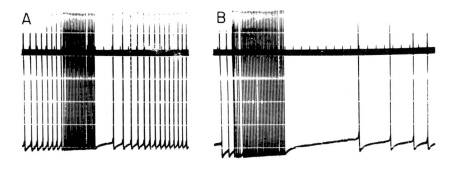

Fig. 1. Overdrive suppression of spontaneous diastolic depolarization occurring at a high level of membrane potential in a canine Purkinje fiber superfused with normal Tyrode's solution. Maximum diastolic potential is −85 mV. In A the first eight action potentials are spontaneous, following which the fiber was driven at a rapid rate for 20 sec. At the end of the period of driven activity the fiber remains quiescent for 10 sec and then gradually resumes the rate seen before the overdrive. In B, a longer period of rapid overdrive (45 sec) is followed by a more prolonged period of quiescence (45 sec) and a far slower return to control rate (time marks occur at 5 sec interval). (From P. F. Cranefield, *The conduction of the cardiac impulse; the slow response and cardiac arrhythmias,* by permission of Futura Publishing Co.)

fibers (853). If one allows a Purkinje fiber that shows phase 4 depolarization in the range of −90 to −60 mV to assume its spontaneous rate and then drives it at a faster rate for a time, cessation of the drive is not immediately followed by a resumption of the prior spontaneous rate; on the contrary, a period of quiescence may ensue after which the automatic fiber will gradually speed up until it once again attains its inherent automatic rate (fig. 1). The inhibitory effect of a period of driven activity on the automatic activity is known as over-drive suppression. The duration of the overdrive suppression is related to both the duration and the frequency of overdrive stimulation (853).

That overdrive suppression in Purkinje fibers is related to electrogenic sodium extrusion has been convincingly argued by Vassalle (853,854). When a spontaneously active Purkinje fiber is subjected to electrical stimulation at a much more rapid rate there is an initial depolarization, followed by a late hyperpolarization: the depolarization has been attributed to an accumulation of potassium outside the cell membrane and the hyperpolarization to a frequency activated electrogenic pump (853). The increase in rate leads to an increase in Na-influx which in turn stimulates electrogenic Na extrusion. This electrogenic sodium extrusion develops comparatively slowly so that its effect to increase resting potential is seen only as a late hyperpolarization. The continued activity of the electrogenic pump after stimulation is terminated results in an increased outward Na current that opposes the time dependent decrease in outward K current and thereby dampens spontaneous diastolic depolarization. Electrogenic Na extrusion gradually de-creases, and as it does the spontaneous rate once again accelerates. Automatic impulse initiation does not cease but is only temporarily arrested.

The effects of premature stimulation on phase 4 depolarization of Purkinje fibers occurring at high levels of membrane potential have also been studied in detail (444). Premature impulses exert a variable effect on such a spontaneous rhythm. Stimuli induced late in the spontaneous cycle length usually lengthen the returning cycle by transiently

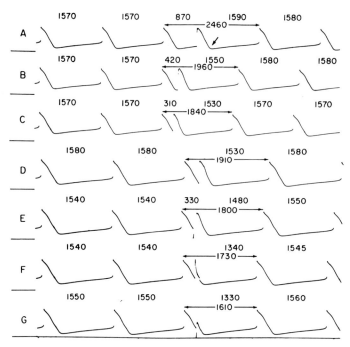

Fig. 2. Effect of stimulated premature extrasystoles on stable rate in automatic sheep Purkinje fiber (spontaneous diastolic depolarization at high level of membrane potential). In A, the extrasystole is followed by a slightly lengthened returning cycle. The duration of the premature action potential is unchanged and phase 4 duration is slightly increased. In B, the returning cycle is shortened because of decreased premature action potential duration and despite increased phase 4 duration. In C, the returning cycle is even more shortened because of a greater decrease in premature action potential duration. In D, the returning cycle is shortened by 50 msec. In E, a 50 msec delay has occurred between stimulus and action potential. If the returning cycle was measured from the stimulus artifact, it would be equal to the dominant cycle. If it is measured from the onset of the action potential, however, the returning cycle is shortened. In F and G, stimuli are of opposite polarity and the premature action potentials are extremely brief. The returning cycle is shortened by more than 200 msec in G. The duration of the conjoined cycles in E-G clearly shows that the pacemaker center has been reset by the extrasystole in spite of the brevity and small amplitude of the action potential. (From H. O. Klein, P. F. Cranefield and B. F. Hoffman (444) by permission of the American Heart Association.)

depressing phase 4 depolarization (fig. 2). This may result from a transient increase in [K] immediately outside the cell membrane. Early premature stimuli may produce shortening of the return cycle because the duration of the premature action potential is markedly shortened (fig. 2). Premature stimulation cannot terminate this type of spontaneous activity nor can it initiate it, if it is not present.

Clinical implications
Certain clinically occurring atrial and ventricular tachycardias respond to electrical stimulation of the heart in a manner which suggests that spontaneous diastolic depolarization in fibers with high membrane potentials is the cause of the arrhythmia (312,906). These tachycardias cannot be induced nor terminated by applied electrical stimuli. The effect of premature stimuli induced during sustained tachycardia is consistent with the predicted behavior of an ectopic pacemaker and overdrive suppression of the ectopic

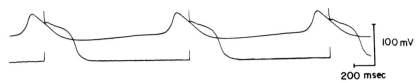

100 mV

200 msec

Fig. 3. Spontaneously occurring action potentials in a subendocardial Purkinje fiber (top trace) surviving in a region of extensive canine myocardial infarction. The fiber in the top trace has a low maximum diastolic potential (about −55 mV), spontaneous diastolic depolarization, and a slow action potential upstroke. The bottom trace shows an action potential recorded from a subendocardial Purkinje fiber in an adjacent, non-infarcted region. Note the large resting membrane potential (about −90 mV) and fast upstroke. This fiber does not show spontaneous diastolic depolarization. The fiber in the top trace with slow response activity appears to be the pacemaker for the preparation; this fiber depolarizes 200 msec before the fiber in the adjacent normal region

pacemaker can be demonstrated. Other clinical characteristics of nonreentrant tachy-cardias are discussed in detail by Goldreyer et al. (312) and by Wellens et al. (906).

Spontaneous diastolic depolarization occurring at low levels of membrane potential

The ionic mechanism for spontaneous depolarization in cardiac fibers with low membrane potentials differs from that in fibers with high membrane potentials (168). At levels of membrane potentials of −60 mV or less the gating variable, s, is fully activated and the i_{K_2} pacemaker current is inoperative (601). Furthermore, when membrane potential is near −60 mV the Na$^+$ channel is nearly completely inactivated (168). Yet spontaneous activity may occur in Purkinje fibers which are depolarized to levels of membrane potential of −60 mV or less. Similar activity may also occur in Purkinje fibers with normal resting potentials but with abnormal repolarization phases of the action potential (168).

An example of sustained rhythmic activity in a partially depolarized Purkinje fiber is shown in figure 3. The fiber is surviving in the subendocardial region of an area of extensive myocardial infarction in the dog (285,474). Maximum diastolic potential is only −55 mV, jet continuous spontaneous action potentials are evident.

The occurrence of abnormal automaticity at low levels of membrane potential, under different circumstances is shown in figure 4. These records were taken from a Purkinje fiber obtained from a pigtail monkey heart and superfused with Tyrode's solution. Initially, when the fiber was impaled with a microelectrode the fiber was quiescent with a resting potential of about −90 mV. When the fiber was stimulated once, it responded with an extraordinarily long action potential. While all phases of repolarization were prolonged, most of the increased duration occurred during the plateau. Fifteen seconds after the initial depolarization phase and during the plateau, when membrane potential had declined to about −25 mV, small oscillations appeared, growing in amplitude as the fiber slowly repolarized until overshooting spikes with a total amplitude of about 70 mV occurred. The maximum amplitude of these spikes occurred when they arose from a membrane potential of around −60 mV, during the plateau. Thirty eight seconds after the initial upstroke of the action potential, the fiber fully repolarized to −90 mV and remained quiescent until stimulated again. The two examples of automaticity at low levels of membrane potential shown in Figures 3 and 4 may be the same; in the latter case the cell was able to regain its normal level of resting potential after a period of time (fig. 4) while in the other, it could not (fig. 3).

A

B

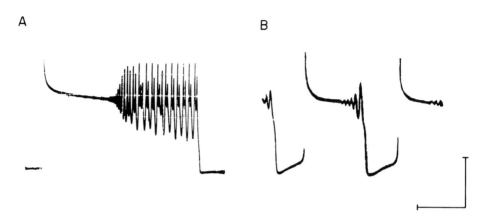

Fig. 4. Two types of spontaneous depolarization in a monkey Purkinje fiber. In A spontaneous depolarizations occurring at low membrane potentials, during the plateau phase of the action potential are shown. These may result from the same mechanism which caused the spontaneous depolarizations of the Purkinje fiber in figure 3, except that the Purkinje fiber in this figure was able to eventually regain its normal resting potential. In B, spontaneous diastolic depolarization in another monkey Purkinje fiber is shown, occurring at high levels of membrane potential after exposure to epinephrine. Some small membrane oscillations are also occurring during the plateau. The spontaneous depolarizations shown in A and B are indicative of the two mechanisms for automatic impulse initiation. Calibrations; vertical = 50 mV horizontal = 10 sec.

Relatively little is known about the mechanism for spontaneous impulse initiation at low levels of membrane potential. Noble and Tsien have indicated that oscillations in membrane potential may occur in the range of −60 to +10 mV, possibly due to variations in a current designated as i_{x_1} (602). Studies by Hauswirth, Noble and Tsien did not determine whether this slow oscillatory current results from a decay in outward current or an increase in inward current (347). Our own speculation is that oscillatory changes in an outward current result in membrane oscillations which trigger the slow inward current, when membrane potential declines to the threshold of the slow channel. Fairly large changes in membrane potential due to only small changes in outward current are favored by the high membrane resistance which occurs at low levels of membrane potential, and the high membrane resistance also favors the occurrence of slow response action potentials.

Evidence suggesting the contribution of the slow inward current to action potentials occurring spontaneously at low levels of membrane potential has been derived from experiments using the slow channel blocking agent, verapamil (168). The effects of verapamil on the type of spontaneous activity occurring during the prolonged plateau phase of a Purkinje fiber action potential is shown in figure 5. These records were obtained during washout of 2 uM verapamil. The events shown occur in the reverse order during initial exposure to the drug. Initially, during exposure to the full concentration of the drug the plateau of the action potential was shifted to a more negative level and no oscillatory activity or slow response action potentials occurred. During the course of washout of verapamil, low amplitude oscillations appeared which increased in amplitude and rate with time. After 30 minutes membrane potential shifted to the more negative level of −90 mV. Spontaneous activity in cardiac fibers with a consistent low level of membrane potential can also be abolished by verapamil (166).

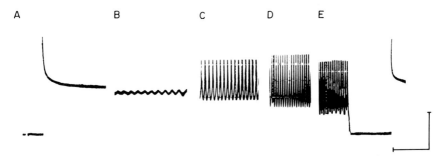

Fig. 5. Effects of verapamil on spontaneous depolarizations occurring at low levels of membrane potential during the plateau of a Purkinje fiber action potential. Panel A shows that spontaneous depolarizations are absent in the presence of 0.1 mg/L verapamil. The panels to the right (B-E) show the return of oscillations which progressively increase in amplitude as the verapamil is washed out of the tissue chamber over a period of 5 min and as membrane potential increases. In panel E after verapamil is washed out, the cell repolarized to its high level of membrane potential. Calibrations: vertical = 50 mV; horizontal = 10 sec.

That the slow inward current is triggered by and superimposed on an oscillation in membrane potential in the range of membrane potential between −60 to −40 mV, which is almost certainly different in kind from normal phase 4 depolarization receives support from the phenomenology of spontaneous activity in depolarized Purkinje fibers in Na-free solutions. These studies have demonstrated that spontaneous impulse initiation at low levels of membrane potential are due to oscillatory after potentials (168). If an action potential is evoked in a quiescent, partially depolarized Purkinje fiber in Na-free solution, the action potential may not terminate by a simple return to the level of membrane potential from which it arose; the action potential is followed by a marked early afterhyperpolarization that carries the membrane potential to a more negative value and this afterhyperpolarization then slowly declines not only to, but beyond the resting level creating a delayed after-depolarization which then slowly declines to the resting level (38, 167) (fig. 6). If the oscillatory after-depolarization following an action potential reaches threshold potential, a nondriven action potential will occur, which will also be followed by an oscillatory after-depolarization which may or may not reach threshold. If the oscillatory after-potential of each action potential reaches threshold sustained rhythmic activity

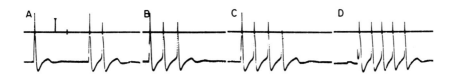

Fig. 6. The effects of single driven impulses on a canine Purkinje fiber that was quiescent when exposed to a Na-free solution containing 16 mM Ca and 128 mM TEA Cl. In A the action potential at the far left occurs after electrical stimulation and is followed by an after-hyperpolarization and a delayed after-depolarization. The second action potential in A is also driven but its delayed after-depolarization reaches threshold and it is followed by a single, nondriven (triggered) action potential. The first action potentials in B, C and D are driven and they are followed by several nondrive (triggered) action potentials. The last triggered action potential in each panel is followed by a delayed after-depolarization which fails to reach threshold potential. (From P. F. Cranefield, *The conduction of the cardiac impulse; the slow response and cardiac arrhythmias*, by permission of Futura Publishing Co.)

will occur. The apparently spontaneous depolarization during phase 4 is actually due to the oscillatory after-potential with the upstroke of the action potential superimposed upon it. Similar oscillatory after-potentials occur in Purkinje fibers which are partly depolarized by toxic concentrations of digitalis (265,677) or in bovine Purkinje fibers exposed to elevated $[K]_o$ and catecholamines (108). This indicates that after-potentials occurring at low membrane potentials are a real property of Purkinje fibers and not an artifact of the abnormal Na^+ free environment. There are several factors which determine whether sustained rhythmic activity occurs in Purkinje fibers with low membrane potentials, whether the low membrane potential is due to Na^+ free perfusion, digitalis toxicity, or possibly even some pathological state such as myocardial infarction. The most important is the level of the resting potential; sustained rhythmic activity only occurs if membrane potential is low enough so the after-depolarization of each action potential reaches threshold (fig. 6, 7). If membrane potential is too high each stimulated action potential may be followed by a delayed after-depolarization but no nondriven activity. At slightly lower membrane potentials the after-depolarization may sometimes reach threshold, and give rise to nondriven activity following a stimulated action potential. At still lower membrane

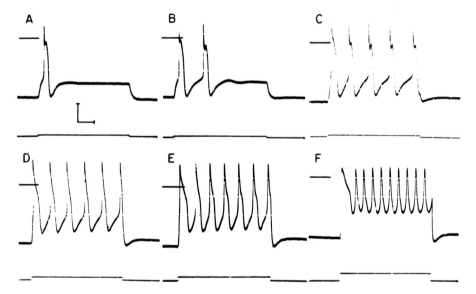

Fig. 7. The effect of membrane potential on the electrical activity of a quiescent canine Purkinje fiber exposed to Na-free solution containing 16 mM Ca. The line at the upper left hand edge of each figure shows zero membrane potential. Maximum diastolic potential is being altered by passing a depolarizing current pulse through a microelectrode, the strength and duration of which is shown in the lower trace on an arbitrary scale. The deflection of the current trace in F corresponds to 2×10^{-7} A. In A a single action potential occurs soon after the beginning of the 12 sec depolarizing pulse. The action potential is followed by a delayed after-hyperpolarization and a slight after-depolarization. In B, a slightly stronger depolarizing pulse results in two action potentials, the second of which is followed by an after-depolarization which fails to reach threshold potential. In C, a larger reduction in membrane potential results in sustained rhythmic activity; membrane potential is decreased enough so that the after-depolarization of each action potential reaches threshold. In D, E, and F passage of stronger currents through the microelectrode result in greater reductions in membrane potential and a more rapid rate of rhythmic activity partly due to the decreased potential difference between maximum diastolic and threshold potential. (From R. S. Aronson and P. F. Cranefield (38) by permission of Pflügers Archiv.)

potentials, after a single evoked action potential, the after-depolarization of each sub-sequent action potential reaches threshold and sustained rhythmic activity occurs. During sustained rhythmic activity phase 4 depolarization resembles phase 4 depolarization at high levels of membrane potential. In fibers which are not spontaneously active, any influence which decreases membrane potential may cause a fiber to become rhythmically active (38, 167). Also any influence which increases the amplitude of the after-depolariza-tion so that it reaches threshold potential may have the same effect.

The effects of electrical stimulation and the phenomenon of triggering
The oscillatory delayed after-depolarization which causes sustained rhythmic activity in Purkinje fibers with low membrane potentials is dependent on the prior initiation of an action potential. When an action potential is evoked by electrical stimulation, and the sub-sequent after-depolarization reaches threshold to cause a nondriven action potential, this nondriven action potential is *triggered* by the driven one (167, 168). The number of non-driven action potentials triggered by a driven action potential can vary from a single action potential to continuous sustained rhythmic activity. Therefore electrical stimulation can initiate nonreentrant sustained rhythmic activity at low levels of membrane potential (167).

We have also indicated that in Purkinje fibers with levels of membrane potential low enough to inactivate i_{K_2}, but yet with a membrane potential which is too high for the delayed after-depolarization to reach threshold, influences which further decrease membrane potential or which increase the amplitude of the after-potential may cause the appearance of nondriven action potentials. Changes in the rate or rhythm of electrical stimulation may exert this effect. In electrically driven Purkinje fibers exposed to toxic concentrations of digitalis, which show delayed after-depolarizations, increasing the rate of stimulation will cause a gradual decline in membrane potential, an increase in the amplitude of the delayed after-depolarization and trigger sustained rhythmic activity (fig. 8) (265). In calf Purkinje fibers superfused with K + rich Tyrode's and catecholamines, an increase in the driving rate will increase the amplitude of the delayed after-depolariza-tion and trigger sustained rhythmic activity (108). In Purkinje fibers exposed to Na-free

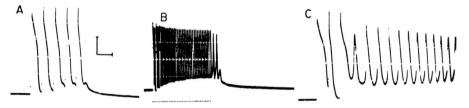

Fig. 8. Effects of driven impulses on the electrical activity of a quiescent canine Purkinje fiber exposed to normal levels of Na and to 0.125 mg/liter of ouabain. In A a period of driven activity leads to a progressive loss of resting potential and the appearance of a small oscillatory after-potential following the third, fourth and last driven impulses. In B, two spontaneous action potentials follow the cessation of a long period of driven activity; the bottom trace shows the time of application of stimuli. The appearance of spontaneous action potentials occurs because of the decline of membrane potential due to electrical stimulation. In C the first three impulses are driven and this leads to sustained spontaneous activity arising from a much reduced level of membrane potential. Calibrations: horizontal 1 second in A, 5 seconds in B, and 1 second in C. vertical = 20 mV. (From P. F. Cranefield and R. S. Aronson (167) by permission of the American Heart Association.)

174   A. L. WIT ET AL.

Tyrode's a single evoked premature impulse may trigger sustained rhythmic activity, presumably because the premature impulse has a delayed after-depolarization of greater amplitude than the basic impulse (167, 168).

Once sustained rhythmic activity has been initiated at low levels of membrane potential, electrical stimulation might have several effects, but unfortunately detailed studies are not yet available. If the Na pump is not functioning such as during digitalis intoxication overdrive suppression will not occur, and in fact overdrive may accelerate the rate by causing a further decline in membrane potential (168). If the Na pump is functioning, overdrive may induce hyperpolarization by the same mechanism described previously and if membrane potential is increased to levels at which the after-depolarization no longer reaches threshold, sustained rhythmic activity may cease (760). A triggering influence which increases amplitude of the after-depolarization or decreases membrane potential is once again necessary to induce rhythmic activity after it has been terminated in this way. Single premature impulses may simply 'reset' the rhythm in the same manner as for phase 4 depolarization, or may sometimes terminate sustained rhythmic activity (168) (fig. 9). The after-hyperpolarization following a premature impulse sometimes increases, and the after-depolarization which follows fails to reach threshold and the rhythmic activity terminates.

Clinical implications
We must be cautious in transferring findings from experimental studies on isolated tissues, many of which were performed in highly abnormal ionic environments, to the whole heart

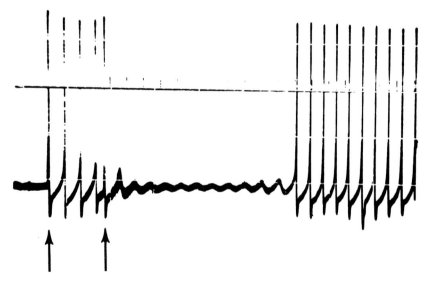

Fig. 9. The termination of sustained rhythmic activity in a Purkinje fiber perfused with a Ca^{++} rich, Na^+ free solution, by a premature electrical stimulus. Maximum diastolic potential is -50 mV. The fiber is initially quiescent but a single stimulus applied at the first arrow triggers rhythmic activity. A second premature electrical stimulus was applied at the second arrow, and this stimulated action potential was followed by a delayed after-depolarization which failed to reach threshold potential. A prolonged period of quiescence ensued but after 11 seconds oscillatory potentials appeared which gradually resulted in the occurrence of sustained rhythmic activity, once again.

in humans. We cannot precisely detail the significance of depolarizing after-potentials in Purkinje fibers to the genesis of cardiac arrhythmias, but we can suggest how the phenomenology described in the previous section might manifest itself in the clinical situation especially in response to electrical stimulation of the heart. Further investigations by both laboratory and clinical electrophysiologists are needed to test our hypotheses.

As we have indicated, the response to electrical stimulation of a ventricular arrhythmia caused by delayed after-depolarizations will depend on the precise level of membrane potential of the fibers in which the arrhythmia arises, and the amplitude of the delayed after-depolarization with respect to the threshold potential. Also the etiology of the low membrane potentials may be important. If membrane potential is at the level where sub-threshold after-depolarizations follow each driven action potential during sinus rhythm, electrical stimulation (either rapid or premature) may induce a tachycardia caused by sustained rhythmic activity by any of the mechanisms described previously. Once induced, this tachycardia may also be terminated either by overdrive or premature stimulation. In this respect it might therefore be difficult to distinguish a ventricular arrhythmia caused by sustained rhythmic activity due to delayed after-depolarizations from one caused by reentry. If membrane potential is low enough so that after a single activation the delayed after-depolarization of each impulse reaches threshold and sustained rhythmic activity per-sists, the resultant arrhythmia might also respond to electrical stimulation in a manner simi-lar to an arrhythmia due to phase 4 depolarization at high levels of membrane potential.

Triggered activity in cardiac muscle fibers of the mitral valve

It is uncertain what the mechanism for automaticity is in cardiac fibers which naturally have low membrane potentials. Although the characteristics may vary from one region of the heart to another, after-depolarizations of the type shown in Purkinje fibers with low membrane potentials may be important.

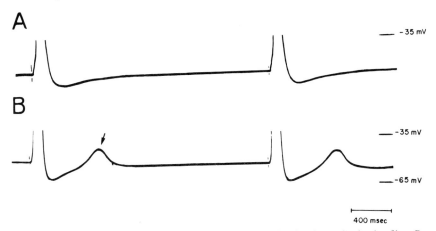

Fig. 10. The effect of epinephrine to elicit a delayed after-depolarization in a mitral valve fiber. Recordings from the same fiber are shown in each panel. Only the lower part of the action potential (more negative than −35 mV) is shown in each panel so that greater amplification could be obtained. In the top panel which is the control there is a prominent after-hyperpolarization; repolarization procedes to a value 10 mV more negative than the membrane potential from which the upstroke arose. The bottom panel shows development of a delayed after-depolarization (arrow) during superfusion with 1.0 ug/ml of epinephrine.

We have recently investigated impulse initiation in a type of cardiac fiber that has a low membrane potential, the atrial fibers in the mitral valve of the monkey (165,940). These fibers have maximum diastolic potentials of -60 to -70 mV, action potential amplitudes of about 80 mV, and upstroke velocities of 5–6 V/sec. The upstroke exhibits all the characteristics of the slow response: 1. catecholamines increase the amplitude of the action potential without affecting the membrane potential from which the upstroke arises; 2. low concentrations of verapamil depress both upstroke velocity and action potential overshoot; 3. the amplitude of the action potential is quite insensitive to tetrodotoxin; and finally 4. the overshoot of the action potential is not dependent on the level of membrane potential from which the upstroke arises and the upstroke of the action potential is not inactivated by membrane depolarization of 30 mV or more.

When these fibers are superfused with Tyrode's solution their action potentials show

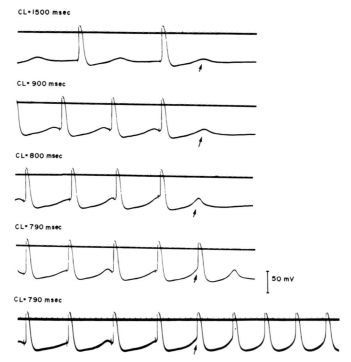

Fig. 11. The effect of decreasing stimulus cycle length on the amplitude of the delayed after-depolarization. Recordings from the same mitral valve fiber are shown in each panel. The preparation was superfused with 1.0 ug/ml epinephrine. In this experiment 15 consecutive action potentials were elicited and the stimulus then turned off; the last several driven action potentials of the series are shown in each panel. In the top panel the stimulus cycle length is 1500 msec and the amplitude of the delayed after-depolarization (arrow) is quite small. In the next two panels stimulus cycle length is decreased to 900 and then 800 msec; each action potential is elicited before complete repolarization of the preceding after-depolarization. There is an increase in the amplitude of the delayed after-depolarization both during stimulation and after the last stimulated action potential (arrow). At a stimulus cycle length of 790 msec the delayed after-depolarization following the last stimulated action potential reached threshold and a nondriven action potential occurs (arrow). The after-depolarization of the nondriven action potential was sometimes subthreshold and nondriven activity ceased, and sometimes reached threshold and sustained rhythmic activity occurred (bottom panel). Time marks in top trace of last panel are at 100 msec intervals.

a marked early after-hyperpolarization following which the membrane potential declines to a steady resting level (fig. 10). If these fibers are exposed to epinephrine or norepinephrine, a delayed after-depolarization develops which may be up to 20 mV in amplitude (fig. 10). The amplitude of this delayed after-depolarization is quite sensitive to the rate of stimulation. Reduction of the stimulus cycle length results in an increase in the amplitude of the delayed after-depolarization, and the amplitude keeps increasing as the cycle length is further reduced. When the cycle length is shortened to a critical value, nondriven action potentials may occur, arising from the peak of the after-depolarization (fig. 11,12). A further reduction in cycle length often triggers sustained rhythmic activity at a rate more rapid than the rate at which the fiber is being driven (fig. 11,12). Sustained rhythmic activity can last from several minutes up to 30 minutes or more but usually subsides spontaneously if no intervention is introduced to terminate it (see below). This sustained rhythmic activity is not reentrant since after the mitral valve leaflet was cut into many small pieces, some no larger than 2 mm², the same phenomenon could be induced in each small piece. When triggered activity was induced in small pieces of valve, the upstrokes of action potentials recorded simultaneously from different cells occurred virtually simultaneously; the pattern of conduction expected from circus movement of excitation was not seen (931).

The occurrence of single nondriven action potentials or sustained rhythmic activity appeared to result from the delayed after-depolarization reaching threshold. This inter-

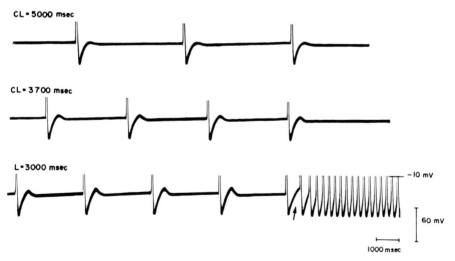

Fig. 12. Triggered sustained rhythmic activity in a mitral valve fiber induced by decreasing the cycle length. Only the lower part of the action potential recorded from the same fiber is shown in each panel. The preparation is being perfused with 0.5 ug/ml norepinephrine. Each panel shows the first driven action potentials after a 30 sec period of quiescence. In the top panel, at a stimulus cycle length of 5000 msec, a small delayed after-depolarization is present. In the middle panel, the cycle length is reduced to 3700 msec and there is an increase in the amplitude of the after-depolarization. In the bottom panel at a shorter stimulus cycle length the amplitude of the delayed after-depolarization is still larger and there is a progressive increase in amplitude of the after-depolarization following the first four driven impulses. The after-depolarization following the fifth driven impulse reaches threshold (arrow) and a nondriven action potential occurs which is followed by sustained rhythmic activity.

pretation is based on the observation that nondriven activity occurred only when the amplitude of the delayed after-depolarization reached a critical value; otherwise the after-potential decayed to the level of constant diastolic depolarization. When sustained rhythmic activity was triggered the after-depolarization of each action potential reached threshold to evoke the next impulse.

If the fibers of the mitral valve are driven at a fixed rate that does not lead to triggering because the delayed after-depolarizations are subthreshold, the delayed after-depolarizations that follow prematurely induced impulses may be larger in amplitude than those following regularly driven action potentials and may trigger nondriven activity (fig. 13). A premature impulse occurring late in the cycle length may be followed only by a slightly larger after-depolarization which is still subthreshold, but as the premature impulse is induced earlier and earlier the amplitude of the delayed after-depolarization becomes progressively greater. Finally, at a critical coupling interval, the after-depolarization following the premature impulse reaches threshold and results in a nondriven action potential. Sustained rhythmic activity may supervene if the after-potential following each subsequent action potential reaches threshold potential. The degree of prematurity needed to induce sustained rhythmic activity is quite variable. In some experiments sustained rhythmic activity was triggered by premature impulses which occurred late in the

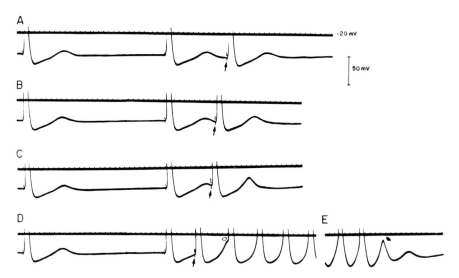

Fig. 13. Triggered sustained rhythmic activity in a mitral valve fiber induced by a premature stimulus. Only the lower part of the action potentials recorded from the same fiber are shown in each panel. The top trace in each panel (100 msec time pips) is at −20 mV. The preparation is being perfused with 1.0 ug/ml of epinephrine and is driven at a basic cycle length of 2700 msec. In A, a premature impulse (arrow) is induced 1200 msec after the last basic impulse, and well after the peak of its after-depolarization. The amplitude of the after-depolarization of the premature impulse is the same as that of the basic impulse. In B and C, the premature impulse (arrows) is induced progressively earlier on the preceding after-depolarization, and the amplitude of the after-depolarization of the premature impulse is increasing. In D, when the premature impulse (solid arrow) is induced prior to the time at which the after-depolarization of the preceding basic impulse would have occurred, a nondriven action potential arises from the peak of its after-depolarization (open arrow) and nondriven, sustained rhythmic activity continues for 15 minutes. Only the first four action potentials of the sustained rhythmic activity are shown.

cycle, well after the peak of the preceding after-depolarization; in other experiments, the premature impulse which triggered sustained rhythmic activity occurred early in the cycle length, prior to the moment at which the peak of the preceding after-depolarization would presumably have occurred. However, a well defined coupling interval for triggering sustained rhythmic activity was present in each preparation.

In addition to inducing nonreentrant, sustained rhythmic activity in mitral valve fibers by electrical stimulation, we were able to terminate it by properly timed premature stimuli (fig. 14). Premature impulses induced early in the cycle length of spontaneous activity occurred while the mitral valve fibers were partially refractory and evoked only an abortive response, following which the after-depolarization did not reach threshold (not shown in the figure). Stimuli which occurred later evoked action potentials with normal amplitude and did not terminate the sustained rhythmic activity but the cycle following the premature impulse was longer than the basic nondriven cycle. Premature impulses which were followed by a lengthened cycle often demonstrated an increase after-hyperpolarization of several mV which resulted in an increase in the time needed for depolarization to reach threshold and initiate the next impulse. Premature impulses which were induced still later in the basic cycle could terminate sustained rhythmic activity. Such impulses

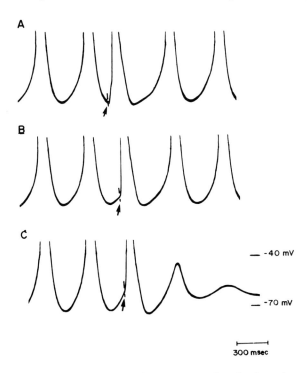

Fig. 14. Termination of sustained rhythmic activity by a premature impulse. In each panel the last two action potentials during sustained rhythmic activity are shown prior to the stimulation of a premature action potential. In A the premature impulse (arrow) is induced early in the cycle length of sustained rhythmic activity and is followed by a slightly lengthened cycle length of spontaneous activity. In B a premature impulse (arrow) induced later in the cycle length also does not interrupt sustained rhythmic activity. In C, a still later premature impulse (arrow) is followed by an enhanced after-hyperpolarization; the following after-depolarization does not reach threshold and sustained rhythmic activity is terminated.

were followed by a slightly increased after-hyperpolarization, the subsequent after-depolarization failed to give rise to an action potential and quiescence ensued.

Exposure of mitral valve fibers to acetylcholine can also terminate sustained rhythmic activity. Acetylcholine increases K+ conductance to such an extent that the increase in outward K+ current can overcome the weak, slow inward current responsible for the upstroke in valve fibers, and prevent excitation of these cells (932).

Sustained rhythmic activity triggered in the mitral valve leaflet could propagate into atrial wall if this was left attached to the valve leaflet in the isolated preparation. Sustained rhythmic activity can also be induced by impulses which propagated from the atrium into the valve.

The ionic mechanism underlying the delayed after-depolarization which causes triggered and sustained rhythmic activity in mitral valve fibers, as well as the factors responsible for the alterations in its amplitude in response to changes in rate and rhythm, are unknown. We have observed that both the delayed after-depolarization and triggered activity are blocked by low concentrations of verapamil, but not by tetrodotoxin, suggesting that the delayed after-depolarization may depend, at least in part, on the slow inward current. The appearance and increase in amplitude of the after-depolarization in response to catecholamines is compatible with the previous observations indicating that catecholamines increase the magnitude of slow inward current in cardiac fibers and increase the level of membrane potential at which it is activated (108,652). The delayed after-depolarization may result from a phasic increase in slow inward current during diastole or it may arise because the slow inward current is not completely inactivated with complete repolarization. Inactivation of slow inward current may lag behind complete repolarization and the magnitude of slow inward current flowing at this time may be increased by catecholamines. The terminal phase of repolarization may be due to a transient increase in K conductance. If the slow inward current persists after K conductance returns to its normal diastolic value, an after-potential might result; in fact, P_K may, after the after-hyperpolarization, fall below the value characteristic of diastole, thus contributing to the delayed after-depolarization. However we do not have data to indicate whether there is a time-dependent decrease in K+ conductance. The mechanism for the increase in amplitude of the after-depolarization in response to an increase in frequency of activation of mitral valve fibers is presently unknown.

Clinical implications

The characteristics of impulse initiation in mitral valve fibers described above are based on studies on isolated, superfused tissues and we have no data to indicate that these events also occur in the *in situ* human heart. Fibers which are anatomically similar to those described exist in the human heart (564) so that triggered activity is at least a possible form of behavior in such fibers. We found it necessary to add catecholamines to the perfusate in order to obtain triggered activity. It is possible that such an addition of catecholamine merely restores the fiber to the state in which it exists *in situ*; it is also possible that such activity occurs *in situ* only in the presence of increased levels of catecholamines or increased activity of adrenergic nerves which richly innervate the valve leaflet (234).

If triggered activity can occur in mitral valve fibers *in situ*, or indeed, if it can occur in some other cardiac fibers that have low membrane potentials and slow response action potentials, careful consideration must be given to the meaning of the induction or termination of cardiac arrhythmias by electrical stimulation. As we have discussed above paroxysmal atrial tachycardia is often initiated by a premature impulse, can be terminated by a premature impulse and is generally regarded to result from circus movement of excitation in a pathway which passes through the AV node (68,309,310). However, some atrial arrhythmias that behave in this way may be triggered since triggered arrhythmias can also be evoked by a single timed premature impulse and can be interrupted in the same way.

It may, therefore, be difficult to distinguish reentrant from triggered arrhythmias in the atrium. Conduction delay should not be prerequisite for a triggered atrial arrhythmia; the primary consideration is that the after-potential of the triggering impulse reach threshold. This may occur when the triggering impulse is initiated either early in the cycle or late in the cycle. If triggered sustained rhythmic activity is induced by a premature impulse which occurs early in the cycle, the triggering impulse may also conduct slowly through the AV node and the onset of tachycardia might be erroneously considered to result from such slowed AV nodal conduction and a reentrant mechanism. If triggered sustained rhythmic activity resulted from a premature atrial impulse occurring late in the cycle length slowed conduction through the AV node would not occur and AV nodal reentry discounted. Similarly, if sustained rhythmic activity was triggered by atrial pacing, it might occur at pacing cycle lengths short enough to produce significant AV nodal conduction delay, or at long cycle lengths which do not produce AV nodal conduction delay.

Recently Wu et al. reported their studies on several cases of paroxysmal supraventricular tachycardia that did not seem to result from AV nodal reentry (949). Even though supraventricular tachycardia could be induced by atrial pacing or premature stimulation, its onset did not correlate with a critical degree of prolongation of AV nodal condution. Atrial activation occurred in an antegrade direction in many of the cases, unlike the sequence of atrial activation during AV nodal reentry, but was occasionally retrograde. Atrial tachycardia could be terminated by atrial stimulation or carotid massage. Although these authors postulated that these arrhythmias were due to reentry within the sinus node or within atrial tissue we suggest that some arrhythmias with these characteristics may result from triggered sustained rhythmic activity arising in mitral valve fibers or in other triggerable fibers in the atrium. The onset and termination of these arrhythmias are compatible with this interpretation. Their termination by carotid massage could easily be explained by the ability of acetylcholine to abort triggerable arrhythmias. The sequence of atrial activation which would occur if impulses originated in the anterior valve leaflet is uncertain but an antegrade sequence is certainly possible. Tiny fiber tracts from Bachmanns bundle course in the anteromedial atrial wall near the origin of the anterior valve leaflet, and impulses arising in the valve may immediately enter these tracts, conduct rapidly through Bachmanns bundle to the right side of the heart and then in a superior to inferior direction. The experimental studies of Waldo et al. support this suggestion (870).

10

THE EFFECT OF ANTIARRHYTHMIC AGENTS ON IMPULSE FORMATION AND IMPULSE CONDUCTION

LEONARD S. DREIFUS, M.D., YOSHIO WATANABE, M.D.,
HENRY N. DREIFUS AND IRANY DE AZEVEDO, M.D.

Since the dawn of modern electrophysiology in the 1950's, many pertinent and useful observations have aided the physiologist and clinical cardiologist in the diagnosis and management of disturbances of impulse formation and conduction (91). While it is generally acknowledged that the precise action of antiarrhythmic agents remains unclear, some important strides have been made in an attempt to understand the electropharmacology of antiarrhythmic agents. Admittedly there is still an incomplete understanding of the mechanisms engendering various cardiac arrhythmias despite the recent contributions by investigators using ultramicroelectrode and His bundle techniques. Too often the clinician, surprised by the actions of a specific agent, may be unable to predict whether the drug will be beneficial or precipitate more hazardous problems. This is particularly true when one antiarrhythmic agent is used in the wake of another since the interactions of various antiarrhythmic drugs still remain unclear (210). Recent reviews have brought into sharp focus both the electrophysiology and pharmacology of anti-arrhythmic agents (210, 302, 675, 681, 877, 935). It is the purpose of this discussion to relate some of the presently available antiarrhythmic agents to their possible modes of action on impulse formation and conduction. Previously documented data will be summarized and newer information presented to define the present state of our knowledge with the hope that this will serve as a basis for future investigation.

For purposes of classification, Hoffman and Bigger have summarized the possible membrane effects of antiarrhythmic agents and have classified these compounds into several groups (372). Group 1, the quinidinelike group, includes quinidine, propranolol, and procaine amide. To the original list can be added antihistamines, a new ester of ajmaline (MCAA), aprindine, disopyramide phosphate, amiodarone, and potassium. These agents

Table 1. Classification of antiarrhythmic drugs.

Group I	Group II	Group III	Group IV
Quinidine	DPH	Bretylium	Verapamil
Procaine amide	Lidocaine		
Propranolol			
Norpace			
17-MCAA			
(Ajmaline)			
Amiodarone			
Aprindine			

are classified together because they appear to decrease automaticity and responsiveness and prolong the refractory period.

A second group of antiarrhythmic drugs includes diphenylhydantoin (DPH), lidocaine, and under certain conditions, the catecholamines. Lidocaine and DPH decrease automaticity and increase responsiveness and the refractory period. However, this last group is far more heterogeneous with respect to membrane action, and several investigators have observed sharp differences in their action, particularly when the drug concentration and potassium concentration have a wide range (615, 766, 877). Bretylium tosylate, a beta blocking agent with potent antiarrhythmic action, cannot be included in these two groups and could possibly comprise a third group (42, 44, 71, 713, 884).

Finally, agents such as verapamil and manganese (387, 440, 633, 678, 725) appear to have a very selective action on the slow response mediated through the calcium/sodium $(Ca^{++}/Na+)$ channels. These agents which appear to slow intranodal conduction and also offer potent antiarrhythmic action, will be discussed as a possible fourth subset of drugs (table 1).

While it is generally acknowledged that antiarrhythmic agents cannot be classified precisely, this tentative format will be used as an approach to this overview. Several anti-

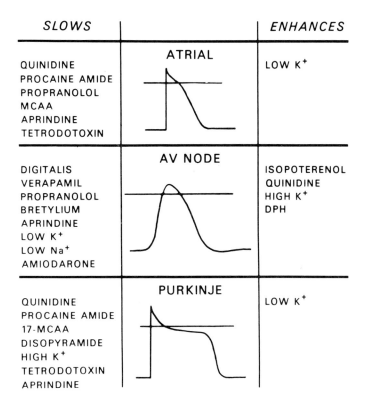

Fig. 1. Effect of electrolytes and antiarrhythmic agents on AV transmission.

arrhythmic drug interactions will be discussed when it is considered of clinical or electro-physiological importance. Finally, it should be emphasized that hypopotassemia may completely nullify the depressive or antiarrhythmic effects of antiarrhythmic drugs while hyperpotassemia or concomitant administration of potassium salts may enhance the development of serious intoxication (615, 766, 877).

METHODS

All ultramicroelectrode experiments described by the authors were carried out on isolated perfused rabbit hearts using the techniques of isolation and perfusion previously reported (883). A modified Chenoweth's solution with the following composition in millimoles per liter: NaCl–119.8; KCL–4.5; $CaCl_2$–2.1; $NaHCO_3$–25.0 and dextrose 10.0. The perfusate was saturated with 95% oxygen plus 5% CO_2 Ventricular electrograms were recorded by 2 small surface electrodes attached to the right ventricular apex and left ventricular base. A bipolar stimulating electrode was placed near the sinus node and the heart was electrically driven at a constant rate 10–15 beats per minute higher than the intrinsic rate. Glass micro-electrodes filled with 3 M KCL with tip resistances of 10–25 megohms were used to record transmembrance potentials from either the AV junctional or ventricular fibers. The poten-tials were amplified by a neutralized input capacity amplifier and Tektronix amplifiers. A Grass camera was used to photograph tracings from a Tektronic oscilloscope.

Catheter electrode studies to test the refractory periods of the atria, AV node, and His-Purkinje system were carried out in intact dogs. The dogs weighed from 18–22 kilograms and were anesthetized with sodium phenobarbitol and maintained on a respirator for the period of the experiment. A tripolar His bundle recording catheter was positioned across the tricuspid valve for the recording of His potentials. The sinus node was crushed and a close bipolar tefloncoated stimulating electrode was placed in the high right atrium near the sinus node for directly stimulating the atrium and introducing premature atrial stimuli. Recordings were made on a multichannel oscilloscope recorder at paper speeds of 100 and 200 mm per second. Atrial stimulation was performed utilizing a programmable stimulator (manufactured by M. Bloom of Philadelphia) using stimuli of 1.5 msec duration at approxi-mately twice disastolic threshold. Refractory periods were determined using the extra-stimulus technique. Beginning late in the cardiac cycle a premature atrial stimulus (S_2) was introduced after every 8th driven beat (S_1) in all animals. The prematurity of the S2 was decreased in 20 msec steps until the atrial refractory period was encountered, so that the entire atrial cycle was scanned. Lidocaine 5 mg/kilogram, procaine amide 5 mg/kg, deslanoside C 0.05 mg/kg, propranolol 0.1 mg/kg, and aprindone 10 mg/kg were adminis-tered after control refractory periods for the AV transmission system were obtained. Measurements of the intracardiac conduction intervals and refractory periods were accomplished according to standard techniques (926).

A_1, and H_1 are the atrial and His electrograms resulting from either spontaneous sinus beats or driven atrial beats, S_1.

A_2 and H_2 represent the atrial and His electrograms resulting from a premature atrial stimulus, S_2.

The refractory periods for the AV conduction system were defined as follows: Atrial effective refractory period (atrial ERP) = longest S_1-S_2 interval not resulting in atrial capture by S_2. Atrial functional refractory period (atrial FRP) = shortest A_1-A_2 interval achievable. AV nodal effective refractory period (AV nodal ERP) = A_1-A_2 interval in which A_2 does not conduct to the His bundle. AV nodal functional refractory period (AV nodal FRP) = shortest H_1-H_2 interval achievable by atrial stimulation. All determinations could not be obtained in all animals, particularly the effective refractory period of the AV node.

DIGITALIS

A. Cellular physiology
While it has been generally accepted that digitalis inhibits the active transport of sodium and potassium across the cell (372,532,798), it appears that the potassium ion is more important than sodium (270,372,851,885). In fact, relative intracellular vs. extracellular potassium concentration may be crucial in the genesis or termination of cardiac arrhythmias (372,454,885). Several recent reviews are available describing the precise electrophysiologic action of digitalis (207,373,681). Extensive studies of the action of digitalis glycosides on transmembrane potentials of ventricular fibers are in general agreement that digitalis shortens the action potential duration (103,798,851,878). On the other hand, the effects on membrane action and resting potentials and the rate of depolarization have been less consistent (214,796,878,945). Digitalis may affect automaticity in excessive doses. The increase in phase 4 depolarization may result in the obtaining of threshold potential and in automatic rhythm (681). A transient sequence of oscillations from membrane potential and subsequent electrical quiescence can occur (183,265,345,376,676,677,681). When this occurs in specialized conducting cells it is referred to as a low amplitude potential (676), a transient depolarization (265), or enhanced diastolic depolarization (183). Rosen et al. (681) have shown that following excessive ouabain administration phase 4 depolarization can be produced. Furthermore, discontinuation of the stimulus can be succeeded by a stable spontaneous rhythm at a slower rate than the drive stimulus. Discontinuation of the stimulus resulted in a subthreshold depolarization succeeded by repolarization and no further electrical activity was seen.

Other investigation has shown oscillatory phenomena due to digitalis administration (183). Aronson and Cranefield (38) demonstrated oscillations or after-potentials in slow cardiac fibers. Depolarization occurs to the extent that the normal mechanism for phase 4 depolarization and the fast inward sodium current are inactivated and only the slow response and its accompanying automaticity remain. These observations follow completion of the action potential repolarization in cells that now have low resting and maximal diastolic potentials (38). Cranefield has identified these observations as delayed after-depolarization. Rosen et al. (681) suggests that this not only is an appropriate description of the oscillatory events that occur during phase 4, but distinguishes them from those oscillations which may occur prior to full repolarization and hence are designated 'early after-depolarization'. It has now been shown that under certain conditions digitalis-induced delayed after-depolarizations can reach threshold potential and initiate spontaneous action potentials (183, 265, 376). Rosen et al. (681) further described that when an appropriate coupling interval or sinus stimulus rate is reached, after-depolarization will reach threshold and initiate a variable number of spontaneous action potentials. These authors further suggested that two distinct types of automatic activity may occur as the result of digitalis toxicity. Either the automatic activity is seen in the ventricular escape beat, or the delayed after-potentials reach thresholds which result in a variable number of propagated action potentials (934). These abnormal automatic responses are much less prone to develop when the potassium concentration is between 4 and 5.5 mM (934). It should be pointed out that manganese and verapamil decreased the magnitude of digitalis-induced-delayed after-depolarization (267, 679).

King et al. (440) showed suppression of ouabain-induced ventricular ectopy with verapamil and reversal with calcium. Rosen et al. (679) showed verapamil counteracted the effects of digitalis on the slope of phase 4 depolarization. Hence, it can be concluded that an inward current carried by calcium could be responsible, at least in some part, for the changes in diastolic membrane potential induced by digitalis. Finally, it has been shown that the interactions between digitalis-induced delayed after-depolarizations and premature action potentials can result in concealment of conduction within the His-Purkinje system and result in complex disturbances of rhythm including reentry (681).

B. The effect of digitalis on AV transmission
Recently, Goodman et al. (315) demonstrated that the electrophysiologic effects of digitalis on atrioventricular conduction in man are most marked in the AV node and appear dependent on cardiac innervation. Both the AV nodal functional and effective refractory periods were prolonged by digitalis and were unrelated to changes in cycle length (315). However, no significant changes were seen in patients with denervated hearts. Prolongation of the effective refractory period in the AV junction is caused partly by vagal activation and partly by direct effect on the nodal fibers themselves (540, 851, 878, 880, 886, 888). Characteristically, digitalis engenders a low amplitude and phase 0 upstroke velocity (V max) of the action potentials from the N region of the AV node (886). The rate rise of phase 0 ($\dot{V}$ max) in nodal His (NH) fibers also appears to be decreased. Hence, a greater decrement and failure of propagation may result within the AV node (886). Furthermore, part of the increase in the so-called effective refractory period of the AV transmission system results from concealment of rapid atrial impulses, especially in the presence of atrial fibrillation and to a lesser extent of atrial flutter, into the AV junction. Hence, in the presence of repetitive concealment, fewer supraventricular impulses will propagate to the ventricles. Partial penetration into, and conceivably reentry within, the AV junction could also inhibit subsequent AV transmission (879, 888).

The interrelationship of digitalis with potassium and propranolol appears most important the management of patients with supraventricular arrhythmias.

C. Interrelationship of digitalis and potassium
It appears that cardiac glycosides and potassium primarily affect different portions of the AV conducting system (880, 882). Lanatoside C almost selectively depresses conduction

across the AV node with little or no delay in the intra-atrial and His-Purkinje transmission (880, 886).

In contrast, high potassium concentration will slow intra-atrial and subnodal conduction and provides protective action for intranodal conduction (882). Hence, elevation of potassium may counteract the depressant action of cardiac glycosides on intranodal transmission, but could cause further delay above and below the AV node. Figure I.

If intranodal conduction is severely depressed by toxic doses of cardiac glycosides, the beneficial effect of elevated potassium concentration may be insufficient to restore 1:1 conduction across the crucial N region of the AV node. Significant prolongation of intra-atrial conduction by cardiac glycosides is seen only in the presence of a high potassium concentration. The delay is attributed to the potassium alone (210, 882).

Since cardiac glycosides increase diastolic depolarization in His-Purkinje fibers (715), and since the resultant loss of membrane potential could cause a decreased rate of phase 0 depolarization ($\dot{V}$ max) and slower conduction velocity (760), suppression of automaticity by a high concentration of potassium may sometimes improve His-Purkinje conduction. However, it has been pointed out that in the presence of a severe conduction disturbance in the more proximal portion of the AV transmission system (e.g., the AV node), such suppression of His-Purkinje automaticity may result in abolition of subsidiary pacemakers and ventricular standstill. For this reason great caution must be exercised in the administration of potassium in patients with AV block and possible digitalis excess.

D. Interrelation of digitalis and propranolol

The combined use of digitalis and propranolol probably represents one of the most significant advances in the control of supraventricular arrhythmias (210, 615). The complimentary action of these agents slows the ventricular rate in the presence of atrial flutter and fibrillation. Propranolol has been shown to depress both intra-atrial and His-Purkinje conduction with little effect on intranodal conduction in rabbit hearts (203, 615) (fig. 1, 2).

Further studies in the dog demonstrated an increase in the functional and effective refractory periods by digitalis with a further increase when digitalis and propranolol were combined (fig. 3). Although the A-H interval and the refractory periods were increased by digitalis and further increased by the addition of propranolol, measurement of these parameters is not sufficient to precisely characterize conduction across the AV node (882). This may, in part, explain the confusion concerning the actions of antiarrhythmic agents and electrolytes on AV conduction.

GROUP I

QUINIDINE

A. Cellular physiology

Agents which decrease automaticity and responsiveness and prolong the refractory period are rather typical of the quinidine or so-called Group I drugs (372). However, there are notable exceptions among the agents listed in table 1. These differences will be discussed subsequently.

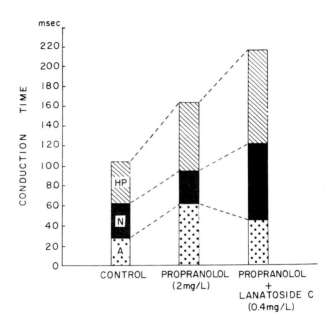

Fig. 2. Site of AV conduction delay in the presence of propranolol and lanatoside C in isolated rabbit heart. Intraatrial conduction (A); intranodal conduction (N); His-Purkinje conduction (HP). Propranolol (2.0 mg/L) increases the A and HP conduction time with only a small increase of intranodal conduction. After administration of Lanatoside C (0.4 mg/L), the intranodal time is increased. (fig. 3) Reference (615).

Fig. 3. Effect of lanatoside C (0.05 mg/kg) and propranolol (0.1 mg/kg) on the AV nodal refractory periods. A_1-A_2 = the interval between the last driven atrial beat and the premature atrial stimulus; H_1-H_2 = the interval between the last driven His bundle deflection, and the His bundle deflection resulting from the premature stimulus. The AV node effective and functional refractory periods are increased after lanatoside C and further increased after the addition of propranolol.

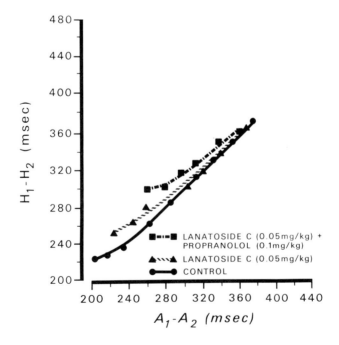

Weidmann, Johnson (414,415), Hecht (352), Gettes et al., (301) and Watanabe et al. (202,876,878) have demonstrated a decrease in the maximal rate of depolarization ($\dot{V}$ max) in the presence of quinidine and quinidine-like agents. Furthermore, suppression of the spontaneous pacemaker activity of the Purkinje fibers by this drug was also reported by Hoffman (363) and Weidmann (898). Other investigators emphasized the importance of the delay in repolarization following the administration of quinidine (363,922). Although the action potential duration was increased by quinidine, recovery of excitability lagged further behind the completion of repolarization (675,877). Restoration toward normal of the action potential amplitude, resting potential and phase 0 depolarization ($\dot{V}$ max) occurred in the presence of a lowered potassium concentration (fig. 4).

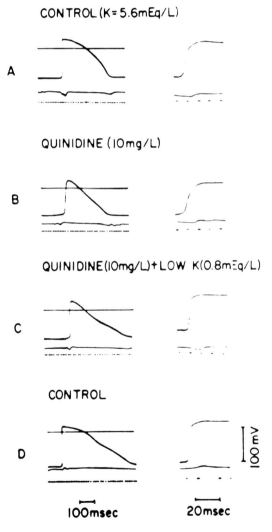

CONTROL (K = 5.6mEq/L)

A

QUINIDINE (10mg/L)

B

QUINIDINE(10mg/L)+LOW K(0.8mEq/L)

C

CONTROL

D

100mV

100msec   20msec

Fig. 4. Effect of lowering of the potassium concentration on phase O depolarization ($\dot{V}$ max). Control (A) Quinidone reduced V max (B), lowering of potassium (K = 0.8 mEq/L) restored phase O depolarization towards normal (C). Control (D) (fig. 1) Reference (878).

B. Effect of quinidine and potassium on atrioventricular conduction

Quinidine, in the presence of normal potassium, markedly prolonged AV conduction time with a further increase by high potassium (414). Quinidine or high potassium concentration prolongs the AV interval by slowing intra-atrial, His-Purkinje, and intraventricular conduction (882). Lowering potassium concentration in the presence of quinidine shortens the AV interval by enhancing His-Purkinje conduction. Hence, different regions of the AV conduction system are selectively influenced by these agents (882). Josephson et al. (418) found that quinidine routinely prolonged His-Purkinje and intraventricular conduction time in man. In addition, the refractory periods of the atria and His-Purkinje system were prolonged while the effective refractory period of the AV node was consistently shortened. They thought that procaine amide had effects similar to quinidine but different from diphenylhydantoin, lidocaine, and propranolol (107, 174, 288, 289, 394, 417). These findings were consistent with those found in rabbit hearts by Watanabe and Dreifus (882). In short, these studies suggest that quinidine has anticholinergic properties which can be of clinical significance. Josephson et al. (418) noted an apparent shortening of the effective refractory period of the His-Purkinje system in one patient. However, when low potassium effects predominated, the AV interval could remain relatively unchanged before second degree block would occur. In short, different portions of the AV conduction system can be selectively influenced by quinidine and potassium. AV conduction in the presence of low potassium and quinidine depends on the net results of their antagonism within individual fibers.

C. Effect of quinidine and propranolol on atrioventricular conduction

While propranolol has similar membrane effects to quinidine in that it decreases automaticity, slows the rate of depolarization, and decreases responsiveness, it has little or no effect on the action potential duration (372). However, the shortening of the action potential duration is probably less marked than the shortening of the refractory period. Further

Table 2. Electrophysiologic effects of combined use of quinidine and propranolol on ventricular fibers.

	Control	Control + Quinidine (5 mg per Liter)	Quinidine (5 mg per Liter) + Propranolol (0.5 mg per Liter)
APA	79.9 ± 4.9	77.2 ± 2.2	74.6 ± 6.8
MRP	60.5 ± 3.4	57.5 ± 3.7	59.6 ± 5.6
OS	19.4 ± 4.9	19.7 ± 3.4	15.0 ± 2.2‡‡
APD	126.0 ± 19.0	149.0 ± 13.7**	165.4 ± 12.8‡
MRD	81.7 ± 17.6	44.5 ± 12.0*	36.2 ± 13.3*

*P < 0.001   APA = action potential amplitude in millivolts
**P < 0.01   MRP = membrane resting potential in millivolts
‡P < 0.02   OS = overshoot in millivolts
‡‡P < 0.05   MRD = maximal rate of phase 0 depolarization in volts/second

Table 3. Effect of propranolol on A-V conduction time (msec).

	Control	Propranolol (2mg/liter)	P % change value
Intraatrial	32.0 ± 4.09	73.8 ± 12.91	+130.6** < 0.05
Intranodal	41.7 ± 6.79	51.8 ± 6.76	+ 24.2* < 0.1
His-Purkinje	37.5 ± 3.07	72.2 ± 5.04	+ 92.5* < 0.01
Total A-V	110.8 ± 10.15	192.7 ± 15.20	+ 73.9* < 0.01

*P < 0.01
**P < 0.05

Table 4. Electrophysiologic effects of combined use of quinidine and propvanolol of AV conduction (in milliseconds).

	Control	Control + Quinidine (5 mg per Liter)	Quinidine (5 mg per Liter) + Propranolol (0.5 mg per Liter)
Intraatrial	18.8 ± 4.4	38.4 ± 13.5‡	54.0 ± 19.2‡
Intranodal	42.4 ± 19.4	69.6 ± 12.1**	109.2 ± 25.7**
His-Purkinje	31.4 ± 9.2	52.2 ± 19.7‡	90.8 ± 51.2**
Total AV conduction	92.6 ± 16.3	160.2 ± 17.8*	254.0 ± 59.9*

*P < 0.01
**P < 0.02
‡P < 0.05

studies of the interaction of propranolol and quinidine show that V max was decreased by quinidine and this change was further exaggerated by the addition of propranolol (table 2). The effect of propranolol alone on AV conduction is shown in table 3. Propranolol significantly increased intraatrial and His-Purkinje conduction without a significant increase in intranodal conduction (615). However, the addition of propranolol to quinidine further depressed intraatrial, intranodal, and His-Purkinje, conduction (table 4). In summary, quinidine and propranolol have been shown to be extremely effective in the management of cardiac arrhythmias presumably because of their additive action on cellular electrophysiology and AV conduction (615, 787–789).

D. Disopyramide phosphate, (norpace)
A new antiarrhythmic agent, disopyramide phosphate, has been successfully used for the treatment of various cardiac arrhythmias including atrial fibrillation and ventricular tachycardia (208,212,710,867). The drug appears to be effective in the presence of paroxysmal atrial and nodal tachycardia. The membrane effects of disopyramide phosphate include an increase in the action potential duration and refractory period with a decrease in phase 0 depolarization (V max) (208,212) (fig. 5). Similar to quinidine and other antiarrhythmic agents (202,876–878), lowering of the potassium concentration tended to

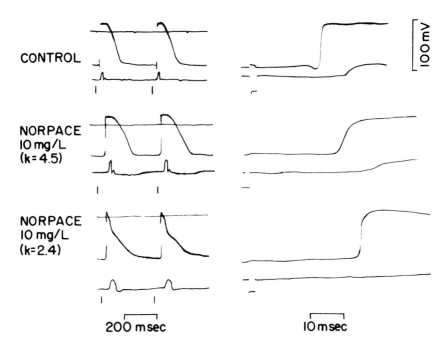

Fig. 5. Effect of disopyramide (Norpace) on rabbit ventricular fibers. Norpace slowed phase 0 depolarization and prolonged the action duration. (Middle curve). Lowering potassium from 4.5 to 2.4 mEq restored phase 0 depolarization towards normal. (Lower)

Table 5. Electrophysiologic effects of disopyramide on ventricular fibers.

	APA	MRP	OS	APD	MRD
Control	91.4 ± 14.9	69.1 ± 15.6	23.8 ± 10.2	125.3 ± 16.8	149.3 ± 57.7
Disopyramide 10 mg/L (K = 4.5)	91.5 ± 17.0	69.6 ± 16.1	20.9 ± 6.1*	164.5 ± 24.0*	46.0 ± 18.1*
Disopyramide 10 mg/L (K = 2.7)	100.4 ± 14.6*	85.5 ± 8.3*	15.0 ± 8.3*	168.5 ± 50.3*	140.5 ± 46.0*

*P < 0.02
For abbreviations, see table 2.

reverse the membrane effects of norpace (fig. 5) (table 5). Disopyramide phosphate appears to increase intraatrial, intranodal, and His-Purkinje conduction time (208, 212) (fig. 6) (table 6). The slowing of conduction within the N fibers of the AV node may contribute to the marked effectiveness of disopyramide phosphate in terminating reciprocating atrial tachycardias.

E. 17-Monochloroacetyl ajmaline hydrochloride (MCAA)

The alkaloids of rauwolfia serpentia have been used for the treatment of cardiac arrhythmias of supraventricular and ventricular origin (100, 101). Ajmaline, the principal alkaloid, has a brief effective duration. Beccari (52) studied the antiarrhythmic action of

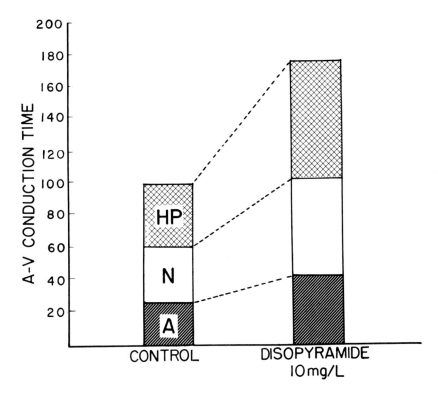

Fig. 6. Effect of disopyramide phosphate (Norpace) on AV conduction. Conduction time is increased in all 3 regions of the AV transmission system. The greatest increases occurred within the AV node and His-Purkinje system.

Table 6. Electrophysiological effects of norpace on AV conduction time (in milliseconds).

	Control	Disopyramide Phosphate (10 mg/L) K + (4.5 mEq/L)	Disopyramide Phosphate (10 mg/L) LOW K + 2.7 mEq/L)
Intraatrial	24.8 ± 3.3	45.3 ± 10.1**	26.2 ± 6.8
Intranodal	32.0 ± 10.2	56.0 ± 9.0**	66.1 ± 37.5
Intra-His-Purkinje	39.2 ± 6.5	74.5 ± 12.6*	46.7 ± 11.2*
Total AV cond.	96.0 ± 8.2	175.8 ± 18.9*	139.0 ± 43.8

*P < 0.001
**P < 0.01

some ajmaline derivatives and concluded that the esterfication of 2-hydroxyls of ajmaline caused a potentiation of the antiarrhythmic action. However, when these compounds are introduced into the organism, the action of the precursor is enzymatically regenerated. From an electrophysiologic standpoint, there is a significant decrease in the action potential amplitude, overshoot, and maximal rate of depolarization ($\dot{V}$ max) as well as an increase in the action potential duration (43). These findings are similar to those of quinidine as far as ventricular fibers are concerned, although studies on Purkinje fibers exposed

Table 7. Electrophysiologic effects of MCAA on ventricular fibers.

	Control	*Control +* *MCAA (3 mg/L)*
APA	84.1 ± 6.0	75.2 ± 5.8*
MRP	61.0 ± 5.8	59.1 ± 6.7
OS	23.1 ± 5.9	16.1 ± 2.9**
APD	119.8 ± 12.6	135.6 ± 25.1**
MRD	63.4 ± 30.8	40.7 ± 19.7*

MCAA = 17-monochloroacetyl ajmaline hydrochloride
*P < 0.01
**P < 0.05

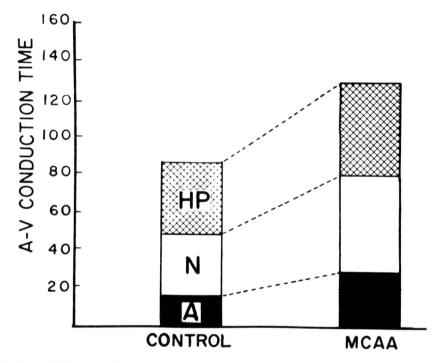

Fig. 7. Effect of MCAA on AV transmission. The intraatrial and intranodal conduction times were significantly prolonged, while the intra-His-Purkinje conduction time was increased to a lesser degree than the intranodal conduction delay. The total AV conduction was markedly prolonged (fig. 3). Reference (43).

to epinephrine were not performed. However, it can be speculated from this data that MCAA probably has antiarrhythmic effects similar to quinidine (table 7).

Intra-atrial, nodal, and total AV conduction times are increased (fig. 7). In contrast to quinidine, the slowing of conduction, especially in the atria and AV node, could offer important therapeutic action in the presence of supraventricular tachycardias, atrial fibrillation, flutter, and tachycardias associated with the Wolff-Parkinson-White syndrome. MCAA may offer potent antiarrhythmic effects and deserves more extensive clinical evaluation.

F. Aprindine

Aprindine is an antiarrhythmic agent with local anesthetic properties similar to lidocaine (648). It appears effective both orally and parenterally (216). Van Durme et al. (216) found aprindine to be superior to procaine amide and quinidine in a crossover experiment in patients with stable ventricular dysrhythmias following healed myocardial infarction. The effectiveness of this agent appears related to the plasma level of the drug. Zipes et al. (962) found a high incidence of ventricular fibrillation in dogs with acute left anterior descending artery ligation. Initiation of ventricular fibrillation was related to a critical myocardium, rapid infusion, and ischemia. The high aprindine concentration preferentially binds to the myocardium immediately after an intravenous dose when the serum aprindine level represents only 1–2% of the total dose. It was further observed that the myocardial aprindine level fell rapidly, and after 1 hour ventricular fibrillation could no longer be produced (962). Hence, rapid infusion rates plus ischemia plus high myocardial aprindine concentrations produced asynchronous ventricular excitation leading to ventricular fibrillation.

The membrane effects of aprindine were studied by Greenspan et al. (323) in normal non-automatic Purkinje fibers. Aprindine depressed the rate of rise of phase 0 with concomitant reduction in action potential amplitude, duration and, at times, membrane potential. With prolonged superfusion, conduction became altered with varying degrees of block and exhibited the clinical counterpart of the Wenckebach structure. In Purkinje fibers rendered automatic by stretch, hypoxia, digitalis, or catecholamines, the slope of phase 4 depolarization was reduced and eventually abolished with aprindine. Conduction depression, and block at high doses, also occurred in muscle with this agent but was less sensitive than Purkinje tissue. Greenspan suggested that the alteration in conduction in association with abolition of automaticity would thus abolish a tachycardia (323). All investigators found that the effects of aprindine persisted with low doses and after long periods of time.

Aprindine significantly prolongs the effective refractory period of the atrium, AV junction and ventricular myocardium. The conduction times of the atria, AV, and H-V were also increased (648). These authors found a return of the functional refractory periods to control values while the relative refractory periods remained above control after 2 hours (648).

GROUP II

LIDOCAINE

A. Cellular electrophysiology

The electrophysiologic and pharmacologic effects of lidocaine have been extensively reviewed by Rosen et al. (682). Consequently, this section will review only the interrelationship of lidocaine, a Group II agent, with procaine amide and propranolol, agents often used clinically in combination.

It appears that lidocaine will produce a concentration-dependent decrease in $\dot{V}$ max and depression of membrane responsiveness (682). This depression of conduction by lidocaine could theoretically convert areas of unidirectional conduction block into bidirectional block, thereby abolishing reentry. This may be of particular importance as lidocaine exerts a differential effect on healthy and diseased tissues (682). Maximum diastolic potential amplitude and $\dot{V}$ max are reduced or further depressed by therapeutic concentrations of lidocaine.

The action potential duration and effective refractory period of Purkinje fibers are decreased by lidocaine (70). The degrees of alteration is related to the location of the particular Purkinje fiber, as the most significant effects of lidocaine are seen at a site close to the insertion of the free running strands into the ventricular myocardium (572,942). Furthermore, lidocaine causes the greatest changes in action potential duration and refractoriness is normal Purkinje fibers in which these parameters are initially longest (942).

Lidocaine suppresses spontaneous diastolic depolarization and automatic impulse formation at membrane potentials between -90 and -60 mV due to a time—and voltage-dependent decrease in an outward $K+$ current (iK_2) (934). This occurs at lidocaine concentrations that do not influence sinus node automaticity.

The action potential amplitude and $\dot{V}$ max are decreased by lidocaine, but to a lesser degree than procaine amide (767). Singh and Hauswirth (767) attributed the effects of lidocaine on V max to a decrease in membrane conductance for Na +.

Recent studies in our laboratory in rabbit ventricular fibers confirm the reduction in $\dot{V}$ max but no significant change was observed in the action potential amplitude, membrane resting potential or action potential duration (211) (table 8). Addition of procaine amide to lidocaine engendered a smaller decrease in $\dot{V}$ max. Table 8. When the drugs were administered in a reverse fashion the effect on phase 0 depolarization ($\dot{V}$ max) was additive (table 9) (fig. 8). There was no further increase in the action potential duration when lidocaine was added to procaine amide (table 9). Han et al. (339) found that both procaine amide and lidocaine were effective in decreasing automaticity since they significantly increased post extra systolic escape intervals of idioventricular beats. Although procaine amide failed to abolish the reentrant beats induced by early premature beats, lidocaine abolished these beats in a considerable number of the dogs studied. These results suggest

Table 8. Electrophysiological effects of combined use of lidocaine and procaine amide on ventricular fibers.

	Control	Control + Lidocaine (10 mg/Liter)	Lidocaine (10 mg/Liter) + Procaine amide (5 mg/Liter)
APA	100.2 ± 12.2	102.5 ± 14.4	99.6 ± 10.4
MRP	72.5 ± 11.1	76.0 ± 11.8	86.0 ± 10.2
OS	28.0 ± 8.9	26.5 ± 6.6	27.7 ± 5.8
APD	127.9 ± 35.8	144.8 ± 17.3	132.3 ± 22.1
MRD	103.1 ± 16.8	44.6 ± 14.2*	41.7 ± 7.5

*P < 0.01

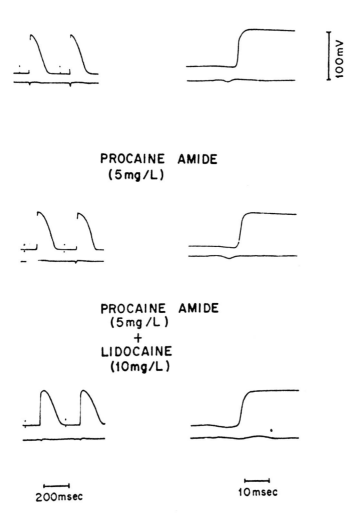

CONTROL

PROCAINE AMIDE (5 mg/L)

PROCAINE AMIDE (5 mg/L) + LIDOCAINE (10 mg/L)

200 msec   10 msec

Fig. 8. Effect of lidocaine on ventricular fibers. Procaine amide increased action potential duration and phase 0. Addition of lidocaine to procaine amide caused a further decrease in the maximum rate of depolarization of phase 0.

that lidocaine is more effective than procaine amide in preventing ventricular reentrant activity induced by early premature beats. Thus, the interrelationship of procaine amide and lidocaine could be useful in the management of resistant cardiac arrhythmias. Kabela (421) noted a lesser sensitivity of atrial fibers to lidocaine and attributed this to a smaller efflux of K from atrial as opposed to ventricular muscle and Purkinje fibers. This may explain the inconsistent effect of lidocaine on atrial arrhythmias.

From earlier studies on the interrelationships of antiarrhythmic agents and potassium, it became apparent that the divergence of effects seen with lidocaine resulted from a wide variation of potassium concentrations in the animal models (202, 208, 876, 877, 882, 885).

Table 9. Electrophysiologic effects of combined use of procaine amide and lidocaine on ventricular fibers.

	Control	*Control* + *Procaine amide* *(5 mg per Liter)*	*Procaine amide* *(5 mg per Liter)* + *Lidocaine* *(10 mg per Liter)*
APA	79.7 ± 5.3	78.6 ± 5.1	75.7 ± 6.7
MRP	58.8 ± 5.4	58.9 ± 5.7	59.7 ± 7.4
OS	20.9 ± 7.6	19.7 ± 6.3	16.0 ± 4.4
APD	126.0 ± 42.7	132.3 ± 42.0**	137.3 ± 44.4
MRD	115.0 ± 23.3	54.0 ± 11.7*	44.8 ± 20.2*

For abbreviations see table 2.
*P < 0.01
**P < 0.05

Studies by Singh and Vaughan Williams (765) indicated that at 5.6 millimolar K^+ concentration, lidocaine reduced the maximum rate of depolarization of phase 0. The potassium concentration compared favorably to those found in the blood of successfully treated patients. However, at lower potassium concentration of 3.0 millimolar, lidocaine did not necessarily change the electrophysiologic parameters. The present studies showed a marked reduction in the maximum rate of depolarization ($\dot{V}$ max) in the presence of a potassium concentration of 4.5 millimoles.

B. *Effect of lidocaine and procaine amide on atrioventricular conduction*
The previous discussion indicated that the effect of lidocaine on AV conduction must necessarily be related to the potassium concentration (668). Previous electrophysiologic studies utilizing His bundle recordings have demonstrated no significant depression of intra-atrial, AV nodal, or intraventricular conduction (118). However, studies using ultra-microelectrode techniques demonstrated a significant increase in intra-atrial and intra-nodal conduction time with a net increase in the total AV interval following lidocaine administration in rabbit hearts (211). (table 10). No further increase following procaine

Table 10. Electrophysiological effects of combined use of lidocaine and procaine amide on A-V conduction.

	Control	*Control* + *Lidocaine* *(10 mg/Liter)*	*Lidocaine* *(10 mg/Liter)* + *Procaine amide* *(5 mg/Liter)*
Intraatrial	20.9 ± 8.3	35.1 ± 3.8*	30.3 ± 11.8
Intranodal	39.0 ± 10.2	53.1 ± 9.3*	54.9 ± 9.7
His-purkinje	27.4 ± 8.6	24.2 ± 6.2	42.6 ± 10.6*
Total A-V conduction	83.3 ± 11.6	112.4 ± 19.6*	127.8 ± 10.0*

*P < 0.01

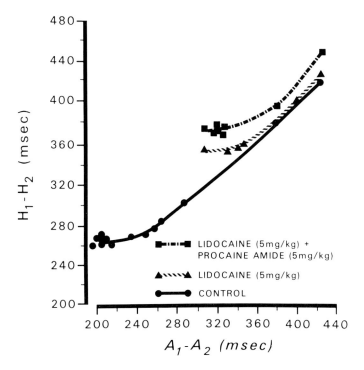

Fig. 9. Effect of lidocaine and procaine amide on the functional and effective refractory periods of the AV node. Addition of lidocaine (3 mg/kg) increased the effective and functional refractory periods. A further increase of the refractory periods was seen following the addition of procaine amide (3 mg/kg).

amide was seen in intraatrial or intranodal conduction time but the usual increase in His-Purkinje conduction was observed. Both the effective and functional refractory periods of the AV junction were increased following lidocaine administration (3 mg/kg) and further prolonged after the addition of procaine amide (3 mg/kg) (fig. 9).

Although lidocaine and procaine amide show several dissimilar electrophysiologic actions, there appear to be significant additive effects when these agents are combined. It is not unusual that lidocaine and procaine amide are used in combination in the presence of resistant cardiac arrhythmias and from the electrophysiologic studies presented it would appear that some beneficial effects could be expected.

DIPHENYLHYDANTOIN

Although diphenylhydantoin (DPH) has been in clinical use for more than 25 years, its precise role in the treatment of heart disease is still unsettled (205). Several clinical reports as early as 1939 suggested that DPH may exhibit antiarrhythmic effects on the heart (923). Although DPH still appears to have only limited value in the therapy of cardiac arrhythmias, its unique electrophysiologic properties render it extremely useful as a pharmacologic tool.

DPH appears to depress automaticity and enhance conduction and responsiveness, thus differing from Group I agents in several respects (66,135,354,615,733).

However, Strauss et al. (791) using higher concentrations of DPH (10^{-5} moles) showed a decrease in the slope of phase 4 depolarization in sinoatrial and venous automatic tissue. Sano et al. (716) demonstrated a decrease in phase 0 over a wide range of concentrations and an increase in the action potential duration in higher concentrations. It appears that any particular action of the drug is essentially related to its concentration. Further studies using ultramicroelectrode techniques with higher concentrations of 10 mg/liter showed an increase in intraatrial as well as His-Purkinje conduction time (205). However, Scherlag et al. (733) noted a decrease in the His-ventricular activation time measured by intracardiac catheters. It is reasonable to suspect that arrhythmias which are mainly a result of reentry due to depressed conduction, DPH in low concentrations may be effective in terminating the mechanism by improving the conduction (615). Like lidocaine, DPH causes abbreviation of the action potential duration. However, the effective refractory period is reduced to a lesser degree and therefore, the ratio of abbreviation of the effective refractory period to action potential duration remains less than 1. Since the rate of action potential propagation depends on $\dot{V}$ max, DPH will increase conduction at voltages where membrane responsiveness is altered (72).

Studies by Sasyniuk and Dresel (718) suggest that DPH prolonged the AV interval. Again it should be stressed that in most studies, DPH enhanced AV conduction. Species variation, drug concentration, and the underlying potassium concentration will vary the effect of DPH on AV transmission time. Our group has occasionally observed slowing of the ventricular rate in the presence of atrial flutter or fibrillation as well as high grade AV heart block. Thus, extreme care must be exhibited when using this agent in the presence of underlying AV conduction disorders.

GROUP III

BRETYLIUM TOSYLATE

A. Cellular electrophysiology

It is difficult to classify bretylium tosylate among the two previous groups of antiarrhythmic drugs because the primary effects of this agent do not appear to decrease automaticity and responsiveness or prolong the refractory period. In fact, automaticity has actually been increased by bretylium, and spontaneous firing in quiescent fibers in preparations of papillary muscle and Purkinje fibers has been observed (71,928). This response is usually transient and is abolished by pre-treatment with reserpine. Wit et al. (928) noted occasional hyperpolarization induced by bretylium, especially when the membrane resting potential was reduced or the tissue was considered hypoxic. They explained such findings by possible release of catecholamines from the sympathetic nerve endings. It is conceivable that this mechanism played a role in the hyperpolarization and increased conduction velocity observed in our previous experiments (71,884). It is unlikely that the same mechanism

Table 11. Effects of quinidine and bretylium on the ventricular fibers of rabbit heart.

	APA	MRP	APD	MRD
Control	90.0 ± 9.1	64.8 ± 10.3	118.0 ± 22.0	57.5 ± 14.6
Quinidine alone	93.0 ± 11.3	69.4 ± 13.1	147.0 ± 25.6*	36.0 ± 8.9†
Quinidine and Bretylium	92.8 ± 13.3	67.1 ± 9.6	135.0 ± 25.2†	42.1 ± 12.1

*P < 0.01
†P < 0.05
APA = action potential amplitude in millivolts
MRP = membrane resting potential in millivolts
APD = action potential duration in milliseconds
MRD = maximal rate of phase 0 depolarization in volts/second

prevailed in the present study of isolated hearts perfused through the coronary system since myocardial oxygenation in this setting should be better than in a tissue bath experiment and recirculation of released catecholamines should not play a major role (884). Absence of this mechanism may explain why the addition of bretylium to quinidine did not change the membrane resting potential or the action potential amplitude and overshoot (42) (table 11).

All the effects of bretylium cannot be attributed to catecholamine release, since this agent shortened the action potential duration, both alone in the tissue bath experiments and in the perfused heart in the presence of quinidine. Furthermore, if catecholamine release were solely responsible for the electrophysiologic action of bretylium, one would not expect significant depression of intranodal conduction by this agent, whether used alone or after perfusion with quinidine. Cervoni et al. (119) showed that bretylium increased the fibrillation threshold in both reserpine-pre-treated and chronically sympathectomized dog hearts, and concluded that the antiarrhythmic effects of bretylium are due to a direct action on the myocardium rather than to its adrenergic blocking action or its ability to release norepinephrine. In their study, the positive inotropic effect of bretylium was apparently not dependent on catecholamine release since it was demonstrated after sympathectomy and in reserpinized dogs. In our experiments using normal potassium concentration (K = 4.5 millimoles), the membrane resting potential, action potential amplitude and maximal rate of depolarization were increased while the action potential duration and effective refractory periods were decreased (42,615,884). These findings were in contrast to those found by Bigger and Jaffe (71) and could be related to the 4.5 millimolar potassium concentration of the perfusate in our experiments (42) as opposed to the 2.7 millimolar concentration employed by other investigators (71).

The important electrophysiologic mechanisms of bretylium may be related directly to its ability of chemical defibrillation (42). Figure 10 shows that bretylium produced a more normal looking action potential following a premature depolarization. As a result, after bretylium administration the earliest premature response arises at a more negative level of membrane potential and conducts at a more rapid velocity than the earliest premature depolarization-evoked after washout of the drug. Improved propagation of premature systoles may not entirely abolish ectopic beating, but may, instead, engender more efficient conduction, and consequently less chance for micro-re-entry and ventricular fibrillation.

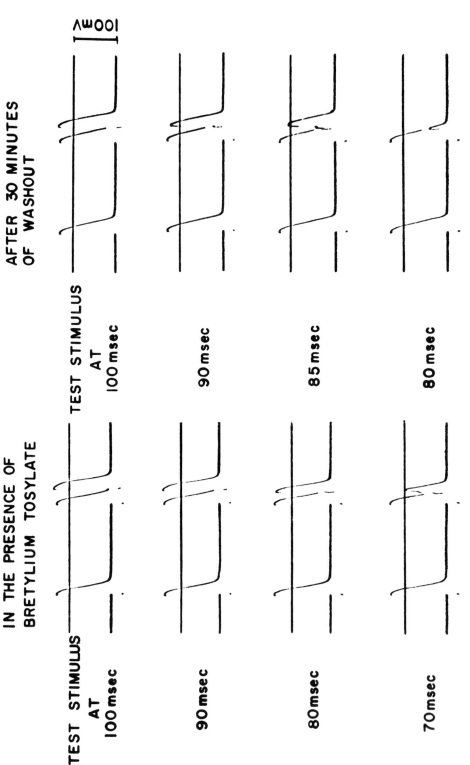

Fig. 10. Effect of bretylium tosylate on the action potential of a premature stimulus. Left column bretylium (20 mg/L) Right column—after washout of bretylium. Premature systole 90 msec following the last driven beat produced a smaller action potential amplitude with a slowly rising phase 0, as compared to the action potential in the presence of bretylium. At 85 msec there is a further deterioration of the action potential configuration after washout, while a rather normal appearing action potential is seen in the presence of bretylium. At 80 msec there is a failure of activation of the fiber while an abortive action potential is seen after the premature stimulus is delivered 70 msec following the last driven beat.

Quinidine alone produced an increase in the action potential duration and V̇ max. Following the addition of bretylium, there was a significant decrease in the action potential duration with no change in action potential amplitude, membrane-resting potential and decrease in V̇ max. Hence, the addition of bretylium to quinidine decreased the action potential duration and, in general, appeared to have the opposite effect as quinidine (table 11).

B. Effect of bretylium tosylate on atrioventricular conduction

Bretylium alone selectively increased intranodal conduction (fig. 11). Furthermore, when quinidine and bretylium were combined, there was an antagonistic effect by bretylium on the increased intraatrial and His-Purkinje conduction time (table 12). Hence, bretylium depresses intranodal conduction similar to low potassium, digitalis and propranolol, with little or no effect on intraatrial or His-Purkinje conduction. However, the combined effect of quinidine and bretylium tended to prolong total AV interval (table 12).

Although bretylium may never gain widespread popular use as a primary antiarrhythmic drug because of its hypotensive effects, it deserves further study to identify its antiarrhy-

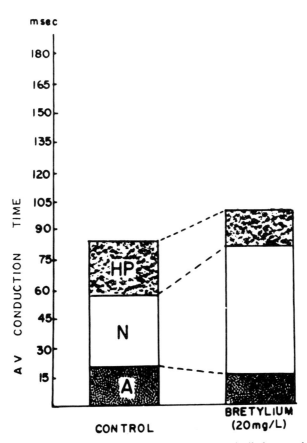

Fig. 11. Effect of bretylium tosylate on AV conduction. Bretylium markedly increased intranodal conduction with no effect on intraatrial or His-Purkinje conduction time.

Table 12. Combined effects of quinidine and bretylium on AV conduction time (means ± standard errors).

	Control (msec)	Quinidine (msec)	Quinidine and bretylium (msec)
Atrial	25.6 ± 11.6	75.0 ± 6.6	63.6 ± 56.6
Nodal	43.8 ± 13.4	69.0 ± 37.5	100.2 ± 52.2**
His-Purkinje	30.2 ± 12.3	70.6 ± 24.7*	69.4 ± 28.8
AV interval	99.6 ± 36.0	214.6 ± 102.8**	233.2 ± 105.4

*P < 0.01
**P < 0.05

thmic and antifibrillatory actions. Its contrasting effects to those of Group I or Group II agents indicate that this drug is a very interesting pharmacologic tool. It is obvious, however, that bretylium should not be used in combination with either Group I and Group II agents, as this combination may completely nullify the antiarrhythmic effects of either agent alone (42).

GROUP IV

VERAPAMIL

Verapamil

In contrast to the other possible classifications of antiarrhythmic agents, verapamil appears to have a rather selective action on fibers dependent on a slow inward current. Wit and Cranefield (938) demonstrated that verapamil reduced the action potential amplitude in the upper and mid AV nodes so that maximum depolarization was below 0, without reducing maximum diastolic potential. However, action potentials in the lower AV node were not affected. Verapamil prolonged the time dependent recovery of excitability and the effective refractory period of AV nodal fibers. Premature impulses would be blocked in the AV node preventing the conduction delay necessary for AV nodal reentry and tachycardia. Verapamil had no effect on the ventricular diastolic threshold or amplitude of atrial or His bundle action potentials. King et al. (440) showed that verapamil blocked the slow ionic current carried by calcium and/or sodium, but not the rapid current carried by sodium alone. Verapamil suppressed ouabain-induced ventricular ectopy and this suppression was reversed by calcium administration. Rosen et al. (678) showed that verapamil, at concentrations of 2×10^{-6} moles, decreased action potential amplitude, resting membrane potential, maximum rate rise of phase 0 and membrane responsiveness. Changes in the effective refractory period were compatible to those in action potential duration. Conduction velocity was slowed only by the higher concentrations of verapamil. Verapamil also suppressed automaticity and calcium-induced low amplitude potentials. These effects on the action potential and low amplitude potentials were partially reversible by increasing calcium concentration (678). Its effects on the action potential plateau were consistent with blockade of an inward calcium current and suggest that verapamil may suppress arrhythmias due to calcium-induced slow potentials. Lower concentrations of verapamil did not alter phase 4 depolarization or conduction, but did suppress low amplitude potentials. These authors suggest that verapamil acts by a mechanism different from other antiarrhythmic agents (678).

Imanishi et al. (387) also found that verapamil-induced suppression was partially restored by increasing extracellular calcium concentration. These authors compared the effects of lidocaine with verapamil and found that slow channel-dependent rhythmic automatic depolarizations in depolarized ventricular myocardium could be suppressed by moderately high doses of verapamil, but not by very high doses of lidocaine. The unique action of verapamil appears to be quite different from those of the other antiarrhythmic agents discussed thus far, suggesting a possible fourth group of antiarrhythmic agents. The clinical effects of verapamil, particularly in suppressing supraventricular arrhythmias and slowing the ventricular rate in the presence of atrial fibrillation and atrial flutter as first reported by Schamroth et al. (725) appear to have electrophysiologic confirmation.

Recent extensive reviews (210, 885, 889) of the interaction of magnesium, potassium, and sodium and tetrodotoxin are available and will not be considered in this overview.

EPILOGUE

The precise action of antiarrhythmic agents still remains unclear, and even less is known of the interactions of antiarrhythmic drugs that are often used in the wake of each other. From this discussion it is obvious that various antiarrhythmic agents available for clinical use have diverse and competing mechanisms of action and it may be impossible to produce the best therapeutic effects under all conditions. Indeed, the clinician must gain enough information to utilize antiarrhythmic agents in combination or alone, while avoiding the pitfalls of antagonistic actions that may prove detrimental to the patient. When one considers the complex interaction of antiarrhythmic drugs, either among the various groups or in the presence of altered serum electrolytes, the number of possible antagonistic and synergistic actions becomes almost infinite. Fortunately, in the clinical setting one is usually operating within the physiologic range for serum electrolytes and many of these observations which have been discussed and demonstrated in the laboratory may not be pertinent in clinical practice. Certainly, correction of serum potassium and magnesium can be done with great efficiency. It should be remembered that when serum electrolyte derangements are present, the usual or expected effects of antiarrhythmic agents may be masked. This could lead to erroneous therapy or to the conclusion that the therapy is either inadequate or useless.

One can also profit from some of the observations made in this discussion that marked beneficial effects can be achieved, particularly by the use of digitalis and propranolol in slowing AV conduction in the presence of supraventricular rhythms. The effect on AV transmission, whether studied by absolute intervals within the atria, AV node and His-

Purkinje system, or by the extrastimulus method, may have different physiologic manifestations. Hence, the functional and effective refractory periods may mean one thing, and
absolute conduction times denote other mechanisms of action. Combinations such as
lidocaine and procaine amide, or lidocaine, procaine amide and propranolol, can be used
to gain significant clinical effectiveness when the action of one drug alone is inadequate.
Bretylium appears to be antagonistic to the other groups of antiarrhythmic agents discussed. This agent, along with verapamil, offers very pertinent and useful pharmacologic
tools for future studies. Finally, it should be stressed that the actual mechanism of antiarrhythmic drugs is probably still unknown and that the observed membrane effects may
have very little to do with their actual antiarrhythmic action. In short, antiarrhythmic
agents are mainly nonspecific protoplasmic poisons. The fact that significant membrane
effects occur in no way implies that this is the precise electrophysiologic action. The future
must resolve the many conflicting results within the so-called groups of various antiarrhythmic agents.

SINUS NODE AND ATRIUM

11
THE SINOATRIAL NODE AND ITS CONNECTIONS
WITH THE ATRIAL TISSUES[1]

RAYMOND C. TRUEX, Ph.D.

> Those who look have learned to doubt;
> those who have never looked are never in doubt!

It will be recalled that during cardiogenesis there is a sequence of pacemaking regions and the first is detected in the primitive ventricle (141, 316, 331, 619). Next, the atrial myocardium becomes the dominant pacemaker and the atrial beat is soon supplanted by a fast

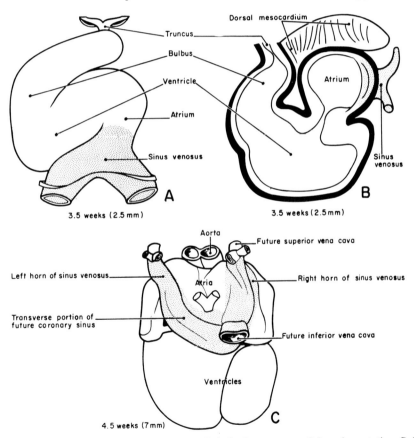

Fig. 1. Diagrams of the developing human heart. A. Tubular heart stage at 3.5 weeks gestation. B. Sectioned chambers of the heart at 3.5 weeks. C. Posterior view of atria and ventricles at 4.5 weeks. SA node arises from primitive caval cells in the right horn of sinus venosus, while the AV node is presumably derived from primitive cells adjacent to the terminus of the left horn.

1. Supported by NIH Grant HL-07047 and Career Award K06-GM-14092.

intrinsic rate that originates in cells of the sinus venosus (fig. 1). Later, the sinoatrial node (SAN) is derived from cells of the right horn of the sinus venosus (i.e., right venous valve) and this structure normally remains as the definitive pacemaker. It should be noted also that large clear atrial cells first make their appearance in both the atrium and sinus venosus regions of the developing heart (fig. 1). Isolated fascicles, as well as individual large clear cells have been illustrated in the atrial regions of fetal, newborn and adult hearts of many mammals (122, 142, 403, 835, 837).

Even though there is no doubt of the existence of large cells scattered throughout the walls of the atria and interatrial septum (IAS), there is considerable controversy as to the fate of the large embryonic cells, as well as to the derivation, distribution and precise function of the large cells observed in atria of the adult heart. Two essential questions remain unanswered: How do large atrial cells fit into the organization of the atrial myocardium, and do they form identifiable pathways between the SAN and atrioventricular node (AVN)? Secondly, do the large atrial cells show the specialized physiologic properties of either fast conduction or a slow diastolic depolarization that are characteristic of pacemaker cells? This communication is directed only toward structural elucidation of the first question—namely, the SAN and its continuity with the atrial myocardium as observed by light microscopy.

Pertinent facts related to the embryonic development, ultrastructure and innervation of the cardiac conduction system are described in chapter 1. This chapter is based on recent and many previously prepared serial microscopic sections cut through the SAN and blocks of atrial tissue of fetal, neonatal, young and adult human hearts. Similar atrial tissues were examined from numerous specimens of the pigeon, rabbit, calf and dog heart in order to provide comparative atrial cell information in these common laboratory animals.

SINOATRIAL NODE

The clear and prophetic printed words by the discoverers of the SAN merit repeating: 'There is a remarkable remnant of primitive fibers persisting at the sino-auricular junction in all mammalian hearts. These fibres are in close connection with the vagus and sympathetic nerves, and have a special arterial supply; in them the dominating rhythm of the heart is believed to normally arise' (431). The atrial location and blood supply still remains as valid macroscopic landmarks for the SAN, while an abundant literature has accumulated on the structural and electrophysiological aspects of the component cells.

It is now known that there is considerable variation in the blood supply to the SAN of different animals. For example, it may have one or more prominent centrally placed nodal arteries, as in the ferret, dog, monkey and man, or the node may not display any arteries of appreciable size, as in the bird, rabbit and calf. There are recognizable differences also in the shape and organization of the SAN in the different species. The node of the pigeon is a small, poorly defined cell mass located at the base of the right venous valve, while that of the rabbit is elongated as it extends cranially into the caval wall. In contrast, the ferret SAN is a gray ovoid cell mass that is discrete and elevated within the sulcus terminalis several millimeters inferior to the caval-atrial junction (846). In dog, monkey, baboon and man, the interwoven, grayish nodal mass of muscle cells and condensed connective tissue fibers is less sharply defined beneath the epicardium of the sulcus terminalis. In spite of these structural variations, the SAN has been identified and described in practically all mammals and in several avian species (92, 142, 178, 180, 391, 392, 395, 485, 635, 655, 656, 659, 699, 835, 838).

In order to visualize the shape of the SAN in three dimensions, an investigator would have to recall a multitude of microscopic relationships observed in several hundred serial sections. If the tissue block is oriented so that the crista terminalis and superior vena cava are sectioned transversely, as recommended by one investigator (382), the SAN is triangular in shape and most of the intrinsic cells appear to be cut in cross section. Serial sections cut parallel to the long axis of the node provide a better microscopic orientation of SAN shape, size and cellular topography. The human node shown diagrammatically in figure 2 was reconstructed from such longitudinal sections. This node exhibits the usual curved myocardial surface (labeled 2 in fig. 2) that faces the superior vena cava. Along this surface numerous bundles of atrial fibers blend with the nodal cells, while distally the atrial cells course into the interatrial septum (IAS) in the location of the muscular tract described by Wenckebach (917). A photomicrograph through the superior portion shows this blending of nodal and atrial muscle cells of Wenckebach's bundle (arrow in fig. 3A) along the myocardial surface of the SAN. Cells leave the tapered superior end of the SAN (labeled 1 in fig. 2) to blend with bundles of muscle cells in the crista terminalis that are presumed to be the atrial bundle described by Bachmann (45). The epicardial blending of nodal elements with the atrial muscle cells in Bachmann's bundle is indicated by the two arrows in figure 3B. From the tapered inferior end of the SAN (labeled 3 in fig. 2), other nodal elements blend with atrial muscle cells in the crista terminalis that presumably descend as components of Thörel's bundle (812). The photomicrograph shown in figure 4 is cut through the inferior tapered end of an SAN to demonstrate the gradual

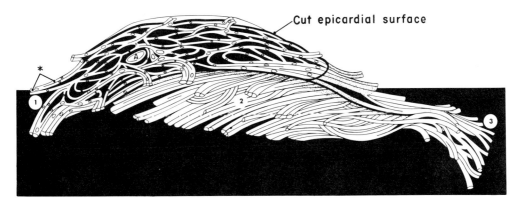

Fig. 2. Wax model reconstruction of human sinoatrial node. Atrial muscle and endocardium are removed to expose the deep concave (2, myocardial) surface of the node as viewed laterally from the superior vena cava. The top of the interatrial septum is to the left of the model, while the inferior vena cava would be located to the right. A cut section through the superior, tapered end of the SAN demonstrates the nodal artery (A), internal cellular organization and modes of continuity (*) between nodal elements and atrial myocardium. Male 41 years of age.

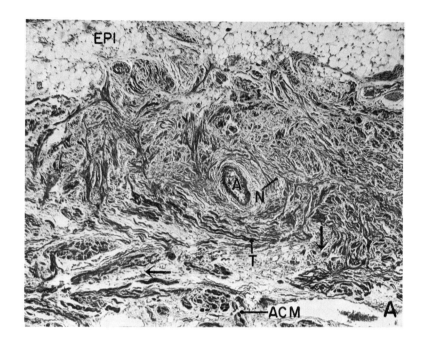

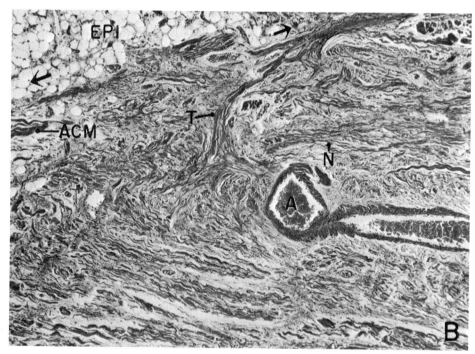

Fig. 3. A. Longitudinal section through superior portion of human SAN and epicardium (EPI). Note bulk of the node is composed of small nodal (N) and more prominent transitional (T) cells that form an anastomotic network around the nodal artery (A). Most of the transitional (T) cells leave myocardial surface of the node to become continuous with atrial muscle (ACM) bundles described by Wenckebach (arrows). Photomicrograph, male 41 years (H16-572-2), hematoxylin-phloxine-saffranin stain. × 40. B. Same SAN specimen and stain, but this section is 1.4 mm inferior to that illustrated above. Note that some transitional (T) cells do leave epicardial surface (EPI) to blend with atrial cells (ACM) within the sulcus terminalis as components of the bundle described by Bachmann (arrows). Section H16-432-1. × 85.

longitudinal blending of nodal elements with atrial cells in the region of the muscle bundle described by Thörel.

Areas of nodal-atrial continuity such as those depicted in figures 2, 3 and 4 represent important structural bridges between the SAN and myocardium. The refractory periods in the cells of such perinodal fascicles provide the anatomic substrate for reentry, as well as entrance and exit conduction blocks of the SAN.

Cell types. Along the periphery and within the SAN of most mammalian hearts, one normally encounters four cells of differing diameter and staining intensity. Their shapes are exceedingly varied as they branch and anastomose with each other to form loose or tightly arranged circular and longitudinal cell strands within the node. In order of their frequency, the four types are identified as typical nodal (N), transitional (T), large pale (P) and atrial cardiac muscle (ACM) cells (fig. 3–7).

Nodal cells are the most numerous, and they have the smallest diameter. These more lightly stained elements demonstrate myofibrils, faint cross striations, and an elongated nucleus that is almost as wide as the cell. In man the nodal cells have a mean cytoplasmic diameter of 5 μm (843). Such tightly packed elements give the SAN of animals a highly cellular appearance that aids in its microscopic identification. As a result of combined

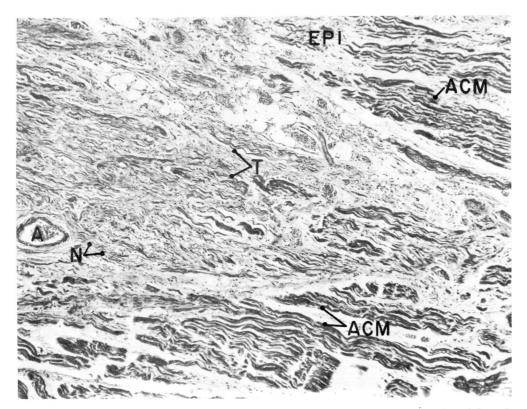

Fig. 4. Photomicrograph from SAN section in 3B. This plane through a more inferior region of the node illustrates the longitudinal mode of continuity between transitional (T) and atrial cardiac muscle (ACM) cells. Note these junctions occur at both the epicardial (EPI) and myocardial surfaces of the node. Hematoxylin-phloxine-saffranin stain (H16-432-1). × 85.

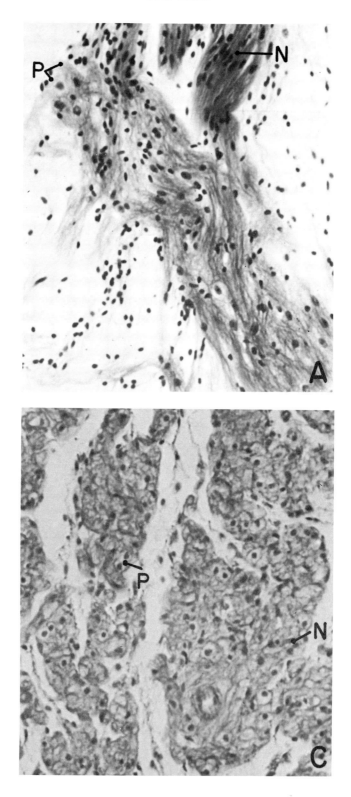

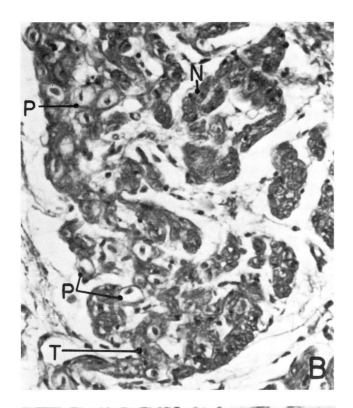

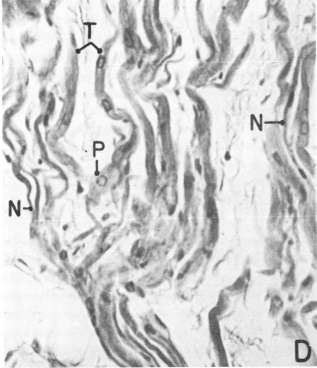

Fig. 5. Photomicrographs of cell types within SAN of the adult pigeon (A), rabbit (B), calf (C) and dog (D) heart. Nodal (N) cells are smallest and most numerous. Large pale (P) cells occur singly or in clusters, and have few or no myofibrils, depending upon species. The pale angular P cells are interposed and continuous with both nodal and transitional (T) cells. All magnifications × 356.

electrophysiologic and anatomic studies, the slender nodal cell was believed by some investigators to show slow diastolic depolarization that is characteristic of a true pacemaker cell (121,830).

Transitional cells are a prominent microscopic feature of the mammalian SAN (T, figs. 3 and 4) as they form intercalated units between typical nodal, pale, and the large darkly stained atrial cells. Such intercalated elements may appear to be either cylindrical units or highly branched cells that vary in cytoplasmic diameter from 6 to 10 μm. They also possess a high complement of myofibrils per unit area, and for this reason the transitional cells are easily identified by routine histologic techniques and also in electron micrographs. This cells type gradually acquires more myofibrils and increases in diameter until it becomes indistinguishable from atrial muscle at the level of light microscopy. The transitional cells are conspicuous components within the bridges as they connect SAN elements to the atrial myocardium (fig. 3,4,7A).

The third nodal element has a large diameter, abundant pale cytoplasm with quantities of glycogen granules, and an oval nucleus. In some animals a sparse or reduced number of myofibrils are present (pigeon, calf, dog, monkey, man), whereas, in other animals there are no myofibrils in these cells (rat, rabbit). In this report such large pale elements, interposed between nodal and transitional cells, are illustrated and identified as pale (P) cells (fig. 3–7). It is the opinion of the author that such pale cells represent the 'clear nodal fibres' of the rat (860), the 'peculiar cells' of the dog SAN (428), the 'poorly developed nodal cells' of the rabbit and monkey (861), and the syncytial or 'pacemaker P cell' described in several mammals including man (296,391,429). The apperances of pale cells in the SAN of the pigeon, rabbit, calf and dog heart can be compared in figure 5. Examination of the P cells in these four animals also reveals that intermediate forms can be identified, inasmuch as the P cells are interposed between the small nodal and larger transitional SAN elements. The mean cytoplasmic diameter of P cells in the pigeon, rabbit, calf and dog SAN was 10.2, 11.7, 10.6 and 13.5 μm respectively. In a four year old child the P cells had a mean diameter of 13.2 μm, while that of the P cells of an adult was 14.2 μm. The appearance and cellular relationships of P cells in these two measured human SAN specimens are illustrated in figure 6.

The angular pale cells comprise an estimated 5% of cells seen in the human SAN and are most often observed as clusters of two or more cells located near the nodal artery (fig. 6A,7A). Such elements also occur singly and may be oriented at any angle in relation to the long axis of the node, including its tapered superior and inferior ends. In some specimens, the P cells formed highly elaborate complexes having multiple junctions with nodal and transitional cells (fig. 7A). A detailed view of this P cell complex at higher magnification (fig. 7B) also reveals that transitional cells are usually interposed between the pale cells and the larger darkly stained atrial muscle cells. As many as three such intricate complexes have been observed in one presumably normal human SAN.

The pale cells remain, for the present, a functional enigma and a challenge to one's curiosity. One day it will be known for certain whether pale cells are merely primitive embryonic remnants or indeed represent specialized pacemaker cells.

The fourth element observed in the SAN is typical atrial cardiac muscle cells that penetrate the margin of the node and ultimately become continuous with transitional cells

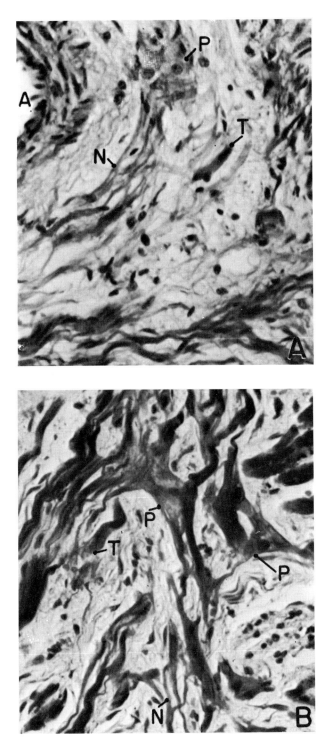

Fig. 6. Photomicrographs of cell types in SAN of infant (A) and adult (B) human hearts. In A, note the cluster of pale (P) cells near nodal artery (A) and their continuity with thin nodal (N) cells. In adult SAN, the pale (P) cells are more angular and can be identified by their sparse myofibril content and light stain. A. Hematoxylin-phyloxine-saffranin stain (H24-105-1). Age 4.5 years. × 356. B. Hematoxylin-phloxine-saffranin stain (H16-593-3). Age 41 years. × 356.

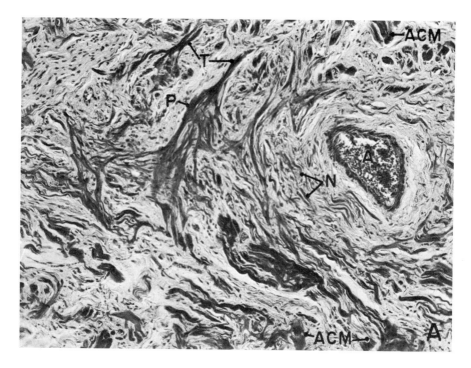

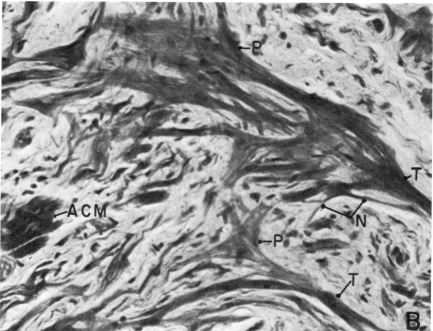

Fig. 7. A. Topography of section in central SAN region to illustrate a complex network of pale (P), transitional (T) and nodal (N) cells adjacent to the nodal artery (A). Note atrial muscle cells (ACM) have penetrated into substance of the node to become continuous with transitional cells. Photomicrograph, hematoxylin-phloxine-saffranin stain (H16-581-3). × 142. B. Photomicrograph of central region shown in A above to demonstrate microscopic appearance and interconnections of the nodal (N), transitional (T), pale (P) and atrial muscle (ACM) cells. × 356.

(fig, 2,3,4). One last point remains to be made concerning continuity between SAN elements and the atrial myocardial cells. Such continuity is actually accomplished in two ways—in one, the atrial cells penetrate into the node for variable distances before blending with intranodal transitional cells (fig. 3,4,7). It is by virtue of such penetration that the atrial cells are considered the fourth cell type found in the human node. The second mode of continuity is established by small fascicles of nodal and transitional cells that occasionally leave the margins of the more compact SAN to become interdigited between adjacent bundles of atrial myocardium for longer or shorter distances before becoming typical atrial cardiac muscle cells. In only a small number of specimens were larger pale atrial cells observed near or along the margins of the human SAN. The above two modes of continuity provide two different structural routes for the cardiac action potential to enter as well as leave the SAN. The electrophysiologic characteristics of the different morphologic atrial cell types have not been established for any animal to date. Appreciation of the final role and mechanism of these anatomic junction sites in the different types of SAN block must await future intracavitary electrode or microelectrode recordings combined with better localization of the recording sites.

  Stroma of SAN. All four cell types are embedded in an admixture of connective tissue fibers (i.e., black intercellular areas in cut superior surface of node in fig. 2). The interstitial fibers are predominantly collagen with lesser amounts of fine elastic fibers. The fibrous stroma of the SAN is gradually increased with age, while there is a corresponding decrease in the number of nodal cells (181,483,759). When disease is superimposed on the aging process within the SAN, it is often difficult to demonstrate more than a few scattered nodal cells embedded in a sea of collagen fibers. Needless to say, the nodal-atrial muscle cell junctions in diseased hearts are largely replaced by intranodal and perinodal fibrosis. This pathologic appearance of the SAN is seen in human necropsy specimens of patients who had demonstrated antemortem bradycardia-tachycardia syndrome and cardiac arrest.

ATRIAL MYOCARDIUM AND INTERNODAL PATHWAYS

It is well established and accepted that atrial muscle cells are variable in diameter, and that they branch and divide as they traverse atrial walls and interatrial septum (IAS) enroute to the atrioventricular node (AVN) or to their insertion into the anulus fibrosus. The myocardium of both human atria and the IAS normally has a heterogeneous cell population that ranges between 8 and 32 μm, with a mean cytoplasmic diameter of 15.8 μm (843). Union between two or more branched atrial cells frequently appears as broadened or triangular shaped complexes (arrows in fig. 8).

  Microscopic observations also demonstrate that single atrial cells, particularly those near the epicardium, may appear to be dilated and then suddenly become continuous with one or more small cells. The human atria may show small collections of large cells that can be followed for several millimeters—then quite rapidly they become transitional in size and soon appear to be continuous with working atrial myocardial

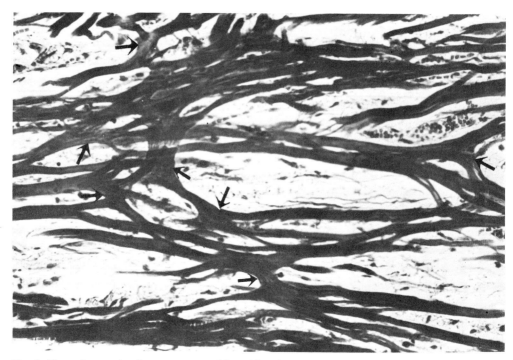

Fig. 8. Photomicrograph of anastomoses and broad junctions (arrows) between cells of human right atrial myocardium. Note loose arrangement and variations in cell diameters within this fascicle of atrial cells. Hematoxylin-phloxine-saffranin stain (H16-250-31). × 243.

cells. Numerous investigators have observed and designated such components of the human heart as large atrial cells (77,142,485,835,836,838,841,843,845), while others have described them under the misnomer of 'atrial Purkinje cell' (296,391,393,403) and 'Purkinje-like' cell (657,659,803,820). These large atrial cells are commonly present in the subendocardium and myocardium of both atria, in the crista terminalis, in the pectinate muscles of the auricular appendages, within many parts of the IAS, in and around the fossa ovalis, and frequently adjacent to the ostium of the coronary sinus (838).

Atrial cells of the avian and rabbit heart have been used extensively for either ultrastructure or electrophysiologic microelectrode studies (80,92,317,366,399,413,567,714, 749,772,866). Figure 9 is included to illustrate for the reader the appearance and frequency of large pale atrial cells that are so characteristic of these two animals. In the pigeon, clusters of large cells accompany the atrial arteries for considerable distances before they become reduced in size (arrow, fig. 9A), acquire a greater number of myofibrils (transitional cells, T in fig. 9A) and become continuous with atrial cells. The pale atrial cells of the rabbit (identified by arrows in fig. 9B) demonstrate transitional stages (T) as they blend with adjacent atrial cells of smaller diameter.

Such large atrial elements of pigeon and rabbit hearts have also been referred to in the literature as 'Purkinje' or 'Purkinje-like' cells. Some investigators have described specialized atrial internodal conduction pathways in the rabbit heart that are presumably

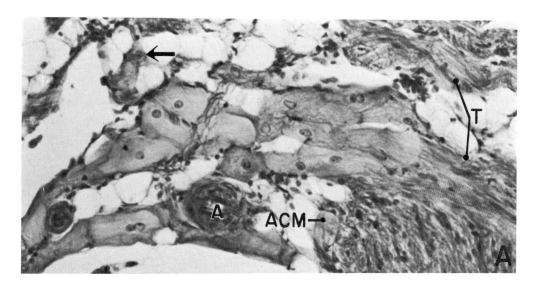

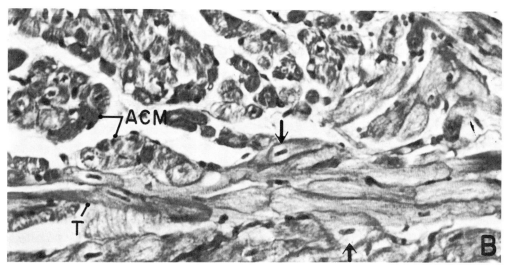

Fig. 9. A. Photomicrograph of large pale periarterial cells commonly observed in the avian atrium. Note the pale cells become small in diameter (arrow), acquire more myofibrils to become transitional (T) cells, and then blend with adjacent atrial muscle cells (ACM). The small atrial artery is identified (A). Right atrium (P2-266-1). Holmes silver stain. × 356. B. Photomicrograph of pale (arrows), transitional (T) and atrial cardiac muscle (ACM) cells in rabbit right atrium. Hematoxylin-phloxine-saffranin stain (R18-767). × 356.

formed of these large cells (247,611,613). Eighteen serially-sectioned adult rabbit hearts were recently studied in an attempt to identify these cells in the sinoatrial ring bundle and internodal pathways. In each specimen we did observe large atrial cells, such as those illustrated in Figure 9B, in the atrial myocardium and IAS. However, in no rabbit heart could we trace a discrete or continuous anatomic tract of large atrial cells that extended between the SAN and AVN.

The presence or absence of specialized atrial internodal pathways in the human heart has been a highly controversial issue since 1909, when Thörel first described a tract of 'Purkinje-like' cells between the SAN and AVN. Individual large atrial elements, as well as fascicles of such large cells, are present in the human atrial myocardium and IAS as noted above. In only two of 32 human specimens have we observed large atrial cells lying along the myocardial surface (labeled 2 in fig. 2) and within the SAN as illustrated in figure 10A. The large atrial cells in this heart establish continuity with the SAN through transitional cells and then continue a short distance as a discrete fascicle into the most superior part of the IAS before blending with regular atrial muscle. This fascicle corresponds to the atrial position described by Bachmann (labeled 1 in fig. 2). However, similar large cells are scattered in areas of both atria, including the pectinate muscles and tip of the right auricle. The large cells shown in figure 10B are far removed from the presumed location of all three internodal pathways. The uninitiated could conceivably designate these cells as 'Purkinje-like,' in view of their large diameter, scanty myofibrils and areas of abundant perinuclear cytoplasm. On the other hand, these enlarged elements cannot be considered normal muscle cells, for they were observed in the 295 gram heart of a 22 year old male drug addict. Note the numerous and abnormally large pyknotic nuclei in the muscle cells (arrows, fig. 10A, 10B). The observed changes reflect only a minimum of cell autolysis, for the coronary arteries of this specimen were perfused with 10% neutral formalin within two hours of established death.

Pertinent anatomic, physiologic and clinical evidence that either discredits or supports the existence of specialized internodal pathways was reviewed recently (128, 247, 393, 404, 410, 845). Neither time nor space permits a complete survey of the crucial literature related to the atrial internodal pathways and the interested reader should consult the above references.

There is no lack of agreement that there are many continuous atrial muscle bundles between the SAN and AVN. It is also recognized that large atrial cells are observed on occasion within these atrial bundles. It is an established fact that the lower IAS myocardium constitutes a vital segment of atrial conduction as the septal muscle fibers converge to blend with the superior, posterior and right endocardial surfaces of the human AVN (389, 840, 842, 844). The thickened muscle bands of the upper IAS around the fossa ovalis also participate in conduction of the atrial cardiac impulse, and such thickened bands can be injured during surgical procedures that involve the atrium and IAS. If a sufficiently large amount of IAS myocardium is interrupted either surgically or under experimental conditions, one could anticipate the now documented atrial conduction dysrhythmias (243, 305, 388) or pacemaker translocation to the AVN region (377). Indeed, the IAS muscle cells located anteriorly (i.e., Bachmann's bundle) could constitute a preferential pathway and have a high conduction velocity (377), for such cells normally form the most direct route between the SAN and AVN. Atrial dilation and myocardial hypertrophy increase individual cell diameters, as well as the length of the internodal route, and these factors may also result in a longer atrial conduction interval.

Some supposed evidence for preferential internodal pathways may depend on the ability of some atrial muscle cell bundles to remain functional in the presence of hyperkalemia, while other atrial myocardial areas become inactive and there is a disappearance of P

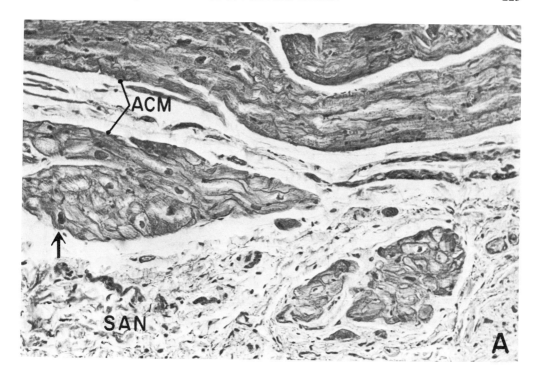

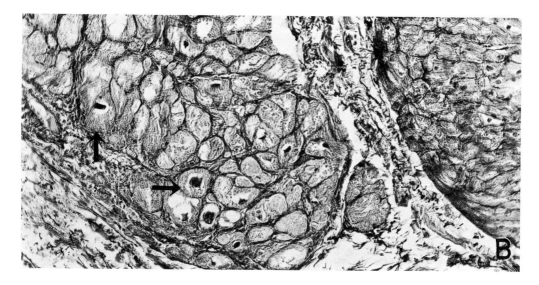

Fig. 10. A. Bundles of large pale atrial cells (ACM) along myocardial border and within periphery of a human SA node (SAN). Note abnormally large nuclei (arrow) in these large pale cells. Hematoxylin-phloxine-saffranin stain (H21-371-3). × 186. B. Photomicrograph of same specimen taken through pectinate muscle at tip of right atrium. Note myofibrillar appearance and large dark nuclei (arrows) of the pale atrial muscle cells, Hematoxylin-phloxine-saffranin stain (H21-306-2). × 142.

waves. One study (377) reported that in four of five dog experiments, once the potassium infusion was adequate, there was no contraction of the atrial muscle fibers, but the bundles comprising the internodal tracts continued to contract. It is most regrettable that no microscopic sections were reported on the structure of the cells within any of the contracting internodal bundles. If, as the present author believes, the above statements related to atrial muscle bundles, large cells and hyperkalemia are all accurate and tenable, wherein lies the controversy?

One of the strongest proponents for specialized tissues and preferential atrial conduction used a dissection technique and subserial sections to identify the three internodal pathways in the human heart (393). In a later paper (404), it was noted that each of the tracts contained not only Purkinje fibers, but also what appeared by light microscopy to be ordinary myocardial fibers. In the same communication, the authors described intermingling and multiple cross-over communications between the internodal tracts above the AVN. They stated also, 'In the human heart the region encompased by the three internodal pathways corresponds directly to the residium of the primitive sinus venosus. Cells of the Purkinje type are a major component of the internodal tracts, and these cells are generally considered to possess latent automatic properties. From these physiologic and anatomic observations it appears that cells possessing automatic properties are located in the internodal and interatrial pathways. When such a latent pacemaker becomes active under certain pathologic or pharmacologic conditions, clinically or experimentally, then the new pacemaker location will influence the normal synchronized deplorization order of the atria, change its electrical vector and, consequently, the form of the P wave.' From a pedagogic viewpoint, these statements seem to provide plausible explanations for some of the events of atrial conduction observed in clinical electrocardiography. However, they are not consistent with the structural information that has emerged over the last few years.

The above quote contains the major points of current anatomic and physiologic disagreement: 1. whether the three internodal pathways correspond to the residium of the sinus venosus; 2. whether Purkinje cells, which the present author prefers to designate as 'large atrial cells,' are a major component of specialized internodal tracts; 3. whether such large atrial cells of man and other mammals indeed possess specialized or latent automatic properties; 4. and whether the normal synchronized depolarization order of atrial conduction occurs through specialized internodal pathways rather than a radial spread over bundles of regular atrial muscle. Some investigators believe the remnants of the primitive sinus venosus in the adult heart are demarcated by the venous valves (410), and their embryologic observations led them to state '. . . the area of septum traversed by the purported anterior and middle tracts is derived from the primitive atrium rather than the primitive sinus venosus.' The definitive boundaries between these two embryonic atrial components are less clearly defined in the minds of some investigators, for no markers have been established that could demarcate the precise limits of mesodermal cell migrations from each of these atrial structures. One of the most dramatic and clear examples of primitive atrial cells we have observed was found to traverse the full length of the human septum primum (i.e., from the posterior superior region of the left atrium to an IAS termination as regular atrial muscle a short distance from the AVN). This most unusual strand of primitive cells occurred in the atrium of a one month human neonate, but we are unable to predict its developmental heritage. Yet, these vestigial cells afford a measure of explanation for the large pale cells that are so often encountered in the region of the human fossa ovalis.

We have already noted that large cells have been described in the atrial myocardium of most birds and mammals. However, these large atrial elements are not the major cell type, and, when present in mammals, the scattered cells never formed discrete or continuous pathways between the SAN and AVN. It should be appreciated that many large atrial cells may be the direct result of hypertrophy, atrial disease, or artifacts in man due to necropsy delay and cell autolysis. In fact, one group of investigators (84,828) indicated the component cells of the caudal end of the rabbit SAN and ring bundle were of smaller diameter than atrial working cells. The same authors emphasized that the two structures did not consist of large, Purkinje-like cells. Indeed, they commented that Purkinje cells were mainly observed in their poorly fixed material, and concluded these large cells probably represented fixation artifacts.

Again it is recommended that the term 'Purkinje cell' be restricted and applied only to the specific cells of the ventricle which Purkinje described originally (646). The indiscriminate use of this term for large atrial cells leads not only to semantic problems, but also connotes a functional pacemaker property that has never been established. Not only is there little experimental data to correlate large cell diameter directly with pacemaker activity, but the evidence on the SAN suggests it is the small cell that has the pacemaker properties (121,830). This problem can only be resolved by intracellular recording, followed by cell marking and histologic or ultrastructural localization of the precise recording site.

The concept of specific internodal tracts is supported by both clinical and experimental electrophysiologic evidence (405,528). However, there are dissenting reports and strong evidence that the propagated wave front during atrial conduction in the canine and human heart spreads diffusely over thick myocardial bands of regular atrial muscle (18,224,314, 410,485,775,777,908).

The present intensive search for anatomic evidence to substantiate the presence or absence of the much publicized atrial internodal tracts has been a tedious and time consuming task. Indeed, we have looked at innumerable SAN and atrial myocardial cells in many hearts of several mammals, but alas, we have failed to delineate the widely acclaimed specific interatrial pathways. Many promising possibilities and unique atrial cellular complexes were identified and traced in serial sections. Yet, we have observed no specific or specialized internodal tracts. It is concluded that bundles of regular atrial muscle cells are the predominant elements that provide cellular continuity between the SAN and AVN. The oft repeated statement that atrial conduction occurs over specialized pathways remains as a plausible but premature assumption that must await additional morphologic, clinical and experimental validation. When, and if, such validation is acquired, we will have attained also a more knowledgable basis to account for 'sinoventricular conduction' and a variety of unusual atrial dysrhythmias.

ACKNOWLEDGMENTS

The author is indebted to Linda Ginsberg, Deborah Rapp, Martha Smythe and Rick Hartman for their valued technical and research assistance. He expresses sincere appreciation to Crystel Passauer for the medical art, and to Otto Lehmann and William Verzyl for their photographic aid.

12
DIRECT AND INDIRECT TECHNIQUES IN THE
EVALUATION OF SINUS NODE FUNCTION[1]

HAROLD C. STRAUSS, M.D., AND ANDREW G. WALLACE, M.D.

Interest in the electrophysiology of the human sinus node began at the turn of this century when techniques became available that provided the clinician with recordings of atrial activity initially as jugular venous pulse tracings (513) and later as electrocardiograms (235). These two techniques enabled clinical investigators to document the presence of atrial premature depolarizations (514), evaluate the effect of premature depolarizations on sinus rhythm (915,916) and document the presence of long atrial pauses which were interpreted as being due to sinoatrial block (258,356,468,488,515,917). Disturbance of sinus node function was initially recognized in the form of sinoatrial block that occurred in a patient who had influenza (515). Later patients with sinus bradycardia (138,442) and sinus pauses or sinus arrest (75,468,623,684) were described. The characteristics of four patients with alternating bradycardic and tachycardic rhythms were described in 1954 (757). In addition, as experience was gained in the use of DC countershock for interruption of atrial fibrillation, it was recognized that normal resumption of sinus rhythm failed to occur in some patients (507). These different electrocardiographic descriptors were recognized as being due to a disturbance of sinus node function and were designated as the ECG criteria that defined the 'sick sinus syndrome' (263).

The bradyarrhythmias that occur in this syndrome were postulated to result from either disturbance(s) of sinus node automaticity and/or sinoatrial conduction (818). The first documentation of a sinoatrial conduction disturbance occurred in an experiment performed by Stannius, when he placed a ligature between the sinus venosus and the auricle of the frog heart and showed that while the sinus venosus continued to beat, the auricle stopped beating for some time. Spontaneous occurrence of second degree sinoatrial block in man was first reported in 1901 (515). Although second degree sinoatrial block was identified in many subsequent patients, it was recognized that lesser degrees of sinoatrial conduction disturbances, namely first degree sinoatrial block, eluded detection (258, 488,917). The effects of atrial premature depolarizations on the rhythm of the heart were analyzed in detail by several different investigators (85,86,169,229–231,249,274,311, 355,358,445,460,495,551,587,620,649,717,753,793,818,915). In the mammalian studies atrial premature depolarizations were followed either by compensatory or less than compensatory responses. Wenckebach postulated that an atrial response to an atrial premature depolarization would be determined by the retrograde and antegrade conduction times between the sinus node and atrium and by the sinus node return cycle (915). This interpretation was criticized by Eccles and Hoff because, in their experiments, where they

1. Supported in part by U.S. Public Health Service Grants HL-15190, HL-08845, HL-05736, the Walker P. Inman Fund, and a N.C. Heart Association Grant-in-Aid.

believed that they were directly stimulating the sinus node, APDs elicited at progressively decreasing coupling intervals were followed by progressively longer atrial return cycles until the return cycles approached some constant value (230). They interpreted the prolongation of the atrial return cycles as indicating depression of sinus node rhythmicity by the APD. Langendorf et al. (460) and Fleischman (274) extended the analysis of the effects of APDs on the spontaneous sinus cycle in patients that had atrial parasystole.

The introduction of catheter electrodes and the techniques of programmed stimulation into the cardiac catheterization laboratory permitted a more detailed analysis of the effects of APDs on sinus cycle length. In graphs where the atrial return cycles (A_2A_3) are plotted as a function of the test cycles (A_1A_2) (fig. 1A), the distribution of data points about the compensatory line and below the compensatory line, forming a 'plateau', seemed to concur with the Wenckebach hypothesis. We postulated, as had Wenckebach (915) and Langendorf (460), that the compensatory response that followed an APD was due to collision of the APD and the emerging sinus node impulse that left the basic sinus rhythm undisturbed (793). Once the APD had gained access to the sinus node and reset it, then a less than compensatory response followed (793,915). Less than compensatory return cycles (A_2A_3) which indicated sinus node capture by A_2 could be used to calculate the 'sinoatrial conduction time' (793). If the captured or reset sinus cycle length is equal to the basic sinus cycle length then by subtracting the A_1A_1 cycle from the A_2A_3 cycle, a value would be obtained that would equal the retrograde conduction time of A_2 to the sinus node and the antegrade conduction time of SAN_3 to the atrium (fig. 2). We also proposed that such an analysis would be best performed on A_2A_3 cycles falling in the last third of Zone II (fig. 1A) (793). The duration of the segment of the A_1A_1 cycle where com-

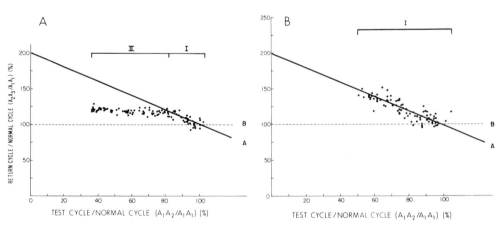

Fig. 1. Return cycles plotted as a function of the test cycles for two patients (793). The return cycles (A_2A_3) and the test cycles (A_1A_2) are normalized by dividing them by the last undisturbed sinus cycle (A_1A_1). Line A is the compensatory line and line B indicates the value of one spontaneous sinus cycle A_1A_1. The mean value of the A_1A_1 cycle in panel A is 1176 msec. In panel A, late in diastole, points fall about line A as compensatory return cycles follow A_2 (Zone I). As A_1A_2 decreases, points fall below line A and form a plateau (Zone II). Points falling in the last third of Zone II (adjacent to Zone I) are used to calculate the mean value of $A_2A_3 - A_1A_1$. In panel B, Zone I is markedly prolonged. The points all fall about the compensatory line, despite the decreasing A_1A_2 interval. This indicates first degree sinoatrial block. (Reproduced by permission of *Circulation*.)

pensatory responses followed APDs (Zone I) would also be expected to be a function of the sinoatrial conduction time. In figure 1B, an example of a markedly prolonged Zone I is shown, which was interpreted as being a manifestation of 'first degree sinoatrial block with interference' (793).

Although these hypotheses seemed to be supported by the published clinical data (311, 587, 620, 649, 753, 793), direct experimental verification of the hypothesis was lacking, Experiments were designed to validate the premature atrial stimulation technique as a means of estimating the 'sinoatrial conduction time'. The isolated rabbit right atrial preparation was selected for these experiments since its electrophysiological properties had been well characterized in previous studies (611, 714, 792). Experiments analogous to those performed in man were carried out on the isolated rabbit atrium with the spontan-

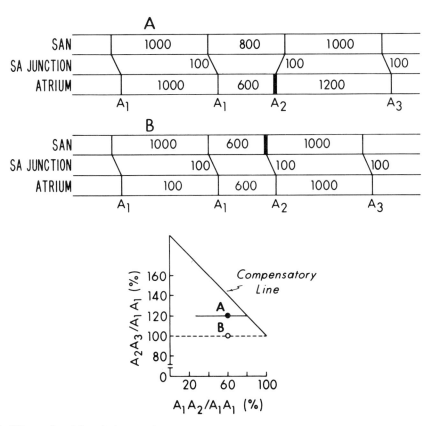

Fig. 2. Effects of atrial and sinus node premature depolarizations on sinus rhythm. Conventional ladder diagrams for an atrial premature depolarization (A) and sinus node premature depolarization (B) are shown along with a graph where A_2A_3 is plotted as a function of A_1A_2. If one assumes that the atrial (A_1A_1) and sinus node (SAN) cycle lengths are equal and the normal antegrade conduction time through the sinoatrial junction is equal to 100 msec, then an A_2 elicited at an A_1A_2 interval of 600 msec would conduct back to the sinus node and reset it. If the sinus node return cycle is equal to the A_1A_1 cycle and the sum of the retrograde and antegrade conduction times equals 200 msec, then A_2A_3 equals 1200 msec, or 120% of the A_1A_1 cycle. If a sinus node premature depolarization occurs at a coupling interval of 600 msec that has a normal sinoatrial conduction time and is followed by sinus node return cycle that is equal to the A_1A_1 cycle, then A_2A_3 should equal the A_1A_1 cycle, and fall on the dotted line projected from the ordinate at 100%. Hence, the technique provides a means of differentiating between atrial and sinus node premature depolarizations.

eous sinus rhythm interrupted by a premature depolarization following every eighth beat. Transmembrane action potentials were recorded from the sinus node and electrograms were recorded from the surface of the crista terminalis using close bipolar electrodes. Stimuli were delivered to the crista terminalis through another set of close bipolar electrodes. Transmembrane potentials recorded from the sinus node had to fulfill certain criteria to be acceptable for inclusion in our study. These criteria were that: a. the interval between depolarization of the sinus node and crista terminalis had to exceed 25 msec; b. there was smooth mergence between phases 4 and 0; and c. the potential recorded had to exceed 50 mv.

In this study, late APDs were followed by compensatory A_2A_3 cycles (fig. 3). As the A_1A_2 interval decreased, the A_2A_3 cycles became less than compensatory and this transition to a less than compensatory response did not coincide with the sinus node

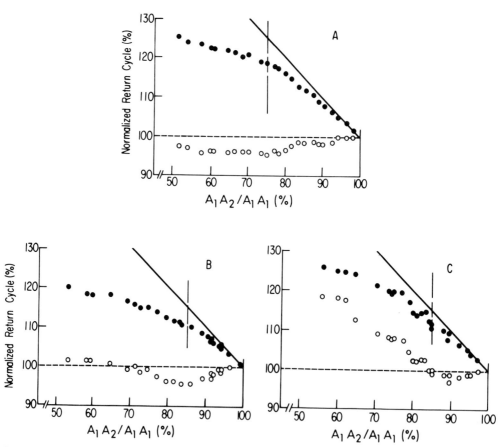

Fig. 3. The normalized atrial return cycle (solid circles) and the normalized sinus node return cycles (empty circles) are plotted as a function of the normalized atrial premature cycle in three different experiments carried out on the isolated rabbit right atrial preparation (551). Although the values of the atrial return cycles in each of the three experiments are similar, the sinus node return cycles differ. As A_1A_2 decreases, sinus node return cycle remains short (A), returns to control values (B) or markedly lengthens (C). The marked lengthening of the sinus node return cycle seen in panel C was an unusual response in this series of experiments. (Reproduced by permission of *Circulation Res.*).

capture. (fig. 3). As the A_1A_2 intervals decreased further, the less than compensatory A_2A_3 cycles usually lengthened, as shown in figure 3, but sometimes reached a constant value forming a 'plateau' in the graph. The departure of the A_2A_3 cycle from the compensatory line prior to sinus node capture was caused by shortening of the SAN_2SAN_3 cycle (551). Alteration in the sequences of depolarization and repolarization of cells between the sinus node and crista terminalis was marked enough to shorten the SAN_2 action potential and the SAN_2SAN_3 cycle. The close correlation ($r = 0.85$) between shortening of the SAN_2SAN_3 cycle and the SAN_2 action potential provided further evidence to support the view that in these experiments we were recording action potentials from the sinus node pacemaker cells (551). Action potentials recorded from cells outside of the cluster of cells functioning as the pacemaker might shorten in response to A_2 but the shortening of SAN_2 would not be expected to closely correlate with the shortening of the SAN_2SAN_3 cycle. Hence, the appearance of less than compensatory A_2A_3 cycles did not coincide with sinus node capture by A_2 and the use of the less than compensatory A_2A_3 cycles in the A_2A_3 versus A_1A_2 graph provided a value that underestimated the sinoatrial conduction time (fig. 4) (551).

The relevance of these observations to the results obtained *in vivo* experiments on cats, dogs and humans can be questioned (229–231, 311,587,620,649,753,793,818). The

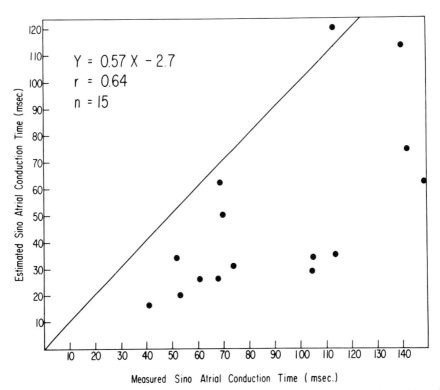

$$Y = 0.57 X - 2.7$$
$$r = 0.64$$
$$n = 15$$

Estimated Sino Atrial Conduction Time (msec.)

Measured Sino Atrial Conduction Time (msec.)

Fig. 4. The estimated sinoatrial conduction time is plotted as a function of the measured sinoatrial conduction time. Values from fifteen different experiments performed on the isolated rabbit right atrial preparation show that when the latest A_2 giving a less than compensatory A_2A_3 cycle is used, the sinoatrial conduction time is almost always underestimated (551).

mean cycle length in the rabbit studies was shorter than those reported in the human studies (551). In the human studies many of the graphs depicting A_2A_3 plotted as a function A_1A_2 showed a sharp transition from a compensatory response to a constant but less than compensatory A_2A_3 cycle, which occurred infrequently in the rabbit studies (85, 86, 311, 445, 551, 587, 620, 649, 753, 793). The sinus node studied in our isolated rabbit right atrial preparation was located on the endocardial surface and these cells do not surround a central sinus node artery (399). In dog and man the sinus node is an epicardial structure that surrounds the sinus node artery (391, 392, 431). In addition, in dog and man the heart is much larger than it is in the rabbit and this difference may mean that conduction between the sinus node and the crista terminalis is markedly different in man and dog than it is in the rabbit. However, comparison of the A_2A_3 versus A_1A_2 graphs obtained from lapine, feline and canine studies have shown a marked similarity in that the transition from the compensatory response to the constant less than compensatory A_2A_3 cycle is gradual, as shown in figure 5. Although the sequence of conduction between the sinus node and crista terminalis has only been studied in the rabbit, the similarities of the A_2A_3 versus A_1A_2 graphs in these different studies (85, 230, 551, 818) strongly suggest that, following A_2, similar electrotonic interactions resulting from altered repolarization sequences are occurring in cats and dogs. In fact, similar curves have been observed in some of the human studies (794), suggesting that this shortening of SAN_2 is probably

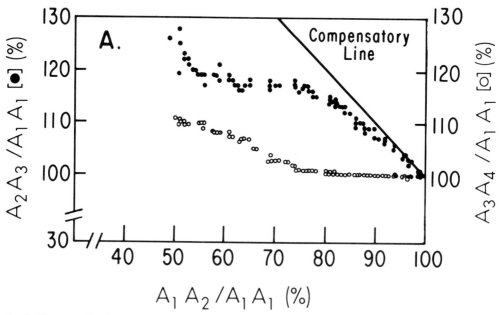

Fig. 5. The normalized return (A_2A_3/A_1A_1) and post return (A_3A_4/A_1A_1) cycles are plotted as a function of the normalized test cycle (A_1A_2/A_1A_1). In this experiment, the dog had a mean A_1A_1 cycle length that was 330 msec (818). Late in diastole A_2A_3 cycles fall on the compensatory line, as A_1A_2 decreases, the A_2A_3 cycles fall below the compensatory line, but as A_1A_2 decreases further, A_2A_3 cycles continue to increase until they reach a constant value and form a plateau. Note the long transition between the compensatory A_2A_3 cycle and the plateau response. (Reproduced by permission of *Amer. J. Cardiol.*).

occurring in man, precluding an accurate estimation of the 'sinoatrial conduction time' in man using the premature atrial stimulation technique.

It has been noted that APDs are followed by prolonged cycles that take two to four cycles to return to the control cycle length (169). This observation, coupled with the studies reported by Eccles and Hoff (230), led investigators to propose that APDs caused depression of sinus node automaticity (169, 230, 311, 587). In studies carried out on dogs, when the A_3A_4 cycle was plotted as a function of the A_1A_2 cycle, it was noted in many experiments that the A_3A_4 interval increased as A_1A_2 decreased (fig. 5) (818). It was proposed that this was indicative of the degree of depression of sinus node automaticity caused by A_2 (818). As shown in figure 3, the differing degrees of depression of sinus node automaticity following A_2 would further complicate the use of the Zone II A_2A_3 cycle in the calculation of the 'sinoatrial conduction time'.

To further analyze the factors underlying the prolongation of the A_3A_4 cycle, and to determine if the A_3A_4 cycle length correlated closely with the recorded SAN_2SAN_3 cycle length, the normalized A_2A_3 cycles were plotted as a function of normalized A_1A_2 cycles in the left hand panel of figure 6. In addition, the normalized A_3A_4 cycles and the normalized SAN_2SAN_3 cycles were plotted as a function of the normalized A_1A_2 cycles in the right hand panel of figure 6. It can be seen that as the A_1A_2 intervals decrease, both the A_3A_4 and the SAN_2SAN_4 cycles prolong. Although the prolongation of the A_3A_4 cycle is

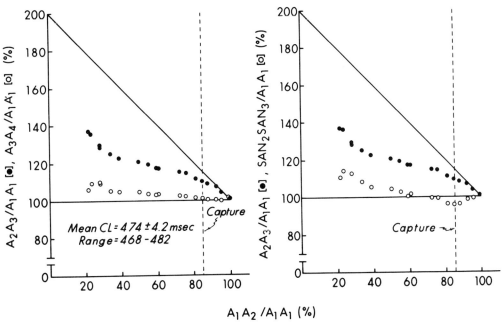

Fig. 6. Effects of an atrial premature depolarization on atrial and sinus node cycle. In the left hand panel, A_2A_3 and A_3A_4 are normalized and plotted as a function of the normalized test cycle A_1A_2/A_1A_1. In the right hand panel, A_2A_3 is again displayed and the normalized sinus node return cycle (SAN_2SAN_3/A_1A_1) is plotted against A_1A_2/A_1A_1. The mean cycle length was 474 ± 4.2 msec in this isolated rabbit right atrial preparation. The distribution of A_3A_4 and SAN_2SAN_3 cycles at each of the different A_1A_2 coupling intervals is remarkably similar.

less marked than the prolongation of the SAN$_2$SAN$_3$ cycle, the curves described by these two sets of points are markedly similar, suggesting that the A$_3$A$_4$ cycle could be used to monitor the degree of depression of sinus node automaticity following A$_2$.

To determine if the A$_3$A$_4$ cycle length reflected the degree of depression of sinus node automaticity following A$_2$, we plotted A$_3$A$_4$ and SAN$_3$SAN$_4$ as a function of A$_1$A$_2$ (figure 7). If, in fact, it is true that A$_3$A$_4$ reflects the depression of sinus node automaticity that follows APDs, then A$_3$A$_4$ and SAN$_3$SAN$_4$ should be very close in value at each of the dif-

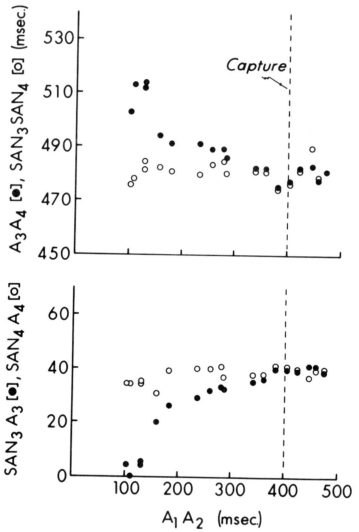

Fig. 7. The post return atrial (A$_3$A$_4$) and sinus node (SAN$_3$SAN$_4$) cycles are plotted against the A$_1$A$_2$ cycle in the top panel and the antegrade conduction times for the first (SAN$_3$A$_3$) and second (SAN$_4$A$_4$) impulses following A$_2$ are plotted against the same A$_1$A$_2$ cycles in the bottom panel. As A$_1$A$_2$ decreases, A$_3$A$_4$ lengthens, but SAN$_3$SAN$_4$ remains relatively unchanged. Over the same range of A$_1$A$_2$ coupling intervals, SAN$_4$A$_4$-SAN$_3$A$_3$ increases to a maximal value of 34 msec, and at each of the A$_1$A$_2$ coupling intervals, the difference between SAN$_4$A$_4$ and SAN$_3$A$_3$ corresponds to the difference between A$_3$A$_4$ and SAN$_3$SAN$_4$. Thus, the prolongation of the A$_3$A$_4$ cycle may not reflect depression of sinus node automaticity following A$_2$.

ferent A_1A_2 intervals. As can be seen in the top panel of figure 7, at A_1A_2 intervals of less than 300 msec, as A_1A_2 decreases, A_3A_4 increases; however, the recorded SAN_3SAN_4 cycles remain relatively unchanged or increase slightly. The reason for this discrepancy between the two cycles is apparent when one analyzes conduction times between the sinus node and atrium for the first and second impulses following A_2 (bottom panel, fig. 7). As A_1A_2 decreases, the SAN_2SAN_3 cycle begins to shorten (fig. 6) as previously described (551), and there is an associated decrease in SAN_3A_3 conduction time from 41 to 0 msec (bottom panel, fig. 7), presumably reflecting a shift in pacemaker site (85, 551). However, over the same range of A_1A_2 coupling intervals, the SAN_4A_4 interval only decreased from 41 to 31 msec, and as A_1A_2 decreased, the discrepancy in values between SAN_3A_3 and SAN_4A_4 increased to a maximum value of 34 msec. Even though the recorded SAN_3SAN_4 cycle is close in value to the SAN_1SAN_1 cycle (mean cycle length 474 $\pm$ 4.2 msec, range 468–482 msec) the difference between SAN_3A_3 and SAN_4A_4 (maximum value 34 msec) due to pacemaker shift means that the A_3A_4 cycle can be prolonged by as much as 7% over the basic A_1A_1 cycle.

The return of the sinoatrial conduction time for the fourth beat toward control values (SAN_1A_1) probably reflects a return of the pacemaker site to the position occupied under control conditions (85). In support of the hypothesis is the close approximation of the values obtained when the SAN_4A_4 conduction times are subtracted the SAN_3A_3 conduction times and compared to the values obtained by subtracting the SAN_3SAN_4 cycles from the A_3A_4 cycles. Hence, either a pacemaker shift or a depression of sinus node automaticity will cause the A_3A_4 cycle to be longer than the A_1A_1 cycle. Thus, the prolongation of the A_3A_4 cycle over the A_1A_1 cycle may not reflect, or may only reflect in part, depression of sinus node automaticity following A_2.

In another series of experiments, subthreshold stimuli were shown to prolong the sinus node cycle length (15). It was proposed that these stimuli caused release of acetyl choline from the multitude of nerve terminals in and around the sinus node (15). In the majority of our experiments we have found no evidence to support the view that the stimulus causing A_2 produced a prolongation of SAN_3SAN_4 or SAN_4SAN_5 cycles. However, in two patients late atrial premature depolarizations falling in Zone I were followed by more than compensatory A_2A_3 cycles, and by A_3A_4 cycles that were greater than the corresponding A_1A_1 cycles (794). This greater than anticipated prolongation of the A_2A_3 and A_3A_4 cycles occurring so late in Zone I would most likely be due to a depression of sinus node automaticity and would not be the result of an extensive pacemaker shift.

Thus, although the premature atrial stimulation technique is our only means of directly assessing sinoatrial conduction in vivo, it can only provide a value that approximates the true sinoatrial conduction time. First, the A_2A_3 cycle is determined by the conduction time between the site of stimulation and the sinus node, the SAN_2SAN_3 cycle, and conduction time back to the crista terminalis. In the sick sinus syndrome, atrial disease is often present and a long intraatrial conduction time would not be unanticipated. This value of the intraatrial conduction time would be incorporated into the A_2SAN_2 and SAN_3A_3 intervals which are determined by subtracting the A_1A_1 cycles from the A_2A_3 cycles. Thus, a disturbance of conduction between the sinus node and atrium could not be differentiated from a disturbance of conduction in atrial tissue. Second, the shortening of the SAN_2

action potential occurring in part of Zone I and adjacent part of Zone II causes the
SAN_2SAN_3 cycle to be shorter than the SAN_1SAN_1 cycle, resulting in an underestimation
of the 'sinoatrial conduction time'. The shortening of SAN_2 is sometimes accompanied
by a variable degree of depression of sinus node automaticity and an increase in the
SAN_2SAN_3 cycle so that it returns to or exceeds the value of the SAN_1SAN_1 cycle
(fig. 3). The marked difference between the SAN_2SAN_3 and SAN_1SAN_1 cycles would
affect the estimation of A_2SAN_2 and SAN_3A_3 intervals. Third, in most instances, we are
unable to detect shortening or prolongation of the SAN_2SAN_3 cycle relative to the basic
cycle length SAN_1SAN_1 (A_1A_1), and therefore would be unable to compensate for the
difference between SAN_2SAN_3 and the basic cycle length. Fourth, a pacemaker shift
that follows A_2 can result in a decrease in the sinoatrial conduction time (SAN_3A_3). In
addition, as the pacemaker returns to the control site as reflected in a return of SAN_4A_4
interval to control values (SAN_1A_1) this causes the A_3A_4 cycle to be longer than the
SAN_3SAN_4 cycle. This difference between the SAN_3SAN_4 and A_3A_4 cycles indicates
that in most instances we would be unable to use the A_3A_4 cycle to monitor different
degrees of depression of SAN automaticity following A_2. Fifth, as the A_1A_2 interval
decreases, the retrograde conduction time into the sinus node increases, prolonging the
A_2SAN_2 interval, and causing a lengthening of the A_2A_3 cycle. This effect is most marked
at short A_1A_2 coupling intervals. Since factors two through five assume increasing importance as the A_1A_2 coupling intervals decrease, any determination of the 'sinoatrial
conduction time' from the A_2A_3 cycle must be made from points as late in the cycle as
possible. Finally, the technique is most accurate at short cycle lengths and least accurate
at long cycle lengths. For example, at a cycle length of 500 msec, a 3% error in measurement of cycle length would result in an error of 15 msec. If the sinoatrial conduction time
(antegrade and retrograde) were 100 msec, this would result in a 15% error in the estimated
value. If, on the other hand, the cycle length was 1000 msec, a 3% error in measurement
of cycle length would result in an error of 30 msec. If the sinoatrial conduction time
were again 100 msec, this could result in a 30% error in the estimated value.

  Although the limitations of the premature atrial stimulation technique have been
discussed in detail, the positive aspects of the technique deserved to be emphasized at
this point. The duration of Zone I, during which a compensatory response follows an
APD, is principally determined by the retrograde conduction time of the APD and
the normal antegrade conduction time between the sinus node and atrium. The patients
in whom a markedly prolonged Zone I is present (753, 793) have first degree sinoatrial
block and the technique has permitted their identification, which was heretofore impossible. The use of the technique in the analysis of sinoatrial conduction times that fall
within the normal range is less satisfactory for the reasons stated above. Part of the
problem is in deciding whether to use the transition between Zones I and II (551) or
the height of the A_2A_3 cycle above the 100% line $(A_2A_3-A_1A_1)$ during the last third of
Zone II (adjacent of Zone I) in the estimation of the 'sinoatrial conduction time'. For
the moment, we favor using the A_2A_3 cycle in the last third of Zone II, as a 'plateau'
response can usually be identified in most patients; the mean value of many A_2A_3 cycles
can be obtained; and, in this portion of diastole there is little likelihood of a significant
depression of sinus node automaticity. In addition to determining the mean value of

A_2A_3 in this calculation, the slope of the line through these points should also be determined. In most instances the values obtained through use of the transition between Zones I and II and the use of the plateau response are in close agreement. Thus, while the technique can only provide an approximation of the sinoatrial conduction time, its use in the analysis of sinoatrial conduction in patients with sinus node dysfunction will provide electrophysiologic data on patients with sinus pauses, sinus arrest, and intermittent second degree sinoatrial block. This data will help characterize the pathophysiology that underlies the syndrome of sinus node dysfunction.

13

STUDIES ON THE EFFECT OF DRUGS ON SINUS NODE-ATRIAL CONDUCTION

IWAO YAMAGUCHI, M.D., AND WILLIAM J. MANDEL, M.D.

Although the mechanism responsible for cardiac rhythmicity has been of interest to physicians since the time of Hippocrates it was not until the late 19th and early 20th century that experiments were designed which identified a pacemaker site (493,536). Clinical disorders of sinus node function have, however, only been the subject of reports over the past several decades (75,225,228,757). Studies were then directed toward the catagorization of the clinical manifestations of sinus dysfunction in man. Ferrer, in her initial description, commented on the multifaceted clinical presentations of sinus node dysfunction in man (263). Subsequently, workers have commented on the varied clinical background and subsets of electrocardiographic diagnoses present during the clinical manifestations of sinus dysfunction (264,522,586,670,706).

Recently, however, attempts were made to define, with electrophysiologic methods, means of evaluating sinus node function in man (311,521,587,793). Initial attempts utilized applications of investigations described by Lange and coworkers utilizing over-drive atrial pacing techniques (311,521,587). In addition, (311,587,793) induced premature atrial systoles were utilized to calculate sinus to atrial conduction.

The purpose of this present study is to expand our present knowledge of sinus node electrophysiology by evaluating node function including sinus to atrial conduction in both experimental preparations and in man.

METHODS

I. Isolated tissue studies

Rabbits weighing 1.5 to 3 kilograms were stunned by a blow on the head. The hearts were rapidly excised and dissected in cool, modified Tyrode's solution. The right atrium, including the sinus node and AV node were dissected free and pinned in a tissue profusion chamber, utilizing the method of Paes de Carvalho et al. (611).

The modified Tyrode solution had a composition, (in millimoles per liter) of: $NACL$ 137, KCL 3, $N_AH_2PO_4$ 1.8, C_ACL_2 2.7, $MgCL_2$ 0.5, Dextrose 5.5, N_AHCO_3 24 in triple-distilled, deionized water. The flow rate for the bath was 8 ml. per minute and the Tyrode solution was equilibrated with 95% oxygen and 5% CO_2. The temperature of the bath was maintained at $35 \pm 0.2°$ centigrade. The isolated tissue experiments were in two parts. In the first series of experiments, microelectrodes were impaled in the area of the sinus node and the crista terminalis. In addition (fig. 1) a closed bipolar silver electrode was placed on the crista terminalis near the area of the microelectrode. This bipolar surface electrode was

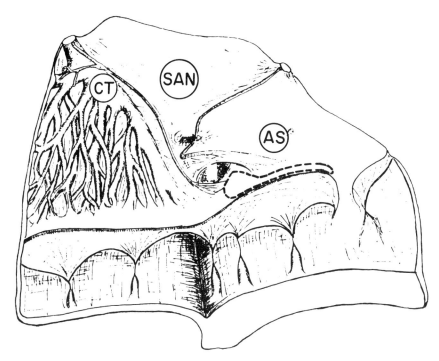

Fig. 1. Endocardial aspect of isolated rabbit right atrial preparation. Circles identify stimulation sites.

used to deliver isolated, variably coupled, premature stimuli to the area of the crista terminalis. These stimuli could be coupled to the preceeding crista terminalis electrogram at variable intervals utilizing syncronization and stimulation circuitry of special design.[1]

Transmembrane action potentials were recorded through machine-pulled glass microelectrodes filled with 3 M KCL having resistances from 20–40 megohms. These electrodes were coupled by a silver-silver chloride wire, to amplifiers with high input impedence and variable capacity neutralization (Bioelectric instruments). The amplified transmembrane voltages were displayed on a dual beam cathode ray oscilloscope (RM-565 Tektronics). In addition these action potentials were also displayed on a slave storage oscilloscope (RM 564 Tektronics). Timemarks were also displayed on the oscilloscopes utilizing a crystal time mark generator (Tektronics). The traces were viewed directly and also photographed on 35 mm film (Grass model C-4 camera).

Recordings were obtained only utilizing preparations which manifested initial activation from the sinus node area. All data was analyzed and expressed as means plus or minus standard error of the means. Statistical analyses were carried out by the T-test for paired samples.

Initial observations were obtained in the control state and subsequently following the administration of lidocaine 1×10^{-5} M, procaine amide 1.1×10^{-4} M or ouabain 3×10^{-7} M.

1. W. Daley, Biomedical Engineer. Cedars/Sinai Medical Center.

The second series of experiments were carried out with a similar preparation differing only in the fact that extrasystoles were initiated from three sites on the endocardium of the right atrium: 1. low right atrium near the area of the coronary sinus; 2. mid atrial septum, and 3. the crista terminalis. All other studies were similar to those previously described.

DATA ANALYSIS

The following measurements were carried out: Basal Sinus Rate (A-1, A-1 intervals), test cycle intervals (A-1, A-2), return cycle interval (A-2, A-3). Data was expressed as a normalized value utilizing the basal heart rate (A-1, A-1) as the common denominator in all measurements. In addition, conduction times from the crista terminalis to the sinus node, and from the sinus node to the crista terminalis were measured as well as the total duration of sinus node action potential duration. Particular attention was made of the effects of late diastolic extrasystoles on sinus node action potential duration.

II. Patient studies

Two series of studies were carried out in patients. In the first series of studies the effects of pharmacologic intervention on sinus to atrial conduction time were evaluated in patients with clinical diagnosis of 'sick sinus syndrome'. Studies were performed in the control state and following administration of Edrophonium, 10 mg by intravenous bolus, isopro-

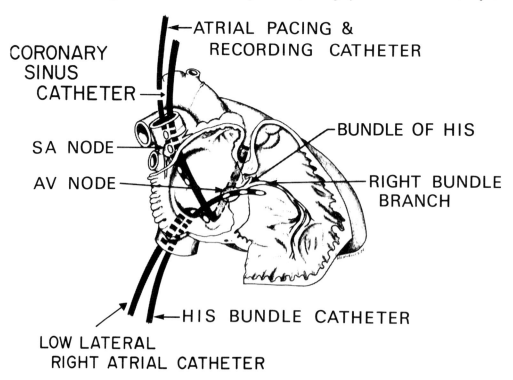

Fig. 2. Artist drawing of catheter positions for stimulation and recording in man.

terenol 1 microgram per minute by infusion and atropine 0.025 mg per kilogram by intravenous bolus. Sinus to atrial conduction was assessed in the control state, using the extra
stimulus technique as previously described by Strauss and coworkers (793). Studies were
repeated following administration of these agents to see the effect of altered autonomic
tone on sinus to atrial conduction.

   In the second series of studies the effects of alterations at the site of origin of the atrial
impulse were assessed by inducing atrial premature systoles from the high right atrium,
low right atrium, and distal coronary sinus following positioning of catheters utilizing
standard techniques (fig. 2). All calculations were formed as previously described. (Vide
Supra.)

RESULTS

I. Isolated tissue studies
Measured sinus to atrial conduction time was evaluated in 15 experiments. (55.0 ± 4.5

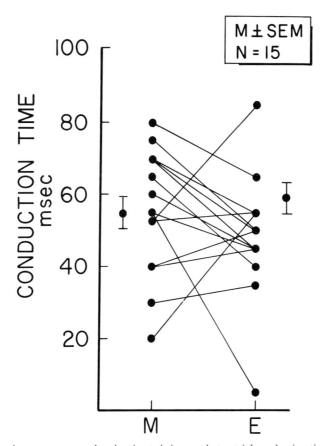

Fig. 3. Comparison between measured and estimated sinus node to atrial conduction time in 15 experiments.
The horizontal axis identifies measured (M) and estimated (E) variables. The vertical axis shows the conduction time in msec. Means and standard errors are shown at the lateral portions of the figure.

Table 1. Conduction characteristics: effects of drugs.

	CL	CT-SAN	SAN-CT	Measured	Estimated
Control	428.7	23.1	33.7	56.8	50.5
	±39.6	±4.0	±5.1	±8.4	±17.5
P.A.	480*	18.1	46.2**	64.4	53.7
N = 4	±42.5	±2.3	±7.2	±7.4	±1.2

	CL	CT-SAN	SAN-CT	Measured	Estimated
Control	440	19.5	30.5	49.5	51.0
	±32.7	±4.7	±5.5	±9.8	±13.2
Lidocaine	485	11.0	40.0***	51.0	46.0
N = 5	±45.1	±1.7	±7.1	±7.1	±3.3

	CL	CT-SAN	SAN-CT	Measured	Estimated
Control	435	35	45	80	65
Ouabain	415	20	45	65	40
N = 1					

*P < 0.05
**P < 0.025
***P < 0.0025

msec; M ± SEM). These data were compared to the data obtained by calculation from plotted responses utilizing the method of Strauss et al. The calculated conduction time was 59.3 ± 4.4 msec and was not significantly different from the measured values. All data is plotted in figure 3. Measured conduction times from crista terminalis to sinus node (19.5 ± 4.8 msec) was compared to conduction times from the sinus node to the crista terminalis (30.5 ± 5.5 msec) and found to be significantly shorter (P < 0.0125).

Subsequently, experiments were carried out to study the effects of drugs on measured and estimated sinus to atrial conduction time (table 1). Lidocaine (N = 4) and Procaine Amide (N = 5) produced no significant change in measured or estimated conduction time. Ouabain, in one experiment, was noted to *shorted* both measured and estimated conduction. A typical experiment is shown in figure 4.

Particular attention was directed at the effects of late atrial extrasystoles on the sinus node firing rate and sinus node action potential duration. These variables were evaluated in the control state and following drug superfusion. A typical example is seen in figure 5. No apparent alterations in these variables were noted following exposure to lidocaine, procaine amide or Ouabain.

Studies were then carried out to see the effects of stimulation site on the calculation of sinus to atrial conduction time. Estimated conduction times were calculated utilizing stimulation from the crista terminalis, low atrium near the coronary sinus and in the mid atrial septal area. The estimated conduction times were 52.5 ± 17.0, 41.5 ± 15.9 and

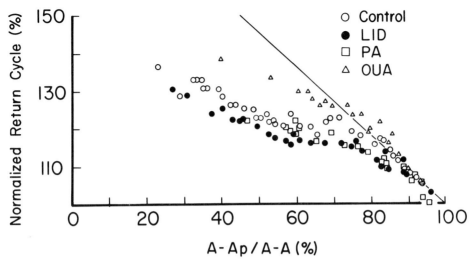

Fig. 4. The effect of drugs on sinus node to atrial conduction time as tested from the crista terminalis. The legend to the right of the figure identifies control symbols and symbols for each of the test drugs. The horizontal axis identifies the normalized test cycle and the vertical axis identifies the normalized return cycle. See text.

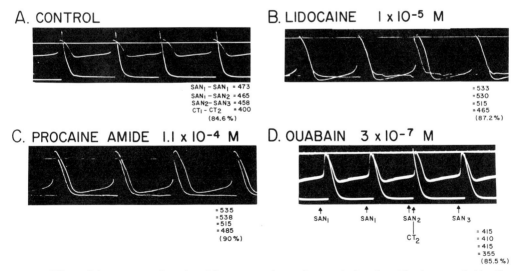

Fig. 5. Effect of late, non-conducted atrial extra systole on sinus node function. The four panels identify the effect of premature systoles originating from the crista terminalis with coupling intervals from 84.6 to 90%. The return sinus action potential is shortened. This reflects in part shortening of the sinus node action potential duration following the test crista terminalis beat. At no time did the crista terminalis beat prematurely depolarize the sinus node.

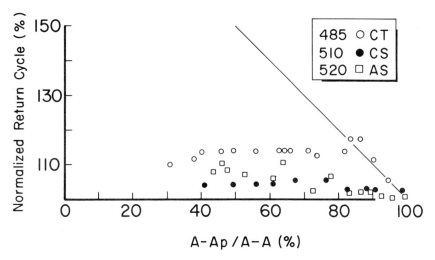

Fig. 6. Effect of different stimulation sites on sinus node to atrial conduction time. The legend to the right of the panel identifies the site of stimulation and the cycle length at the time of study. See figure 4.

37.5 ± 10.3 msec respectively: No statistically significant differences were noted. Figure 6 shows typical curves from a representative experiment.

Studies were then performed utilizing drug superfusion to determine whether these agents would charge the sinus node response to isolated extrasystoles from different atrial sites. Four studies performed utilizing the three above (fig. 7) named sites, before and after lidocaine, again demonstrated no significant changes in the estimated conduction times (CT 51.5 ± 13.2 (c), 46.0 ± 3.3 (L) (NS); AS 41.7 ± 22.4 (c), 30.0 ± 5.8 (L) (NS); CS 40.0 ± 15.0 (c), 42.5 ± 7.5 (L) (NS)). Four studies performed before and after procaine amide (fig. 8) also demonstrated the lack of effect of this drug on calculated conduction time (CT 50.0 ± 17.1 c, 53.7 ± 1.2 PA (NS); AS 57.5 ± 27.5 c, 40.0 ± 0 PA (NS); CS 55.0 ± c, 45.0 PA). Studies were also performed in one experiment with ouabain (fig. 9) and demonstrated apparent shortening in conduction times (CT 85 (CS, 40 (0); AS 85 (c), 25 (0), CS 55 (c), 80 (0)).

II. Patient studies

Sinus to atrial conduction times were assessed in 11 patients with sinus dysfunction before and within 5 minutes following Edrophonium administration. This drug significantly prolonged the estimated conduction time from 283.5 ± 56 to 300.4 ± 52.3 msec (p < 0.05).

In contrast, atropine administration significantly shortened sinus to atrial conduction time in 14 patients from 262.1 ± 46.4 to 141.1 ± 23.3 msec (p < 0.005). Similarly, isoproterenol infusion in 5 patients also significantly shortened sinus to atrial conduction time from 271.6 ± 36.8 to 124.2 ± 19.0 msec (p < 0.01).

An additional series of studies was carried out to assess the effect of various sites of stimulation on sinus to atrial conduction time. These studies compared the calculated conduction times obtained via atrial extrasystoles induced from the high right atrium

EFFECT OF LIDOCAINE (I x I0⁻⁵ M)

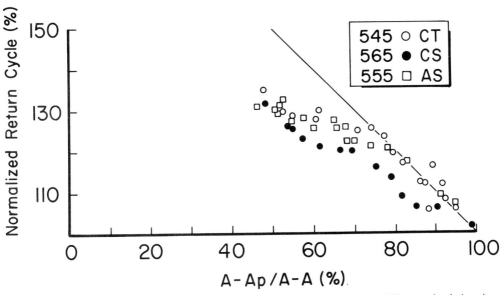

Fig. 7. The effect of lidocaine on sinus node to atrial conduction time utilizing different stimulation sites. See figure 4, 6.

EFFECT OF PROCAINE AMIDE (1.1 x 10⁻⁴ M)

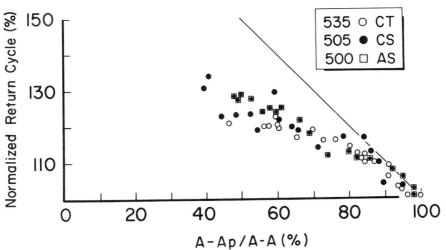

Fig. 8. Effect of procaine amide on sinus node to atrial conduction time utilizing different stimulation sites. See figure 4, 6.

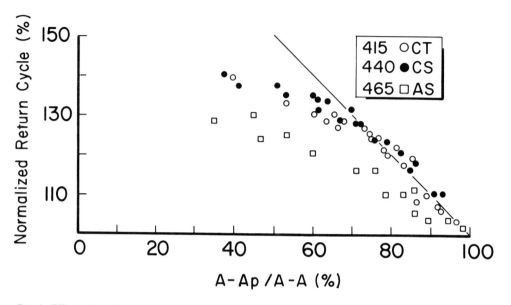

Fig. 9. Effect of ouabain on sinus node to atrial conduction time utilizing different stimulation sites. See figure 4, 6.

with data obtained from the low right atrium and distal coronary sinus locations (fig. 10). Statistically different effects were obtained when comparisons were made between the high right atrial site and the coronary sinus site (165 ± 30vs 192 ± 38 uses (NS). No significant difference was observed between calculated conduction times from the high right atrium and the low right atrial site (270 ± 46 vs 247 ± 90 msec NS).

DISCUSSION

The estimation of sinus to atrial conduction time may prove to be of great clinical significance in the evaluation of patients with historical evidence of syncopal-like attacks. Nevertheless, it has been suggested that presently available techniques are inaccurate in their measurement of this variable (18).

Data previously available from a variety of investigators have defined in detail the methods of analysis utilizing the atrial premature stimulation technique (85,86,126,334, 445,551,793,818). These authors have pointed out that late extrasystoles may influence sinus node rate without causing premature sinus discharge. Our present data confirms these observations. In addition, the variation in conduction time into and out of the sinus node was not considered equal. Our present data also confirms these observations and emphasizes that sinus to atrial conduction is longer than atrial to sinus conduction.

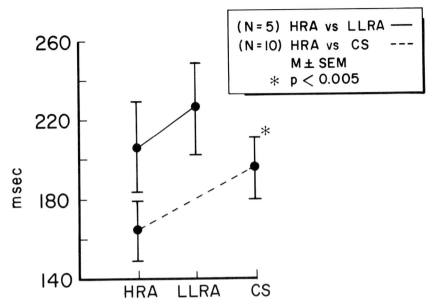

Fig. 10. Effect of site of stimulation on estimated sinus node to atrial conduction time in man. The horizontal axis identifies the test sites. The vertical axis identifies the conduction time in msec. Statistically significant differences were noted between the high right atrial and coronary sinus sites only.

Nevertheless the comparison of measured and estimated conduction did not significantly differ. However, striking individual exceptions were observed thereby expressing a precautionary note with regard to clinical utility of this method in any individual patient.

Pick and co-workers in 1951 emphasized the alteration induced in sinus discharge by premature systoles (626). Subsequently, data has been accumulated in isolated tissue and whole animal experiments as well as in man with regard to the effects of atrial extrasystoles (85, 86, 126, 311, 334, 445, 551, 626, 793, 818). However, only limited data is available as to the effects of the site of origin of the extrasystole on subsequent sinus node rate (818). Our present data has identified that with regard to sites within the right atrium; limited differences are apparent with regard to estimated conduction time. Nevertheless the effects of early extrasystoles failing to conduct if originating close to the sinus node but conducting with delay if located at a distance, may play a role in the development of reentrant arrhythmias involving sinus and perinodal tissues (126, 622, 626).

Our experimental results did moreover identify that some of our available antiarrhythmic agents would not significantly alter the response to induced extrasystoles ... regardless of the site of origin within the atrium. This observation is of interest in light of prior experimental data obtained by Paulay et al. (622). These authors observed that quindine administration could prevent the induction of sinus node reentry in intact dogs. This is in contrast to the observations by Paritzky et al that atropine administration abolished sinus node reentrant arrhythmias in man (618). Therefore, it would seem that as observed in isolated Purkinje fiber preparations, either enhancement or depression of conduction in a reentrant pathway can produce the desired effect, i.e., elimination of tachyarrhythmias. (72).

The availability of measurement of sinus to atrial conduction time in man allows the clinician to explain with more clarity some arrhythmias and conduction disturbances heretofore not elucidated. Intrinsic abnormalities of sinus node function in man have, over the past two decades, been recognized with increasing frequency (75, 228, 255, 263, 522, 706, 757). Our present studies have attempted to define whether intrinsic sinus conduction abnormalities are of significance in the clinical presentation in patients with the 'sick sinus syndrome'. Although the symptomatic manifestations of this syndrome need not be due to sinus dysfunction per se (523) sinus conduction abnormalities appear to be commonplace. Nevertheless our data supports the suggestion that a significant portion of the intrinsic pathophysiologic abnormality in this syndrome is disordered autonomic neural control. This comment is based on the dramatic shortening of sinus conduction following atropine suggesting enhanced parasympathetic stimulation. Nevertheless, the beta receptor function was intact as isoproterenol infusion produced comparable shortening.

Clinically the most commonplace situation associated with disordered sinus function is in the setting of digitalis excess. Our data are incomplete with regard to digitalis' effects on sinus to atrial conduction but in doses used in this study sinus to atrial conduction was, in fact enhanced. This paradoxical response may be a result of rapid heart rate, low exposure time and low concentration.

CLINICAL SIGNIFICANCE

Disordered sinus function in man is being recognized with increasing frequency in the clinical setting. Present methodology is, however, limited in its ability to determine, with a high degree of specificity early stages of conduction abnormality. This latter fact does not therefore allow the clinician to determine the early yet detrimental effects of cardioactive drugs on sinus node conduction characteristics.

14
OBSERVATIONS ON CIRCUSMOVEMENT TACHYCARDIA IN THE ISOLATED RABBIT ATRIUM

MAURITS A. ALLESSIE, M.D., FELIX I. M. BONKE, M.D.,
AND FRANCIEN J. G. SCHOPMAN.

It is well known both from experimental studies as from clinical observations that a premature beat arising in some part of the heart shortly after the end of the refractory period may evoke a sudden burst of rapid repetitive activity (97, 425, 492). Figure 1 gives two examples of this phenomenon. When the heart is regularly paced, as indicated by the white arrows, the application of an early premature stimulus (black arrow) does not induce merely one premature beat, but is followed by a series of depolarizations with short coupling intervals. This spontaneous activity may vary from just one coupled beat

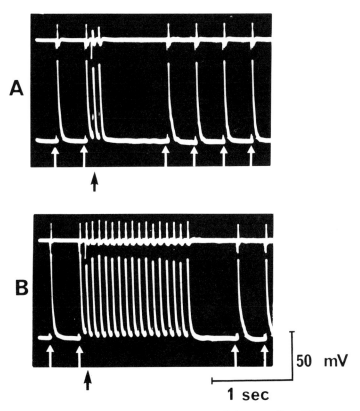

Fig. 1. Upper trace: surface electrogram. Lower trace: intracellular recording. White arrows indicate basic stimuli (interval 333 msec). Black arrows indicate moments of application of the test stimulus. In panel A the premature beat elicited by the test stimulus is followed by one extra discharge. In panel B a train of rapid repetitive activations results from the early premature beat.

(panel A) to a paroxysm of tachycardia of variable duration (panel B). The mechanism underlying this 'vulnerability' of the heart is not fully understood. There are two alternative hypotheses to explain the nature of this spontaneous activity: 1. the premature beat might induce rapid impulse formation in a group of normal atrial myocardial fibers, which then act as an ectopic pacemaker; or 2. the premature impulse might be entrapped in a circuitous route.

A direct approach, allowing a choice between these possibilities, is to map the spread of activation during the onset of tachycardia. In case of an ectopic focus one would expect a radial spread from the site where the spontaneously discharging fibers are located, whereas in case of a circus movement a circulating excitation should be found. A main difficulty of this approach however is the limitation of the number of recordings that can be made simultaneously. To overcome this limitation we developed a method to induce identical tachycardias repeatedly.

INDUCTION AND RECORDING OF TACHYCARDIA

In small segments of the left atrium of the rabbit (15 × 15 mm), containing no gross anatomic obstacle and normally showing no spontaneous activity, the application of a single properly timed premature stimulus can induce a paroxysm of tachycardia (86). However, the vulnerable period in the atrial cycle was very short, often no longer than 1–5 msec. Also the site where the premature stimulus was applied was very critical.

In fact, in most preparations only one or two places could be found where a premature stimulus caused a series of rapid spontaneous discharges, while in other preparations we even failed completely to produce tachycardias in this way. On the other hand, when once the right combination of the exact moment and the favourable place was found, it was possible to start identical tachycardias again and again. During each period of tachycardia the activation times of 10 sites of the atrium were recorded simultaneously. Before reproducing the tachycardia the multiple recording electrode was moved to another position where the next ten recordings were made. By means of a fixed reference lead it was controlled whether the subsequent tachycardias really had the same sequence of activation. In this semi-simultaneous way the moments of activation of more than 300 sites could be measured and the spread of activation during the onset of tachycardia could be reconstructed accurately (13). Since Janse and van Capelle got such excellent results with a 'brush' of 10 microelectrodes impaling in the A-V node (409), we decided to use this technique as well (12). However instead of using a brush of 10 microelectrodes glued together, we used the apparatus as illustrated in figure 2. The microelectrodes were mounted in individual holders, situated on a circle around a central stimulating electrode. By turning the wheel to which the microelectrode holders are attached, all microelectrodes could be moved together, either closer to the stimulating electrode or further away (741). With this equipment it is possible to make simultaneous intracellular recordings to every distance around the site where the induction of a premature impulse results in a paroxysm of tachycardia.

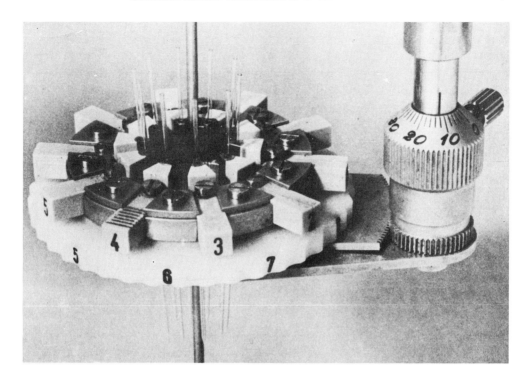

Fig. 2. Top: Photograph of tenfold electrode holder. Microelectrodes are fixed in separate holders which are mounted on a circle. In the center of the microelectrodes a stimulating electrode is placed. By turning the white wheel, the position of the microelectrodes can be adjusted concentrically. The pinion showed at the right is used to change the position of the electrodes radially over an angle of 36 degrees.

Bottom: Close-up of the electrode arrangement on the isolated segment of left atrial muscle.

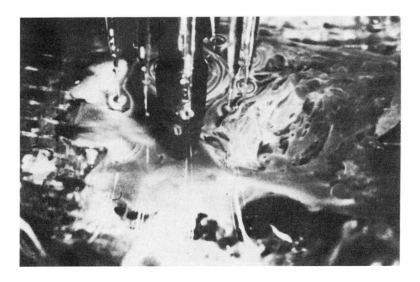

252 M. A. ALLESSIE ET AL.

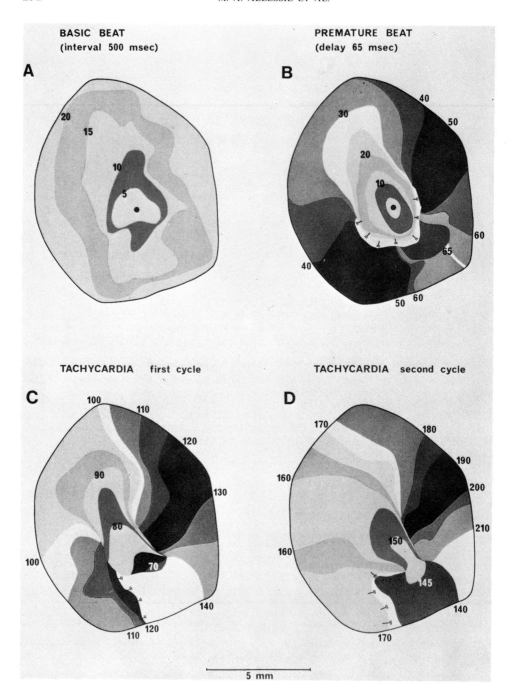

Fig. 3. Maps of the spread of activation during the onset of tachycardia as could be constructed from the intracellular recordings of more than 100 fibers. The site of stimulation is indicated by a black dot in A and B. The parts of the preparation that are activated at about the same moment (within 5 msec) are indicated with different colors. (This figure is a black and white print of a color picture.) The activation times given in the maps are related to the basic stimulus in A and to the premature stimulus in B, C and D. Double bars indicate conduction block. See text for further discussion.

MULTIPLE MICROELECTRODE RECORDINGS DURING THE ONSET OF A PAROXYSM OF TACHYCARDIA

In figure 3, a complete map of the spread of activation during the onset of tachycardia is given, as could be drawn from intracellular recordings of more than 100 fibers. The areas activated at about the same moment (within 5 msec) are indicated by different colors. During basic rhythm the impulse spread more or less radially from the point of stimulation (panel A). During the propagation of the premature impulse, elicited 65 msec after the basic beat, this concentric conduction was completely altered (panel B). First of all, the speed of propagation was diminished considerably. However the most striking change was, that antegrade conduction succeeded only in one direction (upward in figure 3B), while into the other directions the impulse was conducted only for a short distance before it died out completely. The premature impulse then turned around both sides of the blocked area splitting up in two separate wavefronts. About 65 msec after they started, these turning activation waves collided at the opposite side from which they emerged.

However before being extincted, the impulse found an entrance in the region where antegrade conduction was blocked and about 70 msec after its origin the impulse re-entered the area where it was born (see panel C). The impulse, thus entrapped in a circular course, circulated for many revolutions. Only the first two tachycardial cycles are shown in figure 3 (panel C and D). It may seem from this figure that there were actually two circular pathways during tachycardia, each of them extending to an area of no more than half a square cm. However these two circulating wavelets were not really independent since they had a part of their circuits in common. Furthermore the impulse turning in a counter-clockwise direction was blocked somewhere in the circuit (after 120 and 170 msec respectively), evidently because it travelled too fast in a circuit too small for every part of the route to restore its excitability. Only the impulse travelling in a clockwise direction was responsible for the tachycardia. The revolution time of this circulating excitation determined the rate of the arrhythmia.

Figure 4 shows a selection of action potentials recorded from the area where antegrade conduction block occurred. Here the premature impulse was conducted with decrement as indicated by the gradual decrease of amplitude and rate of rise of the early action potentials of fibers A and B. This decay of the stimulating efficacy of the antegrade activation wave continued until the impulse was unable to excite the tissue ahead. Consequently in fibers C and D lying beyond the site of block only a small electronic hump was recorded.

In figures 5 and 6 a period of tachycardia is shown during which the transmembrane potentials of five fibers (A-E) lying along the circular pathway were recorded simultaneously. The exact position of the fibers is indicated by the corresponding letters in the maps of figure 6. Fiber A is lying on the antegrade pathway. Therefore in this fiber the increase of the latency after the premature stimulus (20 msec) compared with the delay in activation after the basic stimulus (12 msec) is caused completely by a decrease in condition velocity. Fibers B and C are located in a part of the atrium where antegrade conduction of the premature impulse failed. In these fibers although situated only a few

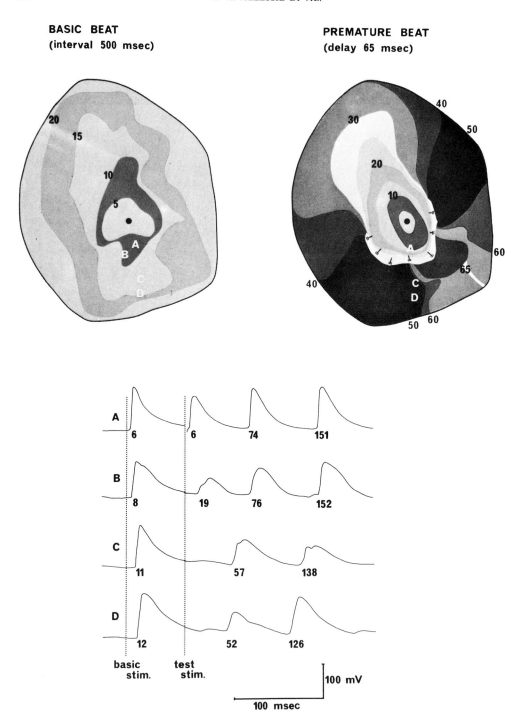

Fig. 4. Maps of the spread of activation during the basic beat and the premature beat of the same experiment as depicted in figure 3, together with the membrane potentials of fibers located in the area of antegrade conduction block of the premature impulse. The site of the fibers is indicated by the corresponding letters in the maps.

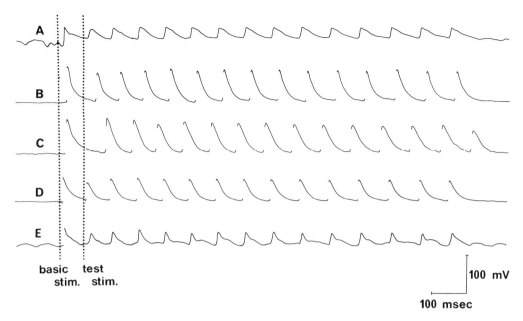

basic   test
 stim.   stim.

100 mV

100 msec

Fig. 5. Simultaneous intracellular recordings of five fibers during a short period of tachycardia. The fibers are lying on the circuit in which the impulse is trapped during the tachycardia. The exact position of the fibers is indicated by the corresponding letters in the maps of figure 6.

mm from the point of stimulation, no trace of antegrade conduction could be detected. The delayed response exhibited by these fibers (41 and 63 msec) is mainly caused by the roundabout way the premature impulse travelled to reach these fibers. Fibers D and E which were proximal to the area of block not only showed an antegrade response (latency 6 and 21 msec respectively) but were also activated retrogradely (delay 74 and 83 msec) by the wave-front travelling from A to B to C. It is in the surrounding of fiber D that re-entry occurred for the first time. This sequence of activation as established during the premature beat was maintained during the rest of the tachycardia. After thirteen cycles, the circus movement was suddenly interrupted. From the recordings in figure 6 it can be seen that the impulse was blocked on its 13th round trip somewhere between fiber C and D.

The last action potential of this period of tachycardia was recorded from fiber C. Compared with the responses of this fiber in an earlier stage of the tachycardia, this last action potential already showed a decrease in amplitude and rate of rise. It may be assumed that this fall in stimulating efficacy of the circulating impulse gradually increased on its way from C to D finally resulting in a failure to excite the tissue ahead. A satisfactory explanation for this spontaneous interruption of the circus movement can not yet be given except that one may suppose that slight spontaneous changes in electrophysiologic properties of the fibers composing the circular pathway, might be enough to disturb the delicate equilibrium between excitation and recovery of excitability which exist when an impulse is travelling in such a small circuit.

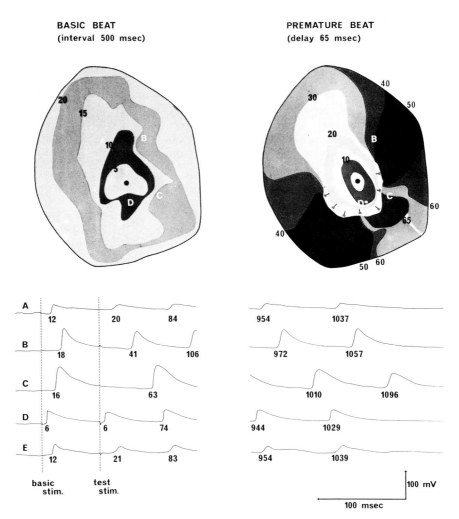

Fig. 6. Simultaneous intracellular recordings of the same fibers given in figure 5. The recording sites are marked on the maps. The activity of these fibers during the onset and the termination of the tachycardia are shown at a larger time scale. See text for further explanation.

SIGNIFICANCE OF NONUNIFORM RECOVERY OF EXCITABILITY FOR THE OCCURRENCE OF UNIDIRECTIONAL BLOCK

Since the occurrence of unidirectional block is a first requisite condition for the initiation of circus movement tachycardia, the question arises what kind of inhomogeneity of the atrium is responsible for the occurrence of local block. At least three possibilities have to be mentioned: 1. variations in membrane responsiveness resulting in differences in stimulating efficacy of a depolarization wave; 2. differences in geometry creating pathways of preferential conduction; and 3. differences in the rate of recovery of excitability. Since the last possibility is exclusively affecting the propagation of early premature impulses, we investigated whether nonuniform recovery of excitability played a role in the initiation of circus movement tachycardia.

The refractory period, defined as the minimal delay between the basic stimulus and a test stimulus (duration 1 msec, strength 4 times threshold) which resulted in a propagated response, was determined at about 50 sites of the isolated left atrium. We found that in most preparations there was a considerable dispersion in recovery of excitability, the difference between shortest and longest refractory period amounting to about 30 msec. In preparations, demonstrating a more or less uniform restoration of excitability, it was very difficult or even impossible to find a place where tachycardia could be induced. On the other hand, if a premature stimulus initiated tachycardia, this was always on the border of two areas where a considerable difference in refractory period could be demonstrated. Furthermore, relating the spread of a premature impulse which initiated circus movement with the dispersion of refractory periods, it was striking that always the premature impulse was propagated into the direction with the shorter refractory period, while it was blocked into the direction where excitability was restored at a slower rate. In figure 7 the results of one of these experiments are shown. This strongly suggests that dispersion of refractory periods plays a key role in the occurrence of unidirectional block and thus in circus movement tachycardia.

WHAT IS HAPPENING IN THE CENTRE OF A CIRCUS MOVEMENT?

Most studies on re-entry and circus movement in cardiac tissue are done, either in the intact heart (221,351,497) or in parts of the heart isolated in such a way that the preparations got a more or less ringlike structure (552,553,931). Other investigators made artificial barriers to facilitate the production of circulating excitations in the experiment (697). In contrast to these studies, the isolated segments of rabbit atrial muscle which we used did not contain any gross anatomical obstacle. This raises the question what is happening in the centre of a circus movement when there is no anatomical obstacle present to serve as an inexcitable centre around which the impulse may circulate. A possible explanation which we suggested before (13) is that the membrane potential of the fibers in the centre is held above threshold by electrotonic influence of the depolarization process which continuously turns around this area. In this way the centre would be functional inexcitable and the activation wave, instead of travelling around an anatomical barrier, then would circulate around a functional obstacle.

However intracellular recordings from the centre of a circus movement made clear that such a functional inexcitability does not exist. We therefore now postulate the model of the 'leading circle'. The leading circle is the smallest possible circuit in which the impulse can circulate. In this pathway the crest of the activation wave always encounters tissue that has restored its excitability just enough to be reactivated by the circulating wavelet. From this leading circle not only the periphery is activated but also centripetal wavelets are emerging which invade the central region. These centripetal wavelets collide to each other in the centre where they are extinguished (see fig. 8). In contrast with a circus movement around an anatomical obstacle, neither the position nor the

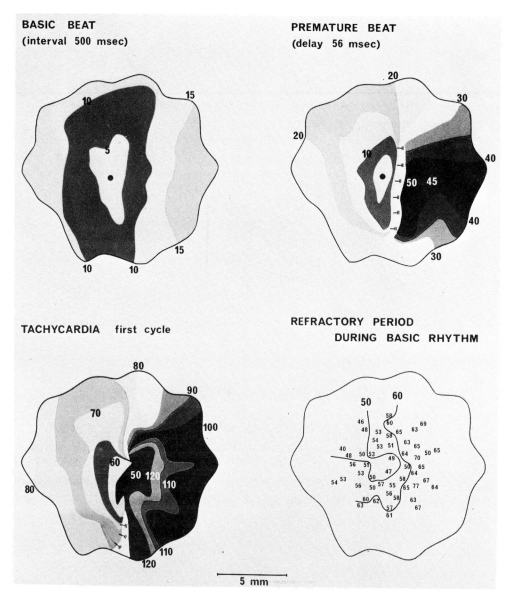

Fig. 7. Map of the refractory periods during basic rhythm together with the spread of activation during the onset of tachycardia as could be induced in this preparation. The site of stimulation is indicated by a black dot. Double bars indicate conduction block. See text for further discussion.

dimension of a leading circle are fixed. One of the consequences of this concept can be described as follows. Suppose that during a circus movement tachycardia the refractory period of the atrial fibers is shortened for some reason, without a change in the conduction velocity of the impulse. In this case the dimension of the leading circle will become smaller and consequently the revolution time will get shorter. As a result the rate of the tachycardia will increase. If, on the other hand, the impulse is conducted around an

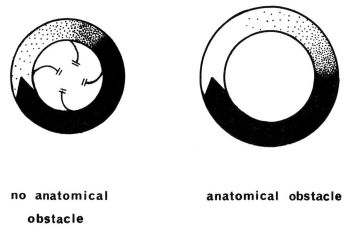

no anatomical

anatomical obstacle

obstacle

Fig. 8. Two models of circus movement of the cardiac impulse. At the right the classical model for circus movement around an anatomical obstacle. The black part of the circuit represents tissue that is in the absolute
refractory state. The dotted area contains fibers which are in the relative refractory period, while in the white
in the white part excitability has restored completely. At the left the model according to the leading circle hypothesis. Here a central anatomical obstacle is absent. In this model there is no white area: the crest of the circulating wave front always encounters tissue which has restored its excitability just enough to be excited. Thus the
leading circle represents the smallest possible pathway in which the impulse can circulate. From this leading
circle both the periphery and the central region are activated. In the centre the centripetal wavelets are colliding
with each other.

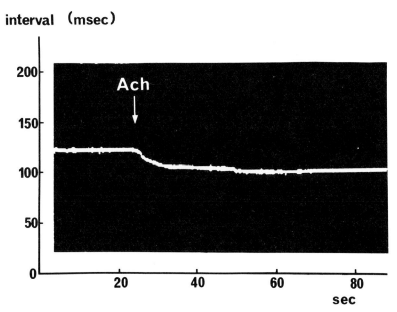

Fig. 9. Effect of Acetylcholine on the rate of tachycardia. After the administration of acetylcholine to the tissue
bath, the revolution time of the circus movement decreased from 125 to 104 msec.

anatomical obstacle, a shortening of the refractory period is not expected to cause any change in the revolution time of the impulse. The only effect will be that the part of the circuit that has completely restored its excitability—the white part in the schematic drawing of figure 8—will enlarge. To test the validity of the leading circle concept, the theoretically expected differences in behaviour between the two models as illustrated in figure 8 have to be tested.

So far we did only some preliminary experiments in this direction. Figure 9 shows the effect of acetylcholine, added to the perfusion fluid during a long lasting tachycardia. The marked decrease of the revolution time as response to the shortening of the refractory period caused by acetylcholine, is in good agreement with the leading circle hypothesis. However further investigation is necessary to elucidate whether the leading circle concept is correct.

The demonstration of micro-re-entry in atrial muscle, as presented in this paper, offers a possible explanation for those cases of supraventricular tachycardia where re-entry in the AV node or SA node is unlikely and also no long circuitous pathway can be detected. Furthermore it gives support to the hypothesis that fibrillation is based on the existence of multiple circulating wavelets (556–557). This is true in spite of the fact that in our experiments we never observed tachycardias turning into fibrillation: under the circumstances of the experiment, fibrillation might be prevented by the small dimensions of the atrial preparation, offering no room for more than one independently circulating wavelet.

THE ATRIOVENTRICULAR JUNCTION, THE BUNDLE
BRANCHES AND THE VENTRICLE

15

MORPHOLOGY OF THE HUMAN ATRIOVENTRICULAR JUNCTIONAL AREA

ANTON E. BECKER, M.D., AND ROBERT H. ANDERSON, M.D.

INTRODUCTION

The nature of the precise morphology and architecture of the human atrioventricular node and its adjacent junctional areas must still be considered a controversial subject. To a great extent this controversy reflects the differences that exist between individual hearts, the changes which take place in the junctional area during growth of the individual and the different techniques employed for their study by different investigators. Moreover, considerable discrepancies exist between the definition of the 'atrioventricular node' as given by morphologists, clinicians and electrophysiologists. Some of the discrepancies relate to the fact that the atrioventricular node, as defined by most modern day morphologists, refers only to part of the original structure described by Tawara (804). For example, the human node recently has been described as a structure composed solely of a network of small fibers (485). However, the 'node' as thus defined corresponds only to the area of 'Knotenpunkten' described by Tawara (804). Indeed, Tawara himself never used the term 'node'. This term was introduced by Keith and Flack (431), who thus attributed this name to only one part of the proximal extensions of the specialized atrioventricular structures described by Tawara (804). Tawara, additionally described cells transitional in form between the area composed of 'Knotenpunkten' and the atrial working myocardium, but this fact is infrequently commented upon by modern day authorities. It is possible that consideration of the atrioventricular node as being composed only of the area of interweaving cells may account for the fact that only a poor correlation could be made between this area and the area defined as the node by electrophysiologists (366).

These latter investigators stated that from a functional point of view the node should be considered as the area producing atrioventricular conduction delay. Recent studies in our laboratories (31), have demonstrated that in the rabbit heart this area of delay indeed corresponds to the tightly packed 'morphological' node, together with an area of transitional cells corresponding to that previously described by Tawara (804). The discrepancies that exist between morphology and electrophysiology, therefore, can be related to differing interpretations of earlier descriptions.

It is also pertinent to consider the statement of Truex and Smythe (840), that in order to comprehend fully the exact arrangement of a complex three dimensional structure such as the atrioventricular junctional area, reconstructions of the area are essential. However, to the best of our knowledge, the study of Truex and Smythe (840), is the only one using the human material that is founded upon this approach. It is therefore right and proper that a recent special article (353), by a group of distinguished American investigators concerning the nomenclature of the atrioventricular node was to a great extent based upon this study. However, other concepts were incorporated into this nomenclature, such as those of James and colleagues (389, 754), which in many respects are in disagreement with those adduced from the investigation of Truex and Smythe (840). This is particularly true with regard to the morphology of the nodal approaches and the existence of so-called 'by-pass fibers'. For these reasons, the present authors, together with their collaborators in morphology within the European Study Group for Pre-excitation, outlined their own concepts of the architecture of the human junctional area, basing their approach, like Truex and Smythe (840), upon three-dimensional reconstructions (33). The views presented in this chapter are a distillate of this work, together with additional findings from ongoing studies in our laboratories.

THE ATRIOVENTRICULAR JUNCTIONAL AREA

The atrioventricular junctional area is defined as the area of the atrioventricular specialized tissues forming the connection between the atrial and ventricular working myocardia. It is composed of cells which are histologically distinct from 'working' myocardium. Its atrial component is localized anteriorly in the base of the atrial septum, mainly on the right atrial aspect of the central fibrous body (fig. 1). The junctional tissue extends

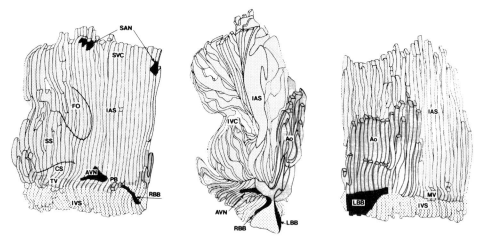

Fig. 1. Reconstruction of the interatrial septum and superior rim of the ventricular septum taken from a young adult of 19 years of age. The superior vena cava (SVC) had been opened, thereby now separating the two portions of the sinoatrial node (SAN). The tissues of the sinoatrial node and atrioventricular junctional area were the only histologically specialized areas. The reconstruction is shown from its right side (left hand drawing), from in front (center) and from its left side (right hand drawing). The atrioventricular junctional area is located anteriorly in the base of the atrial septum, mainly on the right atrial aspect of the central fibrous body. However, as indicated in the text, the atrioventricular junctional area should not be considered a right atrial structure. Only the deep component of the atrioventricular junctional area has been indicated in this reconstruction. FO = foramen ovale. IAS = interatrial septum. SS = sinus septum. CS = coronary sinus. AVN = atrioventricular node. PB = penetrating bundle. RBB = right bundle branch. LBB = left bundle branch. IVC = inferior vena cava. TV = tricuspid valve. IVS = interventricular septum. Ao = aorta; MV = mitral valve.

Table 1. Main differences with definitions of Hecht and colleagues.

Hecht et al.	Presently proposed
Nodal approaches	'Transitional cell zone'
Penetrating part of AV bundle Non-branching part of AV bundle	'Penetrating bundle'
Junctional tissues exclude branching bundle	Junctional area includes branching bundle*

*We would point out that from a morphologic point of view it is hard to exclude the branching portion of the nodal-bundle axis from the junctional tissues. However, we accept the fact that from a clinical and electrophysiologic point of view it may indeed be important to differentiate arrhythmias that occur in this area from those that originate in the compact node or penetrating bundle (629).

through the fibrous body to the ventricles. On the basis of cellular morphology and architecture four different zones can be recognized. These are: 1. a transitional zone between working atrial myocardium and the compact atrioventricular node; 2. the compact atrioventricular node; 3. the penetrating atrioventricular bundle; and 4. the branching atrioventricular bundle. In many ways this nomenclature is in keeping with that proposed by the American investigators (353), but differs in certain respects as indicated in table 1. These differences will be amplified and discussed by elaborating the structure of each of the zones of the area. For ease of comprehension, these will be described in reverse order.

A. Branching atrioventricular bundle
This bifurcating part of the junctional area is situated astride the muscular ventricular septum, related superiorly to the membranous septum (fig. 2F). In our experience, the cells of the left bundle branch cascade as a continuous sheet from the branching bundle upon the septum (fig. 2D and E). The bundle, having given off the left branches continues as the right bundle branch, which usually runs an intramyocardial course. The right bundle branch can therefore be considered as the direct continuation of the branching bundle, as is well illustrated by our reconstruction (fig. 3). In our material, the cells composing the branching and proximal bundle branches are of similar size to working 'cells' and do not approximate in morphology to 'Purkinje' cells.

B. Penetrating bundle
This structure is the proximal continuation of the branching bundle (fig. 2C), the junctional point being that at which the first downgoing left bundle branch fascicle is observed. The cells of the penetrating bundle are enclosed by the connective tissue of the central fibrous body and the membranous septum (fig. 2C). In its distal portion the constituent cells are similar in morphology to the branching bundle, and again we would stress that it is rare in our experience for these cells to exhibit 'Purkinje' characteristics. In its proximal extent, the cells of the penetrating bundle are more heterogeneous, the superficial cells resembling those of the compact node (fig. 4C and D). However, as will be elaborated

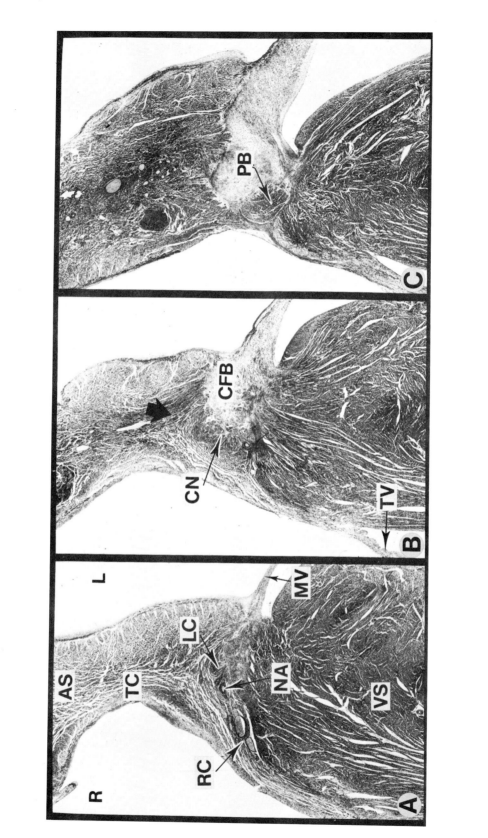

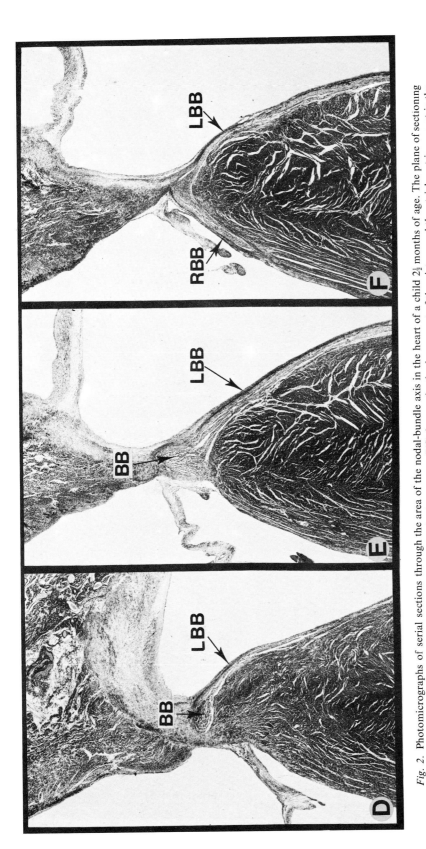

Fig. 2. Photomicrographs of serial sections through the area of the nodal-bundle axis in the heart of a child 2½ months of age. The plane of sectioning is perpendicular to the atrioventricular ring. The ventricular septum (VS) is seen in the lower part of the picture and the atrial part is present in the upper part. R = right side of the heart. L = left side of the heart. All sections are stained with a Masson trichrome stain; ×15. Figure 2A is taken posteriorly, just in front of the ostium of the coronary sinus. The deep nodal component is split into a right-going (RC) and left-going (LC) component. The nodal artery (NA) separates the two components. Both components make contact with superficial transitional cells (TC), with the left-going component still being in contact with the left side of the interatrial septum (AS). Figure 2B is taken more anteriorly. The two components have joined to form the compact node (CN), which makes close contact with both superficial transitional cells and the left side of the septum (arrow). CFB = central fibrous body. Figure 2C is taken through the area of the penetrating bundle (PB). The nodal-bundle axis is now completely encased within the fibrous tissue of the central fibrous body. Figures 2D and E show the branching bundle (BB) on top of the ventricular septum giving rise to a continuous sheet of left bundle branches (LBB). Figure 2F shows the termination of the branching bundle (BB), now astride the ventricular septum, and its continuation as right bundle branch (RBB).

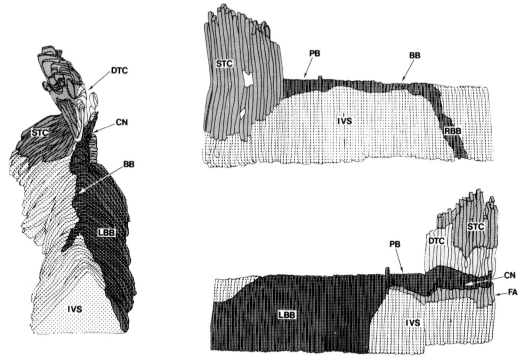

Fig. 3. Reconstruction of the atrioventricular junctional area from the heart illustrated in figure 1. Only the interventricular septum (broadly spaced spots-IVS) and the fibrous anulus (horizontal lines-FA) have been reconstructed apart from the specialized tissues. The bundle branches (RBB, LBB), penetrating bundle (PB) and compact node (CN) are shaded in heavy spots (BB-branching bundle). The superficial (STC) and deep (DTC) transitional cells are demonstrated. Note that the superficial transitional cells descend across the compact node throughout its extent. Note also that the leftward-going component of the compact node receives contributions from the deep transitional cells throughout its extent. The node itself is clearly an interatrial structure rather than a right atrial structure, receiving important contributions from the left side of the septum.

below, as long as the bundle is completely enclosed by fibrous tissue of the central body, we continue to define it as penetrating bundle, irrespective of its cytological characteristics. It is frequent for extensions of the penetrating bundle to be observed which pass into the central fibrous body, particularly in its proximal portions. These extensions are seen in adult hearts as well as infantile hearts (fig. 5). We have not observed them to be the seat of pathological change. When followed through serial sections, particularly in younger hearts, it is possible to trace elongated and tenuous fasciculo-ventricular connections through the fibrous body. However, it is exceedingly rare in our experience to find large, well formed bundles connecting the penetrating bundle to the ventricular septal crest such as exist in embryonic and fetal hearts (411).

C. Compact atrioventricular node

The superficial cells of the penetrating atrioventricular bundle are identical in morphology to those of the compact node (fig. 4). Since the junctional point of these different cellular zones varied considerably in different specimens, and on some occasions extended a

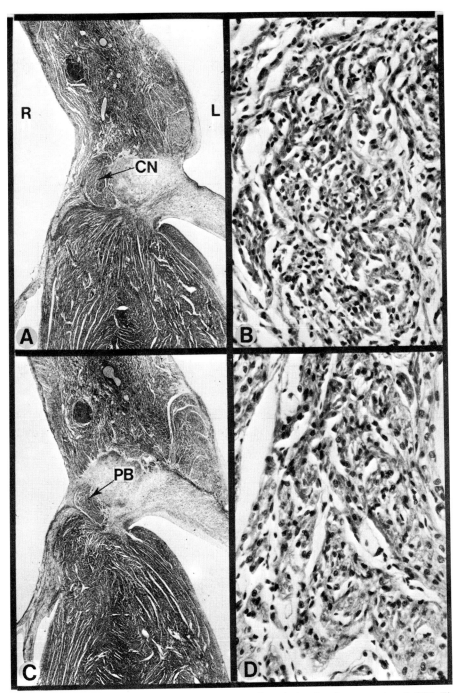

Fig. 4. Photomicrographs of serial sections of the nodal-bundle axis showing the compact node (CN; Fig. 4A) and the penetrating bundle (PB; fig. 4C). Part of the compact node is composed of interlacing cells, forming the 'Knotenpunkten' described by Tawara (804), illustrated in Figure 4B. Figure 4D is taken from the penetrating bundle and illustrates that the area with 'Knotenpunkten' continues into the nodal-bundle axis for a considerable length. Therefore, this cytological feature is an unsuitable criterion for distinguishing the penetrating bundle from the compact node. R = right side of the heart; L = left side of the heart. Masson trichrome stain A,C: ×15; B,D: ×350.

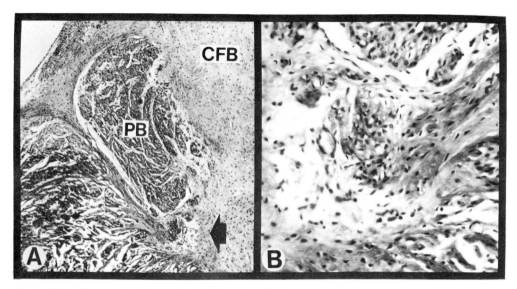

Fig. 5. Photomicrographs of a section in the region of the penetrating bundle (PB). Figure 5A shows the bundle completely encased within the central fibrous body (CFB). Extensions of the penetrating bundle (arrow) are observed passing into the central fibrous body. Figure. 5B shows these extensions at a higher magnification. Pathological changes within these cell nests were not observed. Masson trichrome stain, A: ×50; B: ×350.

considerable distance distally, we considered it an unsuitable criterion on which to base distinction between the compact node and the penetrating bundle. We found a much better criterion to be the point at which the compact node ceased to make contact with transitional atrial fibers, that is to say the point at which it became encircled by connective tissue and did indeed become penetrating (fig. 6). As we will expain below, this point also varied, and contacts with the node were also varied.

However, it is our opinion that this definition is more satisfactory than one based upon cytological examination. For our purposes, therefore, the compact atrioventricular node is that part of the junctional area in contact with the atrial myocardium. The contacting atrial myocardium also for the most part shows specialized features and will be described subsequently as the transitional cell zone.

The compact node as defined corresponds with the area of 'Knotenpunkten' described by Tawara (804); with the interweaving area described by Lev (485) and with the area reconstructed by Truex and Smythe (840). As described by these latter workers, its distal extent can be divided into deep and superficial strata, the whole being surrounded by the half oval cascades of transitional cells (fig. 2B). In our experience, it is rare to find large areas of 'interweaving' cells. The deep strata tends to be composed of small cells oriented in a parallel fashion to the anulus fibrosus (fig. 7). The superficial strata, particularly in infantile hearts, is composed of lattice like bundles, each of the bundles being composed of multiple small cells (fig. 7). These were the cells described by Anderson and Latham (19) as nodal fasciculi. They are much less well seen in older specimens, and indeed the distinction into nodal strata can rarely be made when adult nodes are examined. However, there is no doubt that when both infantile and adult nodes are studied the compact nodal zone

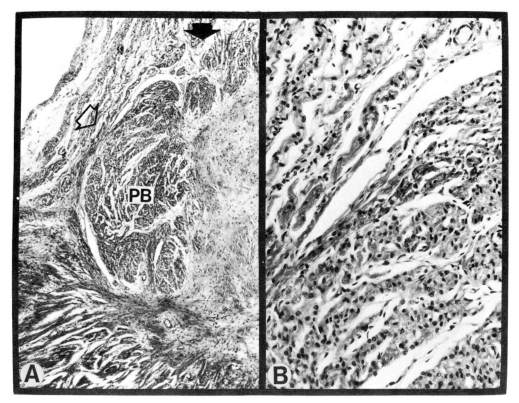

Fig. 6. Photomicrographs of a section which shows the nodal-bundle axis in the area of transition from compact node to penetrating bundle. Figure 6A shows the 'beginning' of the penetrating bundle (PB), since the nodal-bundle axis is now nearly completely encased by fibrous tissue. The deep fibers which previously contacted the compact node are already completely sealed off (closed arrow). In this specimen, the superficial transitional cells are the 'last' fibers to contact the node (open arrow). Figure 6B shows the area of 'last' fiber contact in greater detail. Masson trichrome stain, A: ×50; B: ×225.

can be observed to bifurcate, the two limbs diverging towards the tricuspid and mitral sides of the septal anulus fibrosus (fig. 2A). The cells composing the posterior extensions are small and tightly packed. The fascicle running to the tricuspid anulus approximates to the tricuspid ring tissue observed in human hearts (31), and indeed in fetal specimens the two structures are continuous. It is possible that this structure corresponds to the tract of cells which James (389) described as passing from the posterior 'internodal tract' to the bundle. He suggested it may function as a by-pass tract. However, as we shall describe, we have not observed any such superficial tract contacting the anterior bundle. The fasciculus presently described is a deep structure, is continuous with the posterior aspect of the compact node and is traced into the atrial margin of the anulus fibrosus. The mitral extension from the compact node is again composed of tightly packed, small cells, but these are less readily identified as being specialized. This extension frequently extends into the fibrous tissue of the anulus (fig. 8), and often becomes completely seques-trated from the septum. The bundle may fade out within the anulus, but may also run superficially to re-establish contact with the septum. In one instance we have followed

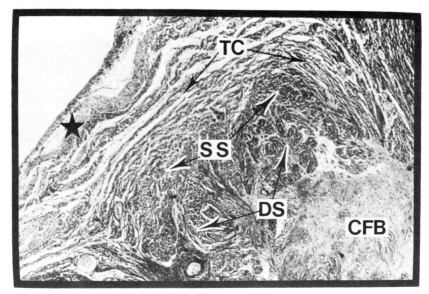

Fig. 7. Photomicrographs through the area of the compact node. The different orientation of the cells in the deep and superficial parts is clearly indicated. The deep strata (DS) tend to be composed of small cells orientated in a parallel fashion to the anulus fibrosis (CFB). The superficial strata (SS) are composed of lattice-like bundles, each of the bundles being composed of multiple small cells. They are surrounded by the half-oval cascades of transitional cells (TC), which in part insert into the tricuspid valve base. Between the superficial layer of transitional cells and the right atrial endocardium a sheet of ordinary 'working' atrial myocardial cells (asterisk) is present. Masson trichrome stain; ×50.

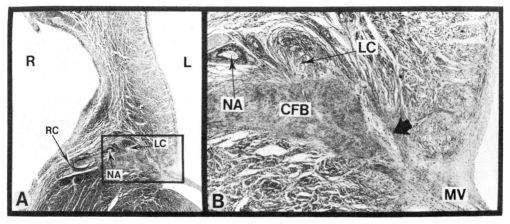

Fig. 8. Photomicrograph of a section through the posterior extent of the nodal-bundle axis. Figure 8A shows both the right-going component (RC) and left-going component (LC) separated by the AV nodal artery (NA). The left-going component is still in contact with deep transitional cells. Figure 8B shows a higher magnification of the boxed area indicated in figure 8A. A strand of specialized cells (arrow) is seen to extend from the left-going component (LC) into the central fibrous body (CFB), close to the mitral valve base (MV). Masson trichrome stain, A: ×15; B: ×50.

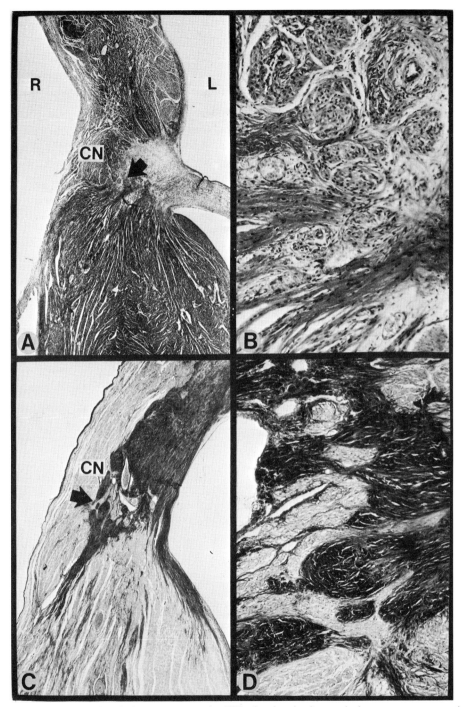

Fig. 9. Photomicrographs of the compact node (CN) showing 'nodo-ventricular accessory connections'. Figure 9A and B show an infantile specimen (Masson trichrome stain); Figure 9C and D show an adult specimen (elastica van Gieson stain). Figure 9B shows a magnification of the area indicated by the arrow in figure 9A. The strands are composed of cells identical to those present in the compact node. Figure 9D shows a similar situation in the adult heart, albeit that the enveloping connective tissue has a more compact appearance. A,C: ×15; B: ×140; D: ×90.

this bundle to make contact with the ventricular septum (300). Such fibers may be comparable with the posterior transient accessory atrioventricular muscle bundles described by Truex et al. (834). However, we would emphasize that such strands extending through the anulus and establishing contact with either atrial or ventricular myocardia are findings in numerous apparently normal hearts (fig. 9). We would hesitate before implicating such structures, to be anticipated on developmental premises (32), as substrates for circus movements and hence sudden death (406). Such fibers, if extending from specialized tissue to ventricle, would be comparable with the fibers described by Mahaim (517). However, since there is some confusion regarding the precise definition of 'Mahaim' fibers, the European Study Group for Pre-excitation has suggested that such fibers should be termed 'nodo-ventricular accessory connections' (33,909). It should also be stressed that in our experience all constituent cells of the compact node were small; 'Purkinje'-like cells were not observed.

D. Transitional cell zone

The transitional cell zone in our definition is the zone occupied by cells we consider to be histologically distinct from atrial myocardium (fig. 10), and which intervene between the atrial myocardium and the discrete cells of the compact node. The transitional cells differ

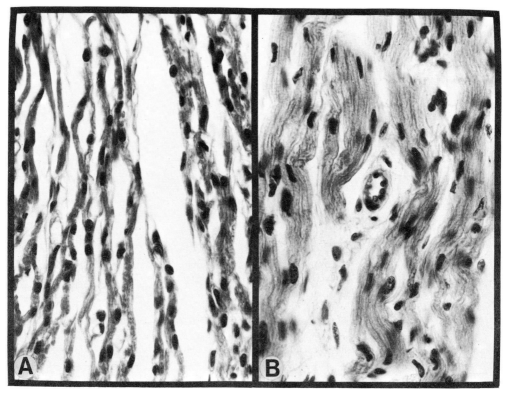

Fig. 10. Photomicrograph demonstrating the histological distinction between transitional cells (fig. 10A) and working atrial myocardium (fig. 10B) in an infantile specimen. Masson trichrome stain, A,B: ×500.

from the cells of the compact node in that they are more widely separated and tend to be arranged individually, being interpersed with connective tissue. At the junction with the compact node the cells coalesce in typical fashion (fig. 7). The zone of transitional cells is comparable with the intermediate area described by Tawara (804) and with the 'nodal approaches' defined by Lev (485). Only the nodal insertions of these cells were reconstructed by Truex and Smythe (840). The transitional cell zone itself could be divided into three groups—posterior, superficial and deep.

The posterior group approached the node both from the sinus septum and from a muscular tract extending beneath the coronary sinus into the posterior atrial wall. This latter approach should not be neglected, since it supplies an important nodal 'input' both in terms of size, embryological development (32), and function, the latter at least being true in the rabbit heart (408). This route has apparently been neglected by James (393) in his concept of spread of the sinus impulse. The cells of this route, and those of the sinus septum, do not exhibit specialized characteristics until close upon the compact node. They then tend to fill the space between the bifurcations of the compact node, and surround the nodal artery (fig. 2A). It follows, therefore, that the specialized cells of the junctional area are not encountered until one is well in front of the coronary sinus. For this reason we consider it fallacious to relate the node to the ostium of the coronary sinus.

The superficial transitional cells sweep forward from the sinus septum and inferiorly from the anterior limbus. Again they do not become recognized as specialized until adjacent to the compact node, usually at a point below but superficial to the Tendon of Todaro (vide infra). The anterior transitional cells hug the compact node in a tight half oval, but then pass on into the tricuspid valve base (fig. 2B). In infantile specimens an additional layer of working cells is observed superficial to the overlay cells, but this is rarely seen in adult hearts. Once the compact node has become the penetrating bundle it is rare, according to our definition of the penetrating bundle, to find the transitional cells contacting the bundle, that is through an anterior defect in the anulus. Indeed, neither this feature nor these cells making contact with ventricular myocardium was observed in our material, but the latter instance was reported by James (389).

The deep transitional cells are an important but short group which connect the left side of the atrial septum to the deep part of the compact node and its mitral limb throughout their extent. The presence of these cells emphasize that the node is an interatrial structure, as pointed out previously by Scherf and Cohen (730). In all our specimens, transitional cells could be traced for only short distances from the compact node before merging and joining with working atrial myocardium. We have defined our compact nodal-bundle junction as the point at which contact with transitional cells is lost. It must be emphasized that this 'last' contact with the atrial myocardium can occur through either superficial or deep transitional cells.

A diagrammatic representation of the atrioventricular junctional area based upon the material described above is given below (fig. 11). Secondary to this concept it is necessary to expand and discuss further topics concerning the area which are of both interest and controversy. Points discussed will be:

I The Tendon of Todaro

II 'By-Pass Tracts'

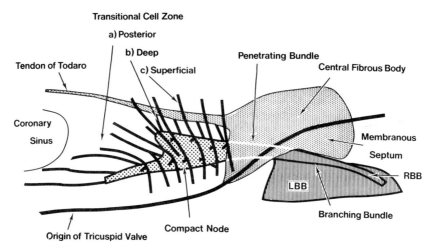

Fig. 11. Diagrammatic representation of the atrioventricular junctional area. The specialized area is divided into four different zones, i.e. the branching bundle, the penetrating bundle, the compact node and the transitional cell zone. The compact node, which is composed of a leftward and rightward-going component, is continuous anteriorly with the penetrating bundle. The compact node is contacted by three groups of transitional cells; superficial, passing superficial to the tendon of Todaro and partly extending over the compact node into the tricuspid valve base; deep, connecting with the left side of the septum and a posterior group. The last group connects with the myocardium both above and below the ostium of the coronary sinus. LBB = left bundle branch. RBB = right bundle branch.

III 'Mahaim Fibers'
IV Atrial Pathways
V Vascular Supply
VI Innervation
VII Ageing changes

I. THE TENDON OF TODARO

This structure is important both as a landmark to the position of the compact node and a fibrous partition subdividing the transitional cell zone. Although eponymously referred to as Todaro's Tendon, much credit for its full description must go to Orsos (610). The tendon originates in the central fibrous body, directly above the point of junction between the compact node and the penetrating bundle. When traced posteriorly, it passes intramuscularly through the atrial septum, separating deep and superficial transitional cells, and becomes subendocardial on the sinus septum, where it continues with the Eustachian valve. If tension is placed upon the Eustachian valve, a triangle is produced between the Tendon of Todaro and the tricuspid anulus (fig. 12). The apex of this triangle is a landmark to the position of the compact node. It should be emphasized that the structure is fibrous throughout its length (fig. 13). It is possible that James (393) was referring to this structure when he described a 'false tendon' as the continuation of the Eustachian valve.

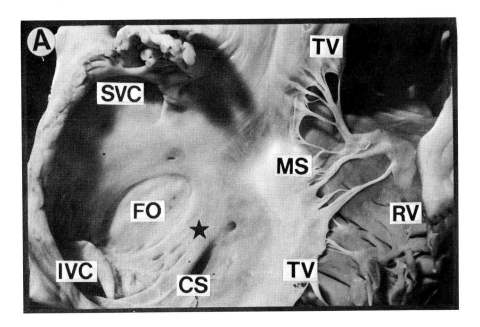

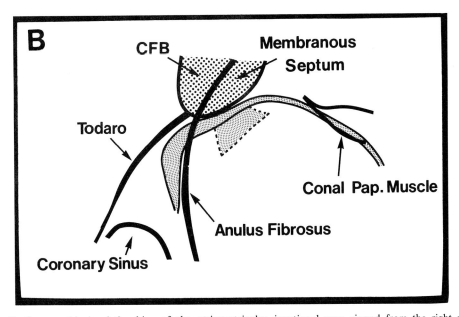

Fig. 12. Topographical relationships of the atrioventricular junctional area viewed from the right side. Figure 12A shows a heart specimen, in which the right atrium has been opened. The membranous septum (MS) is transilluminated. SVC = superior vena cava. IVC = inferior vena cava. FO = fossa ovalis. CS = coronary sinus. RV = right ventricle. The Eustachian ridge is indicated by an asterisk. For comparison, figure 12B shows a drawing of the main structures involved, viewed from a similar angle. The tendon of Todaro which runs in the Eustachian ridge inserts into the central fibrous body. The area of the compact node is delineated by the tendon of Todaro, the central fibrous body and the tricuspid valve base. The apex of this triangle is a landmark to the position of the compact node. This is a better landmark for the position of the 'node' than the ostium of the coronary sinus.

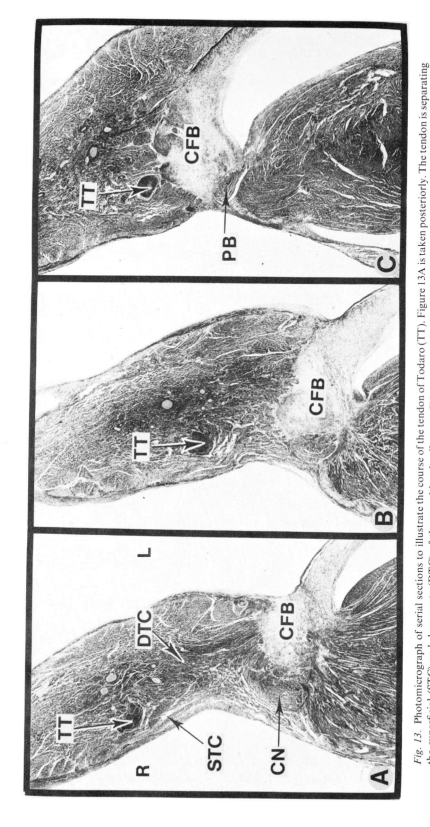

Fig. 13. Photomicrograph of serial sections to illustrate the course of the tendon of Todaro (TT). Figure 13A is taken posteriorly. The tendon is separating the superficial (STC) and deep parts (DTC) of the transitional cell zone. CN = compact node. Figure 13B, taken more anteriorly, shows the tendon of Todaro approaching the central fibrous body (CFB). The nodal-bundle axis shows the transition from compact node to penetrating bundle. Figure 13C shows the insertion of the tendon of Todaro into the central fibrous body. At this point the penetrating bundle (PB) is deeply embedded within the central fibrous body. R = right side of the heart. L = left side of the heart. Masson trichrome stain; × 15.

II. 'BY-PASS' TRACTS

The concept of the 'by-pass tract' was introduced by James (389) on the basis of morphological studies to provide an explanation of some abnormalities of atrioventricular conduction which could be distinguished electrophysiologically. In our opinion, it is a dangerous manoeuvre to extrapolate directly from morphological findings to function. However, there is undoubtedly considerable variation in the manner in which the transitional or nodal approach fibers make contact with the compact node. As presently indicated, we consider it preferable to define the division between compact node and penetrating bundle as the point at which transitional fibers cease to make contact with the nodal-bundle axis. The penetrating bundle can therefore be considered as the 'final common pathway'. From this definition we would define a morphological by-pass tract, without implying any functional significance, as an atrial fiber contacting the nodal-bundle axis distal to the point of origin of the penetrating bundle, that is inserting into the final common pathway distal to the compact node. Such a tract was described by Brechenmacher et al. (88) in a case exhibiting electrophysiological abnormalities. It is true that there are also variations in insertion of transitional fibers to the compact node which could influence the route to the final common pathway. In our experience, the 'last' transitional fibers to make contact with the compact node can be derived either from the superficial overlay fibers or from the deep, left atrial side of the septum. It must be emphasized that in our opinion the anterior overlay fibers originate directly from the anterior limbus and pass to the compact node. We were unable to identify a tract of cells coursing from the posterior part of the atrial septum, as described by James (389). If these variations are of significance to nodal function, then we would consider them as variations in nodal structure and term them intranodal pathways rather than considering them as 'by-pass' tracts. If such fibers are indeed of significance, which is yet to be proven, then account must also be taken of the arrangement of the posterior extensions of the compact node. Variations in these fibers could also affect the route taken to the 'final common pathway'. The connection between the left going extension of the compact node and the left atrial side of the septum is particularly noteworthy. As Scherf and Cohen (730) have pointed out, the node is an interatrial structure and *NOT* a right atrial structure.

III. 'MAHAIM FIBERS'

These fibers, also described as paraspecific fibers, connect the penetrating bundle and the deep part of the node directly to the ventricular septal crest. As described in an earlier chapter (32), they can be considered to represent 'rests' of the embryonic anlagen of the conducting tissues. Indeed, evidence of these 'rests' which remain in the central fibrous body are identifiable in both infantile, adolescent and adult hearts, albeit in a decreasing frequency. Whether these fibers have functional significance cannot be determined from microscopic examination alone. As indicated above, we have studied an embryonic human heart in which multiple atrioventricular connections of this type were present, but in which conduction was normal (32). However, Lev and his colleagues have studied specimens in which the fibers were considered to be of significance (486). In our material we have never encountered pathological changes in these structures. The significance of this finding has already been discussed (32). We consider that it is also justifiable to divide potential 'Mahaim' connections which originate from the compact node from those taking origin from the distal junctional area. In our opinion, it is preferable to term the former fibers 'nodo-ventricular connections' and the latter fibers 'fasciculo-ventricular connections' (33).

IV. ATRIAL PATHWAYS

Recently, Janse and Anderson (410) reviewed the vast literature from both morphological and electrophysiological sources relative to the existence of specialized atrial pathways connecting the sinus node with the atrioventricular junctional area. They concluded from their review and from their personal studies that morphologically discrete internodal specialized pathways have yet to be demonstrated. This conclusion had previously been reached by several distinguished German morphologists in the early twentieth century. However, no proper mention was made of these studies by investigators who have recently propagated once more the concept of specialized internodal pathways. Thus, the views of the protagonists of specialized tracts have become so widely accepted that a recent atlas of the heart (597) has indicated the so-called specialized tracts in the atrium in a fashion analogous to that in use for the delineation of ventricular specialized tissues. Nonetheless, not all modern day investigators have been convinced of the existence of well defined specific internodal pathways (94, 224, 775, 776).

How can this controversy still exist? In part it may relate to the fact that the anatomy of the atria is complex, so that it is easy for investigators to lose perspective. If it is desired to pass through atrial tissues from the sinus node to the junctional area, then the choice of route is limited. In fact, a considerable proportion of the right atrium consists of 'holes', which are the ostia of the superior vena cava, the inferior vena cava, the coronary sinus and the fossa ovalis. The latter is an embryological 'hole', being sealed off in post-natal life by a valve-like structure, the septum primum.

If one considers the anatomy delineated by these 'holes', it is evident that four distinct pathways are present which connect the sinus node to the junctional area (fig. 14). These may then be termed 'preferential pathways'. However, such terminology should not imply that the pathways are actually composed of specialized tissues. It is interesting to note that James, when promoting the existence of such specialized tracts, stated that he was not investigating *whether* the tracts existed, but *where* the tracts were localized, since he considered the existence of the tracts to be supported by unequivocal electrophysiological evidence. The latter statement, however, is not yet justified since unequivocal electrophysiological evidence of the existence of discrete specialized tracts within the 'preferential pathways' has not yet been produced (410). Nevertheless, electrophysiological studies have indicated that the spread of excitation of the sinus impulse is through the 'preferential pathways'. The evidence used by James (393) to establish the histological specificity of the tracts was, firstly, the presence of Purkinje cells and, secondly, the belief

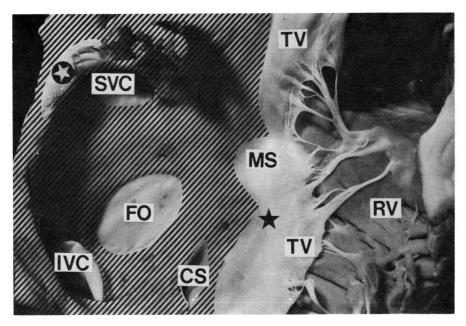

Fig. 14. Specimen of heart (compare with fig. 12A), in which the right atrium has been opened, to show the complex architecture with various 'holes'. The myocardium is hatched, showing the routes through which the atrioventricular junctional area (closed asterisk) can be reached from the sinus node area (open asterisk). These pathways may be termed 'preferential pathways'. However, such terminology should not imply that the pathways are composed of histologically specialized tissues. SVC = superior vena cava; IVC = inferior vena cava. FO = fossa ovalis. CS = coronary sinus. MS = membranous septum. TV = tricuspid valve.

that the area containing the tracts was derived from embryonic sinus venosus. It has repeatedly been indicated that the presence of Purkinje-like fibers in the atrial myocardium is not in itself conclusive evidence for the existence of a specialized tract (39,563,835). Moreover, the embryological premise is not supported by recent studies (32,53,410).

We ourselves have completely serially sectioned the interatrial septum in numerous specimens both infantile and adult in order to see whether or not tracts of specialized tissue could be detected between the sinus node and the atrioventricular junctional area. In no instance did we succeed in identifying such tracts. Ordinary 'working' myocardium was always present between the sinus node and the transitional zone of the AV junctional area. We prefer, therefore, to describe 'internodal atrial myocardium' and state once more that such a description merely endorses views expressed by previous morphologists who also examined these tissues in great detail.

V. VASCULAR SUPPLY OF THE JUNCTIONAL AREA

The atrioventricular junctional area receives its arterial blood supply from two different sources. The first is the atrioventricular nodal artery, which originates from that coronary artery which crosses the crux cordis. In approximately 90% of cases this is the right coronary artery. The AV nodal artery runs a straight course over the top of the ventricular septum towards the AV junctional area. During its course it may give off smaller branches that supply part of the working myocardium of the atrium. In the region of the AV junctional area the artery gives off several small branches and it may continue in close approximity to the penetrating bundle for a variable distance. The second source of arterial blood supply is derived from the first and second penetrating septal arteries, themselves derived from the anterior descending coronary artery. These arteries supply the penetrating bundle and the distal part of the junctional area over a variable distance.

It is of functional significance that the various components of the atrioventricular junctional area have a dual blood supply. Frink and James (287) have recently studied 10 specimens from which they concluded that the 'His' bundle received a dual supply in 9 instances. In only one specimen was the blood supply to the 'His' bundle derived from the atrioventricular nodal artery only. The right bundle branch received a dual blood supply in 5 instances, while both the posterior and anterior radiations of the left bundle branch showed dual supplies in 4 hearts each. In the remaining hearts, when only one artery supplied the area, the posterior radiation of the left bundle branch was mainly supplied by the AV-nodal artery, whereas the right bundle branch and anterior division of the left bundle branch were mainly supplied through the septal arteries. Our own investigations (53), largely endorse this view. Selective post-mortem injections of either the AV-nodal artery or the major septal artery derived from the anterior descending artery revealed that extensive individual variations exist (fig. 15). Isolated injection of the AV-nodal artery led in one instance to filling of the vessels in the transitional zone and compact node only (fig. 15A), whereas in other instances all of the atrioventricular junctional area was reached (fig. 15B). On the other hand, isolated injection of the first or second septal arteries led to filling of only the proximal segments of the right bundle branch and anterior division of the left bundle branch in some cases (fig. 15C), whereas in other cases all of the atrioventricular junctional area was filled (fig. 15D). Knowledge of the existence of such individual variations may enhance the understanding of functional disturbances of the atrioventricular junctional area, particularly in the setting of ischemic heart disease. Another feature which may have clinical significance, is the fact that the AV-nodal artery originates from the terminal part of a main coronary artery, whereas the penetrating septal branches are derived at the very beginning of a main coronary artery. These facts may also bear significance relative to the sequela of coronary atherosclerosis, particularly with regard to conduction disturbances, complicating acute myocardial infarction.

VI. INNERVATION

Details of the nerve supply of the junctional area is abundant in animal preparations, however little reliable material is available concerning the topic in human material. This is an important point since our own investigations have shown a considerable species variation in innervation pattern (21,22,269), as have those of Bojsen-Moller and Tranum-Jensen (83,84). Thus, in guinea pigs the entire ventricular specialized tissue is profusely supplied with cholinesterase (ChE) containing fibers, but less well supplied with adrenergic

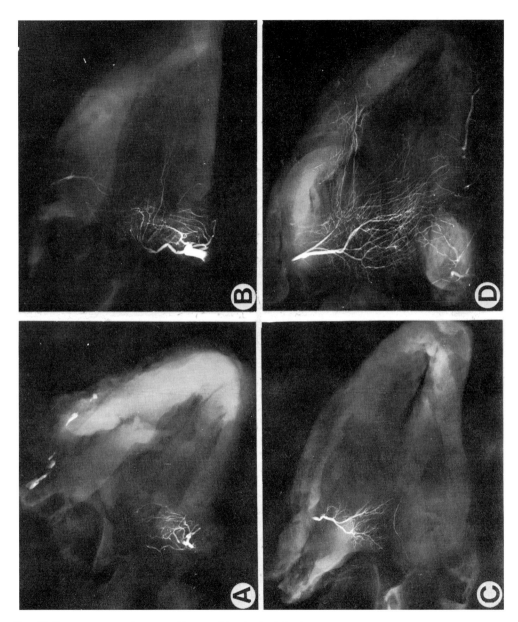

Fig. 15. Post-mortem angiograms of hearts with selective injection of arteries that supply the atrioventricular junctional area. Figures 15A and B show specimens with isolated injection of the AV nodal artery, whereas Figures 15C and D represent hearts with isolated injection of the major anterior septal artery. The individual variations in the extent of 'blood' supply to the AV-junctional tissues is demonstrated. Isolated injection of the AV nodal artery in some cases has led to filling of only the most proximal parts of the AV-junctional tissues (fig. 15A), whereas in other specimens all of the atrioventricular junctional area is reached (fig. 15B). Isolated injection of the major anterior septal artery, on the other hand, has led to filling of only the proximal segments of the right bundle branch and anterior division of the left bundle branch in some cases (fig. 15C), while other cases show filling of all of the atrioventricular area (fig. 15D).

fibers. A similar situation is observed in the pig and rat, but in contrast the rabbit ventricular conducting tissue is well supplied by adrenergic fibers but less well supplied by ChE containing fibers. A further contrast is found in canine material, in which the specialized tissue is itself ChE positive, but appears to be devoid of nerve fibers (unpublished observations). These findings illustrate the complexity of the subject. Further problems arise from the fact that presence of cholinesterase is not unequivocal proof of the parasympathetic nature of a nerve fiber, while adrenergic fibers can only be identified with either fluorescence or ultrastructural techniques in ultrafresh tissues. Such studies to the best of our knowledge have yet to be performed in the human. James and Spence (397) described a study using cholinesterase techniques, and more recently a similar study has been reported (435). However, we have grave reservations regarding the validity of such techniques performed using autopsy material, particularly in the nature of the so-called 'nerves' reported in the latter study. Our own findings on mid-term human fetuses (23,805) show that the transitional cell zone is well supplied with ChE containing nerves, but that the compact node and penetrating bundle are devoid of such nerves, although they are ChE positive. It is of course possible that nerves subsequently grow into the conducting tissues, but this seems unlikely since at the mid-term stage the remainder of the heart, including the coronary arteries, is supplied with ChE containing nerves. Elucidation of this problem will only come from application of ultrastructural techniques such as those of Thaemert (808) or those such as Tranum-Jensen (829) has reported elsewhere.

VII. AGEING CHANGES IN THE JUNCTIONAL AREA

It is our experience that the junctional area shows its fullest degree of cellular differentiation at term. At this stage the compact node is a well formed cellular mass and is encapsulated by layers of transitional cells with little intervening connective tissue. Thereafter the cellular content of the node decreases in relative terms so that in the adult the compact node is a small structure, is extensively infiltrated by fibrous tissue and the transitional cells are dispersed with much intervening adipose tissue (fig. 16). The overall architecture of the junctional area in the adult is comparable with that seen in the infant, but the arrangement is much less obvious. A further important point is that so-called 'Purkinje' cells are, in our experience, encountered much more frequently in adult than infantile specimens. This is not only true of the junctional area. During the discussion of Thorel's presentation at the Erlangen meeting of the German Pathological Society (813), Thorel himself stated that he observed 'Purkinje' cells only in adult tissue. Truex (835) has commented at length on the significance of such cells in the atria. It is our experience that large, vacuolated cells are rarely encountered anywhere in infantile specimens including the bundle branches. It may well be that they are a consequence of poor fixation. Certainly such cells were encountered in greater frequency by Tranum-Jensen and Bojsen-Moller (828) in the presence of poor fixation.

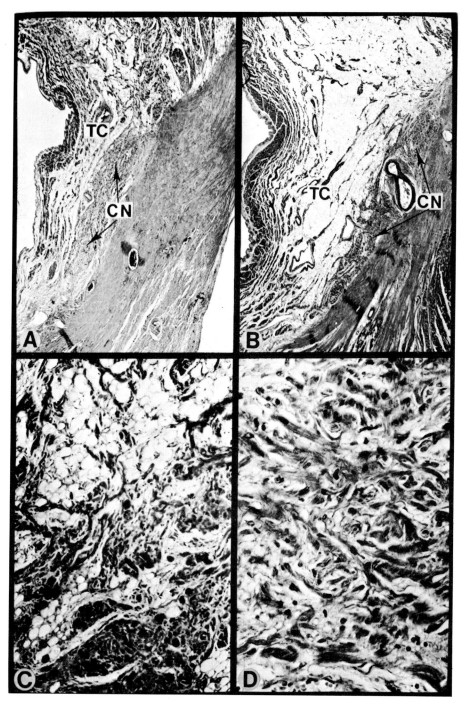

Fig. 16. Photomicrographs illustrating ageing changes in the junctional tissues. Figures 16A and B show considerable infiltration by adipose tissue of the transitional cell zone (TC). The compact node (CN), however, is still recognizable. Figures 16C and D show, at a higher magnification, the separation of the transitional cells by adipose tissue (fig. 16C) and the interposition of fibrous tissue in the compact node (fig. 16D). Hematoxylin-eosin stain, A,B: ×15; C: ×90; D: ×350.

CONCLUSIONS

On the basis of our morphological studies we have divided the atrioventricular junctional areas into four zones. These are the transitional cell zone, the compact node, the penetrating bundle and the branching bundle. The distinction between the first two and the last two is made using morphological criteria. The distinction between compact node and penetrating bundle is difficult to make using histological criteria alone. We have therefore designated the junction between these two zones as the point at which transitional fibers cease to make contact with the nodal-bundle axis. We have been able to trace transitional fibers for only a small distance into the atrial myocardium. We have found no evidence to support the concept of histologically specialized internodal tracts. Following our definition of the penetrating bundle, we define a 'by-pass tract' as composed of atrial fibers which make contact with the penetrating bundle distal to its point of origin. We find considerable variation in the precise mode of junction of transitional fibers with the compact node. The important variations are with respect to superficial or deep insertions of the 'last' transitional fibers to make contact with the compact node. We would emphasize that the junctional area is an intra-atrial structure, and not a right atrial structure.

16

PATHOLOGICAL BASIS OF CONCEPT OF LEFT HEMIBLOCK

H. E. KULBERTUS, M.D., AND J. Cl. DEMOULIN, M.D.

I. INTRODUCTION

The electrocardiographic manifestations of conduction blockade within the atrio-ventricular junction and along the main stems of the right and left bundle branches have long been recognized and accepted by cardiologists.

The concept of fascicular or divisional blocks involving only part of the left bundle branch fibers was first mentioned by Rothberger and Winterberg in 1917 (702). It was not until the late sixties that Rosenbaum et al. introduced this concept into clinical electrocardiography (686). These authors described the left branch as divided into two fascicles along which the transmission of impulse could be blocked separately. In their terminology, conduction delay along the left anterior or posterior subbranches are referred to as anterior or posterior hemiblock. These abnormalities can easily be diagnosed by the dramatic frontal axis shifts which they produce.

In recent years, the concept of left hemiblocks has given rise to some controversy. Different authors have questioned the bifascicular nature of the left branch (353, 700, 849, 871). In support of their opinion, they quoted older and more recent publications written mostly by anatomists who described the left bundle branch as a fanlike structure (871) or as composed of three, rather than two main radiations (49, 200, 658, 702, 748).

In addition, several histopathologists have insisted that they were unable to confirm the specific location of the left bundle branch lesions responsible for left anterior hemiblock (78, 700).

The purpose of the present report is to review these criticisms and to discuss them on the basis of data gathered in our Institution relating to the normal anatomy of the left bundle branch and the pathological significance of left hemiblocks.

II. NORMAL ANATOMY OF THE LEFT BRANCH

a. Techniques and results

The anatomy of the left branch was studied in 26 canine and 49 human hearts.

In the dog, detailed pictures of the peripheral conducting system may be obtained with relative ease by means of iodine staining of the specific fibers (848). In the pictures which we obtained by this method, (fig. 1), the origin of the left bundle branch always appeared as a ribbon which quickly broadened out to form a wide open angle limited by the anterior and posterior radiations. These two subbranches headed towards the corresponding

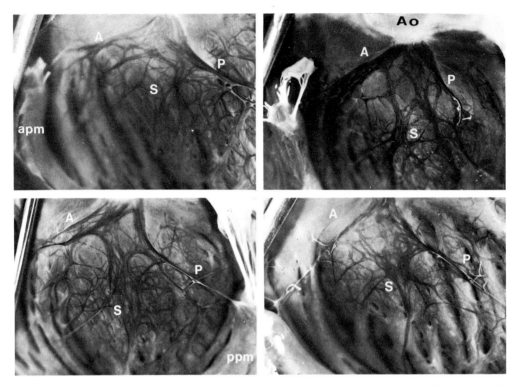

Fig. 1. Photographs of the left bundle branch, stained by iodine, in four canine hearts. The anterior (A) and posterior (B) subdivisions are easily identified in each case. These two ramifications travel towards the corresponding anterior (apm) or posterior (ppm) papillary muscle. In the first instances (left upper corner), the midseptal area (S) is covered by a complicated network of interconnected fasciculi emerging from the two external subbranches. In the other 3 cases, a third central ramification is observed. It is formed by the meeting of rami given off by the anterior and posterior radiations. In the 3rd example (left lower corner), the contribution of the anterior fasciculus seems to be predominant. In the last instance, the midseptal ramification comes mainly from the posterior offshoot. Ao = aortic valve.

papillary muscle; they frequently gave rise to false tendons, and continued, across the papillary muscles, onto the left ventricular free wall. Individual variations were observed as regards the distribution of the septal fibers running inside the angle formed by the two external radiations. In 11 cases, the septum was covered by a complicated network of highly interconnected fasciculi emerging from both the anterior and posterior ramifications. In the 15 remaining hearts, the anterior and posterior fascicles gave off, more or less distally, one or several fairly large rami which joined over the midseptal surface to form a third central subdivision. The latter produced in its turn numerous small strands covering the septum. In seven of these cases, the contribution of the posterior subbranch to the midseptal fascicle was clearly predominant. Extensive anastomoses between the various structures were consistently observed at the periphery.

In the human, it is unfortunately almost impossible to perform similar staining of the conducting tissue and one has to resort to the method of serial histological studies (774, 847). In our laboratory, the septum is sectioned serially in a plane parallel to the atrio-ventricular ring (188). Such an angle of cutting provides transverse sections of the peripheral

Type I

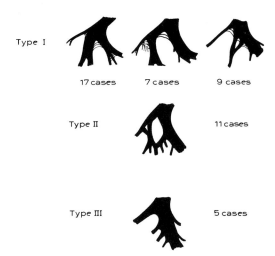

17 cases   7 cases   9 cases

Type II   11 cases

Type III   5 cases

Fig. 2. Distribution of the left bundle branch fibers in 49 human hearts (see text for detailed description).

portions of the left branch and therefore makes it easier graphically to reconstruct their geometry. Every 40th section (6 μ thickness) is routinely stained with hematoxylin-eosin and studied. A drawing of each is made to represent, as closely as possible, the location and width of the various left bundle ramifications. A diagrammatic sketch is finally constructed which describes the modes of subdivision of the left-sided conducting system.

To date, forty nine hearts have been studied by this technique. Twenty of them have been previously reported (188). The results obtained (fig. 2) confirmed the consistent existence of a thin, elongated anterior radiation and of a wider posterior one. The latter frequently gave off smaller branches running posteriorly.

In thirty three instances, a third division could easily be identified (type I). This structure which was sometimes larger than the other two, travelled to the midseptal surface and emerged either directly from the common left bundle (17 cases) or from the anterior (7 cases) or posterior radiation (9 cases). In eleven further instances, the anterior and posterior subbranches produced one or, more frequently, several fasciculi which formed a network of interwoven strands supplying the septal coverage (type 2). In the five remaining cases, the septal conducting fibers came from ramifications directly given off by the posterior radiation (type 3). It should be stressed that we did not trace the conducting fibers down to the more peripheral areas of the septum. It was apparent that the various structures of the left bundle branch system showed multiple peripheral anatomoses in all cases.

b. Comments

The assumption of the bifascicularity of the left bundle branch has wonderfully served the purpose for teaching the concept of left hemiblocks. However, at closer scrutiny, this description seems to be somewhat oversimplified. The existence of a considerable contingent of centro-septal fibers cannot be disregarded. In spite of the individual variations and of the numerous distal anastomoses, the general picture which now emerges is that the left ventricular Purkinje network is composed of three main, widely interconnected, parts depending upon the anterior subdivision, the posterior subdivision and a centro-septal subdivision or plexus of ramifications distributed over the midseptal area. Such a description fits in very well with the electrophysiological results obtained by Myerburg et al. (575) in the dog and by Durrer et al. (224) in the human. These authors found that the depolarization of the endocardial surface of the left ventricle simultaneously starts at three widely separated islands which may reasonably be assumed to correspond to the ending points of the three main parts of the left bundle branch system. According to Myerburg et al. (575), the two islands of early endocardial activation on the high para-septal free wall are likely to play, in the overall pattern of excitation, a minor role in the dog than in the human. In our opinion, the presence of numerous centro-septal fibers in both species is not incompatible with the physiological concept of left hemiblocks. These conduction disturbances are electrocardiographically characterized by conspicuous QRS axis deviations which are thought to result from an asynchronism of depolarization between the antero-superior and postero-inferior aspects of the left ventricle. This as-sumed electrophysiological mechanism appears just as reasonable whatever the mode of distribution of the median specific fibers.

However, the existence of the midseptal fibers and of the rich interconnected network justifies the two following comments. First of all, if one considers the fact that the activation seeks entrance to the left ventricle by three, rather than two routes, the term hemiblock which implies the bifascicularity of the left branch is debatable, and we agree with Hecht et al. (353) that the denomination fascicular or divisional block is to be pre-ferred. Furthermore, the distribution of the left-sided conducting fibers is such that one can hypothesize that the classical hemiblocks are not the only forms of partial left bundle branch blocks which may occur. They were the first to be identified because of the easily recognized frontal axis shifts which they produce on the standard electrocardiogram. Nonetheless, on theoretical grounds, conduction delay within anterior or posterior seg-ments of the left Purkinje network might also exist and, possibly, result in shifts of the horizontal QRS axis (453). There is no doubt that the future will bring forth new data, and probably further controversies, in this interesting field of electrocardiology.

III. HISTOPATHOLOGICAL FINDINGS IN CASES OF LEFT HEMIBLOCKS

a. Techniques and results
At the present time, general consensus has not yet been reached as regards the histopatho-logical lesions responsible for the pattern of left hemiblocks. In 1967, Entman et al. (251) studied fifteen cases of left anterior parietal block. They reported that anatomical ab-normalities were not always present and that no particular region of the myocardium or conduction system seemed more frequently involved than any other. Two abstracts published in 1965 (348) and 1967 (236) reached a different conclusion and stated that the electrocardiographic pattern of left anterior hemiblock was related to damage of the anterior division of the left branch. Further studies were devoted to the association of left anterior hemiblock with right bundle branch block (78, 797). There again, the results were very discordant, some papers indicating a predominant involvement of the anterior fibers (797), others being unable to confirm the specific location of the left-sided lesions (78).

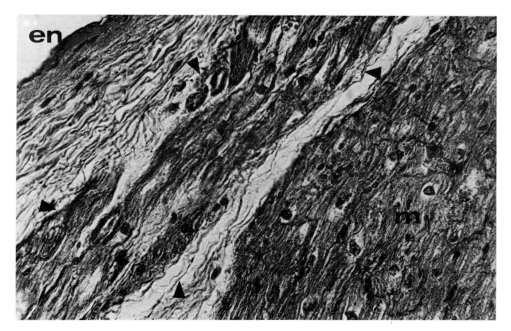

Fig. 3. A. Section through a portion of a normal left anterior subdivision. The conducting tissue, which only shows minimal fibrosis, is easily identified between the endocardium (en) and the common myocardial cells (m). Hematoxylin-eosin = 250 ×.

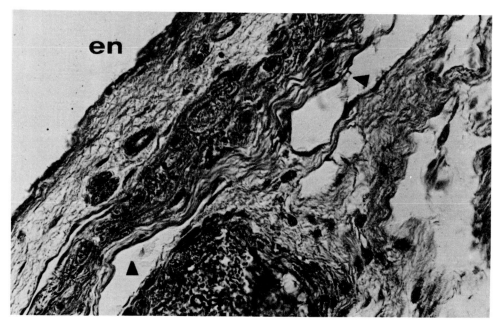

Fig. 3. B. Case of chronic left anterior hemiblock. The anterior subdivision is surrounded by fat tissue and dissected by fibrotic strands. In the lower left corner, the wall of a small coronary artery is visible. Hematoxylin-eosin; 250 ×.

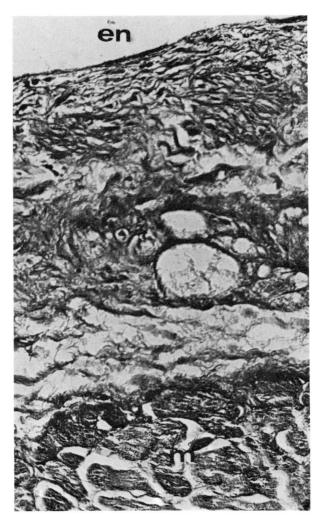

Fig. 3. C. Other case of chronic left anterior hemiblock with total replacement of the specific tissue by fibrosis. Only a few vacuolated Purkinje cells can still be observed. Masson's trichrome; 250 ×.

In 1972, our group reported data on ten cases of chronic left anterior hemiblock (188). The histological features (fig. 3) indicated that this electrocardiographic abnormality was related to severe alterations of the left bundle branch in 9 out of 10 cases. The anterior subdivision was almost totally interrupted in five instances. The lesions were however much more widely distributed than expected from the electrocardiographic terminology: disseminated degenerative or necrotic changes were seen throughout the left conduction system in eight out of the ten cases.

More recently, an attempt was made to approach the problem on a quantitative basis by using a stereological technique, i.e. the point counting technique (896). This method of investigation, described at length in another paper (189), permits the calculation of the relative volumetric density of fibrosis present at a given level of any of the subdivisions of

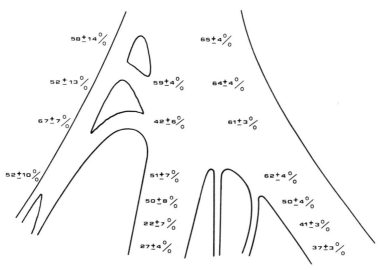

Fig. 4. Diagrammatic sketch of the left bundle branch in a patient with chronic left anterior hemiblock. The relative volumetric density of fibrosis ($\pm 2\sigma$) is indicated at each level where it was measured by the point counting technique.

the left branch. By combining the topographical reconstruction with the stereological approach, it is possible to map out the geometry of the left bundle ramifications and to indicate, at each level, the corresponding relative density of fibrosis (fig. 4). Using this approach, a comparison was made between eight hearts from patients with chronic degenerative left anterior hemiblock and eight hearts from patients of the same age group, who did not exhibit conduction abnormalities (189). It should first be mentioned that the macroscopic examination failed to reveal any significant difference between the two groups of patients as regards the magnitude and frequency of fibrocalcific altera-tions of the left side of the cardiac skeleton or the presence of major coronary artery disease. It was readily apparent that the hearts of patients with left anterior hemiblock showed, throughout the conducting system, a higher density of fibrosis than the hearts from subjects without conduction disturbances (mean values: control: 24.4%; left anterior hemiblock: 51.6%; $p < 0.001$). In a recent study of thirteen hearts from individuals with a normal electrocardiogram and without known cardiac disease, Demoulin showed that with increasing age, a certain amount of fibrosis develops in the left-sided conducting tissue. Figure 5 points out that, in the hearts from our 8 patients with left anterior hemi-block, the relative density of fibrosis was clearly above the normal range.

When treating altogether the data from these 8 patients, it could be demonstrated that the density of fibrosis tended to increase progressively and significantly from the posterior ramification (mean value 43.0%) to the midseptal fibers (mean value 51.3%) and finally to the anterior fasciculus (mean value 63.5%; $p < 0.001$).

However, the statistical analysis performed on each case separately indicated that in four hearts, fibrosis was evenly distributed throughout the three groups of fibers. In one instance, the lesions were significantly more severe along the anterior and midseptal fibers without any demonstrable difference between these two groups. In the remaining three instances,

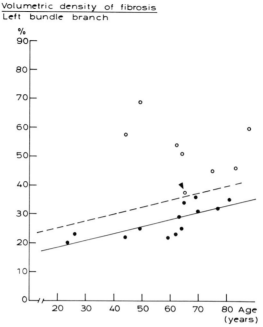

Fig. 5. This figure illustrates the observation that, with increasing age, some fibrosis develops throughout the left bundle branch structures, even in the absence of any conduction disorder or cardiac disease. The regression line calculated from the stereological measurements made on 13 control hearts (black circles) is v (%) = 13, 6 + 0, 24 × age in years; r = 0.77; σ = 3, 3 (Demoulin, unpublished data). The data obtained in the 8 hearts from patients with chronic left anterior hemiblock (open circles) indicate that the latter cases all showed a mean density of fibrosis falling above the normal range. One of these patients (arrow) was found to have a severe calcific alteration of the left side of the cardiac skeleton in addition to the peripheral fibrotic involvement.

the density of fibrosis was higher along the anterior fasciculus than in the other two, and the midseptal fibers were, in their turn, more severely damaged than the posterior offshoot.

b. Comments

The present data first confirmed that the pattern of left anterior hemiblock is associated with significant histopathological alterations of the conducting tissue and that it may therefore be considered as a reliable sign of left bundle branch disease.

Secondly, they show that in the presence of left anterior hemiblock, there is, on the whole, some tendency for the anterior fibers to be more severely damaged than the rest of the left branch. However, the lesions are widely scattered throughout the left-sided conduction structures and, on an individual basis, it is frequently difficult to demonstrate a clearcut predominance of the anterior involvement.

In our opinion, these findings also remain in perfect accordance with the general concept of left hemiblocks. Indeed, in the presence of widespread lesions involving the whole left-sided conducting system, one may anticipate that the functional disorder will primarily involve the much thinner anterior subdivision. In addition, these results bring support to two hypotheses which have recently appeared in the literature. On the one hand, in their experiments on dog hearts, Myerburg et al. (575) showed that discrete lesions in the anterior division of the left branch had little or no influence on the sequence of activation. To produce changes consistent with anterior hemiblock, they had to couple discrete lesions in the anterior division with a vertical cut interrupting many of the interconnecting fibers between the major subbranches. On the basis of their observations, these authors predicted that, if the human heart behaves similarly, 'the mechanism of hemiblock patterns must be related to very diffuse and probably peripheral lesions'. Our data are in agreement with this view. On the other hand, recent surgical experiments on dogs (537) as well as computer studies simulating cardiac excitation (452) have yielded rather unexpected data. They showed that electrocardiographic complexes fulfilling the diagnostic criteria of isolated left anterior hemiblock could, in some particular instances, be associated with conduction disturbances involving not only the anterior ramification but also centroseptal or posterior fibers. Should these data be confirmed by further investigations, they would bring a nice agreement between the histological and physiological findings.

The histopathological basis of left posterior hemiblock will not be considered in the present paper. There are several reasons for this. To start with, it seems that this conduction disorder is extremely rare. Furthermore, the criteria which permit its diagnosis are not as well established as those of its anterior counterpart. Even with the help of non-electrocardiographic data, mistakes remain possible and the selection of cases is therefore extremely difficult. At the present time, the authors have examined only two hearts from patients with an electrocardiogram compatible with left posterior hemiblock. These two patients both showed lesions of the posterior fibers; they also both had a sequelae of postero-inferior necrosis which had remained unnoticed in the clinical history.

IV. CONCLUSIONS

Mauricio Rosenbaum's outstanding contribution to the field of electrocardiography has provided a much better understanding of intraventricular conduction disturbances. When an idea like the concept of left hemiblock is to be introduced into the clinical field, things at the beginning are often kept fairly simple for the sake of clarity. Minor alterations or corrections of the initial theories may be expected at a later stage when the concept becomes more mature.

The present report indicates that the basic structure upon which the concept of left hemiblocks was based is somewhat more complex than initially described. A constant bifascicularity of the left bundle branch cannot be readily accepted. Indeed, in addition to the wellknown anterior and posterior subdivisions, the left branch also comprises a group of central fibers either bunched into a third radiation or appearing as a complicated network over the midseptal area. These fibers cannot be ignored.

Furthermore, the morphological studies failed to confirm the specific anterior location of the lesions responsible for left anterior hemiblock. The alterations of the left bundle branch are rarely limited to an anterior locus and appear much more widely scattered than expected from the electrocardiographic terminology.

In spite of this, careful analysis of these data reveals that they remain perfectly consistent with the original concept of hemiblocks and only bring forth refinements of the initial hypothesis.

17

ELECTROPHYSIOLOGY AND STRUCTURE OF THE ATRIOVENTRICULAR NODE OF THE ISOLATED RABBIT HEART

MICHIEL J. JANSE, M.D., FRANS J. L. VAN CAPELLE, Ph.D., ROBERT H. ANDERSON, M.D., PAUL TOUBOUL, M.D., AND JACQUES BILLETTE, M.D.

The purpose of this chapter is to summarize some of the work on the atrioventricular (AV) node performed in our department.[1] This work was characterized by the following experimental approaches.

1. the simultaneous recording of transmembrane potentials of several AV nodal cells.
2. the construction of maps, giving a two-dimensional impression of the sequence of AV nodal activation, and of areas showing typical potentials in a variety of circumstances.
3. the correlation of nodal electrophysiology with nodal morphology and architecture.

A 'brush' electrode, consisting of 10 microelectrodes glued together enabled us to record acceptable action potentials from 2 to 8 cells simultaneously in the nodal area of the isolated rabbit heart preparation (409). Extracellular electrodes were used to stimulate and to record from atrium and His bundle.

By moving the 'brush' electrode along known coordinates, recordings were made at as many sites as possible during different situations, such as antegrade conduction, retrograde conduction, the Wenckebach phenomenon, conduction of premature impulses, collisions of antegrade and retrograde wavefronts, and reciprocal rhythms. The recorded potentials were stored on magnetic tape. By playing these back, at low speed, and by printing the complexes on a multichannel inkwriter, accurate time measurements could be made. The preparations were photographed through a dissecting microscope with the 'brush' in different positions. After the experiment the 'brush' was dipped into molten beeswax, to obtain an imprint of the configuration of the different microelectrode tips. Finally, two-dimensional maps were constructed, on which data such as moments of activation, or action potential configuration were indicated. In some instances the preparations were fixed for histological studies, and for the purpose of making three-dimensional reconstructions of the nodal area based on serial sections.

NORMAL ACTIVATION

Figure 1 shows the spread of excitation in the AV nodal area of the rabbit heart during spontaneous sinus rhythm. Each symbol indicates a site were a transmembrane potential was recorded, and depicts the activation time in 20 msec intervals (an extracellular complex close to the sinus node was taken as time zero). The main features of normal, antegrade AV nodal activation are clearly demonstrated:

1. The department of Cardiology and Clinical Physiology, University of Amsterdam, Wilhelmina Gasthuis, Amsterdam.

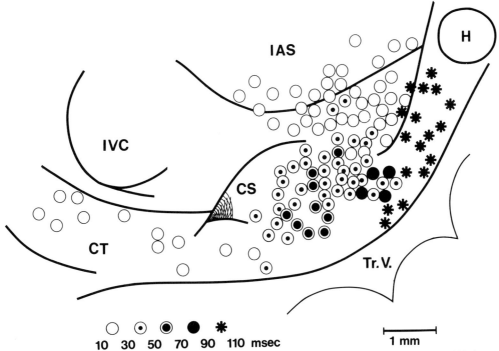

○   ⊙   ◉   ●   ✳
10 30 50 70 90 110 msec   ⊢————————⊣
                                                        1 mm

Fig. 1. Sequence of normal antegrade AV nodal activation. Map shows AV nodal area of rabbit heart. IVC – ostium of inferior vena cava. CT = crista terminalis. IAS = interatrial septum. CS – ostium of coronary sinus. TrV = triscuspid valve. H = position of electrode on His bundle. Symbols indicate position of AV nodal cells of which action potentials were recorded, and also in which 20 msec interval these cells were activated. Note the dual input into the AV nodal area. See text for further discussion.

1. there is a dual input to the AV node (the zones activated between 10 and 30 msec): a posterior input via the crista terminalis, entering the node beneath the coronary sinus ostium, and an anterior input entering the node as a broad wavefront anterior to the ostium of the coronary sinus.
2. The speed of activation in the central part of the node (the zone activated between 30 and 90 msec) is slow, and the pattern is difficult to follow. The latter is partly due to the fact that in this area the activation sequence is a three-dimensional event. Thus, superficial cells may be activated up to 40 msec earlier than deeper cells at the same surface site.
3. In the last part to be activated (at 90 to 110 msec), activation is rapid and synchronous. In this region there is a sharp boundary between cells activated early and cells activated late: the anterior input does not short-circuit the central part of the node to excite the late part directly, but curves in a posterior direction, to merge with the posterior input before jointly activating the central nodal area. We never found electrophysiological evidence for 'bypass tracts' carrying the excitatory wave from atrial input to the distal part of the node.

For retrograde conduction, the activation pattern of the node is essentially reversed. However, the earliest 'exit' to the atrium is the interatrial septum, anterior to the ostium of the

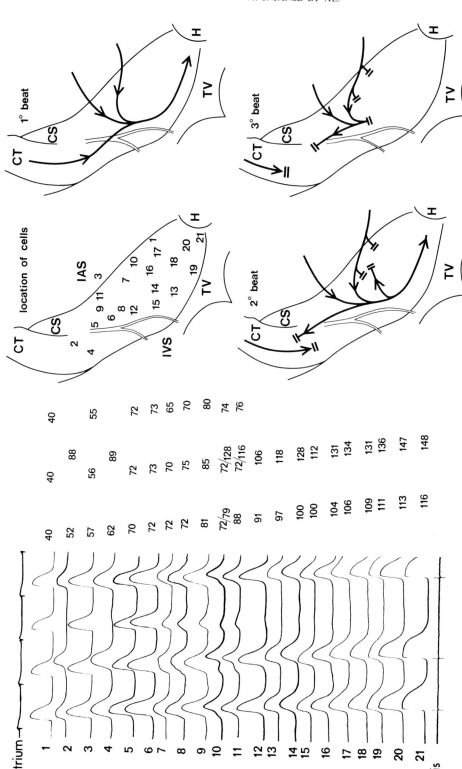

Fig. 2. Superimposed action potentials of AV nodal cells during a 3:2 Wenckebach phenomenon elicited by rapid stimulation of the atrium at a site close to the sinus node. Upper trace: atrial electrogram, lower trace-electrogram of His bundle. In the middle portion the moments of activation of the different AV nodal cells are indicated in msec during the first, second and third beat. Note that block occurs in cells which are activated late in the atrium—His bundle interval. On the right hand side maps of the AV nodal area are shown, in which are indicated the position of the cells from which the action potentials were recorded, as well as a schematic representation of the general spread of activation during first, second and third beat. The activation sequence was reconstructed based on timings of over a hundred impaled AV nodal cells in this experiment. Double bar indicates conduction block. CT = crista terminalis. CS = coronary sinus, IAS = interatrial septum. IVS = interventricular septum. TV = tricuspid valve. H = electrode on His

coronary sinus, the crista terminalis being excited much later. As a consequence, atrial excitation during His bundle stimulation, or ventricular pacing, is not the mirror image of excitation during sinus rhythm, since the interatrial septum is activated much earlier than the crista terminalis.

AN-, N-, and NH-zones

The terms AN-, N- and NH-zone, introduced by Paes de Carvalho and de Almeida (612) are in such widespread use that we will continue to use them. However, we will first define these terms according to the response of the different AV nodal cells during a Wenckebach phenomenon evoked by rapid stimulation. Figure 2 is a composite record in which selected action potentials recorded at different times during a single experiment are superimposed during an antegrade 3:2 Wenckebach phenomenon. More than 100 fibers were impaled during this experiment.

AN cells are proximal to the zone of block. They show fully developed actionpotentials, the upstrokes of which always occur after the same interval following the atrial complex, regardless of the presence of conduction delay or block further downstream (cells 1, 3, 5, 6). In late AN cells (such as cell 5) the actionpotential may be shortened in the presence of block, due to the polarizing electrotonic currents generated by the unexcited region downstream (545).

N cells have actionpotentials with slow upstrokes. The actionpotential-configuration changes with each beat of the Wenckebach cycle: the upstroke becomes slower, more slurred, while the amplitude becomes smaller, until finally a non propagated local response is present. N cells, in other words, produce the typical increment in conduction time and the block (cells 7, 8, 9).

NH cells are distal to the site where block is produced. They generally have faster upstrokes than N cells, although the transition is gradual (cells 12 through 21).

Some cells do not quite fit into this simple scheme. Thus, cells 2 and 4 are activated unexpectedly late during the second beat, and show no response at all during the third beat. Similar behavior is shown by cells 10 and 11. We believe that *longitudinal dissociation*, leading to concealed re-entry is responsible for these events. Local antegrade block in the posterior input during the second beat sets the stage for re-excitation of these cells by a retrograde wavefront, coming from the center of the node, which has been excited exclusively via the anterior input. This retrograde wavefront does not give rise to an atrial echo, hence re-entry is concealed. Similarly, concealed re-entry may be responsible for the unexpectedly late components in cells 10 and 11 during the second activation. The complex activation patterns, indicated on the right hand side of figure 2 were constructed on the basis of data obtained from over 100 impaled nodal fibers. Although concealed, and some times manifest re-entry, can be associated with the Wenckebach phenomenon, it is in our experience not a constant feature.

Figure 3 shows superimposed action potentials derived from an experiment in which a retrograde Wenckebach phenomenon was elicited by stimulating the His bundle at a rapid rate. In this experiment, over 60 different action potentials were recorded. During the retrograde Wenckebach phenomenon the NH cells are proximal to the block. Note the prolongation of the second action potential of cell G, associated with prolongation of

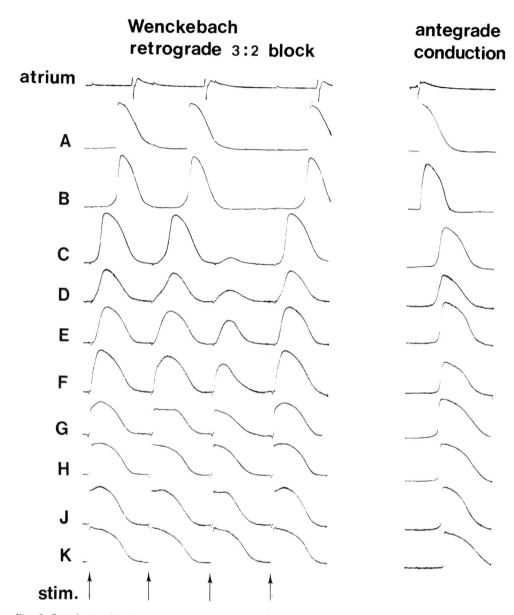

Fig. 3. Superimposed action potentials during retrograde 3:2 Wenckebach phenomenon induced by rapid stimulation of His bundle. Note that block occurs in cells activated early in the His bundle-atrium interval.

conduction time, and the shortening in the third beat, associated with block. N cells show the same characteristics as during antegrade Wenckebach, and AN cells are distal to the block.

Figure 4 is a schematic representation of action potential configuration of the different nodal cells during both antegrade and retrograde Wenckebach phenomenon. Also indicated are the areas from which the potentials were recorded and the moments of activation of the cell group. To indicate moments of activation, the results of 4 experiments were

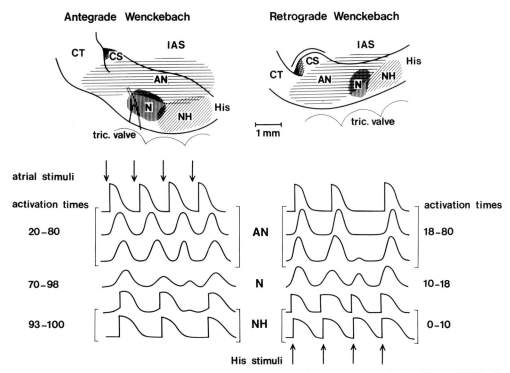

Fig. 4. Schematic representation of action potential configuration and timing of AN-, N-, and NH-cells during antegrade and retrograde Wenckebach phenomenon. Activation times are pooled from different experiments, and are expressed as percentages of total A-H or H-A time. In the upper panel diagrams of the AV nodal area are shown, indicating the zones where AN-, N-, and NH-potentials were recorded (two different experiments). Note the central position of the relatively small N-zone.

pooled: total conduction time during the first beat of a Wenckebach cycle (either A-H time, or H-A time) through the node was taken as 100%, and the moment of activation of a given cell (measured at 50% of the action potential upstroke) was expressed as a precent of total A-H or H-A time.

SITE OF NODAL DELAY

It is important to stress that for normal activation (i.e. the first beat of both the antegrade and retrograde Wenckebach phenomenon) a large part of the nodal delay takes place in the AN zone (20 to 80% of A-H time, 18 to 80% of H-A time). The time taken to activate the NH zone is only some 10% of total conduction time, and the time to cross the N zone normally takes about 20%. However, the N zone is responsible for the increment in conduction time, and for the conduction block in the successive activations of the Wenckebach cycle, both during antegrade and during retrograde conduction.

The detailed studies of Billette et al. (74) have shown that the N zone is also responsible for the other types of cycle length dependent increases in conduction time through the AV node. Thus, whereas the large AN zone during normal conduction accounts for the greater part of nodal delay, it is the small N zone which increases the nodal conduction time upon shortening of cycle length, and which produces block.

The main difference between our subdivision of the AV node and that of Paes de Carvalho and de Almeida (612) is that the latter authors depicted the node as a three layered structure (arranged in parallel with the fibrous annulus) with the AN-, N- and NH-zones all of identical length. In contrast, by our definition the N zone is confined to a small, central area, surrounded at its anterior, superior and posterior margins by the AN zone while inferiorly making contact with the NH zone.

DEAD-END PATHWAYS

There are AV nodal cells which, although excited, do not participate in transmitting the impulse from atrium to His bundle and vice versa (104). These so-called dead-end pathways cells can be detected by comparing their moments of activation during both antegrade and retrograde conduction. For a cell belonging to the AV nodal "mainstream", the sum of antegrade and retrograde activation times should be approximately 100, when both moments of activation are expressed as a percent of total conduction time. Thus, an early AN cell, activated at 20% of total A-H time, can be expected to be excited during retrograde conduction at 80% of total H-A time. For dead-end pathway cells this sum is far greater than 100; during both modes of conduction these cells are activated 'too late'. Identification of dead-end pathways could be performed in the following way (104).

During regular atrial stimulation, the His bundle was stimulated at a faster rate. This resulted in two wave fronts entering the node simultaneously and colliding in the node. With a special stimulation program, the collision site could be moved successively from the level of the His bundle to the atrium—traversing the node in 'steps' of 10 msec. By looking at the activation times it could be decided for any nodal cell at which collision level it switched from being influenced by the antegrade wavefront (long interval) to being influenced by the retrograde wavefront (short interval). Since dead-end pathways branch off the mainstream, all cells in a particular dead-end pathway switch from antegrade influence to retrograde influence at the same collision level. Moreover, the sequence of excitation in a dead-end pathway remains the same during both antegrade and retrograde conduction. In this way, schematically indicated in figure 5, we have identified two different dead-end pathways, one in an anterior position, the other more posteriorly (104).

BLOCK AT DIFFERENT LEVELS WITHIN THE AV NODE

It is well known that succesive blocked atrial impulses, for example during rapid atrial stimulation, may in a given AV nodal cell give rise to local responses of varying amplitudes and configurations (568, 881).

Thus, it can be concluded that block may occur at different levels within the node. In our department, Touboul (826) carried out extensive mapping experiments to plot the responses of nodal cells during various blocked premature atrial impulses. During regular

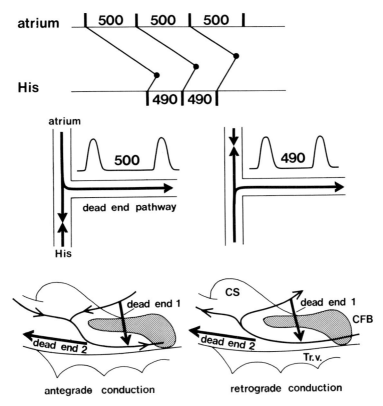

Fig. 5. Identification and localization of dead-end pathways. *Upper panel*: stimulation pattern, in which the His bundle was stimulated at a cycle length of 490 msec, the atrium at 500 msec interval. Collisions of both wavefronts occur at different levels in the AV node with subsequent combinations of atrial and His bundle stimuli. Cells in a dead-end pathway are activated in the same sequence both when under influence of antegrade wavefront (interval between action potential 500 msec) and when under influence of retrograde wavefront (interval 490 msec). The interval between action potentials of all cells in a dead-end pathway switch at the same collision level. *Lower panel*: schematic representation of AV node with the position of the two different dead-end pathways. Arrows indicate activation sequence during antegrade and retrograde activation. Central fibrous body (CFB) is represented by a shaded area. CS = coronary sinus. TrV = tricuspid valve.

atrial stimulation, a premature impulse was evoked after every tenth basic beat, at three different coupling intervals. All three premature ('late', 'intermediate', and 'early') impulses were blocked before reaching the His bundle. The concealment zone in these experiments varied from 30 to 70 msec.

Figure 6 shows superimposed actionpotentials, recorded at 12 representative sites (the number of successful impalements per experiment varied from 70 to 120). It can be seen that the 'late' premature impulse still elicits a local response in the cells close to the electrode on the His bundle. The earlier premature impulses fade away in the area closer to the atrial margin. Because of the difficulty of indicating a precise 'moment of activation' for the small premature responses, no maps were made to indicate the spread of activation, Instead, the amplitude of each premature response was expressed as a percent of the amplitude of the basic actionpotential.

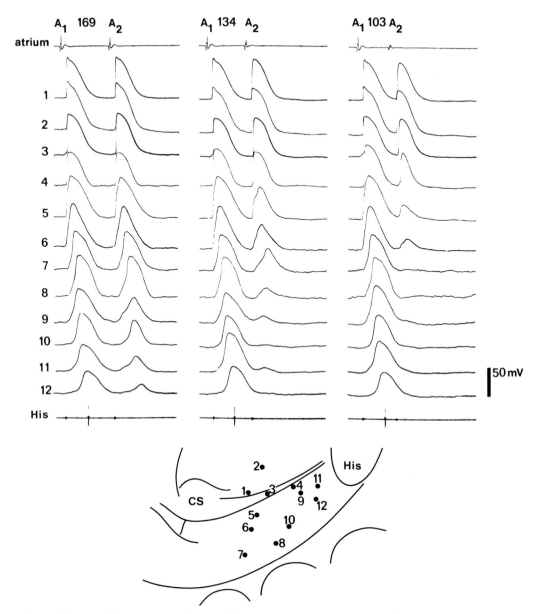

Fig. 6. Block at different levels within the AV node. Superimposed action potentials recorded in one experiment during a 'late' (coupling interval 169 msec), an 'intermediate' (interval 134 msec) and an 'early' premature beat (interval 103 msec). All premature beats are blocked before reaching the His bundle (lower trace is His bundle electrogram). Note that the premature action potentials during the 'late' and 'intermediate' premature beat arise out of the same level of membrane potential as the basic action potential, but have nevertheless a reduced amplitude and rate of rise of the upstroke (cell 5, 6 etc.). See texts for further discussion.

In figure 7 these amplitudes are shown for the various premature beats. With the 'late' premature impulse, the responses throughout most of the node have an amplitude of more than 80% of the basic actionpotential, and very small local responses were found only close to the His bundle. On shortening the coupling interval, the area showing

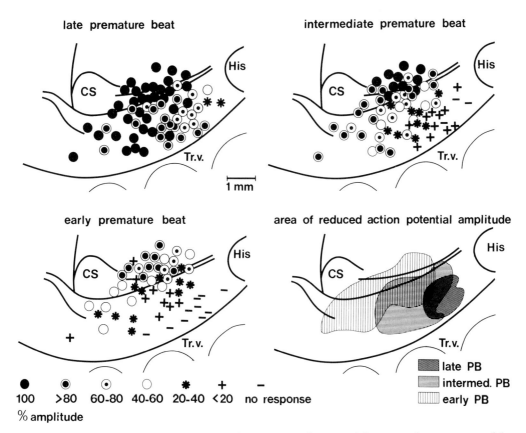

late premature beat

intermediate premature beat

early premature beat

area of reduced action potential amplitude

● ⦿ ⊙ ○ ✱ + −
100 >80 60-80 40-60 20-40 <20 no response
% amplitude

Fig. 7. Maps of AV node showing amplitude of premature action potentials expressed as percentage of the amplitude of the basic action potential. See text for further discussion.

diminished potentials is now considerably enlarged. With the earliest premature beat, practically all nodal cells show either no response, or responses of about half the amplitude of their basic action potentials. In fact, cells in the interatrial septum, which seem well outside the AN zone, also showed a diminished amplitude. Later mapping experiments of atrial excitation demonstrated that during the earliest possible premature beat, the majority of atrial cells show actionpotentials of diminished amplitudes. Thus, for very early premature beats, the boundary between areas with normal and reduced response cannot be ascertained, but certainly includes atrial tissue.

Although no morphological reconstructions were made in these experiments, the area showing local responses during the 'late' premature beat corresponded well to our previously defined N zone; while the earlier responses were blocked in the AN region.

The earliest premature responses were elicited at a moment when repolarization was incomplete (fig. 6 A_1-A_2 103 msec, cells 1,2,3,4). The occurrence of blocks in these instances is probably a consequence of the voltage dependency of the action-potential: a response arising out of a reduced membrane potential will have a lower rate of rise (dV/dt) and a smaller amplitude (897) and consequently will be less effective as a stimulus for cells in the pathway ahead.

In contrast, the premature actionpotentionals in cells 5,6,7, etc of figure 6 during the intermediate and late premature beat occurred at a time when repolarization was complete, and the explanation given above does not hold. That the premature action potentials are smaller than the basic action-potentials, although both arise from the same take-off potential, may be due to the fact that in nodal cells recovery of excitability lags behind full repolarization (548). This would apply not only for N cells, but also for AN cells, since cell 5 of figure 6 for example is clearly an AN cell.

DUAL NODAL INPUT

Earlier experiments showed that the crista terminalis in preparations *in vitro* is the dominant nodal input, because the pattern of AV nodal activation was the same during spontaneous rhythm as during stimulation of the crista terminalis, but changed when the interatrial septum was stimulated (104,408). The site of the atrial pacemaker is a decisive factor in determining which of the two inputs excites the node earlier (410). In the isolated rabbit atrium, the earliest endocardial breakthrough during sinus rhythm occurs in the crista terminalis, about halfway between the ostia of superior and inferior caval vein (410). It is quite possible, however, that in the intact animal the pacemaker site is located more towards the septal branch of the crista terminalis, thus increasing the importance of the septal input. Also, autonomic nervous influences may be shifting the pacemakersite after and thus alter the AV nodal input.

Some consequences of the dual AV nodal input will be illustrated in the following paragraphs.

NODAL ECHOES

A dual AV nodal input seems to predispose for the occurrence of reciprocal rhythms. Unidirectional block in one of the inputs may set the stage for re-entry, since the wavefront from the other input may retrogradely invade the blocked route, and a circus movement may be set up, with the ostium of the coronary sinus serving as an obstacle around which the excitatory wave circles. It is well known that properly timed premature atrial stimuli may give rise to AV nodal circus movement tachycardia (409,544,903). The re-entry circuits, however, are not always confined to the AV node. Re-entry may occur in the sinus node (334), and, as the studies of Allessie et al. (13) have shown, a circus movement tachycardia can be initiated in the isolated left atrium, where no large anatomical obstacle is present, and where no specialized tissues are involved in the circuit.

Thus far we have been unable to initiate a sufficiently reproducible AV nodal circus movement tachycardia to allow mapping of the complete circuit. From our incomplete maps of tachycardia circuits, or echo pathways, we have learned that many different pathways may exist. The experiment to be described, therefore, indicates only one of many possible re-entry circuits involving the AV node. The preparation illustrated in figure 8D differs from the preparations we normally use in that the vena cava superior

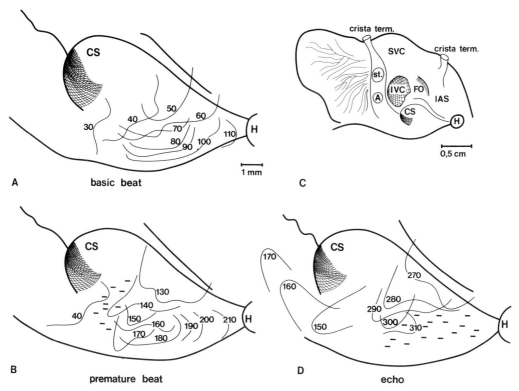

A   basic beat
C

B
premature beat
D   echo

Fig. 8. AV nodal echo. Maps of AV node showing isochrones during basic beat (A), premature beat (B) and echo beat (D). Bars indicate no response. The wave front elicited by the premature stimulus is blocked in the posterior input (B, 40 msec isochrone) and reaches the anterior input zone after a long delay (B, 130 msec isochrone). The posterior input zone is re-excited (D, 150 msec isochrone) and reactivates the crista terminalis in a retrograde fashion. In D, the preparation is shown, in which the crista terminalis is cut. St = stimulating electrode. A = recording electrode on crista terminalis, SVC = superior vena cava (opened). IVC = ostium of inferior vena cava. CS = ostium of coronary sinus. FO = fossa ovalis. IAS = interatrial septum. H = electrode on His bundle.

was opened, thus severing the septal branch of crista terminalis. This implies that when stimulating the posterior crista terminalis, the interatrial septum was activated later, than would have been the case were the connection between posterior crista and septal branch intact. Nevertheless, as shown in figure 8A, during a basic beat the AV node receives a dual input. A premature impulse, however, is blocked in the posterior input, and the AV node is excited exclusively via the interatrial septum, where the wavefront reaches the AV node after a considerable interatrial conduction delay, 130 msec after the stimulus artifact (fig. 8B). This wavefront re-excites the posterior input, and travels along the crista terminalis in a retrograde direction (fig. 8C and fig. 9). In fact, a circus movement tachycardia ensued, with a cycle length of circa 150 msec. Only 50 msec were needed to cross the superior part of the AV node in an antero-posterior direction. The wavefront leaving the AV node via the posterior input arrived at the anterior input some 100 msec later. The exact course of the atrial part of the circuit remains unknown, but it is of interest to note that the sequence of atrial activation along the interatrial septum occurred in the

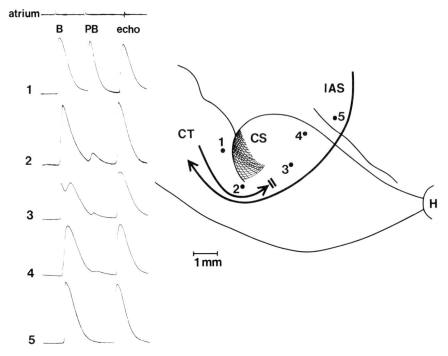

Fig. 9. AV nodal echo beat. Superimposed action potentials of same experiment as figure 8 showing block in posterior input during premature beat, and re-excitation of the posterior input zone.

same direction as during normal sinus rhythm. Therefore, a normal, antegrade sequence of activation along the interatrial septum does not rule out involvement of the AV node in the re-entrant circuit.

SUMMATION

It has been suggested that excitation of a nodal cell would normally result from activity arriving more or less simultaneously over different afferent pathways (159). Several experimental findings support the concept that summation of inputs plays an important role in AV nodal conduction. Thus, stimulation of the interatrial septum at a rapid rate resulted in 2:1 AV block, whereas stimulation of the crista terminalis at the same rate lead to 1:1 conduction (408). By keeping the stimulating frequency constant, a change in refractoriness of AV nodal cells was ruled out. The 2:1 block during stimulation of the interatrial septum could only have been due to a less effective input, presumably because the septal front was less homogeneous, and gave rise to less summation than the wave front initiated in the crista terminalis. Merideth et al. (548) showed that intracellular stimulation could result in a fully developed action potential in an N cell which was not conducted to either His bundle or atrium: lack of summation prevented propagation. Watanabe and Dreifus (879) showed several examples where conduction failure could be attributed to inhomogeneous conduction within the node. Zipes et al.

(957) separated both nodal inputs by making a cut through the roof and the floor of the coronary sinus. Premature stimulation of each input separately gave rise to a local response in a nodal cell, while simultaneous stimulation of both inputs resulted in a full actionpotential, which was conducted to the His bundle.

In the following experiments, some of the conduction disturbances shown can be explained by failure of summation of the two nodal inputs.

In figure 10, the simultaneously recorded action potentials of three nodal cells are

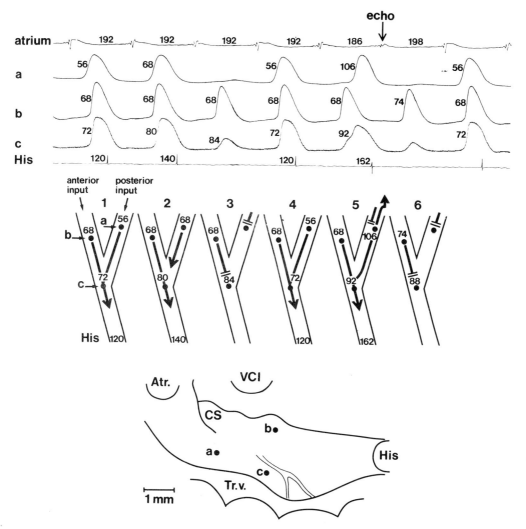

Fig. 10. Abnormal Wenckebach phenomenon. Three simultaneously recorded action potentials in posterior input (cell a), in anterior input (cell b) and in junctional area of these two inputs (cell c). Note the difference in timing and configuration of the action potentials of cells a and c and of the His bundle complex during the first and fifth beat. Double bars in diagram indicate block. Numbers are activation times in msec. Atr. = recording electrode on crista terminalis from which the electrogram in the upper trace was recorded. His = position of electrode recording electrogram of His bundle (lower trace).

shown. Cell a belongs to the posterior input, cell b to the anterior input, and cell c to the junctional region of these inputs. A peculiar type of Wenckebach phenomenon was elicited by rapid atrial stimulation: the moments of activation of the His bundle were 120 msec, 140 msec, block, 120 msec, 162 msec, block, and this sequence repeated itself. Thus, alternation in the conduction time of the second beat of a 3:2 Wenckebach cycle was present. Although the diagram of figure 9 is an oversimplification in view of the intricate structure of the AN zone, the events can to a certain extent be explained as follows: In beat 1, the synchronous arrival of activity along the two inputs at cell c leads to summation, and hence to relatively rapid conduction to the His bundle. In beat 2, cell a is activated later (68 msec after the atrial complex instead of 56 msec), while the moment of excitation of cell b remains unchanged: the two wavefronts arrive slightly asynchronously at cell c and summation is less effective. As a result the action potential of cell c shows a slightly slower rate of rise and is therefore less effective as a stimulus to downstream cells, producing slower conduction to the His bundle.

Beat 3 is blocked at the posterior input, and lack of summation at cell c is one of the reasons for the occurrence of conduction block at the level of cell c. Beat 4 is identical to beat 1. In beat 5, however, activity is blocked somewhere along the posterior input. From cell c activity spreads in two directions: antegradely towards the His bundle and retrogradely into the posterior input zone. The action potential of cell c has to provide excitatory current for two pathways, and consequently its configuration is greatly changed with amplitude and rate of rise of the upstroke being diminished, resulting in a prolonged conduction time to the His bundle (162 msec, as compared with 140 msec in beat 2). The retrograde wavefront excites the crista terminalis as an echo: note the different configuration of the atrial complex (arrow) occurring at a slightly shorter interval. During beat 6, the wave front set up by the stimulating electrode close to the sinus node, probably excites the AV node only via the anterior input, since the preceding echo along the crista terminalis and this new wavefront collide with each other somewhere in the crista. As in beat 3, cell c receives only one input, which is one of the factors accounting for the dropped beat.

We have tried to demonstrate summation by stimulating both nodal inputs, without, however, making a cut through the roof and the floor of the coronary sinus. In these 'intact' preparations, we were unable to demonstrate summation as clearly as Zipes and colleagues (957). When a single premature impulse initiated in one of the inputs was blocked, simultaneous stimulation of both inputs did not result in conduction. We did observe from time to time that, when the single premature inpulse was conducted to the His bundle, simultaneous stimulation of both inputs resulted in a slightly shorter conduction time. Very often, the occurrence of echoes, or partial echoes, complicated the results, particularly when actionpotential configuration was considered: thus, it was often impossible to decide whether a larger actionpotential, occurring when both inputs were stimulated at the same time, was due to summation resulting from the simultaneous arrival of two convergent wavefronts, or due to summation produced by collission of one wavefront travelling in an atrium-His bundle direction and another wavefront returning to the atrium as an abortive echo activation.

An example of the complexity of the wavefronts in the AV node set up by simultaneous stimulation of two atrial inputs is shown in figure 11. The basal stimuli were applied

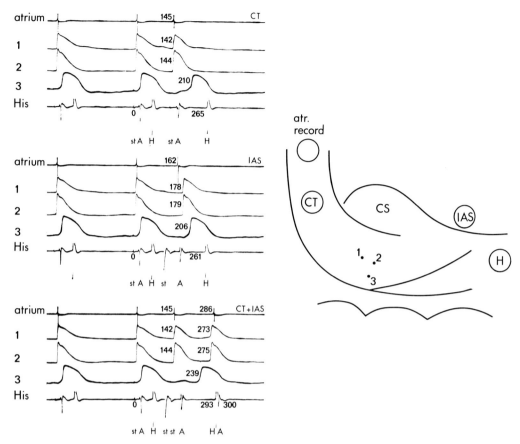

Fig. 11. Cancellation of wavefronts during simultaneous stimulation of both AV nodal inputs. Basic stimuli are delivered through an electrode on the crista terminalis (CT). Premature stimuli are applied to electrode on crista terminalis (CT, upper panel), to an electrode on the interatrial septum (IAS, middle panel), and to both electrodes (CT + IAS, lower panel). Note that, although the coupling intervals of the premature stimuli remain unchanged, the His bundle is activated much later when both inputs are simultaneously stimulated, and that an atrial echo occurs. (The atrial complexes in the lower panel have the same configuration during basic, premature and echo beat, as a consequence of the position of the recording electrode (atr. record) and stimulating electrode (CT)). St = stimulus artifact. A = atrial deflection in His bundle electrogram. H = His bundle spike in electrogram. Numbers are in msec (t = O: last basic stimulus).

to the crista terminalis, and the last basal stimulus served as time zero. Single premature impulses, applied to crista terminalis and interatrial septum arrived at the AV nodal cell no. 3 and the His bundle at about the same time in both instances (210 and 206 msec, and 265 and 261 msec respectively after the last basal stimulus). When both inputs were stimulated simultaneously, at the same intervals, cell no. 3 and His bundle were excited much later (293 and 300 msec), and an atrial echo occurred. Apparently, in the upper node some cancellation of colliding wavefronts must have occurred, resulting in a 'weaker' wavefront which eventually excited the elements closer to the His bundle. Lack of normal summation may have accounted for the longer total conduction time. The pathways over which a tortuous excitatory wave eventually re-excited the atrium are uncertain.

CORRELATION BETWEEN NODAL MORPHOLOGY AND ELECTROPHYSIOLOGY

Previous studies had shown that three cell types can be distinguished within the rabbit AV node: transitional cells, midnodal cells and lower nodal cells (20). By making three-dimensional models, based on enlargements of serial sections, the nodal architecture was reconstructed (31). The node was found to be divided by a fibrous collar into an open and an enclosed part.

The fibrous collar is a posterior extension of the central fibrous body. The larger open node is in contact with atrial myocardium via three groups of *transitional cells.* These cells are smaller than atrial cells, stain more palely and are separated by numerous strands of connective tissue. The posterior group of transitional cells contacts atrial myocardium beneath and behind the coronary sinus. The large middle group connects with atrial fibers from the sinus septum (the area between the ostium of the coronary sinus and the inferior vena cava) and with the deeper myocardium on the left side of the interatrial septum, as well as with the atrial myocardium anterior to the coronary sinus. This myo-cardium is also in contact with the anterior group of transitional cells; part of these fibers pass superficially over the fibrous collar and overlie the enclosed node, without making contact with the underlying tissues of the node. These overlay cells terminate in the tricuspid valve base. The transitional cells merge at the entrance of the enclosed node and surround a small knot of *midnodal cells.* These midnodal cells are small, spherical, tightly packed and are not separated by much connective tissue. The midnodal cells, together with the circumferential transitional cells, abut against a well formed bundle of *lower nodal cells.*

The lower nodal cells are orientated in a direction parallel to the fibrous annulus, and are continuous anteriorly with the His bundle. They also form a thinner, posterior extension that extends to beneath the coronary sinus. Within the enclosed part, the AV node has a trilaminar appearance (see fig. 12). A correlation between the electrophysiology and morphology of the AV node was made in two ways (31). Firstly, a comparison between activation maps and three-dimensionally reconstructed nodes gave an overall correlation between AN-, N-, and NH zones on the one hand, and areas of transitional cells, midnodal cells and lower nodal cells on the other hand. Both in the mapping studies of the Wencke-bach phenomenon, and in the studies of Billette et al. (74) on other forms of cycle length dependent increases in AV nodal conduction time, the functional N zone corresponded well to the small enclosed node, where transitional cells merge with midnodal cells. The AN zone was equivalent to the transitional cell groups of the posterior node and the NH zone to the anterior lower nodal cells.

Secondly, to arrive at a more precise correlation, single microelectrodes, containing cobalt chloride, were used to mark single cells from which action potentials had been recorded (31). From experience acquired in extensive mapping experiments, the single microelectrodes were impaled at sites where typical responses were expected. In each experiment only a few cells were impaled. After recording the action potentials during antegrade and retrograde conduction, and during the antegrade Wenckebach pheno-menon, current was applied to the microelectrode to deposit cobalt in the cell. The pre-

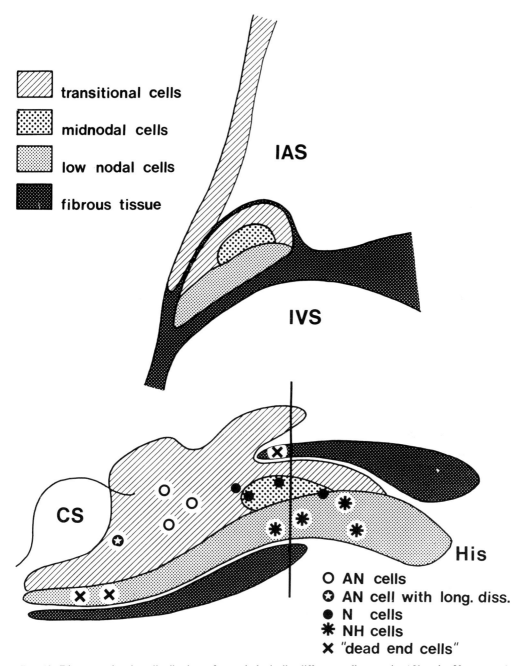

Fig. 12. Diagrams showing distribution of morphologically different cell types in AV node. Upper panel is a transverse section showing the trilaminar appearance of the anterior part of the node. The level of sectioning is indicated by a bar in the lower panel. Lower panel is diagram of the AV node indicating the different cobalt spots identified histologically after recording of typical action potentials.

paration was then serially sectioned and the cobalt spots were identified. In about 50% of the attempts a single, intracellular spot was found at the expected site. In the other cases either no cobalt was found (missing or folded sections, or too little cobalt) or there were multiple cobalt spots, mostly extracellular (due to leakage of cobalt out of the electrode when the tip broke or when it was pulled out of the tissue, leakage directly through the shaft when using strong currents). These latter cobalt deposits were not accepted as reliable indicators of electrode tip position. The results of this cobalt marking technique can be summarized as follows. The AN cells were localized in transitional cells. The NH cells were confined to the anterior portion of the bundle of lower nodal cells. Typical N cells were found at the junction of midnodal cells with the circumferential transitional cells, but were also found in transitional cells located more posteriorly. Dead-end pathway cells were found in the posterior extension of the lower nodal cells (twice) and once in the anterior overlay cells, overlying the fibrous collar.

Thus, a morphological counterpart is present for all functionally distinct cell types. However, neither action potential configuration, nor functional behaviour (i.e. increase in conduction time with shortening of cycle length) seems to be determined by cellular morphology alone. For example, N potentials can originate from both transitional cells and midnodal cells; the configuration of AN action potentials ranges from those with a fast upstroke to those with slow upstrokes and smaller amplitude; although block occurs most easily in the N zone (during Wenckebach phenomenon and late premature beats) it can also occur in the AN zone. Therefore, we believe that nodal architecture, as well as cellular morphology per se, contributes to nodal electrophysiology. Thus, the fact that transitional cells form small strands separated by connective tissue, and branch frequently, may play a role in the gradual decline of action potential upstroke velocity as the impulse penetrates deeper into the AN zone, since the synchronicity of the wave front is diminished by this arrangement. Also this architecture seems ideally suited for phenomena such as summation, and longitudinal dissociation, both of which alter action potential configuration.

On the other hand the bundle like arrangement of the lower nodal cells may be a factor accounting for the rapid and synchronous excitation in that part of the node. The architecture of the anterior overlay cells makes it quite clear that these cells function as dead end pathways and the thin posterior extension of the lower nodal cells tract seems equally fit to serve as a cul de sac. That this posterior extension, which is in contact with transitional cells, cannot serve as a bypass tract from the transitional cells directly to the anterior portion of the lower nodal cells is demonstrated by figure 13. This cell fulfilled the criteria of a dead end pathway cell (excited 'too late' during both antegrade and retrograde conduction). During antegrade Wenckebach it showed a fully developed action potential in the presence of block in the distal node (NH zone). The cobalt deposit was found in the posterior extension of the lower cell tract. Thus, the excitatory wave set up in this posterior extension evidently had insufficient strength to excite the anterior portion of the tract.

In contrast to the transitional cells, midnodal cells are not separated by connective tissue strands but are tightly packed. It is possible therefore that in these fibers special membrane characteristics are primarily responsible for their functional behavior.

A further characteristic of midnodal cells seems to be a nearly complete absence of

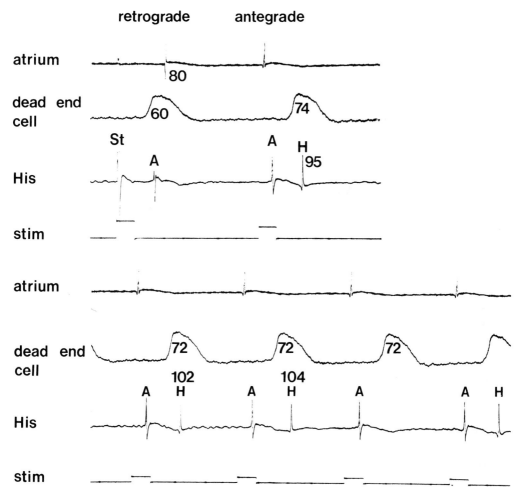

Fig. 13. Action potentials of a dead-end pathway cell. Note that this cell is activated late both during ante-grade and retrograde conduction (upper panel). In lower panel is shown that his cell exhibits a normal action potential in the presence of block during a Wenckebach cycle. See text for further discussion.

nexuses (829). As already indicated, typical N potentials could be recorded from transi-tional cells, and also from the area where transitional cells merge with midnodal cells (31). At this stage it is impossible to state with certainty that midnodal cells, which at the level of the electronmicroscope are not connected with each other via nexuses, do generate typical N potentials. Whether this area is an essential link in the AV nodal transmission, or whether it is responsible for some functional characteristic such as the increase in conduction time with shortening of cycle length, cannot be ascertained before correlation between electrophysiology on the one hand, and light microscopy and electronmicroscopy on the other hand, are made.

That AV nodal action potential configuration, and some disturbances in AV nodal conduction, might to a large extent be determined by the complex geometry of the net-work of transitional cells, will be illustrated in the following chapter (105).

18

INFLUENCE OF GEOMETRY ON THE SHAPE OF THE PROPAGATED ACTION POTENTIAL

FRANS J. L. VAN CAPELLE, Ph.D., AND MICHIEL J. JANSE, M.D.

INTRODUCTION

The configuration of action potentials of AV nodal cells sometimes changes markedly when the activation pattern is altered. For instance, the rate of rise of the upstroke and the amplitude may be very different for antegrade (AV) and retrograde (VA) conduction. The configuration changes are very outspoken in the slowly conducting nodal tissue, whereas they are minor in the fast conducting Purkinje system (104, 777). Furthermore, double components are frequently observed in the AV nodal action potential. The dissociation of the two components usually depends on the refractory state of the fibres. Typically, dissociation is more prominent at higher driving rates. However, quite frequently also the direction of activation plays an important rôle. For instance, during the same basic driving rate, a fibre may display double components when the activation enters the node from the interatrial septum, but not when the Crista Terminalis is the main entrance to the node (408). Similarly, double components may be present during retrograde activation, and absent during antegrade conduction.

These phenomena suggest, that the shape of the AV nodal action potential is determined to a large extent by the nodal geometry and by the activation sequence, rather than by the local ionic membrane mechanism alone. To demonstrate the effect of geometrical factors on the action potential, a simple analog model was built, consisting of 48 regenerative elements, which could be coupled by resistances in various ways. The elements consisted of a capacitor, coupled to a variable potential by a conductance, and of a voltage sensor (Schmitt trigger). As soon as the voltage over the capacitor exceeded a certain adjustable voltage level, the driving potential and the conductance were instantaneously switched from the resting value to an active value, whereafter an exponential decay to the resting potential occurred.

This model, in which the mechanism for the generation of the action potential was chosen to be very simple, was used to test the various geometrical configurations. For instance, the elements could be arranged to form a convergent or divergent structure, and the effects on the shape of the action potential could then be observed. Wavefronts could be made to arrive asynchroneously at a junctional point, giving rise to double components. Elements could be made passive by inhibition of the regenerative mechanism, resulting in an inexcitable 'gap' in a cable geometry.

As a complement to the changes in geometry, which could only be achieved in the model, it was attempted to bring about local excitability changes in the isolated rabbit AV node by application of polarizing current. Significant changes in action potential configuration as well as in A-H conduction time were observed. In the model, similar changes in action potential shape could be obtained in just this way, i.e. by rendering a few elements in a converging geometry more or less excitable.

Generally, the waveforms observed in the model simulation were strikingly similar to the ones recorded from the rabbit AV node. The model demonstrates the consistency of the shape of the nodal action potentials with an electrically tightly coupled system displaying a low margin of safety for propagation and a complex geometrical structure.

METHODS

a. Isolated rabbit heart
The preparation and the recording techniques are described in the chapter by Janse et al. in the present volume. A more detailed description can be found in ref. 104, 282. Extracellular polarizing current was applied using a method suggested by Dr. Jacques Billette from the university of Montréal. 5 broken tip microelectrodes were glued together in such a way, that the broken tips were close together in a line. Each microelectrode was connected with a common current source by a 2 MOhm resistor. This resulted in an even distribution of current over the 5 microelectrodes. The electrodes were placed under a shallow angle with the horizontal plane, and brought close to the tissue with a micromanipulator under microscopic control. This arrangement made it possible for a recording microelectrode 'brush' to be positioned relatively close to the broken tips of the current injecting microelectrodes.

b. Analog model
The analog model used in this study consisted of 48 elements, built according to the principle depicted in figure 1. The passive membrane (switch in left position) was represented simply by a resting potential (E_O), a resting membrane resistance (R_O) and the membrane capacitance C_m. When the membrane was passively depolarized to an adjustable threshold potential E_{th}, a comparator was activated, switching off E_O and switching on an active state driving potential E_1. Repolarization was introduced by permitting the active driving potential E_1 to decline exponentially, once activation had occurred, towards the resting potential E_O. However, this repolarization sequence was not related to the refractory period, which was arbitrarely fixed at 300 msec. For this reason, the model is not suitable for simulation of rate depending conduction disorders, such as first or second degree AV block. Nevertheless, the excitability of the individual elements could be adjusted by the setting of E_{th} or of R_O and R_1. In addition, E_{th} could also be changed for all elements simultaneously, resulting in an overall increase or decrease of excitability. The comparator consisted of a precision Schmitt trigger, followed by a one-shot univibrator which produced a 300 msec voltage gate. The resulting square wave was differentiated using an RC filter with a time constant of 50 msec, followed by a unity gain buffer amplifier which yielded the active membrane driving potential. The resting membrane time constant τ was set to 5 msec.

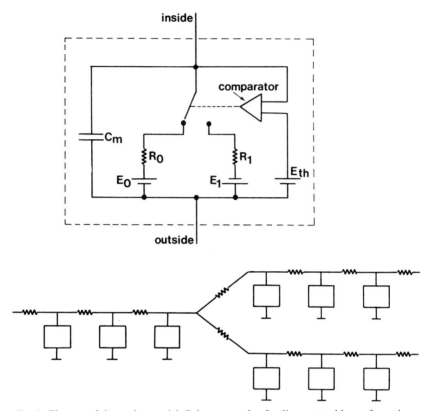

Fig. 1. Element of the analog model. Below: example of a divergent cable configuration.

All elements were connected to a patchboard which permitted a convenient setup for various geometrical configurations, by simple insertion of the appropriate resistors between the elements. Stimulation of the model was done by a conventional electro-physiological current stimulator.

THEORETICAL CONSIDERATIONS

In order to examine the influence of propagation on the configuration of the action potential, it is instructive to consider a continuous cable, in which the ionic mechanism is represented by the simplified model depicted in figure 1. Under the assumption of uniform undisturbed propagation of the action potential the cable equations, together with the ionic mechanism of figure 1, yield the following equations for the foot (V_f) and the crest (V_c) of the propagated action potential:

$$(1) \quad \frac{\lambda^2}{\vartheta^2} \ddot{V}_f - \tau \dot{V}_f - V_f = 0 \qquad (t < 0)$$

$$(2) \quad \frac{\lambda^2}{\vartheta^2} \ddot{V}_c - \tau \dot{V}_c - \frac{V_c - 0.1 \exp{(-t/T)}}{R} = 0 \qquad (t \geq 0)$$

where λ and τ are the length and time constant of the passive cable, ϑ is the conduction velocity, R is the ratio between active state membrane resistance R_1 and resting membrane resistance R_0, and T is the repolarization time constant. For convenience, the resting membrane potential E_0 is set to 0 and the initial value of the active driving potential E_1 is set to 100 mV. Activation occurs at t = O. Equations (1) and (2), together with the boundary conditions V = O at infinity and the requirement of continuity of V and $\dot{V}$ when t = O, can readily be solved analytically.

The propagated action potentials, calculated from these equations, must be compared with the intrinsic or space-clamped action potential associated with the same membrane mechanism. Space clamping, which is unfortunately impracticable in actual AV nodal tissue, would make the intracellular potential identical all over the clamped region. No current can flow under this condition from one region of the fiber to another. As a consequence, all inward ionic current is used exclusively to discharge the local membrane capacitance. The corresponding action potential, which has been called 'membrane' action potential (360) in contrast to the propagating or 'free' action potential, can easily be calculated also for the ionic mechanism of figure 1. Differences in shape between propagated and spaceclamped action potentials reflect the excitatory load imposed upon the action potential by the not-yet depolarized areas downstream.

Three propagating action potentials, calculated from equations (1) and (2) are shown in figure 2, together with their space-clamped counterparts. In all panels of figure 2, the larger action potential is the space-clamped one. The resting membrane time constant was set at 5 msec, the repolarization time constant at 50 msec and the passive length constant of the cable was set at .5 mm. Using the threshold and active state conductance settings indicated in the figure, the conduction velocity of the propagating action potential in the upper panel was 1 m/sec, corresponding to 10 length constants/time constant. In both lower panels, the conduction velocity was reduced to 10 cm/sec by the use of higher settings for the threshold potential and the active state membrane resistance, respectively.

None of the propagating action potentials in figure 2 can quite reach the same amplitude and rate of rise as the correspondent intrinsic membrane response. Still, in the upper panel the discrepancy is only very slight, whereas it is much more outspoken in the slowly conducting action potentials. In these cases, a relatively large proportion of the inward current is required in order to maintain propagation. This current is not available to charge the membrane capacitance and consequently a diminution of rate of rise and amplitude occurs. In the bottom panel, however, the predominant effect is the reduction in amplitude of the space-clamped action potential, due to the reduction of available inward current. In the present model, inactivation (bottom panel) depresses the action potential amplitude to a much larger degree than a high threshold setting (middle panel), even if both result in an equal reduction of the velocity of propagation. Separation of these factors is easy in the model, because neither voltage nor time dependent inactivation mechanism has been included. In actual tissue, a higher threshold setting would probably ensue an increase of inactivation during the time needed for reaching the higher threshold. The sensitivity of biological tissue for changes in threshold or conductance might therefore be much larger than in the model.

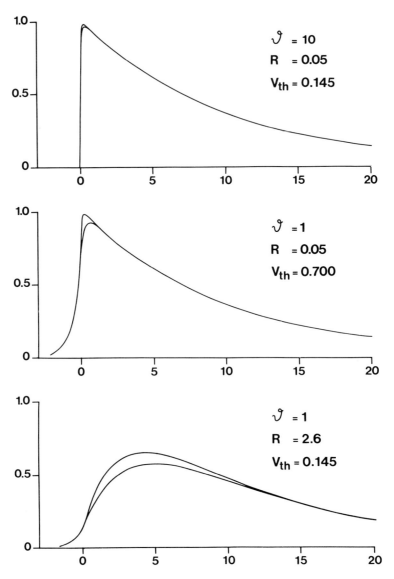

Fig. 2. Comparison of propagated and space-clamped action potentials. The conduction velocity is expressed in length constants/time constant. R is the ratio between active and passive membrane resistance. Abscissa: time expressed in time constants of passive cable. Ordinate: membrane voltage, resting potential corresponds to 0, initial driving potential corresponds to 1.

The question arises, how far conducting velocity can be diminished in the model with conservation of stable conduction. In figure 3, the conduction velocity is shown as a function of V_{th} for various values of the ratio R between passive and active state conductance. As expected, high conduction velocities result from a low threshold setting. In addition, there is no stable propagation when the threshold voltage is raised above a certain value, determined by the setting of R. The corresponding minimal conduction velocity is about 2.5 cm/sec, when τ is set to 5 msec and λ is .5 mm. The lower limb of the curves strikes one as quite paradoxical, because a higher threshold setting is ac-

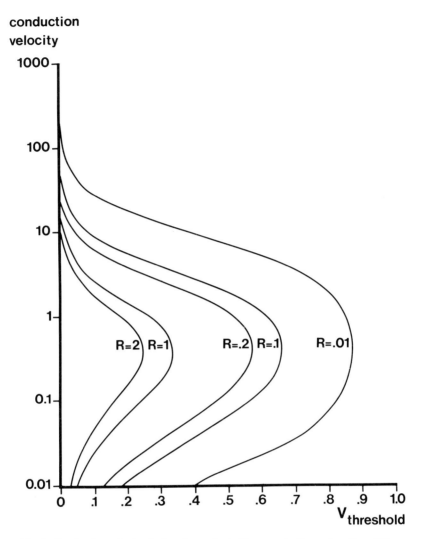

Fig. 3. Conduction velocity (in length constants/time constant) as a function of V_{th}.

companied by a higher conduction velocity. This limb represents unstable 'threshold' propagated responses, which can either decay and die, or grow into full-blown action potential belonging to the upper limb of the curve at the same threshold potential. Such 'threshold' responses have also been described in other models (386,582), but are unlikely to be observed experimentally because of their inherently unstable nature. The separation between the upper and the lower limb of the curve may be thought of as a kind of representation of the 'safety factor' for the maintenance of conduction.

ANALOG MODEL AND EXPERIMENTAL RESULTS

The simplified regeneratieve membrane behaviour, used in these calculations can easily be simulated using analog electronic elements. In this way, situations more complex than uniform conduction through the linear core-conductor model can be handled conveniently. It will be noted, that now we have a lumped model, in contrast to the essentially continuous mathematical model presented above. However, care was taken to keep the resistances between the elements relatively low. In this way, a reasonable approximation of the continuous case was obtained. Specifically, to build one length constant of passive cable, at least four to six elements were used.

In the next sections, some specific instances of actual AV nodal action potential behaviour will be compared with results obtained with this model. Notwithstanding the undoubtedly much more complicated nature of the regenerative mechanism in actual fibers, the potential importance of pure electrotonic interactions on the shape of the action potential will be illustrated in this way.

COLLISIONS OF WAVEFRONTS

Action potentials were recorded from the isolated AV node of the rabbit. Collisions of antegrade and retrograde wavefronts were set up in the AV node using the stimulus

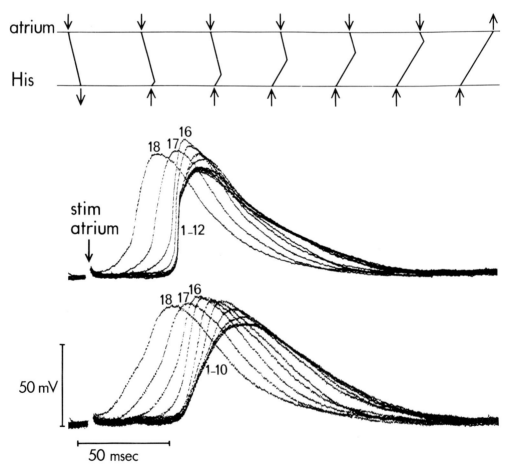

Fig. 4. Two AV nodal action potentials during transition from antegrade to retrograde activation.

pattern depicted in figure 4. First, only the atrium was paced for 10 beats, resulting in stable antegrade conduction of the impulse through the AV node to the His bundle. Then the His bundle was also paced. This resulted in a collision of the antegrade wavefront, set up by the atrial stimulus, with the retrograde wavefront set up by the His bundle stimulus. The first stimulus on the His bundle was given just before the arrival of the antegrade wavefront. Consequently, a collision took place close to the His bundle. The second stimulus on the His bundle was given 10 msec earlier with respect to the atrial stimulus. This resulted in a collision which took place at a slightly higher level in the node. This procedure was repeated for subsequent stimuli, until the collision had moved into the atrium, and all of the AV node was activated in a retrograde way. Then, the atrial stimulus was stopped and pure retrograde conduction was maintained for a few beats before the whole sequence started again. Figure 4 shows the action potentials of two AV nodal cells during this stimulus pattern. Consecutive action potentials have been superimposed, using the atrial stimulus as a time reference. The first 12 action potentials of the first fiber are quite superimposable, which indicates that they were all activated in the same antegrade way. As the collisions moved closer to the recording mictroelectrode, however, notable changes in the action potential configuration occurred. The action potential increased in both amplitude and rate of rise, until the collision took place very close to the impaled fiber (action potential 16). Action potentials number 17 and higher were evoked progressively earlier in time, indicating that the cell was now activated by the retrograde wavefront. Neither the gradual changes in shape nor the increment in amplitude are found in cells from the His bundle (104, 777). This suggest that these phenomena might be accentuated by a low safety factor.

As discussed earlier the amplitude of the propagating action potential is expected to be smaller than the amplitude of the space clamped action potential. The situation during collision is comparable to space clamp because no excitatory current can flow from the

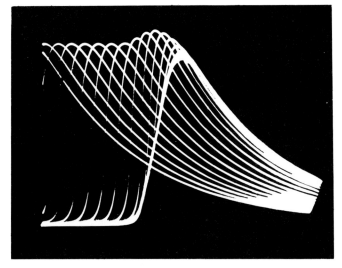

Fig. 5. Simulated action potential during transition from antegrade to retrograde activation in diverging geometry.

collision site to other areas. As a matter of fact, during the larger part of the upstroke, current is supplied to the collision site, rather than extracted from it. This results in rate of rise even faster than that of the intrinsic action potential. Consequently, in those cases, in which the propagating action potential is significantly smaller than the intrinsic one, enhancement of the action potential amplitude may be expected during collision.

By allowing the strands to converge or diverge, an asymetrical situation, which results in a difference in amplitude between antegradely and retrogradely conducted action potentials, can easily be introduced into the model. In a converging geometry less current will have to be supplied by the elements already excited: the 'load' on the active region is diminished. In a diverging geometry the load will be greater, which results in a further reduction in amplitude and rate of rise. A diverging geometry was set up in the model in the way shown in figure 1. Antegrade stimulation was applied to the single left hand branch, retrograde stimulation was applied to both right hand branches simultaneously, resulting in synchronous arrival of both retrograde wavefronts in the branching point. A superposition of action potentials derived from this junction is shown in figure 5. The stimulus sequence was the one explained before. The completely superimposable set of antegrade action potentials is smaller than the retrograde ones. During collision, the amplitude is maximal. These differences became less significant when the overall excitability of the elements was increased.

AMPLITUDE AND RATE OF RISE

In principle, what has been said about the amplitude of the action potential, would also be expected to hold for the rate of rise. It may therefore seem surprising, that many AV nodal fibers behave in the way illustrated in figure 6 (see also ref. 957). With antegrade activation, the action potential is smaller than with retrograde activation. But the rate of rise is clearly much larger antegradely. Part of the explanation may be, that the rate of rise depends more than the amplitude on synchronous arrival of the converging wavefronts. This is illustrated in figure 7. The model was alternately stimulated from S1 (antegrade) and from both S2 and S3 (retrograde). The excitability of the antegrade input branch was set somewhat higher than the two exit branches. An action potential was recorded from the antegrade input path close to the junction. During retrograde stimulation, the synchronicity of the arrival of both retrograde wavefronts was at first disrupted by the introduction of a 15 msec delay between S2 and S3. As a result, the antegrade action potential was smaller but also steeper than the retrograde one. When synchrony between S2 and S3 was restored, the amplitude of the retrograde action potential remained the same, but the retrograde rate of rise became larger than the antegrade one. Thus, the initially discordant relation between rate of rise and amplitude became concordant when the retrograde inputs became more synchronous. In the right hand panels of figure 7, a fourth branch, consisting exclusively of inexcitable elements was added. These elements merely represented a passive load on the junctional elements. This resulted in a clear difference in shape between antegrade and retrograde action potential, to be compared with figure 6. Again, a discordance between amplitude and rate of rise was present, which became smaller when retrograde activation became synchronous.

antegrade

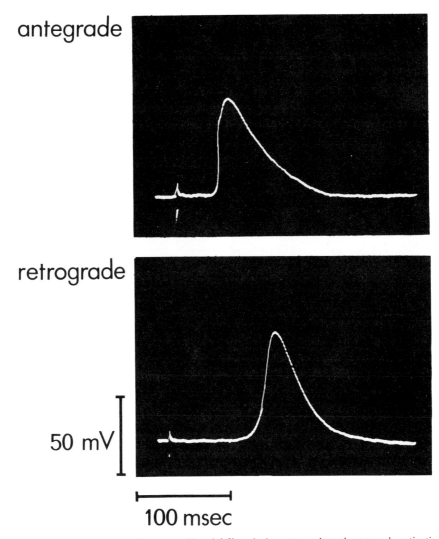

retrograde

50 mV

100 msec

Fig. 6. Action potentials of the same AV nodal fiber during antegrade and retrograde activation.

DOUBLE COMPONENTS

Action potentials, consisting of two or even more components are also observed frequently in the AV node. It is interesting that the occurrence of double components is
sometimes dependent on the direction of the activation front. An example is shown in
figure 8. The action potentials were recorded simultaneously from sites close to one
another. The stimulus sequence is the same as in figure 4. The first 9 antegrade action
potentials are not shown. Both fibers show a clear double configuration when activated in
the retrograde direction. The upper one exhibits a prepotential or foot, the lower trace
shows a double crested action potential. It is noteworthy, that during the transition from
antegrade to retrograde activation (action potential 13 to 18) the first component bears

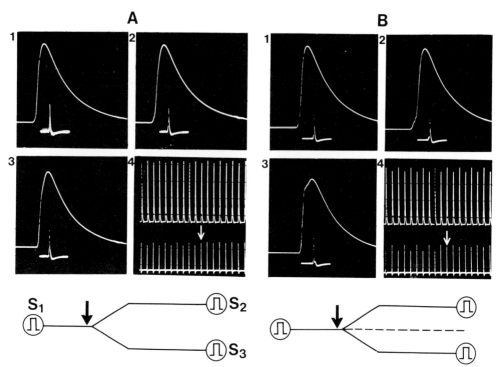

Fig. 7. Simulated action potentials and dV/dt in divergent geometries as shown in the lower part of the figure. A: Synchronous (panel 1) and asynchronous (panel 2) retrograde activation and antegrade activation (panel 3). In panel 4, alternate antegrade and retrograde activation is shown. The retrograde activation was at first asynchronous, resulting in discordance between amplitude and dV/dt. At a certain moment (arrow) retrograde activation was made synchronous, resulting in concordance between amplitude and dV/dt. B: Same as A, after addition of a passive branch.

already a fixed relation to the His bundle stimulus, when the second component still occurs at a constant time after the atrial stimulus. Thus the first component seems to be retrogradely activated at the same time that the second component of the same action potential still belongs to the antegrade wavefront. A possible explanation will be given in the following paragraphs.

UNIDIRECTIONAL BLOCK AND DOUBLE COMPONENTS

When the excitability is reduced far enough, unidirectional block will occur in asymetrical structures. An example is shown in figure 9. Two strands merge into a common exit path. In this case, the threshold setting was so high, that none of the strands could by itself excite either the other strand or the exit path. Only when both strands were stimulated, the exit path could be excited. In case of a time lag of 60 msec between the arrival of the two wavefronts, the exit path could still be excited. Yet now, the action potentials in the two input branches showed double components. The action potential recorded at position 1 showed a second hump in the repolarization phase. This hump is a purely electronic re-

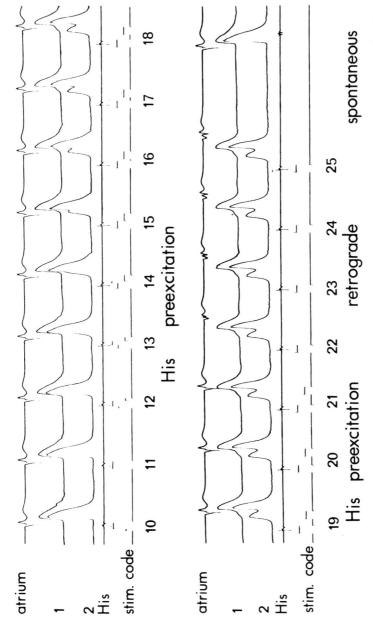

Fig. 8. Two simultaneously recorded AV nodal action potentials during transition from antegrade to retrograde activation. Leading edge of stimulus markers correspond to atrial and His bundle stimuli.

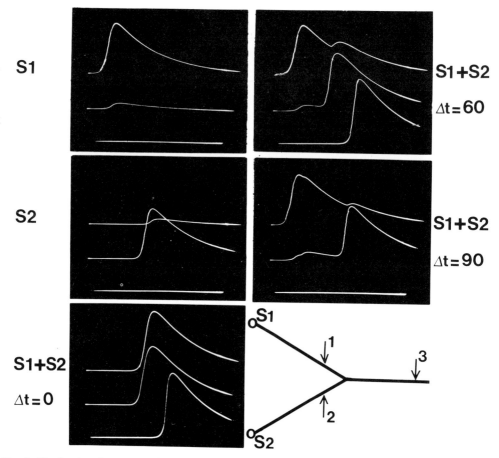

Fig. 9. Simulated action potentials in a converging geometry. Only when S1 and S2 were both stimulated, propagation to the exit path occurred.

flection of the second action potential from the other strand. In a similar way, the pre-potential in 2 is an electrotonic reflection of the earlier action potential from 1. When the time lag was increased to 90 msec, excitation of the exit pat no longer occurred, but the action potentials in 1 and 2 still showed double components.

It is clear from this example that double components in the action potential may be caused by asynchronous arrival of wavefronts at a point where one or more of these wavefronts separately would be blocked. The different branches converging upon each other need not have the same characteristics. Consider for instance the geometry shown in figure 10. The beginning and the end of a long tortuous path come close together, at a point where a small strand can act as a short cut. Due to its small dimensions, this short cut does not conduct as easily as the main pathway: its length constant is shorter and per-haps its regenerative ionic mechanism is more or less inhibited. As a result, conduction through the short cut can occur only up to the point where it rejoins the main pathway. Here conduction block occurs, because the main pathway represents a load too heavy for the activity in the small strand. Recordings of point A and B in figure 10 are shown

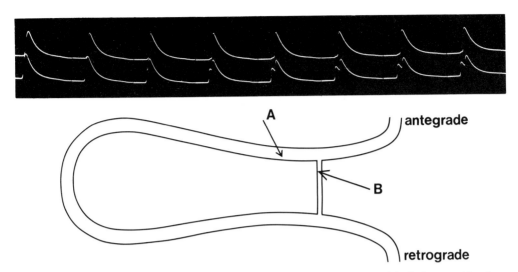

Fig. 10. Gradual development of double components in simulated action potentials during transition from antegrade to retrograde activation. Upper trace corresponds to position A, lower to B.

during the transition from antegrade to retrograde activation. Action potential 1, which is completely antegradely activated, does not show any double components. Action potential 8, which is partly retrograde, shows a clear double configuration. The earliest hump in B and the foot in A reflect the early arrival of retrograde activation through the small strand. This activation front is subsequently blocked at the junction of the two pathways. Thus the early component of B is active, but relatively small because of the block occurring in the junction, whilst the foot in A is a passive response. The second component reflects the arrival of the massive activity through the main pathway; it is active in A and it is a passive reflection in B. When both ends are stimulated in the way described before, collisions are produced in both pathways. Yet as the retrograde stimulus becomes earlier with respect to the antegrade one, the retrograde activation will first reach B by way of a small strand. The early component B will thus become fixed in time with respect to the retrograde stimulus, while the late component stays linked for several more beats to the antegrade activation through the main pathway. In this way action potentials 3–5 show double components, the first of which belongs to the retrograde wavefront, whereas the second one reflects the antegrade activity. This is exactly the situation found in the preparation shown in figure 8.

INEXCITABLE GAP

Double components could also be obtained from the model in a different way. When a few elements in a cable geometry were made inexcitable, consequently behaving as a segment of passive cable, the action potentials of elements close to or in the gap showed double components. Action potentials 1 and 2 in figure 11 were proximal to the gap, 3–6 were in the inexcitable region, and 7, 8 and 9 were distal to the gap. The inexcitable gap

normal conduction   inexcitable gap

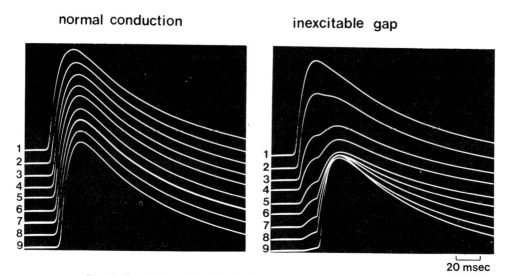

20 msec

Fig. 11. Conduction of simulated action potentials over an inexcitable gap.

has been discussed extensively in the recent literature (502,807,921), and our results were not at variance. Delays of about 15 msec could be obtained over the inexcitable gap. It seems unlikely that much larger delays than twice the membrane time constant can be obtained over a completely unexcitable gap. The length of the gap must be limited to one or two length constants of passive cable in order to maintain conduction and this does not result in excessive delays. Still, if the gap were not completely inexcitable, the resulting decremental activity could conceivably bridge a much larger gap. In addition, the properties of a similar structure would be likely to be rate-dependent, possibly giving rise to the Wenckebach type of partial block.

Asymmetry in a region of depressed excitability can result in undirectional block. For example, a progressively heavier row of shunt conductances over the successive elements of a cable in antegrade direction, resulted in block in antegrade direction only (see figure 12). Block did not occur in retrograde direction, because the healthy action potential arriving from the undepressed distal end of the cable could bridge the adjacent maximally depressed segment. The antegrade wavefront, arriving at this segment, had already been depressed too much to cross it. This situation simulates the experimental results on cooled Purkinje fibers by Downar and Waxman, reported in Chapter 22.

LOCAL POLARIZATION IN THE AV NODE

Unlike the model, actual AV nodal tissue does not permit separate evaluation of intrinsic and electrotonic factors in a simple way. It appears to be possible, however, to influence just the intrinsic factor locally by application of the polarizing current to the cell membranes. Although earlier investigators were unable to demonstrate any influence of polarization on the shape of the action potential in the rabbit AV node (368), Shigeto and Irisawa (756), using a suction electrode for current application, demonstrated recently

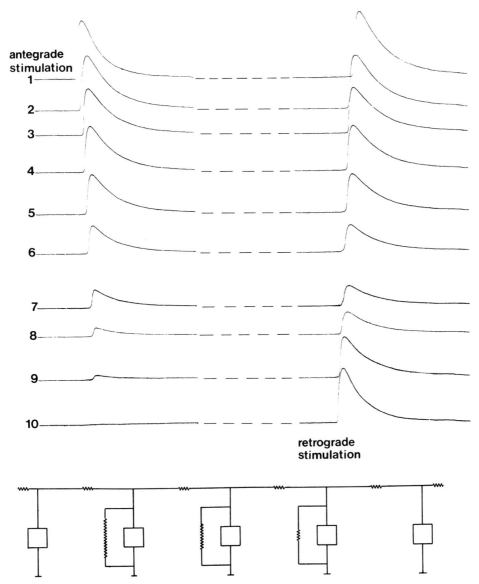

antegrade
stimulation

retrograde
stimulation

Fig. 12. Simulated action potentials showing unidirectional block due to addition of a progressively heavier row of shunt conductances over the elements. The cable consisted of 48 elements. The 20 middle elements were shunted with resistance ranging from 560 KOhm to 18 KOhm.

a definite enhancement of the rate of rise of the AV nodal action potential of the cat when hyperpolarizing current was applied.

Our method of application of positive (anodal) current results in a local hyperpolarization of the cell membrane, because part of the applied current enters the intracellular compartment from the extracellular space. However, this current must also leave the intracellular compartment, resulting in a slight depolarization of the membrane elsewhere. In the same way, cathodal current depolarizes the region under the current injecting electrodes, but results also in a slight hyperpolarization further away.

int. 250 msec   int. 210 msec

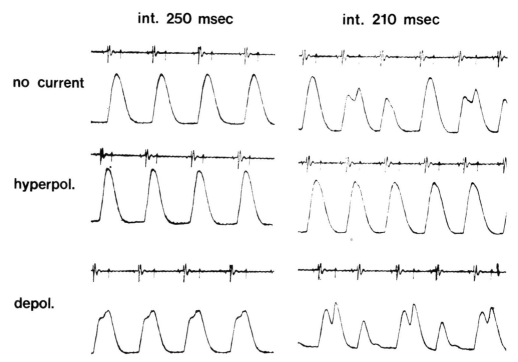

no current

hyperpol.

depol.

Fig. 13. AV nodal action potentials during application of polarizing current. Upper trace shows His bundle spike and atrial deflection.

Definite effects of current application on the Atrium-His conduction time and on the shape of the action potentials in the rabbit AV node could be demonstrated. Yet, only a small area, corresponding more or less to the N region (31), was sensitive to the application of currents in the order of 80 uA. Results are shown in figure 13.

An action potential is shown which was recorded from a site close to the current applying electrodes. When the preparation was paced from the atrium with a basic cycle length of 250 msec, 1:1 conduction to the His bundle resulted. Application of hyperpolarizing current resulted in a definite shortening of the A-H interval, while the action potential became larger and steeper. Application of depolarizing current had the opposite effect.

When the preparation was paced with a basic cycle length of 210 msec, 3:2 block occurred when no polarizing current was present. Hyperpolarizing current now restored 1:1 conduction, but when depolarizing current was applied, conduction became still more impaired and 2:1 block developed. Concomitant changes in the action potential were observed.

The occurrence of double components in the action potential was favoured by depolarizing current. If any changes in the shape of the action potential could be noted at all, usually a second component developed or became more prominent. Hyperpolarizing current acted in the opposite way.

The amount of actual hyperpolarization in the impaled cells was small. It was measured by application of a square-wave on/off current, during withdrawal of the recording microelectrode from the fiber. Comparison of the amplitude of the resulting square-wave voltage in the intracellular and the extracellular compartment yields the amount of local membrane polarization. This was usually less than 2 mV in the cells we impaled. This probably indicates that we were not able to impale cells very close to the site of current injection.

The effect of local excitability changes can easily be mimicked in the model. Reduction of the exitability of one or more elements in a linear cable configuration results in the same kind of conduction disturbances as have been described in the section on the inexcitable gap. More interesting results were obtained from the configuration depicted in figure 14. The overall excitability of the elements was reduced to the point where each of the two inputs alone failed to excite the other input as well as the exit path. Under these conditions conduction was much more sensitive to excitability changes of elements close to the junction than to excitability changes of other elements. The excitability of only the junctional element was changed in figure 14. The two input branches were stimulated asynchronously, resulting in a double component action potential in 1, and relatively late activation of 2. When the excitability of the junctional element was increased, the second component in 1 disappeared and electrode 2 was much earlier activated. The reason for this was, of course, that the earlier wavefront was now conducted across the junctional

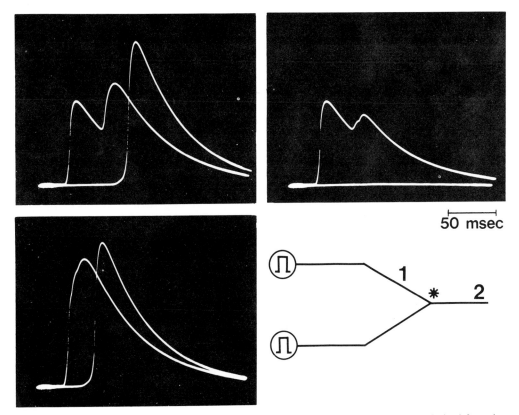

Fig. 14. Simulated action potentials in a converging geometry. The action potentials are derived from sites 1 and 2. The excitability of the junctional element only (asterisk) was changed, resulting in the changes in action potential configuration shown.

element both to the exit path and retrogradely into the other input branch. Depression of the excitability of the junctional element resulted in complete block at the junction. The variations in shape of action potential 1 do not directly reflect the changes in excitability. They do reflect changes in spatial interaction of wavefronts in a complex geometry, brought about by excitability changes of an element further away. One might speculate whether a similar mechanism could be responsible for the large variability in action potential configuration in experiments such as the one described in figure 13, since no actual depolarization or hyperpolarization of the impaled fiber could be demonstrated.

DISCUSSION

The configuration of the propagated cardiac action potential is determined by two factors: 1. the intrinsic generator properties of the local membrane (the intrinsic factor); and 2. the electrical interaction of the local membrane with distant areas (electrotonic factor). The two factors cannot easily be studied separately in heart muscle. The electronic factor describes the distortion in the shape of the action potential, caused by the fact that the membrane potential is not identical everywhere. Spatially uniform depolarization of a certain area of membrane (space clamp) is more difficult to realize experimentally in heart muscle than it is in the heaven-sent giant axon. Since space-clamping is a pre-requisite for voltage-clamp experiments, a reliable description of the ionic mechanism is also much harder to obtain, especially on the slowly conducting nodal fibres.

The ionic mechanism, used in the present model, is certainly much too primitive. No provisions have been made for voltage-dependent inactivation of the regenerative inward current, and the repolarization mechanism is rather artificial. Still, it may be significant, that with so simple an ionic mechanism so many anomalities of AV nodal action potentials can be simulated. Furthermore, since no reliable information is present about the actual ionic mechanism, and since we are concerned only with qualitative modelling, a very simple approximation does not seem out of place. We do not feel that arbitrary inference of a detailed ionic mechanism derived from vastly different tissues, would be of much help.

It is often assumed, explicitly or tacitly, that the shape of the propagated action potential does not deviate strongly from the configuration of 'membrane' (space clamped) action potentials. This assumption is reasonable when the excitatory current, depolarizing the downstream areas, is only a small fraction of the total ionic current of the active area. In this case most of the regenerative inward current is used to charge the membrane capacity, and propagation will not greatly influence the shape of the action potential. This is the case when the margin of safety and the conduction velocity are high. A low margin of safety means that a considerable part of the regenerative inward current is needed to depolarize areas downstream. Under these conditions the influence of propagation on the shape of the action potential may be expected to be considerable. A direct comparison between propagated action potentials and membrane action potentials cannot be made in AV nodal tissue. Still, the influence of propagation on the shape of the action potential is clearly shown when a collision of two wavefronts occur. In the slowly conducting tissues of the AV node the configuration of the action potential may change dramatically during collision, whereas the influence of collision on the shape of the action potential of Purkinje fibers is much less outspoken.

Clearly, the electronic interaction between two regions will depend on the geometric disposition of the fibers. Branching or converging cell strands, for instance, would have opposite effects on the configuration of the action potential. The magnitude of the effect depends on the importance of the electrotonic influence relative to the intrinsic membrane generator. Whereas the effect of the electronus of the action potential can frequently be neglected when conduction is rapid, it is very important in the slowly conducting tissues. So the question arises, whether the shape of the intracellular action potential can give us information about the geometrical arrangement of the fibres (see also ref. 104 and 957).

The present model simulation indicates, that action potential amplitude rather than the rate of rise should be selected as a criterium for possible convergence or divergence. However, in the biological tissue, the ionic mechanism is much more complicated than in the model, and interactions between the electronic phenomena and the regenerative mechanism may be very significant. Extrapolation of the model results to the actual tissue must be made carefully.

Double component action potentials could essentially be simulated in two ways, both of which were associated with depression of excitability. An inexcitable gap, or a segment of cable too much depressed to maintain unimpaired conduction, gave rise to two components in the action potential. The smaller component was either a 'foot' or a hump in the repolarization phase. The configuration of figure 10 or 14 with two clearly separated peaks could not be evoked in this way. On the other hand, asynchronous arrival of activity could yield such a configuration. Yet, in such cases excitability had to be sufficiently depressed to produce block when only the earlier wavefronts arrived at the junction. Otherwise, it would simply cross the junction and be conducted backwards into the other input branches, colliding there with the other, later, input wavefronts. In our opinion, it is not likely that an inexcitable region alone could account for the large variety of double component action potentials observed in the AV node.

Our results indicate, that the variability, as well as many of the anomalies observed in AV nodal action potentials, can be explained straightforwardly by electrotonic interaction in a geometrically complex system with a reduced excitability. On the other hand, there is no proof, that these anomalies do not reflect some intrinsic membrane property. Still, interpretations of the shape of the action potential only in terms of intrinsic membrane mechanisms should be made with great caution.

19

ELECTROPHYSIOLOGY OF ENDOCARDIAL INTRAVENTRICULAR CONDUCTION: THE ROLE AND FUNCTION OF THE SPECIALIZED CONDUCTING SYSTEM

ROBERT J. MYERBURG, M.D., HENRY GELBAND, M.D.,
AGUSTIN CASTELLANOS, JR., M.D., KRISTINA NILSSON,
RUEY J. SUNG, M.D., AND ARTHUR L. BASSETT, Ph.D.

When a cardiac impulse propagates from the A-V node to ventricular muscle, it must excite in temporal sequence: 1. the bundle of His; 2. the bundle branches; 3. the peripheral ramifications of the specialized intraventricular conducting system; 4. the terminal sub-endocardial Purkinje network; and 5. the junctions between Purkinje fibers and ventricular muscle cells (i.e., PF-VM junctions) (572,575). Impulses cannot excite muscle cells lateral to the orientation of the specialized conducting fibers unless PF-VM junctions are present (575), thereby limiting spread in the system to a functionally longitudinal orientation. Thus, the pattern of intraventricular conduction, and the functional electrophysiologic properties of the specialized intraventricular conducting system, are determined at least partially by the following factors: 1. the anatomy of the various portions of the intraventricular conducting system; 2. the functional relationship between intraventricular specialized conducting fibers and the ventricular muscle (PF-VM junctions); 3, the electrophysiologic properties of single units at various levels of the system; and 4. the interactions of groups of cells within the specialized conducting system. Each of these interactions and influences must be considered as one attempts to determine the mechanisms of normal and abnormal impulse conduction, and the nature of functional and pathologic intraventricular block.

ANATOMIC AND PHYSIOLOGIC INTERACTIONS IN THE INTRAVENTRICULAR CONDUCTING SYSTEM

The right bundle branch is an anatomically and physiologically isolated structure along the endocardial surface of the right side of the intraventricular septum (2,14,47,365,366, 482,575,795,833). Anatomic isolation results from the presence of a dense connective tissue sheath surrounding the structure (2,47,482,575,833), and the physiologic isolation has been demonstrated both experimentally (365,366,575), and by inference from clinical electrocardiographic and human surgical studies (14,795). Impulse input directly from the right bundle branch along the upper and mid-right ventricular septal surface does not occur (fig. 1 and 2). Rather, initial activation occurs in the right ventricular apical endocardium,

1. Portions of the work presented were supported by Institutional Research Funds of the Miami Veterans Administrations Hospital; NIH, NHLI Contract #N01-HV-22975; Florida Heart Association Grant-In-Aid #72A25 and 73AG1 (funded by the Heart Association of Palm Beach County); and Grants-In-Aid from the Broward County Heart Association and the Heart Association of Greater Miami.

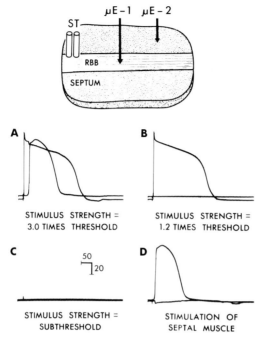

Fig. 1. Physiological isolation of the right bundle branch from the septal muscle. Septal muscle and right bundle branch (RBB) were transected proximal to fibers which reflect back to the lower septum. Surface stimulating electrodes were used (ST), and microelectrodes impaled cells in RBB (μE-1) and septal muscle (μE-2). In A, RBB was stimulated at a current density high enough to also stimulate nearby muscle directly, and propagation occurred through both RBB and septal muscle. In B: stimulus strength was such that the current density could excite only the local cells (RBB). In C, stimulus strength was subthreshold for even RBB and the entire preparation remained quiescent. In D, surface electrodes were moved to the septal muscle, and excitation of the entire muscle mass occurred without depolarization of RBB. The same results were observed with intracellular stimulation, except that simultaneous activation of RBB and muscle with high current densities was not possible. Cycle lengths from 400 to 1000 msec were used. (Reprinted by permission of The American Heart Association, Inc., from Myerburg et al. (575)).

and spreads from that site to the lower portion of the interventricular septum, as well as to the endocardial surface of the free wall of the right ventricle via the moderator band. Specialized conducting fibers from the free-running false tendon at the base of the antero-septal papillary muscle of the dog heart deliver impulses to much of the free wall endo-cardial surface almost simultaneously, resulting in activation of most of the right ventricular endocardial surface area within a time frame of a few milliseconds. The major exception is the most basal portion of the endocardial surface of the right ventricle, near the tricuspid valve ring, where there is somewhat delayed activation. This occurs presumable because of the absence of specialized conducting fibers in the area, and the resultant dependence on slower conduction through true ventricular muscle cells. While the endocardial surface of the right ventricular free wall is being activated, the lower portion of the right ventri-cular side of the interventricular septum is activated by a group of fibers reflecting back from the apical collection of specialized conducting fibers. From the lower portion of the septum, impulse propagation occurs exclusively through the ordinary ventricular muscle of the septal endocardium from apex to base. Since conduction is dependent upon ordinary

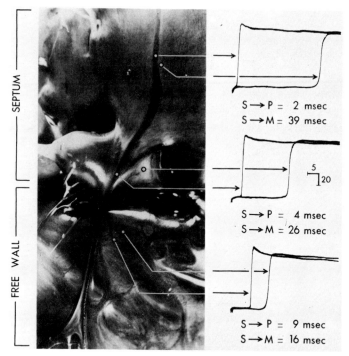

Fig. 2. General sequence of activation of the right ventricular conducting system and muscle. Preparation is of right septum, apex, and free wall in continuity and separated only at the junctions of the anterior and posterior free walls with the anterior and posterior septum. Two microelectrodes were used to simultaneously record mid-bundle branch and adjacent septal muscle (top pair of transmembrane action potentials, TMP's), from the bundle branch crossing the base of the papillary muscle and adjacent muscle cells (middle TMPs), and from an apical subendocardial Purkinje fiber and adjacent muscle (bottom TMP's). Proximal bundle branch was stimulated intracellularly. The sequence of depolarization was from proximal to distal in conducting system, and distal to proximal in muscle. Initial muscle activation was in the region of apical endocardial muscle. The free wall endocardium followed, then papillary muscle, and finally the septal muscle from apex to base. Horizontal calibration = 5 msec; vertical, calibration = 20 mv. (Reprinted by permission of The American Heart Association, Inc., from Myerburg et al. (575)).

ventricular muscle, it occurs more slowly than conduction along the right bundle branch or on the free wall endocardial surface (fig. 2).

The anatomic and physiologic interrelationships on the left side of the interventricular septum are distinctly different from those on the right ventricular septum. The left intraventricular specialized conducting system consists of a main left bundle branch which penetrates the membranous portion of the interventricular septum beneath the aortic ring and divides into two relatively discrete collections of specialized conducting tissue fibers which have been labeled the anterior (superior) and posterior (inferior) divisions of the left bundle branch. These two specialized conducting fiber bundles, plus the right bundle branch, form the components of the trifascicular concept of the intraventricular conducting system. However, physiologic studies on the canine left intraventricular conducting system have demonstrated a profuse network of interconnections on the septal endocardial surface between the anterior and posterior divisions (473,575). Anatomic studies in the human suggest a similar characteristic (188), and it has even been suggested that the

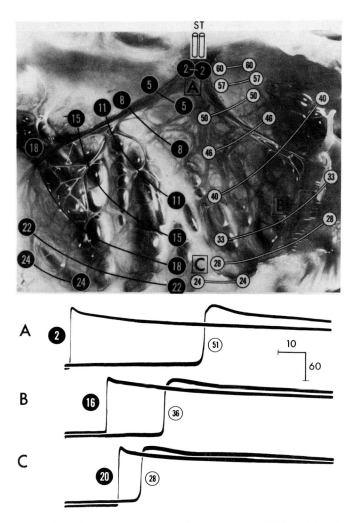

Fig. 3. Impulse input to the left ventricular septum. Preparation is of left ventricle from aortic ring to beginning of the lower third of the septal surface. Anterolateral papillary muscle (PM) is on the left, and posteromedial PM is on the right. Surface electrodes (ST) stimulate the left bundle branch close to threshold at a cycle length of 1000 msec. Isochronic lines on the left connecting the white numbers on black backgrounds represent the sequence of activation of the conducting system tissue. Similar sequence applies to conducting tissue on right of septum. Isochronic lines on the right connecting black numbers on white backgrounds represent the sequence of activation of ventricular muscle. The same sequence applies to true muscle tissue on left side of the septum. The numbers represent time in milliseconds from the onset of the stimulus to activation. The general pattern of activation of the upper two-thirds of septum is from the bundle branch along the major divisions and subendocardial Purkinje fibers, to the junction of the middle and lower thirds of the septum, at which point muscle activation begins and travels back toward the base through ordinary muscle. Action potentials labeled A, B, and C were recorded from sites A, B, and C. The first of each pair is from a Purkinje cell and the second from adjacent muscle. Numbers give activation times. Horizontal calibration = 10 msec; vertical calibration = 60 mv. (Printed by permission of The American Heart Association, Inc., from Myerburg et al. (575)).

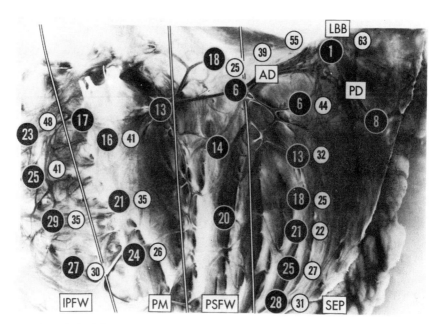

Fig. 4. Excitation of the left intraventricular conducting system and endocardial muscle. The photograph shows most of the left ventricular endocardium stained with Lugol's solution to demonstrate the conducting system. The ventricular cavity has been opened by an incision through the paraseptal free wall between the posteromedial papillary muscle and posterior border of the interventricular septum, the incision extending from the base of the ventricle to the region of the apex. When the ventricle is opened in this way, one views (from right to left) the septum (SEP), anterior paraseptal free wall (PSFW), the anterolateral papillary muscle (PM), the free wall between the papillary muscles or interpapillary free wall (IPFW), and the posteriomedial papillary muscle (not shown). The vertical lines are intended to separate each of these regions for illustrative purposes only. In the experimental preparations represented by this photograph, the left bundle branch (LBB) was stimulated close to threshold by bipolar electrodes or intracellularly, and the intraventricular conducting system and endocardial muscle were mapped for sequence of activation. The rate of stimulation in the experiment shown was 75 impulses/min. The white numbers on black backgrounds are the intervals from stimuli to depolarization of conducting cells at the sites indicated, and the black numbers on white backgrounds are the intervals for ordinary muscle cells at the sites indicated. The impulse originating in the left bundle branch propagates simultaneously along the anterior division (AD) and posterior division (PD) of the LBB, and down the subendocardial conducting tissue network of the SEP. The earliest site of muscle activation (22 msec) occurs at the junction of the middle and lower thirds of the SEP. Muscle is then activated independently of conducting tissue by conduction through ordinary muscle back up the SEP toward the base (25,32,44 msec, etc.). In the meantime, the impulse continues to propagate down the subendocardial conducting tissue network on the lower SEP toward the apex, providing impulse input to the adjacent muscle in the wake of conducting system excitation. Thus, the interval between the excitation of Purkinje fibers and of adjacent ventricular muscle is relatively constant at 1 to 3 msec long the lower SEP and apex, but progressively increases from the junction of the middle and lower thirds of the SEP back to the basal muscle. It is longest between the LBB cells and immediately adjacent muscle. While these events are occurring on the SEP, the impulse continues to propagate along the AD and the conducting tissue on the PSFW, with impulse input to muscle occurring again only at the lower portions of the PSFW, and then propagating through ordinary muscle towards the base of the heart. The exception to this generalization, the high paraseptal island of limited early input described in the text, is seen at the top of the PSFW. When the impulse in the AD reaches the region of the PM, it begins to spread down the conducting tissue on the anterior PM toward its base, and also continues across the PM to the IPFW. At approximately the same time that the impulse reaches the base of the anterior PM from the conducting fibers descending from the upper part of this structure, the impulse propagating in the conducting fibers from the PSFW and apex reaches the base of the PM, providing a dual input. Muscle cell excitation then begins at the base of the PM and propagates through ordinary muscle toward its apex (26,35,41 msec). As the impulse continues along

septal fibers may coalesce into a third division on the left septum (188, 296, 353, 849), resulting in a "quadrifascicular" intraventricular conducting system. In any event, much of the
recent physiologic data indicates that the intraventricular specialized conducting system
is more complex from both a functional and an anatomic point of view than a simple
trifascicular system in which each fascicle can be considered to serve independently an
area of myocardium, in a sense analogous to nerve and skeletal muscle. The right bundle
branch does appear to serve a clearly defined anatomic area of the heart, but the interconnections in the left system makes its functional interpretation much more complex.

   Stimulation of the isolated left ventricular endocardial preparation (575), and mapping
of subsequent impulse propagation through specialized conducting tissue and ordinary
ventricular muscle, has demonstrated that most of the upper portion of the left ventricular
endocardium is devoid of functioning junctions between specialized conducting tissue
and ordinary ventricular muscle (fig. 3) in canine and primate hearts (575, 576). This
appears to be true both on the left septum and the left ventricular free wall endocardium
(fig. 4). Moreover, the upper portion of the papillary muscles of the left ventricle also
appear to be devoid of junctions between specialized conducting fibers and ventricular
muscle (fig. 5), and therefore one could visualize the cylindrical left ventricular cavity as
having sources of impulses input only in the lower one-half to two-thirds of its circumference. The propagation of impulses through the upper one-third of the endocardial
surface occurs later; and appears to occur exclusively through ordinary muscle spread.
The terminations of the anterior and posterior 'divisions' appear to join on the endocardial surface of the free wall of the left ventricle to complete a ring of tissue forming the
upper (basal) border of the specialized conducting system of the left ventricular free wall
(575, 577) (fig. 6 and 7). It is noteworthy, and probably of some significance, that the interconnections of the divisions occurring between the papillary muscles on the free wall are
anatomically broad and diffuse, as shown in figure 7. Physiologic studies of isolated
preparations reveal that the specialized conducting tissue in the area labeled 'intercon-

---

Caption 4 continued

the AD of the LBB past the anterior PM to the IPFW, it excites that portion of the AD on the IPFW which
meets the corresponding portion of the posterior division in the uncut heart, this merger completing the
conducting system 'ring' referred to in the text. We have labeled this portion of the anterior division the
interpapillary Purkinje fiber tract (IPPF in fig. 7), and find it to be activated somewhat earlier than the
rest of the IPFW conducting tissue. The IPFW has impulse input from three sources: 1. the anterior division
conducting fibers, 2. the posterior division fibers, and 3. the subendocardial conducting system from the
apex (see text for details). However, the only area of impulse input into muscle on the IPFW is, again, the
lower (apical) portions of the region with ordinary muscle conduction occurring toward the base. This is
suggested by the sequence of muscle activation times in the illustration (30, 35, 41, 48 msec), and the divergence
of intervals between conducting tissue excitation and ordinary muscle excitation from the apical to the basal
portion of the IPFW (3, 6, 16, 25 msec). The impulse propagating through the profusely interconnecting
subendocardial conducting system network from upper (basal) to lower (apical) ventricle occurs earliest
along the septum and follows sequentially along the paraseptal free walls, papillary muscles, and interpapillary
free wall. The time sequences in this last-named area are made more complex by intermingling of impulses
ascending from the apex with impulses arriving from the major divisions of the LBB. The subendocardial
network described has multiple interconnections with the ring formed by the anterior and posterior divisions.
(Reprinted by permission of Grune and Stratton, from Myerburg et al. (577)).

342

R. J. MYERBURG ET AL.

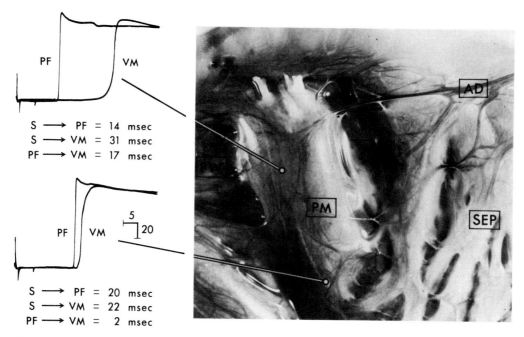

Fig. 5. Excitation of papillary muscle in the left ventricle. Anterior septum (SEP) and anteriolateral papillary muscle (PM) are separated by paraseptal free wall. To the left of the PM is the interpapillary free wall (FW). The anterior division (AD) of the left bundle branch courses toward the upper part of the PM, and conducting fibers from the septal subendocardial Purkinje network cross the paraseptal free wall to the base of PM. Fibers from the AD course down the longitudinal axis of PM toward the base. Action potentials were recorded from Purkinje fibers (PF) and adjacent ventricular muscle (VM) at apical portion of PM (top) and at base PM in the locations indicated. Pairs of electrodes for recording PF and VM were within 0.5 mm of each other. Stimulation on the left bundle branch was at a cycle length of 100 msec. Depolarization of PF on upper part of PM occurred 6 msec before the PF at the base, while VM cells at the base were depolarized 9 msec before VM cells at the upper site. The PF-VM interval at the base was only 2 msec, and at the apical site was 17 msec. Horizontal calibration = 5 msec; vertical calibration = 20 mv. (Reprinted by permission of The American Heart Association, Inc. from Myerburg et al. (575)).

nections of the divisions' in figure 7 is either completely isolated from the surrounding endocardial muscle or has only a relatively few connections, as compared to the density of junctions in the area labeled 'subendocardial conducting tissue network'.

Propagation of impulses is normally balanced along the collections of fibers referred to as the anterior and posterior divisions of the left bundle branch, when studied in isolated tissue preparations (578). Figure 8 demonstrates the results of a mapping study performed on a canine tissue preparation consisting of two parts. The upper half of the preparation is composed of the main left bundle branch and proximal portions of the anterior and posterior divisions in a septal block of muscle. The lower half consists of the terminal interconnections of the anterior posterior divisions on a block of muscle from the upper portion of the left ventricular free wall. The two blocks of muscle are connected only by the major false tendons, extending from the proximal portions of the anterior and posterior divisions to the apices of the two papillary muscles on the free wall block. In the illustration shown, conduction from the point of stimulation on the main left bundle branch, to the point on the free wall at which impulses from the two segments collide, requires approxi-

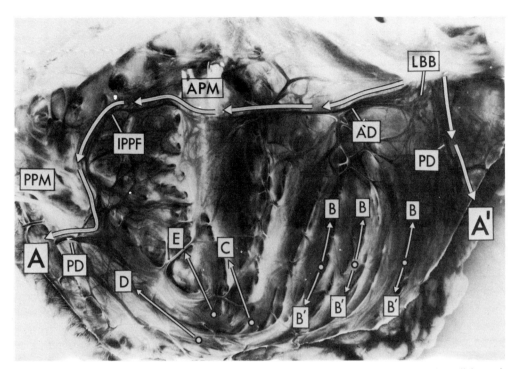

Fig. 6. Intraventricular conducting system ring of the left ventricle and the pattern of endocardial muscle excitation. The entire left ventricular endocardium, stained with Lugol's solution to show the conducting system, is demonstrated, as described in figure 4. The left bundle branch (LBB) divides into the anterior division (AD) and posterior division (PD). The AD crosses the anterolateral papillary muscle (APM), continues across the interpapillary free wall as the interpapillary Purkinje fiber tract (IPPF), and merges with similar fibers from the PD that have crossed the posterior medial papillary muscle (PPM). In the intact preparations, A and A' join to complete a ring of conducting tissue around the upper portion of the left ventricular cavity. The tissue contributing to this ring lies below the arrows on the upper portions of the ventricle. The segment of the ring on the interpapillary free wall is rather diffuse in some preparations, but its functional continuity is clearly demonstrable. The three points at the junction of the middle and lower thirds of the septum and paraseptal free wall, from which arrows B and B' diverge, indicate the earliest regions of muscle cell excitation during stimulation of the left bundle branch. The arrows labeled B indicate the direction of propagation from this site toward the base of the septum and paraseptal free wall through ordinary muscle; B' indicates propagation toward the apex of the ventricle through conducting tissue and muscle. Muscle activation then occurs from base to apex of the anterolateral papillary muscle (C) and posteromedial papillary muscle (D), and finally up the interpapillary free wall (E) from the apex of the ventricle toward the base. The regions from which the arrows to C, D, and E originate imply sites of impulse into muscle from conducting tissue. (Reprinted by permission of Grune and Stratton, from Myerburg et al. (577).

mately 21 msec. It is noteworthy that in the undamaged preparation, conduction to the point of collision of propagating impulses requires approximately the same length of time along each of the divisions, the collision therefore occurring on the mid-free wall. When one of the pathways of conduction is locally damaged, however, (fig. 8B) conduction continues through the usual area of collision, retrogradely onto the opposite division of the bundle branch, and thence to the point of injury. The retrograde conduction time from the mid-portion of the free wall to the point of injury is approximately the same as

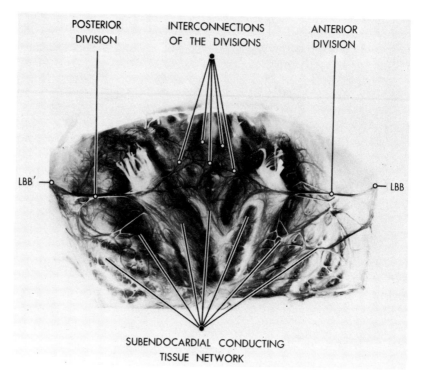

Fig. 7. Interconnections of the divisions of the left bundle branch. The preparation consists of the entire left ventricular endocardial surface stained with Lugol's solution to highlight the specialized conduction tissue. The left ventricular cavity was opened by an incision through the interventricular septum dividing the left bundle branch proper into two portions, LBB' (left side of the illustration) and LBB (right side of the illustration). The two halves of the left bundle branch give rise to the collections of fibers labeled the 'posterior division' and 'anterior division'. Note that the divisions continue across the apices of the two papillary muscles, after giving off fibers which travel longitudinally down the papillary muscles, and the remainder of the divisions interconnect freely on the upper portion of the left ventricular endocardium. Between the divisions and the lower (apical) portion of the left ventricular endocardium, there is a profusely interconnecting sub-endocardial conducting tissue network. Physiologic studies, in which the lower half of the endocardium has been removed, and LBB or LBB' has been stimulated, demonstrate that conduction of the propagating impulse is favored through the specialized conducting tissue, with limited or no input into the upper portion of the endocardial muscle.

the antegrade conduction between these two points in the undamaged preparation. Clearly, conduction through intact hearts, or even intact endocardial preparations, is quite different from that observed in the demonstration preparation shown in figure 8. However, this type of preparation does serve the purpose of illustrating the functional continuity between the two divisions of the bundle branch as their fibers merge on the upper portion of the free wall of the left ventricle.

The earliest site of impulse input from the specialized conducting tissue to the true ventricular muscle on the left ventricular endocardial surface is in the mid-portion of the left ventricular septum. In addition, there are two smaller islands of early activation above the apices of the two papillary muscles (575). Endocardial muscle spread occurs rapidly from the site of earliest activation on the left ventricular septum, through the remainder of the lower portion of the left ventricular endocardium, and finally in an apicobasal orienta-

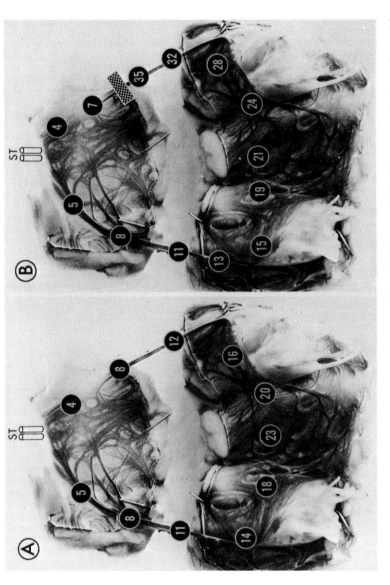

Fig. 8. The functional continuity of the 'divisions' of the left bundle branch. The upper half of the preparation in each panel is composed of the main left bundle branch, the collection of fibers forming the anterior and posterior divisions, and the interconnections between the two divisions on the upper portion of the septum. This complex of specialized conducting tissue overlies a small area of left septal muscle. Bipolar stimulating electrodes are represented by 'ST'. The lower half of each preparation consists of the basal portion of the left ventricular free wall endocardium and the apices of the two papillary muscles. The upper and lower portions are connected by two free-running false tendons. The interconnections of the anterior and posterior divisions are demonstrated by Lugol's solution, staining the conducting tissue. In the unstained state, stimulation of the left bundle branch (panel A) demonstrated balanced conduction along the proximal anterior and posterior divisions, and across the two free running false tendons, to the conducting tissue of the apices of the papillary muscles. Note that conduction time along the two divisions is such that the propagating impulses collide at approximately the midpoint of the left ventricular free-wall endocardium. In panel B, the cross-hatched area along the proximal portion of the free-running false tendon from the posterior division represents an area in which damage was induced by crushing the false tendon. Note that the conduction time from the midportion of the free-wall to the area of damage is approximately the same as it was during antegrade conduction between these two points (panel A). In both conditions, muscle activation on the free wall always lagged by a few milliseconds behind specialized conducting tissue activation. The limitations of the preparations, and the significance of the time relationships of conduction in the free wall specialized conducting tissue, are discussed in the text.

tion towards the base of the septum and free wall. The endocardium of the papillary muscles are activated initially at the bases of these structures shortly after activation of the paraseptal free walls, and propagation occurs towards the apices.

In the isolated endocardial preparation, small lesions through the anterior or posterior division of the left bundle branch cause only minor delays distal to the lesions (fig. 9), and minimal distortion of the normal pattern of endocardial excitation (575). This is consistent with electrocardiographic observations in dogs (894). However recent studies by Gallagher et al. (291), using the intact canine heart and sensitive techniques for recording delays of intramural activation and epicardial surface excitation, have demonstrated that small lesions which cause minimal endocardial delays and minor ECG changes, may cause changes in intramural, epicardial, and vectorcardiographic activation patterns. Extension of the lesions, causing interruption of septal subendocardial Purkinje fibers in addition to one of the divisions of the bundle branch, amplified the conduction delays in endocardial mapping studies (575) (fig. 9), electrocardiographic studies (894), and vectorcardiographic and epicardial mapping studies (291). Studies in our laboratory, using endocardial preparations obtained from primate hearts (baboons), and dissected,

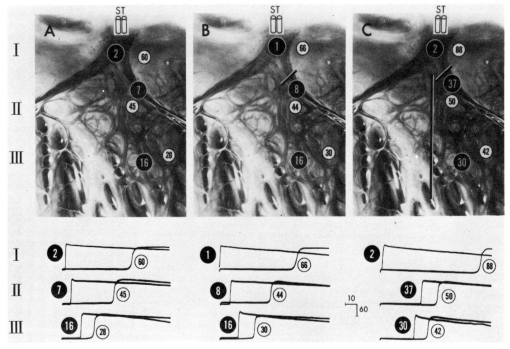

Fig. 9. Influence of lesions in the left conducting system on patterns of activation. Preparation as described in figures 3 and 4. Panel A shows the normal sequence of activation. The pairs of action potentials at levels I, II, and III were recorded from the corresponding levels on the photographs. The first of each pair is recorded from a conducting cell and the second from an ordinary muscle cell. The numbers represent intervals from stimulus to response at each site. In B, the activation is re-mapped after an incision across the posterior division of the left bundle branch. In C, mapping after another incision made vertically through the interconnecting subendocardial Purkinje fibers. Horizontal calibration = 10 msec; vertical calibration = 60 mv. (Reprinted by permission of the American Heart Association, Inc., from Myerburg et al. (575)).

mounted, and studied similarly to the canine hearts (575), indicate that small lesions through the specialized conducting tissue bundles referred to as the anterior and posterior divisions did *not* cause greater delays in activation than those observed with similar lesions in canine preparations (576). We concluded that the species differences reported by Watt et al. (894) may relate to the anatomic difference in the specialized conducting system in the baboon when compared to that of the dog, or to the different positions of the heart in the chest in the two species.

THE GATING MECHANISM AND CONFINEMENT OF IMPULSES

Action potential duration and local refractory periods vary along the course of the intra-ventricular conducting system from the level of the left or right bundle branch to the distal terminations (566, 572). The duration of action potentials from the level of the bundle branches, toward the termination of specialized conducting fibers in muscle, progressively

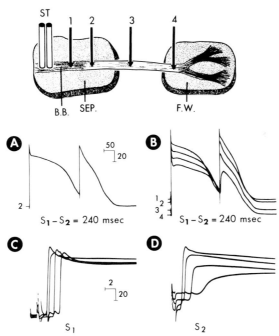

Fig. 10. Refractory periods along the length of the conducting system proximal to the gate. Four micro-electrodes have been used to impale cells from the bundle branch (BB), along a false tendon, to conducting tissue on the free wall of the ventricle just proximal to the gate. In panel D, a time expansion of the simultaneously recorded premature responses from panel B, the premature upstrokes arise at progressively lower membrane potentials, have progressively decreasing upstroke velocities, and the premature impulse is conducted somewhat more slowly than the driven response. Panel C is a time-expanded recording of the driven response in panel B. The sweep speed in panels A and B is 50 msec/division, and in panels C and D is 2 msec/divison. Progressive shortening of the coupling interval of the premature impulse increased the magnitude of the difference between the four premature responses, until conduction failed. (Reprinted by permission of Grune and Stratton, Inc., from Myerburg et al., in Schlant and Hurst, Editors, *Advances in Electrocardiography* 1972).

increase (566,572). Conversely, durations from the most distal branches of the Purkinje fibers, through a sequence of transitional cells, to true ventricular muscle fibers progressively decrease (546,572). Therefore, a map of action potential duration along the length of a strand of specialized conducting tissue obtained from canine endocardium reveals that the durations progressively increase to a point proximal to the termination of the conducting cells in muscle, reach a maximum, and then progressively decrease (572). Local refractory periods parallel the changes in action potential durations, reaching a

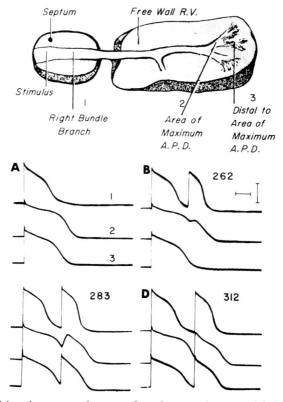

Fig. 11. Conduction of impulses across the area of maximum action potential duration. Panel A shows simultaneous driven action potentials recorded from three sites in the right ventricular conducting system: 1. right bundle branch, 2. area of maximum action potential duration, and 3. Purkinje cell distal to the area of maximum action potential duration. Both the driving impulse (S_1) and the test impulse (S_2) were delivered through small surface electrodes situated on the right bundle branch (drawing). Action potential upstrokes are retouched for clarity where necessary. Top, middle, and bottom records in B, C, and D correspond to 1, 2, and 3. In panel B, the S_1-S_2 interval was 262 msec. The cell in the top record was almost fully repolarized at this time and responded to S_2 appropriately. The cell at the area of maximum action potential duration was still refractory, however, and showed only a minor graded response. Since the impulse was not conducted, the distal cell showed no response to S_2. In panel C, the S_1-S_2 interval was 283 msec, the minimum value at which conduction across the area of maximum action potential duration will occur, i.e., the functional refractory period of the system. Repolarization was complete in the right bundle branch cell and almost complete in the distal cell, and the premature action potentials have appropriate configurations. Repolarization was much less complete in the middle cell, however, and the premature action potential configuration has a very slow upstroke. In panel D, the S_1-S_2 interval was 312 msec and the premature upstroke velocity clearly was much more rapid at site 2. It was still more rapid at sites 1 and 3, although this is not evident in the illustration. (Reprinted by permission of the American Heart Association, Inc. from Myerburg et al. (572).

maximum at the region of maximum action potential durations, and progressively decreasing thereafter (572,573). The general area of maximum action potential duration and maximum local refractory period along a tract of specialized conducting tissue beginning at the level of the bundle branch and terminating in the transitional cells, which go on to form the PF-VM junctions, has been termed a 'gate'; and the function of the collective areas of maximum action potential duration, the gating mechanism (572–574). In preparations of canine tissue originating at the level of the bundle branch and terminating in free wall septal muscle, the area referred to as the gate has been shown to function as a determinant of the functional refractory period of the preparation (572,573) (fig. 10 and 11). However, in isolated preparations which include the bundle of His and bifurcation of

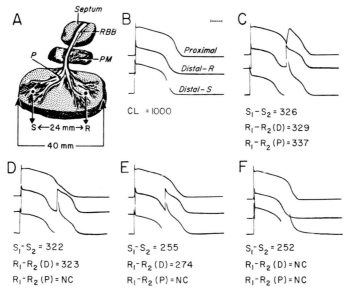

Fig. 12. Normal confinement of premature impulses distal to the gate. The preparation (A) consists of the right bundle branch (RBB) and multiple peripheral false tendons serving a segment of the free wall of the right ventricle. All muscle fibers between the septum and papillary muscle (PM) and ventricular free wall have been severed and the only connection between the septum and the free wall is conducting tissue. 'P' represents the location of a recording microelectrode proximal to the gate, 'R' is the site of a recording microelectrode in a conducting cell distal to the gate, and 'S' is another distal microelectrode used both for intracellular stimulation and recording. In panel B, representative action potentials are shown from each these three sites at a basic cycle length of 1,000 msec (surface stimulation of the distal tissue). In this and subsequent panels the proximal cell is on the top and one distal cell is in the middle. The other distal cell, used for intracellular stimulation, is on the bottom. The time calibration is 100 msec in 20 msec subdivisions. The break in the inscription of the bottom cell during phase 3 is caused by relay system (intracellular stimulation). Panel C shows that the minimum S_1-S_2 interval at which conduction will occur across the gate to proximal conducting tissue was 326 msec. R_1-R_2 (P) is the measured R_1-R_2 interval of the proximal cell at this S_1-S_2 value and R_1-R_2 (D) is that of the distal cell not being directly stimulated. In panel D, the S_1-S_2 interval is decreased just 4 msec to 322 msec and R_2 is not conducted to the proximal cell (R_1-R_2 (P) = NC). At an S_1-S_2 interval of 255 msec, conduction is still occuring between the two distal cells (panel E), but stimulation of cell S finally fails at 252 msec (panel F). Thus the difference between the S_1-S_2 interval at which conduction across the gate to the proximal tissue fails and that at which stimulation of the distal conducting cell fails is 70 msec. (Reprinted by permission of Cardiovascular Research (British Cardiac Society), from Myerburg et al. (580)).

the bundle branches, in addition to the more distal tissue described above, the limiting area for antegrade conduction of premature impulses appears to be located higher in the intraventricular conducting system—at a level in the right bundle branch or one of the fascicles of the left bundle branch (238,477). Similar observations have been reported in intact canine hearts (559,963). The differences in functional observations of these preparations are at least partially understandable on the basis of the data of Harrison et al. (344), who demonstrated that the progressive increase in action potential duration along the length of the right side of the interventricular specialized conducting system accelerated rapidly toward the end of the true (septal portion) right bundle branch and the beginning of the free running false tendon (moderator band). These abrupt changes are more likely to result in block of appropriately timed premature impulses. The more gradual increases in local action potential duration and refractory periods observed distal to the right bundle branch would be more likely to favor slowed conduction—but not necessarily block—resulting in the possibility for sufficient time to elapse to allow repolarization to occur in the wake of the propagating action potential toward the distal end of the conducting system. The group of observations referred to could explain the tendency of the gating mechanism to exert its influence: 1. at a higher level during antegrade conduction of premature beats in the totally intact A-V conducting system; 2. in the distal few millimeters

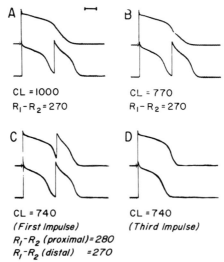

Fig. 13. Confinement of a spontaneous premature impulse arising distal to the gate. The preparation was similar to that shown in figure 12. The top tracing is from a cell proximal to the gate and the bottom a cell distal to the gate. The time calibration is 100 msec. In panel A, at a basic cycle length of 1000 msec with stimulation of the bundle branch, a spontaneous premature impulse was arising distal to the gate and was confined to the distal tissue. The coupling interval was 270 msec. In panel B, the basic cycle length had been decreased to 770 msec, and the coupling interval remained unchanged. When the basic cycle length was further reduced to 740 msec, the first premature impulse (still at a coupling interval of 270 msec) crossed the gate and entered the proximal tissue. The second cycle at this basic driving rate was lost on the back-sweep of the oscilloscope. The third cycle (panel D), and all subsequent ones, failed to demonstrate the premature activity. (Reprinted by permission of Grune and Stratton, Inc., from Myerburg et al., in Schlant and Hurst, Editors, *Advances in electrocardiography*, 1972).

of the preparation consisting of the distal portion of the right bundle branch plus the more peripheral tissues; and 3. under either condition, to confine premature impulses in specialized conducting tissue and muscle distal to the area of the gate (580).

The data demonstrated in figure 12 describes the function of distal confinement of premature impulses. Within a range of approximately 70 milliseconds, premature impulses may be initiated in the specialized conducting system distal to the gate (i.e., the terminal few millimeters of the specialized tissue), propagate through this tissue and adjacent muscle, but fail to propagate back into the specialized conducting tissue proximal to the gate. Figure 13 demonstrates that premature impulses which have been generated *spontaneously* distal to the gate may be similarly confined. Such observations as that shown in figure 13 also provide some indirect evidence for the possibility that re-entrant loops may be generated in relatively small areas of cardiac tissue; and, more specifically, may not necessarily require propagation through proximal tissues.

Regional dysfunction may cause failure of distal confinement due to failure of function of the area of action potential duration in one false tendon. Figure 14 and 15 demonstrate

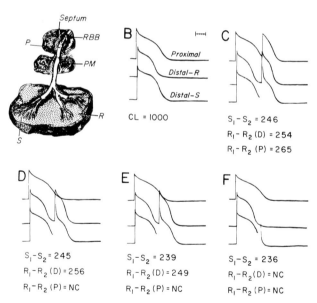

Fig. 14. Failure of the gating mechanism. The preparation (panel A) is similar to that shown in figure 12. However, the proximal microelectrode (P) in this experiment was at the level of the RBB Panel B demonstrates the representative action potentials at a basic cycle length of 1000 msec with surface stimulation of RBB. The time calibration is 100 msec in 20 msec subdivisions. In panel C, retrograde conduction to the proximal conducting system occurs at an S_1-S_2 interval of 246 msec, significantly lower than the functional refractory period of 300 to 330 msec usually seen at a cycle length of 1000 msec in these preparations. In panel D, retrograde conduction has failed at an S_1-S_2 interval of 245 msec. In panel E, conduction between the two distal cells is occurring at an S_1-S_2 interval of 239 msec, but stimulation of the bottom cell fails at an S_1-S_2 interval of 236 msec (panel F). Thus the difference between the S_1-S_2 interval at which proximal conduction failed and that at which stimulation of the distal cell failed only 9 msec, compared with 70 msec in the preparation shown in figure 1. One false tendon of this preparation was found to have an abnormally short refractory period (see figure 15). (Reprinted by permission of Cardiovascular Research (British Cardiac Society), from Myerburg et al. (580)).

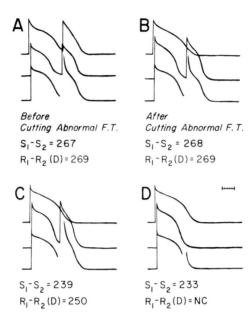

Fig. 15. Restoration of a gate by cutting an abnormal false tendon. The preparation is that shown in figure 14. Panel A demonstrates the absence of a gate at an S_1-S_2 interval of 267 msec, 22 msec longer than the S_1-S_2 interval at which conduction failed in the control measurements (fig. 17). Immediately after cutting the abnormal false tendon, a functioning gate is restored and retrograde conduction is blocked at an S_1-S_2 interval of 268 msec. Panels C and D demonstrate that there has been no change in the functional state of the distal cells as a result of cutting the abnormal false tendon. (Reprinted by permission of Cardiovascular Research (British Cardiac Society), from Myerburg et al. (580).

this phenomenon. The preparation shown in figure 14, which was similar to that demonstrated in figure 12 failed to demonstrate a significant range of coupling intervals at which confinement of premature impulses initiated in the distal tissue could occur. With careful mapping procedures one false tendon was found to have very short action potential durations along most of its length, and local refractory periods were much shorter than those in the other false tendons of the preparation in the region of the gate. Figure 15 demonstrates that cutting the abnormal false tendon restored the gating function, and blocked retrograde conduction of premature impulses originating in the distal tissues at much longer S_1-S_2 intervals than could be achieved before the abnormal false tendon was cut.

Figure 16 diagramatically illustrates the concept of physiologic compartments of the distal A-V conducting system on the basis of data collected in our laboratory (580), as well as the observations of other investigators (238, 344). This hypothesis is consistent with the concept of a limiting segment for propagation of antegradely conducted premature impulses at a level within the right or left bundle branch, or one of the divisions of the left bundle branch; but for retrograde block at more distal levels for premature impulses originating distal to the gate. An elongation of the limiting segment, resulting from differential rates of change of action potential duration (344, 572), is conceptualized.

The interconnecting fibers between the anterior and posterior divisions of the left bundle branch, which we have referred to as the subendocardial Purkinje fiber interconnections (575), and Lazzara et al. have referred to as the interior fibers (473), have variable

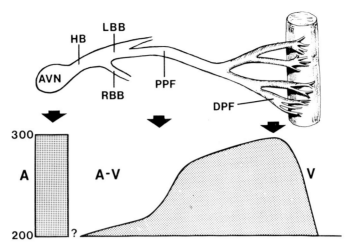

Fig. 16. Electrophysiologic compartments. The diagram at the top represents the A-V node (AVN), bundle of His (HB), bundle branches (RBB, LBB), and a tract of conducting tissue from the bundle branch to ventricular muscle, subdivided in proximal (PPF) and distal (DPF) Purkinje fibers. The shaded areas at bottom represent refractory periods (ordinate = 200 to 300 msec) along the length of the conducting system. Maximum local refractory periods occur at the AVN (first arrow) and the collective gates (third arrow) a few millimeters proximal to the junctions of Purkinje fibers with centricular muscle cells. Functionally, antero-gradely conducted premature impulses that are conducted across the A-V node but blocked proximal to ventricular muscle tend to be blocked at the levels of the second arrow, probably because of the rapid rate of change of action potential duration and local refractory periods in the area. Two electrophysiological compartments are the region proximal to the A-V node (i.e., the atrium (A)) and the region distal to the gates (third arrow), which includes distal specialized conduction tissue and ventricular muscle (V). The A-V compartment, between the first and second arrows, probably includes the His bundle and proximal bundle branches. The '?' symbol at the level of the His bundle and most proximal bundle branches indicates the current limitation of knowledge of local functional properties in this region. (Modified and reprinted by permission of Grune and Stratton, Inc., from Myerburg et al., in Schlant and Hurst, Editors, *Advances in electrocardiography*, 1972).

action potential durations at most of the anatomic levels of the septum. This raises a question as to whether the fibers with shorter action potential duration function as 'short circuits' normally (477), thereby becoming the limiting factor in propagation of premature impulses in either antegrade or retrograde directions. In an earlier study, it was noted that the pattern of action potential duration along the length of the specialized conducting tissue was related to the distance from the level of the left bundle branch to the termination of a conducting fiber tract in an area of left or right ventricular endocardium (572), rather than absolute length of a tract. In order to re-test this question, we have carried out detailed mapping studies to determine the relationship of action potential duration in a Purkinje fiber tract on the lower septum to its point of termination in ventricular muscle. In order to do this, action potential durations were mapped, and correlated with corresponding Purkinje fiber-ventricular muscle junction intervals. The data from a typical experiment is demonstrated in figure 17. In the region of interior fibers, long action potential durations were consistently found in tracts of tissue that were *not* close to their point of termination in muscle, as visualized anatomically, and as reflected physiologically by PF-VM intervals. On the other hand, short action potential durations in the same regions were found in the more delicate twigs of Purkinje fibers which, from previous studies, have been demon-

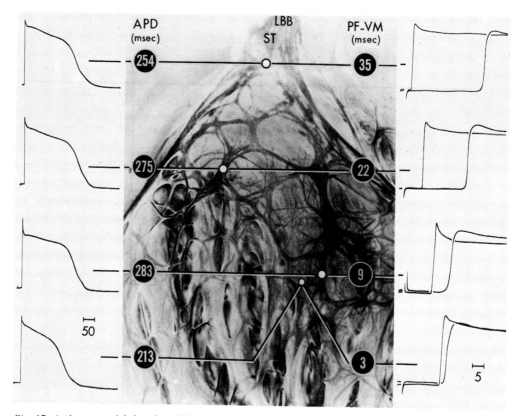

Fig. 17. Action potential durations, PF-VM intervals, and the gating mechanism. As one maps from the level of the left bundle branch distally, action potential durations (APD) increase and PF-VM intervals decrease. The decreasing PF-VM intervals result from progressively later specialized conducting tissue activation, concomitant with earlier ventricular activation, as one approaches the regions of earliest impulse input from conducting tissue to ventricular muscle. On the mid- and lower portion of the septum, subendocardial specialized conducting tissue tracts at greater or lesser distances from their points of termination in muscle may be identified. It is assumed that tracts on the lower septum which are at some distance from their points of termination have PF-VM intervals in excess of 4 or 5 milliseconds (e.g., APD = 283 msec and PF-VM = 9 msec), while those close to their points of termination have PF-VM intervals of 1 to 3 milliseconds (e.g., APD = 213 msec and PF-VM = 3 msec). PF-VM in excess of 4 to 5 milliseconds are associated with action potentials durations of greater length than the PF-VM intervals of shorter duration at the same level of the apico-basal axis of the septum. It is probable that the combination of long action potential durations and relatively long PF-VM intervals identify tracts of tissues relatively remote from their sites of impulse input, while the converse is true for short APDs. Thus, the model of the specialized conducting tissue in the subendocardium composed of gradually lengthening action potential durations, once one is recording beyond the proximal portion of the left ventricular specialized conducting system, is consistent with the model of the gating mechanism described in the text (see fig. 16). Stated alternatively, patterns of action potential duration must be analyzed in the context of the proximity of a tract of conducting tissue to its termination in muscle.

strated to be the terminal ramification of Purkinje network. In these studies, they were shown to be physiologically close to their terminations by the presence of short PF-VM intervals. We conclude from these experiments that, insofar as PF-VM intervals can be used as an indication of proximity of Purkinje fibers to termination in ventricular muscle cells (and this must still be considered a tentative hypothesis), the intermingling of short and long action potential durations relate to physiological proximity of Purkinje fibers to their terminations rather than an intrinsic random variability in action potential duration in the interior fibers, causing 'short circuiting' of the gating mechanism. Nonetheless, in the left ventricular conducting system, as was the case in the right ventricular conducting system (demonstrated in fig. 16), the greatest changes in action potential duration occur proximally; and beyond the left bundle branch and proximal third of the anterior and posterior divisions and proximal interior fibers, action potential durations increase at a much less dramatic rate. The functional implications are likely the same as those described for the right intraventricular conducting system.

CHANGES IN RATE ON THE FUNCTION OF THE DISTAL A-V CONDUCTING SYSTEM

The duration of action potentials of cardiac tissue decrease as the frequency of stimulation is increased (366). Since most normal cardiac tissues recover excitability as a function of transmembrane voltage, increasing rate with concomitant shortening of action potential durations results in a decrease of the refractory period of the tissue. However, since certain normal cardiac tissues (e.g., the A-V node) have a time dependent, as well as a voltage dependent, component for the recovery of excitability, and this may also be true for other (voltage-dependent) tissues under pathologic conditions or pharmacologic interventions, changes in action potential duration alone are not always sufficient to predict changes in refractory period. In regard to the A-V nodal cells, action potential durations are less responsive to rate changes than are tissues of the His-Purkinje system. Similarly, the tissues of the proximal portion of the His-Purkinje system are also less responsive to rate changes than are cells in the region of the gate (572,573). Thus, as the rate of stimulation increases, changes in the refractory period across the AV junction operate within a more narrow range than do the tissues in the distal portions of the specialized conducting tissue. This is consistent with the demonstration by Moe et al. (559) that, at high rates of stimulation, the refractory period of the A-V node exceeds that of the His-Purkinje system, while at slower rates of stimulation the reverse is true. Figure 18 demonstrates this property diagramatically. Since the major refractory period adjustment at a cellular level follows the first beat of a change in frequency of stimulation (and minor changes continue for a period of time thereafter) (407), electrocardiographic phenomenon such as the tendency for aberrant ventricular conduction to occur more often with slow irregular basic rates (525) than with rapid rates seem to have a foundation in the experimental observations described above. Despite the greater sensitivity of tissues in the area of the gate to changes in rate than is the case with proximal or more distal tissues, the gate continues to function at high rates of stimulation (573). However, it does so in a less predictable and less uniform manner (see figure 19). In addition, the difference between the functional refractory periods of the left and right ventricular systems decreases, reverses, or disappears at rapid rates of stimulation.

Certain speculations concerning clinically observed phenomena are relevant to the observation that some segments of the conducting system may show delayed conduction, or 2:1 conduction, at slower rates than others (fig. 19). Aberrant interventricular conduc-

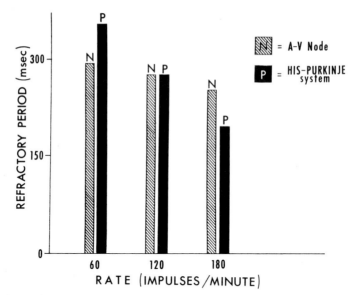

Fig. 18. Effect of rate changes on the refractory period of the A-V node and the His-Purkinje system. Both the A-V node and the His-Purkine respond to increasing rates of stimulation by decreasing their refractory periods. However, the responsiveness of the His-Purkinje refractoriness to changes in rate is much greater than corresponding changes in the A-V node. Thus, based on data from a study of Moe et al. (28) the differential rate responsiveness results in a situation such that the refractory period of the His-Purkinje system exceeds that of the A-V node at slow heart rates, and the reverse is true at fast heart rates. In Moe's study, the point at which the refractory period of the A-V node approximated that of the His-Purkinje system was about 120 impulses per min. in canine tissue. (Reprinted by permission of F. A. Davis Inc., from Myerburg and Lazzara, *Cardiovasc. Clin.*, 5 (3): 1–19, 1973).

tion during supraventricular tachycardia does not follow a fixed pattern in all patients. The degree of aberration is variable, as is the sequence of depolarization. The development of delayed conduction across some false tendons, with normal rates of conduction across others (fig. 19), and the apparent absence of evident electrophysiologic predetermination of the tracts of tissue which will show delayed conduction (573), seems to provide a possible explanation for some of the features of this form of aberration. In addition, however, nonspecific delayed activation of portions of the ventricular muscle mass could also account for rate-dependent alterations in QRS morphology which do not follow a classical bundle branch or 'fascicular' pattern. The occurrence of 2:1 conduction across some portions of the intraventricular specialized conducting tissue at rapid rates of stimulation (fig. 19), concomitant with 1:1 conduction across others, presents one possible mechanism for bidirectional tachycardia, although it is certainly not the only plausible mechanism (110,687,731).

TRANSVERSE SPREAD AND LONGITUDINAL DISSOCIATION IN THE INTRAVENTRICULAR CONDUCTING SYSTEM

The explanation for a number of clinical electrocardiographic phenomena have been based on the presumption of the occurrence of functional longitudinal dissociation in

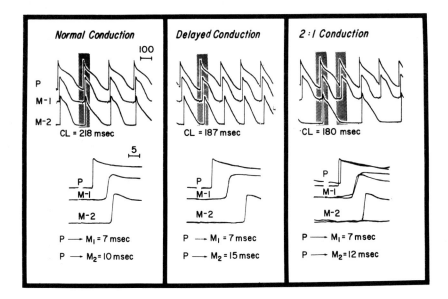

Fig. 19. Conduction of responses across distal false tendons at rapid rates of stimulation. The upper half of all three panels show action potentials recorded from a Purkinje cell proximal to the branching of the false tendon (P) and from muscle cells in each of the two separate segments of free-wall muscle (M-1 and M-2), photographed at a sweep speed of 100 msec/division on the oscilloscope screen. The bottom half of each panel is a time expansion of the shaded areas in the top halves, photographed at a sweep speed of 5 msec/division. As the rate of stimulation is progressively increased, normal conduction continues to occur across one of the false tendons, while there is first delayed conduction (center panel) and then 2:1 conduction (right panel) across the other. (Reprinted by permission of The American Heart Association, Inc., Myerburg et al. (573)).

the specialized A-V conducting system (425). Studies in recent years have supported the hypothesis that functional longitudinal dissociation may occur in the A-V node as a mechanism in the genesis of echo beats, or during the onset or perpetuation of supraventricular tachycardias (309,409,550,560,722,936). However, functional longitudinal dissociation in the more distal tissue of the specialized conducting tissue is more difficult to define and to interpret. Recent studies from this laboratory, using isolated segments of specialized conducting tissue of dog hearts, has demonstrated that delayed transverse spread and longitudinal dissociation of conduction occurs in the distal tissues (bundle branches and false tendons) under carefully defined and limited circumstances (579). Eccentric stimulation of the bundle branch, or of the false tendons, may set up a wavefront of eccentric propagation over a distance of only a few millimeters in normal tissue. However, during early premature stimulation, or during slow regular stimulation of damaged tissue, further delays in transverse spread, and longitudinal dissociation over significant lengths of the specialized conducting system, may occur. The anatomic relationships between the conducting elements and supporting tissue in the specialized conducting system, in conjunction with functional and anatomic characteristics of transverse connections between specialized conducting units, are the probable explanation for this observation. The transverse connections between longitudinal oriented elements have smaller diameters, and therefore are more likely to fail to conduct weak or early premature impulses, than are the longitudinal elements. Thus, under appropriate conditions, failure of transverse conduction may occur before longitudinal conduction fails. We have demonstrated a few instances of total longitudinal dissociation, in which premature conduction occurs along one pathway within a false tendon and fails to conduct along another pathway less than one millimeter laterally. Other investigators have also published data which pertains to the question of functional longitudinal dissociation, and its significance in specialised conducting tissue distal to the A-V node (16,46,777). This is an area of active basic investigation currently, and the clinical significance of these observations must await both further clarification of the basic properties and methodology for clinical interpretation.

DELAY OF CONDUCTION OF PREMATURE IMPULSES ACROSS THE GATE

When a preparation is stimulated prematurely at a coupling interval well in excess of the refractory period at the gate, the conduction velocity of the premature response is approximately equal to that of the driven responses (573). However, when the coupling interval of the premature impulse is short enough to result in an impulse arriving at the region of the cells of the area of maximum action potential duration before they have repolarized to the extent of -75 to -80 millivolts, some delay of conduction of the premature response may be expected to occur. In healthy, rapidly conducting tissue, progressive shortening of the coupling interval generally results in minimal conduction delay prior to block (573). In other preparations, however, greater degrees of conduction delay of the premature response may occur prior to block. This can occur in normal tissue, but it is more often seen in depressed tissue (573). Moreover, if the tissue is sufficiently depressed, refractory periods may dissociate from action potential duration, and intraventricular conduction delay or block may occur long after the completion of electrical repolarization. It follows, therefore, that under normal and some abnormal conditions, the coupling interval achieved distal to the gate must be at least as long as, or exceed, the duration of refractory period at the area of maximum refractory period. The exception to this statement has been described earlier. That is, under certain abnormal conditions, as yet not clearly defined, regional damage to conducting tissue may result in shortening of action potential durations with concomitant shortening of local refractory periods, rather than dissociation between action potential duration and refractory periods. Under these conditions, the minimum coupling interval achieveable distal to the gate will be less than the maximum action potential duration in the distal specialized conducting tissue. These variable response to injury and/or disease processes must be further clarified in order to reach a better understanding of the various mechanisms by which rhythm and conduction disturbances become manifest in the setting of the focal disease processes which underlie many clinical disturbances.

CONCEALED EXTRASYSTOLES

The term concealed extrasystoles has been used in two contexts: 1. Langendorf and Mehlman (456) described concealed A-V nodal impulses, the presence of which was inferred by an unexpected delay or block of conduction of the succeeding sinus beat; and 2. Schamroth and Marriott (720) discussed the concept of concealed ventricular extrasystoles as an explanation for the electrocardiographic finding of intermittant bigeminy. The assumption was that the bigeminy was persistent, but a large number of the ectopic impulses had undergone exit block and not become manifest. Both of these phenomenae can be explained by confinement of premature impulses originating at a level between the A-V node and the proximal end of the gates, with physiologic block occurring at both sites. That such phenomenon can occur in man has recently been demonstrated by His bundle electrocardiography (114). In addition there is one case report (284) which shows both phenomenon in the same patient. This suggests, although it does not prove, that the mechanism of both forms of concealed extrasystole may be the same.

20

THE EXPERIMENTAL EVIDENCE FOR THE ROLE OF PHASE 3 AND PHASE 4 BLOCK IN THE GENESIS OF A-V CONDUCTION DISTURBANCES[1]

MARCELO V. ELIZARI, M.D., ALEJANDRO NOVAKOSKY, M.D.,
RICARDO A. QUINTEIRO, M.D., RAÚL J. LEVI, M.D., JULIO O. LÁZZARI, M.D.,
AND MAURICIO B. ROSENBAUM, M.D.

Clinical (237, 692, 694) and experimental (240, 241) studies have demonstrated two types of rate dependent conduction disturbances. In one of these, the conduction disturbance occurs when the heart rate is accelerated (phase 3 block) and in the other, the conduction disturbance appears after long diastolic intervals or when the heart rate is slowed (phase 4 block). The term 'phase 3 block' has been used since it is assumed that the blocked impulse reaches the injured fibers of the involved region during phase 3 of abnormally prolonged action potentials (237, 240, 692, 694). Phase 4 block has been attributed to a loss of maximum diastolic potential (hypopolarization), enhanced spontaneous diastolic depolarization (SDD), and a shift in threshold potential towards zero (692, 694, 760).

Phase 3 and phase 4 block are commonly observed in patients with intermittent bundle branch block separated by an intermediate normal conduction range. All of these conduction disturbances often coexist in the same affected fascicle. These two varieties of block may also be responsible for atrioventricular (A-V) conduction disturbances whenever the same underlying electrophysiological alterations involve a fascicle which is the only available connection between atria and ventricles (for example one bundle branch in the presence of complete block of the contralateral branch). Thus, two varieties of paroxysmal A-V block (PAVB) have been documented: 1. Phase 4 PAVB, which is commonly precipitated by slowing of sinoatrial rate, and in which A-V conduction is reestablished only after a ventricular escape beat when a subsequent P wave falls on the normal conduction range (147, 693): 2. Phase 3 PAVB which is usually precipitated by sinoatrial acceleration and in which, after the asystole period, A-V conduction is resumed without the need of an intervening ectopic beat (246, 693).

The purpose of this study is to describe *in vivo* and *in vitro* experimental evidences of A-V conduction disturbances due to phase 3 and phase 4 block.

MATERIAL AND METHODS

In vivo experiments
Twenty mongrel dogs weighing 10 to 20 kg were anesthetized with intravenous injection of sodium pentobarbital (30 mg/kg). The animals were intubated and placed under controlled respiration. The chest was opened through a midsternal incision. The pericardium was

1. This work was supported in part by the Comision Para el Estudio Integral de la Enfermedad de Chagas, School of Medicine, Buenos Aires University and by the Fundacion de Investigaciones Cardiologicas Einthoven, Buenos Aires, Argentina.

partially cut at the level of the apex and base of the right ventricle. A pair of plunge teflon coated wire electrodes was placed on the bundle of His to record His bundle electrograms. A unipolar lead similar to V1 was connected to the remnants of the parietal right ventricular pericardium. Atrial and ventricular pacing were achieved through plunge teflon coated wire electrodes inserted in the right atrial appendage and apex of the left ventricle respectively. A pulse generator (Medtronic 5837) was used to stimulate or to overdrive the atria or the ventricles. The right cervical vagosympathetic nerve was exposed and left intact in the neck. Faradic current was used to achieve vagal induced cardiac slowing. Leads I, III and VI were recorded simultaneously along with the His bundle electrogram and displayed on a four channel photographic recorder. Control recordings during normal sinus rhythm, vagal stimulation and atrial pacing were obtained before the production of transient injury of the intraventricular conducting fascicles.

Transient injury of the intraventricular conducting fascicles
The right bundle branch (RBB), left bundle branch (LBB) and divisions of the LBB were reached according to techniques previously described (686). Of the three fascicles, two were more severely damaged while the remainder was slightly injured in order to only partially or transiently affect A-V conduction. A blunt needle was used to press down the fascicles. After the initial injury of the three intraventricular conducting fascicles, complete A-V block occurred. At this time, when needed, the heart was paced through the bipolar electrode placed in the left ventricle. Ventricular pacing was repetitively interrupted until A-V conduction had returned to 1:1 or 2:1 conduction at the spontaneous sinus frequency. At that moment overdrive of the atria as well as vagal stimulation provoked phase 4 and phase 3 A-V block.

In vitro experiments
Ten mongrel dogs of either sex weighing 10 to 20 kg were anesthetized with sodium penthobarbital (30 mg/kg). The heart was rapidly removed through a right thoracotomy and a block of tissue containing the atrioventricular junction, the bundle of His and both bundle branches was excised and placed in a 50 ml Lucite muscle chamber bath. The interventricular septum was split by a saggital cut from the bottom of the block to within 3–4 mm of the summit of the muscular septum. The left septal surface was excised, the LBB cut at its origin and a thin layer of the whole right septal surface was retained. The bundle of His and the proximal right bundle branch were exposed according to the method previously described (233), perfused continuosly with oxygenated Tyrode solution and maintened at a temperature of 35° C. Bipolar extracellular stimulating electrodes were placed on the proximal bundle of His or NH region of the A-V node and on the false tendons of the terminal RBB at the level of the anterior papillary muscle of the right ventricle. Thus, the preparation could be stimulated when desired in either orthograde or retrograde direction at different rates and at 1 to 2 times threshold intensity. Two transmembrane action potentials were simultaneously recorded using standard glass microelectrodes filled with 3 M KCl. One microelectrode (the proximal electrode) was impaled 1 cm from the origin of the RBB and the other (the distal electrode) was impaled near the anterior papillary muscle. A bipolar electrogram was recorded from the beginning of the RBB by means of

teflon coated silver wires. Figure 1 illustrates schematically the preparation and the position of stimulating and recording electrodes. The electrogram along with the transmembrane action potentials were displayed on monitoring and recording oscilloscopes (Tektronix 502 A and 564 B). Calibration of the recording system was achieved by introducing a 100 mV direct current calibration pulse of 200 miliseconds duration into the bath via ground. Photographic recordings of the oscilloscope face were obtained by means of 35 mm moving film in a Grass C4 oscillographic Camera. Conduction disturbances were produced by gentle pressure applied over the RBB with the tip of a thin plastic catheter. This mechanical injury of the RBB was provoked at about 1 cm from its origin in the bundle of His. The proximal recording microelectrode was rapidly impaled in the injured region after complete interruption of conduction through the RBB. This preparation may be considered equivalent to those clinical or experimental conditions where A-V conduction is preserved only via one injured fascicle in the presence of complete interruption of the remaining fascicles.

RESULTS

Phase 4 block was obtained in 6 out of 10 *in vivo* experiments and in 3 of 5 *in vitro* experiments. Phase 3 block occurred in 4 out of 10 *in vivo* experiments and in all of the 5 *in vitro* experiments. Two varieties of PAVB were documented, one related to phase 4 block and the other to phase 3 block. These will be described in detail first and other forms of lesser degrees of phase 4 and phase 3 A-V block will be commented upon later. In addition, reference will be made to the occurrence of concealed and manifest escapes of the injured fascicles, which were another of the important findings of this study.

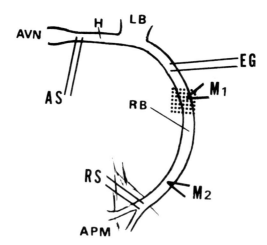

Fig. 1. Sketch of the preparation used for the electrophysiologic studies. The bundle of His and the beginning of the right bundle branch have been dissected. AS = electrodes for orthograde stimulation. RS = electrodes for retrograde stimulation. AVN = A-V node. H = His bundle. LB = left bundle branch. RB = right bundle branch. APM = anterior papillary muscle. M1 = proximal microelectrode. M2 = distal microelectrode. The dotted area indicates the site of injury in the right bundle branch.

PHASE 4 PAVB

In vivo experiments
Figures 2, 3 and 4 describe a typical example of phase 4 PAVB provoked in the intact canine heart. Figure 2 shows tracings before (A) and after injuring the 2 divisions of the LBB (B), illustrating the development of left bundle branch block (LBBB). Figure 2C shows complete A-V block recorded immediately after slight additional injury of the RBB. This stage of complete A-V block lasted only 5 minutes, before changing into 3:1 and 2:1 A-V block. After a few Wenckebach periods, A-V conduction returned to 1:1 conduction at the spontaneous sinus rate as illustrated by the first three beats in figure 3. However the HV interval had increased from 39 msec in the control (fig. 2A and B) to 60 msec. The QRS complex of these three conducted beats showed the pattern of RBBB and left anterior hemiblock, indicating that A-V conduction was occurring through the posterior division of the LBB. A long paroxysm of A-V block is then precipitated by sinus slowing induced by a short vagal stimulation (arrow). The fourth P wave is blocked at the level of the A-V node due to vagal effect. After a diastolic pause of 930 msec, an early escape (E1) is recorded. The fifth P wave, falling after the escape, is also blocked in the A-V node, as shown by the absence of His bundle potential. The next P wave (P6) is blocked below the level of the His bundle because, being too late, it falls upon the phase 4 block range of the injured tissue of the posterior division of the LBB. The following P wave (P7) is again blocked in the A-V node, probably as a consequence of some residual effect of the previous vagal stimulation. After P7 all subsequent P waves are blocked below the bundle of His. A ventricular escape occurs after a diastolic interval of 5340 msec (E2) and the first P wave after the escape is blocked because it is 'too late' (RP interval of 420 msec), and hence falls on the phase 4 block range. After the third escape (E3), the next P wave (P19) is again blocked because of being too late. Finally, after the fourth escape (E4) the subsequent P wave (P21) resumes 1:1 A-V conduction because it falls within the normal conduction range. The critical diastolic interval for phase 4 block in the posterior divisions is extremely short (400 msec), the normal conduction range is very narrow, and the phase 3 block range was considered to be within normal limits. It has been shown that both the shortest RR interval for phase 4 block and the narrowest normal conduction range occur precisely at the moment when rate-independent block changes into rate-dependent block (241). Several episodes of PAVB, as shown in figure 3 were initiated by induced slowing of the sinoatrial rate. Transition between normal conduction and phase 4 PAVB was always abrupt and normal conduction preceded complete A-V block and vice-versa as stated in previous clinical studies

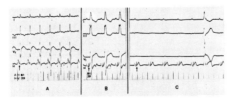

Fig. 2. A: leads I, III, V1 and His bundle electrogram (H) simultaneously recorded (control tracing). B: same leads, after injury of the 2 divisions of the left bundle branch. The tracing shows left bundle branch block pattern. C: complete A-V block recorded after slight injury of the right bundle branch.

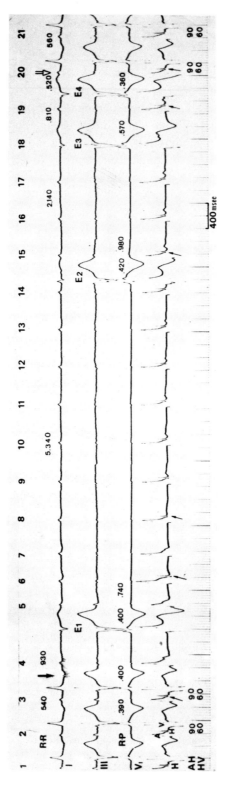

Fig. 3. Phase 4 paroxysmal A-V block. Same leads as in figure 2. There is 1:1 conduction with RR intervals of 540 msec. The arrow indicates a short vagal stimulation which by slowing the sinoatrial rate provokes a long paroxysm of phase 4 A-V block below the His bundle. After the fourth escape (E4), A-V conduction is reestablished. See text for details. Figures are in miliseconds.

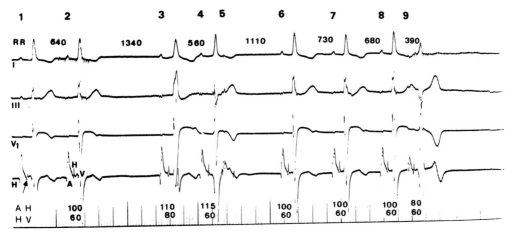

Fig. 4. The effects of varying degrees of multifascicular injury. Recording obtained 2 minutes after figure 2. There is phase 4 block in both right and left bundle branches (but of a lesser degree in the right) and phase 3 block in the right bundle branch and anterior division of the left bundle branch. The prolongation of the HV time after the RR interval of 1340 msec indicates phase 4 conduction delay in the right bundle branch. See text. All figures are in miliseconds.

(147,693). A characteristic finding was that A-V conduction was consistently blocked at a critical RP interval and when a single P wave fell on the phase 4 block range, A-V conduction was totally interrupted and was never resumed unless a ventricular escape intervened. It is worth noting that in all the experiments where PAVB was obtained, the paroxysms could only be provoked during a short period of a few minutes, denoting rapid changes in the basic electrophysiologic mechanisms. The transient nature of these alterations is illustrated in figure 4 which was recorded 2 minutes later than figure 3. Figure 4 also illustrates the effects of varying degrees of multifascicular injury at a moment when the effects of the lesions are probably subsiding at different rate in each fascicle. With RR intervals between 640 msec and 1110 msec, A-V conduction takes place through both bundle branches. The prolonged HV interval as compared with the control implies slower conduction in both, right and left bundle branches, and the fact that the QRS pattern shows a small degree of LBBB reveals greater delay in the LBB. Since this pattern of bilateral bundle branch block (incomplete LBBB and prolonged HV interval), occurs at different RR intervals it was related more to a certain degree of hypopolarization rather than to prolonged recovery (692,694). After a diastolic pause of 1340 msec, the first sinus conducted beat (beat 3) shows a longer HV interval and LBBB pattern. This indicates phase 4 block in the LBB and a conduction delay in the RBB, also related to phase 4 block of a lesser degree. A premature beat (beat 4) shows phase 3 block in the anterior division of the LBB, and a more premature beat (beat 9) adds phase 3 RBBB. An even more premature beat (beat 5) exhibits bilateral bundle branch block as indicated by the His electrogram (RH interval of 280 msec). Summarizing, figure 4 is representative of the following underlying electrophysiological alterations: a. prolonged recovery in the RBB and left anterior division; b. phase 4 depolarization in both bundle branches (more in the left) responsible for phase 4 block; and c. a small degree of hypopolarization, which probably causes both phase 3 and phase 4 block. Phase 3 block in one bundle branch and phase 4 block in the other are

occurring at the same moment in accordance with the diastolic interval. A few minutes
later, A-V and intraventricular conduction were normal at any heart rate.

In vitro experiments
Figures 5 and 6 show the *in vitro* equivalent to the phase 4 PAVB described in figures 2 to 4.
Conduction through the RBB before and after the production of slight mechanical injury at
its middle third was investigated at rapid and slow rates of stimulation. Stimulating and
recording electrodes were positioned as shown in figure 1. Once complete interruption of
conduction was provoked, the proximal microelectrode was impaled in cells of the injured
region. At that moment, severe hypopolarization was recorded (resting potentials of about
−40 to −50 mV) and non propagated local responses were seen at a rate of stimulation
(not shown). After a few minutes, hypopolarization became less severe in the same cells
(resting potentials of −65 to −75 mV), allowing conduction through the injured tissue at
high rates of stimulation. SDD was absent when hypopolarization was severe but it was
present (either normal or enhanced) in cells showing slight injury as illustrated in figures 5
and 6. In figure 5, 1:1 orthograde conduction is observed (left) in three consecutive impulses with an S-S interval of 650 msec. The proximal transmembrane action potential
recorded in the damaged area (M1), shows a resting potential of −75 mV. Following abrupt
interruption of the His bundle pacing, a His bundle escape (arrow) shows complete block

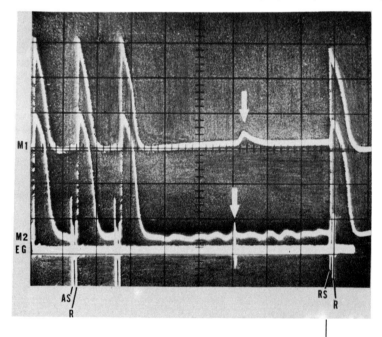

Fig. 5. Phase 4 block in the right bundle branch. M1: microelectrode impaled in the injured area; M2: intracellular recording at the distal end of the right bundle branch. AS = stimulus artifact of orthograde stimulation
recorded in the electrogram. R = right bundle branch potential recorded after the stimulus artifact. There
is 1:1 conduction at relatively high rate of stimulation (left). A late His bundle escape (bottom arrow) is blocked
in the injured area (top arrow). A retrograde impulse (RS) propagates normally through the injured area and the
electrogram shows normal activation of the right bundle branch (R). Calibration: (bottom right) vertical
bar = 25 mV; horizontal bar = 500 msec.

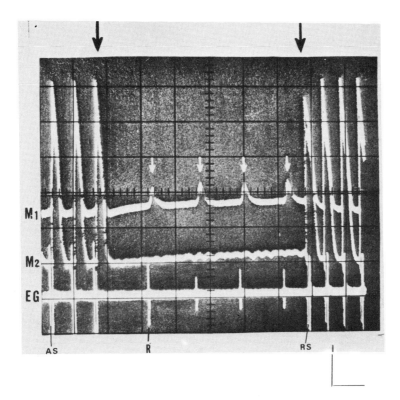

Fig. 6. Same experiment as in figure 5. Paroxysm of phase 4 block recorded at slower sweep speed. The first black arrow indicates the abrupt interruption of orthograde stimulation and the second one the beginning of retrograde stimulation. Abbreviations as in figure 5. Calibration: vertical bar = 25 mV; horizontal bar = 1000 msec. See text for details.

between proximal and distal microelectrodes (M1 and M2 respectively) and the local response in M1 is the only evidence of partial penetration in the damaged area. The loss of resting potential in M1 is minimal and insufficient to explain phase 4 block. Thus, it is inferred that a more marked loss of resting potential due to SDD must exist in more proximal cells. At the end of the long pause (right) the distal end of the RBB is stimulated. The retrograde stimulus penetrates normally the injured area reaching the proximal end of the RBB, explored by the electrogram, demonstrating unidirectional phase 4 block in the injured tissue. In figure 6, the proximal microelectrode (M1) was moved to a more proximal cell in the injured area. The resting potential is about −80 mV and phase 4 SDD is more marked than in the cell shown in figure 5. Again, there is 1:1 orthograde conduction at the same rate of stimulation as in figure 5. Sudden interruption of the His bundle pacing gives rise to a long paroxysm of phase 4 block. Four consecutive His bundle escapes (with HH intervals from 1200 to 1300 msec) are blocked in the injured region showing small local responses. A progressive loss of the resting potential during the long diastole is observed (the slope of SDD is more marked at the beginning of the diastolic pause), and again retrograde stimulation propagates normally through the damaged tissue as observed in the last 4 transmembrane recordings of figure 6 (right). The first action potential after the long pause exhibits lower amplitude as a consequence of the reduced level of the resting potential at the time of stimulation. Note that the electrogram precedes the slow upstroke of the local responses in the proximal microelectrode (M1) in figures 5 and 6, indicating that the escape actually arises in the His bundle. The results obtained in our *in vitro* experiments disclose more direct evidences of the mechanism proposed in previous clinical (147,693) studies of phase 4 PAVB. Moreover, unidirectional block was a constant finding in all the experiments as depicted in figures 5 and 6.

PHASE 3 PAVB

In vivo experiments

Figures 7 and 8 illustrate a typical example of phase 3 PAVB. Figure 7A shows the control tracing and 7B shows LBBB pattern after injury of the 2 divisions of the LBB. Additional injury of the RBB produced complete A-V block (not shown here) which lasted for 8 minutes. During a period of 3 minutes, different forms of second degree A-V block were recorded until 1:1 conduction was observed. In figure 8, the first two beats show sinus bradycardia and first degree A-V block due to prolonged AH and HV intervals. Abrupt shortening of the atrial cycles from 1380 msec to 520 msec, results in a long paroxysm of complete A-V block below the His bundle. A late capture after a ventricular diastolic pause of 9360 msec ends the long period of ventricular asystole. The prolongation of the HV interval in the late capture is of importance because it suggests concealed conduction of one of the preceding P waves in the injured region of the fascicle responsible for A-V conduction (the RBB in this case). Thus, if concealed conduction is present in the last beats following such a long pause, it is reasonable to assume the existence of repetitive concealed penetration of the previously blocked impulses into the injured region. A characteristic

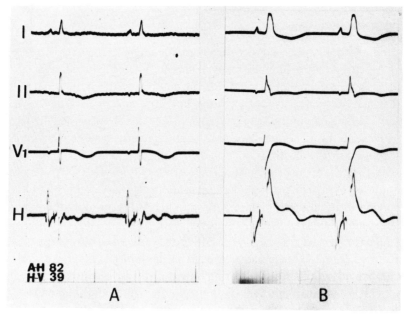

Fig. 7. A: control tracing. Leads I, III, VI and His bundle electrogram. B: same leads as in A showing left bundle branch block after injury of the two divisions of the left bundle branch. The QRS widened from 45 msec to 85 msec.

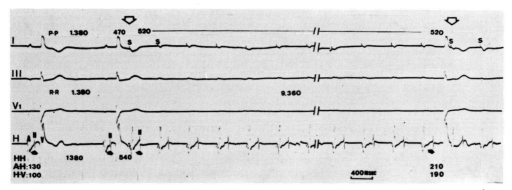

Fig. 8. Production of phase 3 paroxismal A-V block. Same leads as in figure 6. The record illustrates a long paroxysm of A-V block occurring below the His bundle in the right bundle branch, induced by rapid atrial pacing. See text for details.

finding was that the paroxysms were obtained more easily by abrupt rather than by gradual increase of the atrial rate. The critical rate for phase 3 PAVB changed from one minute to the next and further shortening of the atrial cycles were needed to induce paroxysmal tachycardia dependent block. In all cases A-V conduction was resumed without the need of intervening ectopic beats. Another consistent finding was that A-V conduction could be resumed any time a longer HH interval (below the critical rate) occurred either by slowing or interrupting the atrial pacing. Another experiment showed physiologic A-V nodal Wenckebach block which determined lengthening of the HH interval and A-V conduction was observed after the longer HH pause. It has to be mentioned that phase 3 PAVB was much easier to provoke when a widespread lesion was performed by repetitive and more severe injury.

In vitro experiments
Figures 9 and 10 illustrate typical examples of phase 3 PAVB in the RBB of the preparation. The LBB has been cut at its origin in order that the only avilable connection between the A-V junction and ventricular muscle is the RBB. The position of stimulating and recording electrodes is indicated in the sketch of figure 1. The recordings in figure 9 were obtained one or two minutes after complete transient interruption of conduction in the RBB, at a moment when a spontaneous His bundle rhythm (of 60 beats per minute), showed 2:1 block at the level of the injured region. The conduction time between proximal (M1) and distal (M2) microelectrodes is markedly prolonged indicating very slow conduction through the damaged area. This is a consequence of the acute injury of the conducting tissue, where hypopolarization is moderate or severe. It was observed that, although the action potentials of the injured region were always of normal or short duration, the refractory period was significantly prolonged. Rapid orthograde stimulation with SS intervals of 500 msec elicited paroxysmal A-V block. The proximal microelectrode impaled in the injured region shows low maximal diastolic potential, low amplitude and slow rate of rise of phase 0 without conduction toward the distal microelectrode in the RBB beyond the area of injury. The electrogram in figure 9 (bottom tracing) exhibits the stimulus artifact followed by the RBB electrogram, and both preceding the upstroke of the proximal action potential recorded with microelectrode 1. Thirteen consecutive stimuli were blocked until

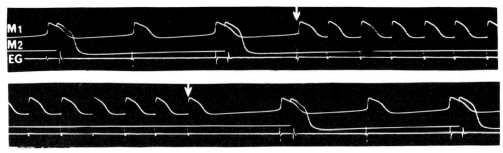

Fig. 9. Continuous strip of intracellular recordings and electrogram illustrating phase 3 paroxysmal block in the right bundle branch. Position of the microelectrodes and symbols as in figure 1. The arrows indicate the beginning and end of the His bundle pacing. Calibration: vertical scale 100 mV; horizontal scale 200 msec.

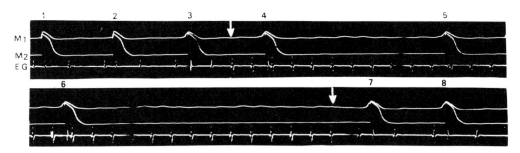

Fig. 10. Continuous recording showing phase 3 paroxismal block in the right bundle branch. Symbols and position of electrodes as in figure 1. Two late captures during the overdrive are indicated with numbers (5 and 6). After abrupt interruption of the His bundle pacing, immediate resumption of conduction through the right bundle branch is observed. Calibration as in figure 9.

His bundle pacing was stopped, the latter resulting in immediate resumption of 2:1 A-V conduction. During a period of 5 minutes several paroxysms of variable length could be provoked any time the preparation was paced at the critical rate. Figure 10, obtained from another experiment, shows similar results as those shown in figure 9. The microelectrode impaled in the injured area shows action potentials of very low amplitude and slow up-strokes in the conducted impulses through the damaged area, as a result of marked hypo-polarization. At rapid rate of stimulation only tiny local responses are recorded by the same microelectrode indicating a higher degree of decremental conduction responsible for repetitive concealed conduction at the site of lesion in the RBB. As in the *in vivo* experiment shown in figure 8, late captures were observed at variable diastolic pauses. The His bundle pacing is stopped (second arrow) and thus a longer cycle occurred resulting in immediate resumption of 2:1 conduction. Again as in the *in vivo* experiments, it was observed that phase 3 paroxysmal block was obtained more easily when the conducting fascicles had been injured several times producing a more widespread lesion.

Phase 4 first degree A-V block

Figure 11 illustrates a typical example of phase 4 first degree A-V block obtained in one of the *in vivo* experiments. The RBB and the divisions of the LBB were injured, and after a short interval of complete A-V block, A-V conduction resumed with normal HV interval (40 msec) and the pattern of RBBB as is shown in the first two beats. After a short vagal

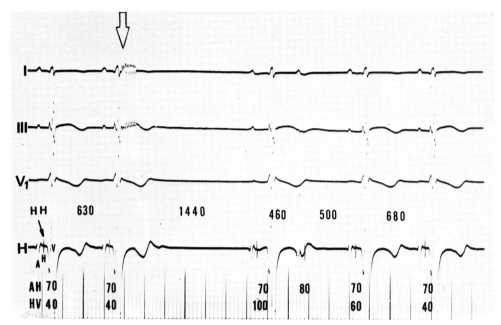

Fig. 11. Phase 4 first degree A-V block (after a long diastolic phase 1440 msec) obtained after a short vagal stimulation. See text for details.

stimulation a diastolic pause of 1440 msec is recorded and the first sinus conducted beat after the pause shows an HV interval of 100 msec indicating conduction delay in the LBB due to phase 4 SDD. The fourth P wave shows phase 3 block after a short PP interval. The fifth P wave again shows a prolonged HV interval of 60 msec. This conduction delay may be interpreted in two different ways depending on the fact as to whether the fourth P wave, which was blocked below the His, has penetrated or has not penetrated the area of injury. If there is penetration, concealed conduction may be responsible for the prolongation of the conduction time in the LBB, and so the prolonged HV interval must be considered as a form of first degree phase 3 block. If there is no penetration at all at the site of lesion, the prolonged HV interval could be attributed to phase 4 first degree A-V block. In the same experiment, a long strip of 2:1 A-V block was recorded (not shown here) and the same tentative explanations were postulated. After a critical PP interval, progressively increasing degrees of first degree A-V block were seen due to prolongation of the HV interval. Further lengthening of the PP interval gave rise to complete A-V block. Since the slope of SDD (responsible for phase 4 block) is rather slow, it was assumed that once it reaches critical levels for abnormal conduction and thereafter, the conduction disturbance will increase gradually. Figure 4 also illustrates phase 4 first degree A-V block.

Manifest and concealed escapes from the injured fascicle
The study of escapes arising from injured fascicles has been a matter of detailed analysis in previous studies (241,693), and the possibility that concealed or abortive escapes may occur in the injured region was postulated on the basis of clinical and experimental observations. Figure 12 illustrates escape beats arising from the intraventricular conducting fascicles. The first two beats show normal HV intervals at the spontaneous rate of the

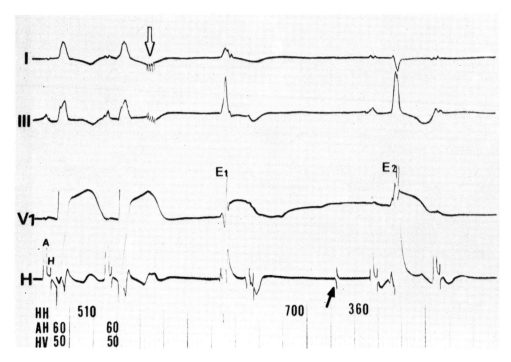

Fig. 12. Manifest and 'concealed' escapes arising from the injured conducting fascicles. Sinoatrial slowing after a short vagal stimulation (open arrow). Two ventricular escapes with different QRS configuration are shown. The black arrow shows a His bundle potential without A and V waves. See text.

dog and LBBB pattern. After a short vagal stimulation a ventricular escape (E1) occurs at a relatively short diastolic interval showing RBBB pattern. After the escape a P wave with an RP interval of 200 msec is blocked below the His bundle. A His bundle deflection is recorded 700 msec after the blocked impulse (black arrow), without A and V waves indicating that the impulse is unable to propagate to the ventricles and to the atria. Changes in shape and duration suggest retrograde invasion of the Bundle of His and the absence of QRS complex is indicative of phase 4 orthograde block. It is remarkable that the coupling interval for the manifest escape (E1) is practically the same as the coupling between E1 and the His electrogram showing phase 4 block. If conduction is totally interrupted in the LBB and phase 4 block exists in the RBB, an escape arising in any of the injured fascicles during the phase 4 block range of the RBB will not be able to reach the ventricles. However, the fact that retrograde conduction is usually preserved, allows retrograde conduction toward the proximal segments of the intraventricular conducting system and hence, recording of the His bundle potential. Obviously, the conventional electrocardiogram can not show direct evidence of the escape.

The fact that slight or moderate injury may produce enhanced SDD and escapes has been pointed out in previous reports (241, 693, 760) and was confirmed in the present study. In 2 out of 5 *in vitro* experiments, at a time when phase 4 block was obtained, escapes arising in the injured area of the RBB were observed. Figure 13 illustrates a typical example. The stimulating and recording electrodes were placed like a figure 1. A continuous strip shows 1:1 conduction through the RBB during orthograde pacing, with SS intervals of 630 msec.

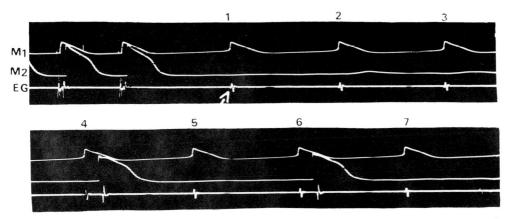

Fig. 13. Continuous strip showing escapes from the injured area. Symbols and position of the electrodes as in figure 1. The arrow shows the first escape (after interruption of the His bundle pacing) which exhibits ortho-grade block. The timing between the microelectrode impaired in injured cells and the electrogram recorded at the beginning of the right bundle branch indicates that the escape is arising in the injured tissue. See text for discussion.

When the His bundle pacing is interrupted, escapes arising in the injured area of the RBB are recorded showing different degrees of orthograde block. The timing between the microelectrode in the injured area (M1) and the electrogram (EG) recorded a few mili-miters above it, indicates that the site of origin of the escape is in the injured tissue. If the escape had arisen above that area, the electrogram would have been recorded before or at least simultaneous with the upstroke of the action potential recorded in the injured area. If the escape had arisen below the damaged area, the impulse would have been normally conducted toward the distal electrode (M2). The fourth escape shows orthograde conduc-tion as indicated by the action potential recorded at the distal microelectrode (M2) and muscle electrogram. Thereafter, a period of 2:1 orthograde conduction and 1:1 retrograde conduction was recorded. Again, these results show clear evidences of unidirectional block within the injured area.

DISCUSSION

Our results in this chapter illustrate that phase 3 and phase 4 block may occur in the same fascicle under similar pathological conditions. However, some differences in the basic electrophysiological mechanism could be determined because in some instances we could obtain only phase 4 block and in others phase 3 block. The production of phase 3 or phase 4 block, in our experiments depended principally on the amount of injury imparted to the conducting fibers and hence on the degree of hypopolarization. It is known that one of the most important determinants of conduction velocity is the rate of rise of the action potential (dV/dT), which in turn depends on the level of the resting potential at the time of stimulation (366,897). Moreover it has been demonstrated that conduction will be more and more impaired at progressively lower levels of the membrane potential as occurs when SDD is present. Our *in vitro* experiments showed that phase 4 PAVB could be obtained only when hypopolarization was slight or moderate, (resting potentials of -85 to $-75\,\mathrm{mV}$).

Conversely, phase 3 PAVB was obtained when the degree of hypopolarization was much more severe and when resting potentials of about −60 mV or less were recorded all over the injured area. Consequently, phase 4 A-V block was related to a lesser degree of injury while phase 3 block to a greater degree of injury. The extension of the lesion was also a decisive factor in the production of phase 3 or phase 4 block. Phase 4 block was always obtained after linear and very circumscribed lesions of the conducting fascicle. Conversely a more widespread lesion generally precluded the production of phase 4 block and favored phase 3 block. In summary, phase 4 PAVB was related to less severe and circumscribed lesions while phase 3 PAVB to more widespread and more severe lesions.

The pathophysiological basis for phase 4 and phase 3 A-V block
It has been stated that phase 4 block is related to hypopolarization, SDD and a shift of the threshold potential toward zero (692). Hypopolarization was a consistent finding in all *in vitro* experiments as a result of the mechanical injury. Under such conditions, it was observed that the transmembrane potential recorded in the injured cells showed lesser and lesser degrees of hypopolarization as the minutes were passing. Up to resting membrane potentials of about −60 mV, block through the injured area was totally rate independent. At this moment SDD was minimal or absent. At resting potentials of around −65 to −70 mV, the conduction disturbance rapidly became rate dependent. Simultaneous with this change phase 4 SDD was recorded in the same injured cells either with normal or enhanced slope. After long diastolic intervals, SDD produced further lowering of the membrane potential needed to cause a significant conduction disturbance. At the control stages, SDD did not produce conduction disturbances. Under such circumstances SDD gave rise to spontaneous firing once the threshold potential was reached. Conversely, when SDD was related to or accompanied slight or moderate hypopolarization it gave rise to conduction block after appropriate diastolic pauses. Although we did not investigate the threshold potential of the injured cells, it has been pointed out (760,692,694) that for SDD to give rise to a conduction disturbance, it is essential that the threshold potential shifts toward zero. Under such condition SDD may reach critical levels for conduction without reaching the threshold potential.

In our experiments, and in accordance with previous clinical observations (147,693), once phase 4 orthograde block occurs, conduction should no longer happen unless an escape beat or any other form of retrograde stimulation brings back the membrane potential to greater resting values after active depolarization of the damaged area (fig. 5 and 6), indicating that retrograde activation of that region takes place at a time when orthograde conduction does not occur. Previous *in vitro* observations (160, 760) have also demonstrated unidirectional block in depressed segments of Purkinje fibers.

Our experimental observations show 2 types of phase 3 block: a. phase 3 block of single impulses and b. phase 3 block of repetitive impulses. The first type was seen in experiments where the injury was small and circumscribed. The prolongation of recovery was very small and high rates of stimulation gave rise to 2:1 block or Wenckebach periodicity but never to repetitive A-V block. In the other type, usually observed after more extensive and severe injury of the conducting tissue, recovery was markedly prolonged. Two to one block or Wenckebach periodicity was observed even at slow rates of stimulation as shown in figures 9 and 10. Acceleration of the rate of stimulation provoked repetitive block. The intracellular recordings in phase 3 PAVB showed markedly depressed cells and slow response action potentials (162) with very slow conduction. The action potentials resembled those of the A-V node and like in this tissue, the diseased segment of the conducting fascicle was very prone to repetitive concealed conduction (367,558). The premature impulses block within the injured area creating refractoriness that blocks the next stimulus and so on. It has been reported that in depressed Purkinje fibers showing low resting potentials the time required for complete recovery of excitability far exceeds the time needed for complete repolarization (160,259). The fact that refractoriness outlasts repolarization and that excitability and conduction are not completely recovered after the end of the action potential supports the idea that phase 3 PAVB is due to tachycardia-dependent repetitive concealed conduction in the area of injury of the conducting fascicle responsible for A-V conduction. Repetitive concealed conduction has been shown to occur in Purkinje (163) and His bundle cells (475). Our results indicate that it may and does occur in any of the intraventricular conducting fascicles.

The two varieties of PAVB
Clinical studies demonstrated two varieties of PAVB, one was bradycardia-dependent (693) and the other tachycardia-dependent (246). Experimentally (246) it has been shown that tachycardia dependent PAVB may occur in the bundle of His. Our experimental study shows for the first time that both types of PAVB may occur in any of the intraventricular conducting fascicles under appropriate circumstances. We have also demonstrated that one type is bradycardia dependent (phase 4 PAVB) and the other tachycardia-dependent (phase 3 PAVB). In phase 4 PAVB, like in clinical cases (693), A-V conduction was only re-established after escape beats or retrograde stimulation, indicating that during phase 4 orthograde block, retrograde conduction in the injured area tends to be preserved (147,237,240,241,692–694). Our in vitro experiments showed direct evidence of unidirectional block in the damaged tissue as illustrated in figures 5 and 6. Thus, retrograde stimulation, as escape from the injured area or from any other region brings back the transmembrane potential to its maximal resting value (fig. 5 and 6). Figure 3 shows that when the appropriate RP interval occurs, after the escape, A-V conduction is resumed. As it was pointed out (693), the preservation of retrograde conduction in phase 4 PAVB must be considered the essential mechanism for the recuperation of orthograde conduction. If retrograde activation in the damaged tissue would be precluded A-V block would become permanent.

In phase 3 PAVB, A-V conduction is re-established without the need of ectopic beats. During rapid pacing late captures were always observed, as shown in figures 8 and 10, indicating that orthograde conduction although very much impaired was still preserved. Moreover, it has been shown in figures 9 and 10 that abrupt interruption of the overdriving determined immediate resumption of conduction through the damaged tissue.

The role of phase 3 and phase 4 in other forms of A-V block
In our experiments, phase 3 block was invariably observed at the moment when rate independent block changed into rate dependent A-V block. As stated, phase 3 block was

attributed to hypopolarization and accordingly, the phase 3 block range was short or long depending on the degree of hypopolarization. It was stated that slight and localized injury did not significantly prolong the refractory period. Under such circumstances, phase 3 block could be obtained only with very short RR intervals, resulting in 2:1 or Wenckebach periodicity but never in PAVB. Conversely, in more widespread and severe lesions the refractory period was markedly prolonged and first degree A-V block, 2:1, 3:1 or Wenckebach periods could be seen even with RR intervals of 1000 msec or more as shown in figures 8 and 9. In these cases, heart rate acceleration may give rise to PAVB. Phase 3 first degree A-V block occurring at the transition between the phase 3 block range and the normal conduction range (237, 240, 241, 692, 694), was considered equivalent to incomplete degrees of block in cases of intermittent bundle branch block (237, 240, 241, 692, 694). It is assumed that in this form of phase 3 A-V block, the impulses are falling on the relative refractory period. Acceleration of the rate of stimulation induced greater degrees of block while slowing of the heart rate tended to normalize A-V conduction.

Phase 4 first degree A-V block was commonly observed in our experiments as shown in figures 4 and 12. Since the slope of phase 4 SDD is very gradual, it is reasonable to assume that once the transmembrane resting potential attains critical levels for conduction delay, and thereafter, the conduction disturbance must increase very gradually. In our experiments, the intraventricular conducting system was transformed into a monofascicular system, and hence the progressive impairment of conduction appeared as an increment of the PR interval. Phase 4 block cannot produce by itself second degree A-V block because once a P wave (or stimulus) is blocked, the next one will have probabilities of being blocked as a consequence of the longer RP (or S-S) interval. Consequently, regarding A-V conduction, phase 4 SDD can only be responsible for first degree A-V and PAVB.

SUMMARY

Phase 3 and phase 4 A-V block was investigated in 20 *in vivo* experiments after transient injury of the intraventricular conducting fascicles, and in 10 *in vitro* experiments using microelectrode techniques. Phase 4 A-V block was provoked in 6 out of 10 *in vivo* experiments and in 3 of 5 *in vitro* experiments. Phase 3 paroxysmal A-V block occurred in 4 out of 10 *in vivo* experiments and in all of the 5 *in vitro* experiments. Phase 4 paroxysmal A-V block was obtained by slowing the heart rate, normal A-V conduction being re-established only after a ventricular escape beat. It was assumed that the escape beat penetrated the critically injured region and produced retrograde activation, thus re-setting the whole mechanism of phase 4 block. Such a mechanism was obtained after slight and circumscribed injury of the conducting fascicle and was related principally to hypopolarization plus normal or enhanced spontaneous diastolic depolarization. Phase 3 paroxysmal A-V block was obtained after acceleration of the heart rate and normal A-V conduction was re-established without the need of an intervening ectopic beat. Phase 3 block was obtained after extensive and more severe injury. It was related to repetitive concealed conduction at the level of the damaged area. It was demonstrated that retrograde conduction was usually preserved at a time when orthograde block was present. Manifest and concealed escapes arising in the injured area were documented in the *in vitro* experiments.

21

VENTRICULAR ACTIVATION IN HUMAN AND CANINE BUNDLE BRANCH BLOCK

RUDOLF TH. VAN DAM, M.D.

INTRODUCTION

Ever since the first experiment by Eppinger and Rothberger (252), on the effect of inter-ruption of the bundle branches on the electrocardiogram, there has been a great deal of controversy on the subject of bundle branch blocks. This confusion partly has been due to the extrapolation of the results of acute animal experiments to the findings in chronically affected human hearts. The longstanding argument about the exact interpretation of the bundle branch blocks, described by Lewis (494) was resolved in 1932 by Wilson (924), who on the basis of his experimental evidence designated clearly what should be called a left and a right bundle branch block.

Several years later some more confusion has been created by the experimental studies of Sodi-Pallares and his group (664), who concluded that in bundle branch block most of the time-delay in activation of the controlateral ventricle was due to a 'barrier' between the right and the left ventricular parts of the intraventricular septum, and also that the activation-process, once having passed the septum, was carried further in an almost normal way by the peripheral part of the affected bundle branch. These results seemed question-able from the onset and have not been confirmed by others, notably by Erickson et al. (256) and Becker et al. (54).

In more recent years, the concept of fascicular blocks has been advanced by Rosenbaum et al. (688) and was taken up by many investigators because of the important clinical implications in human patients. Unfortunately, the distribution and consequently the functional properties of the human intraventricular conduction system are somewhat different from those in the dog heart, the experimental model most commonly used for conduction studies.

Myerburg (575) demonstrated the close functional interrelationship between the main divisions of the left ventricular conduction system that caused Watt et al. (895) to resort to a rather drastic but ingenious technique in order to experimentally study the left fascicular blocks in canine hearts. All the experiments on bundle branch block mentioned above, have been performed in the acute stage. They should be interpreted with some caution, because in experiments with acute interruption of the conduction system at least three factors are present that may obscure the results:
1. acute injury to the myocardium.
2. ectopic impulse formation in the periferal end of the freshly cut bundle branches.
3. a marked depression of the circulatory condition of the animal that often occurs in acute experiments on bundle branch blocks and may impair myocardial conduction.

378 R. TH. VAN DAM

For this reason we decided to experimentally study the bundle branch blocks in a chronic situation.

METHODS

During a sterile thoracotomy, in the canine hearts a complete right bundle branch block (CRBBB) or a complete left bundle branch block was produced by cutting the right bundle branch or the main stem of the left bundle branch by a superficial incision of the right or left surface of the interventricular septum by means of specially designed scalpels with a curved blade.

Following recovery of this operation, the animals with a chronic and complete bundle branch block were sacrificed 6 to 8 weeks later in an acute experiment, in which an epicardial map was made and the heart isolated and perfused according to the Langendorff procedure that has been described in our studies on isolated human hearts (224). In some experiments, the modified Tyrode solution was replaced by blood from a donor dog; the arterial blood from the donor was led into the aortic canula of the Langendorff-system and the used blood was collected and returned to the femoral vein of the donor. Following the suspension of the heart in the perfusion-system, a period of about 20 minutes was allowed for its recovery of the transient effects of anoxia.

The recording technique has been described earlier (234).

All activation times were measured from the rapid deflections in unipolar leads and related to the onset of the cavitypotential in the ventricle where no bundle branch block was present.

An epicardial activation map was carried out in situ or during the perfusion. Intramural activation was studied by recording uni- and bipolar complexes from a large (±64) number of electrodeneedles inserted in several planes into the heart. Throughout the experiment, control records were taken from intramural terminals in order to exclude possible variations in activation sequence. All hearts were beating in sinusrhythm.

After the experiment, the hearts were deep frozen and cut into slices; photography of these served for the correlation between anatomy and activation.

Human hearts with chronic bundle branch block were explored, during surgical exposure, by means of epicardial mapping and intramural leads recorded from a few needle electrodes.

RESULTS

In ventricular activation during complete bundle branch block, three phases can be roughly distinguished:

phase I: normal activation of the unaffected ventricle and excitation of the interventricular septum, breakthrough at the endocardium at the side of the block.

phase II: spread of activation in the anterior and posterior wall across the insertions of the interventricular septum, continued septal activation.

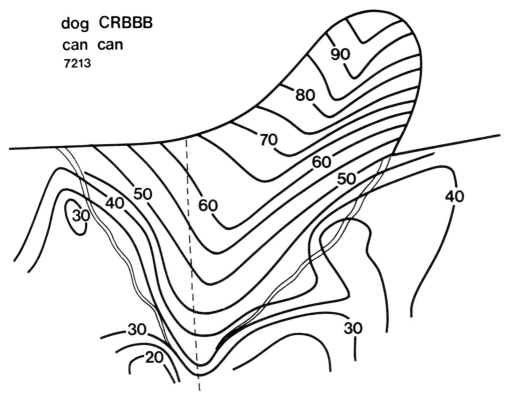

Fig. 1. Epicardial activation map in a donor perfused canine heart with a chronic right bundle branch block. Times: msec after the onset of left ventricular cavity potential; undulating double line indicates border between right and left ventricles. Discussion in text.

phase III: activation of the lateral part of the affected ventricle and of the top part of the interventricular septum.

COMPLETE RIGHT BUNDLE BRANCH BLOCK (CRBBB)

A. Canine CRBBB

1. *Epicardial activation* (fig. 1)
During phase I (0 – ±40 msec), epicardial breakthrough occurs in 3 areas of the left ventricle; on the anterior and posterior surface. The resulting activation fronts rapidly expand and merge; they result in two wavefronts invading the right ventricular surface both anteriorly and posteriorly, and together form a V-shaped front. During phase II (40 – ±55 msec), these wave fronts advance into the right ventricle at an almost equal speed.

During phase III (±55 – ±100 msec) the V-shaped activation front further advances and reaches the pulmonary conus, where the latest activation occurs. The isochrones are more

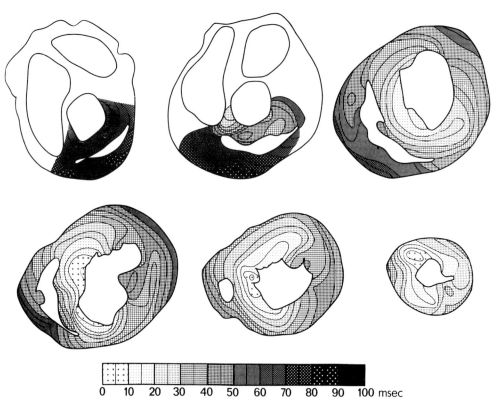

Fig. 2. Intramural activation in the same heart as illustrated in figure 1. Horizontal sections approximately 1 cm apart, from basis to apex. Discussion in text.

widely spaced on the posterior side of the right ventricle than anteriorly, indicating a more rapid spread in the posterior wall.

2. *Intramural activation* (fig. 2)

During phase I, left ventricular activation begins and proceeds according to the normal pattern of left ventricular excitation. The interventricular septum is activated entirely from left to right without any local delay. Activation reaches the right ventricular endocardium at approximately 25 msec, in the posterior lower half of the right septal surface.

Those parts of the septum and the right ventricular wall that during normal conduction are excited early (i.e. 10–15 msec after the onset of the left ventricular cavity potential), are now being activated late, by spread of activation from the neighbouring myocardium and across the interventricular septum. During phase II and III, excitation moves into the free right ventricular wall along its anterior and posterior insertions to the interventricular septum. In the middle sections, activation proceeds slower in the anterior wall presumably by myocardial conduction, than in the posterior part where the isochrones are separated more widely, and show an isolated area of relatively advanced excitation at 40–50 msec. This arrangement of isochrones suggest the secondary involvement of a local

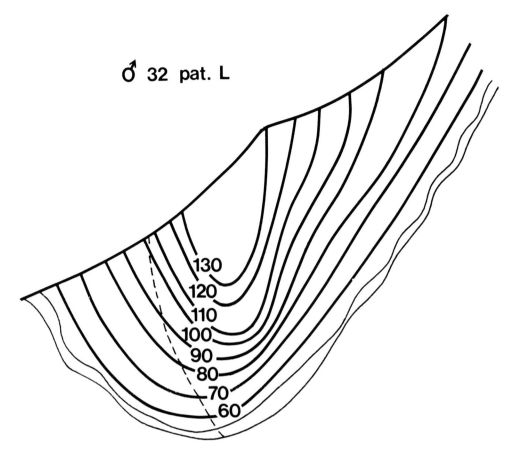

Fig. 3. Right ventricular epicardial activation sequence in a human heart with CRBBB; undulating double line indicates border between right and left ventricles.

Purkinje system. However, no direct proof for this possibility has been found in the recordings from the needle-electrodes situated in this area. In main, the right ventricle appears to be activated by myocardial conduction originating in the left ventricle. Conduction along the crista supraventricularis contributes to late activation of the pulmonary conus.

B. *Human CRBBB* (fig. 3)
In the heart of 32-year old male patient with CRBBB, undergoing pulmonary surgery, we observed a similar epicardial sequence of activation spreading anteriorly and posteriorly from the left into the right ventricle as in the canine heart (fig. 3). The main differences with the canine CRBBB as illustrated in figures 1 and 2, are the later arrival of excitation in the right ventricle which may be ascribed to the larger diameter of the left ventricular wall, and the about equal spacing of isochrones in the anterior and posterior wall of the right ventricle, resulting in a more lateral localisation of the latest area of excitation.

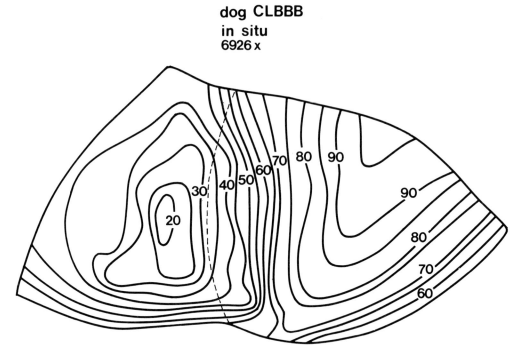

Fig. 4. Epicardial activation in a canine heart with, chronic CLBBB in situ. Activation times in msec measured after the onset of right ventricular cavity potential. Discussion in text.

COMPLETE LEFT BUNDLE BRANCH BLOCK (CLBBB)

A. Canine CLBBB

1. *Epicardial activation* (fig. 4 and 6)
An essentially identical excitation pattern is displayed by the two epicardial maps illustrated. During phase I (0 − ±45 msec), following normal right ventricular epicardial breakthrough, activation spreads out in both the anterior and posterior surface, and enters the left ventricle. In phase II, further double activation occurs of the left ventricular epicardial surface. The isochrones are relatively closely spaced and parallel to each other. The two activation fronts meet in the apical region and together form a V-shaped front. During phase III, this front moves out in a basolateral direction and reaches the area of latest activation near the AV-groove at approximately 100–110 msec. During this latter phase, the isochrones are more widely spaced than during phase II.

2. *Intramural activation* (fig. 5 and 7)
During phase I, activation starts in the right ventricle according to the normal pattern of right ventricular depolarization, i.e. in the anterior papillary muscle and the adjoining areas of the ventricular wall and the right surface of the interventricular septum. From there, activation spreads into the right ventricular wall and into the interventricular wall and the right ventricular wall and into the interventricular septum, where activation occurs

6926×

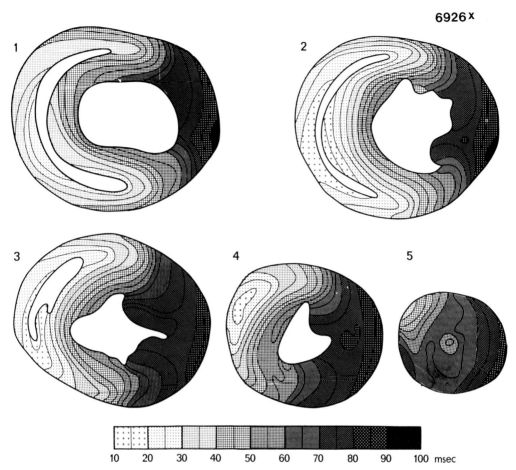

Fig. 5. Intramural activation of the same canine heart with chronic CLBBB as illustrated in figure 4, during donor perfusion. Discussion in text.

entirely in a right to left direction, and without any delay at the junction between right and left ventricular parts of the septum. Excitation traversing the septum reaches the left ventricular cavity lining at about 45 msec. after the onset of right ventricular depolarization. During phase II (±45 – ±70 msec), activation of the septum continues. According to the regular and parallel arrangement of the isochrones, propagation at first is more or less uniform, with the exception of some areas high in the septum (fig. 7, section 2) and near the apex (fig. 5, sections 4 and 5), where a more irregular spread of activation occurs.

In the same time-interval, activation moves from the right into the left ventricular wall via the anterior and posterior septal insertions, in a directional tangential to the epicardial surface. In the paraseptal parts of the left ventricle, the isochrones are more or less crescent-shaped and appear to be a direct continuation of right ventricular activation pattern. Here, activation in the middle layers of the ventricular wall generally is 5–10 msec advanced on epicardial excitation and 15–20 msec on activation in the sub-endocardial layer. During phase III, late activation occurs of the remaining part of the

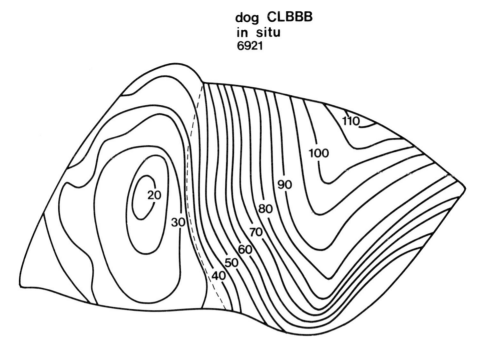

Fig. 6. Epicardial activation of a canine heart with chronic CLBBB in situ.

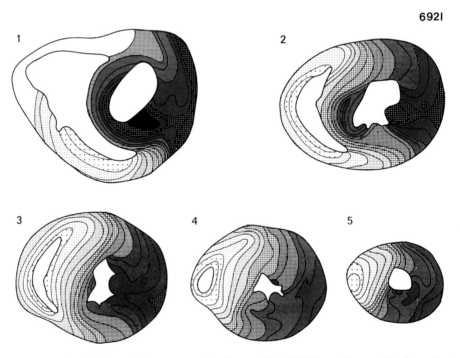

Fig. 7. Intramural activation of the same canine heart with CLBBB as illustrated in figure 6, during Langendorff perfusion (excitation is 15–20% faster than in situ). The area of late activation in the basal anteroseptal region is probably due to the scar caused by the incision for producing the CLBBB. Same time scale as in figure 5. Discussion in text.

left ventricle. Isochrones are more widely spaced and irregularly arranged. In some areas, excitation in the subendocardial partsi is more advanced than in the middle or outer layers (fig. 5, sections 2 and 5; fig. 7, sections 1 and 4). Ultimately, the activation fronts progressing in the anterior and posterior left ventricular wall meet in the lateral part of the left ventricle, the latest in the basal area.

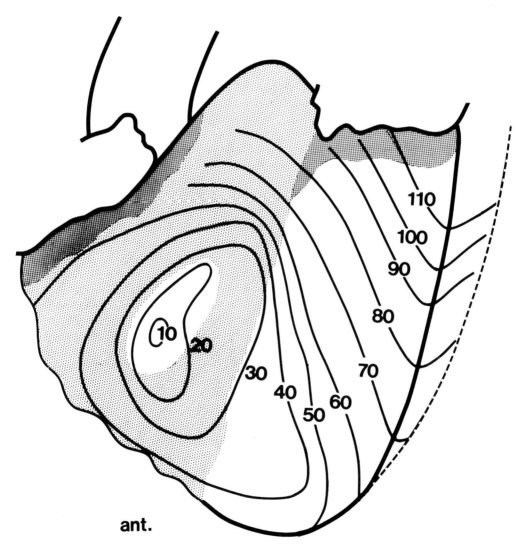

Fig. 8. Epicardial activation sequence on the anterior surface of a human heart with chronic CLBBB, explored during cardiac surgery. Activation times are measured in msec from the onset of right ventricular cavity potential. Greyish shaded areas indicate epicardial fat deposits. Discussion in text.

B. *Human CLBBB*

During surgery for advanced aortic stenosis, we explored the heart of a 57 year old male patient with CLBBB and left ventricular hypertrophy. Epicardial exploration was somewhat hampered by the presence of epicardial fat-deposits; we had to restrict the intramural exploration to the insertion of two needle-electrodes.

1. *Epicardial activation* (fig. 8 and 9)

During phase I, activation moves out into the left ventricular surface, following epicardial breakthrough in the pretrabecular area of the right ventricle and the formation of a radially expanding activation front in the right ventricle. During phase II ($\pm40 - \pm60$ msec), the activation waves progressing on the anterior and posterior surfaces merge near the apex at the lateral border of the left ventricle. At the anterior surface, the isochrones are relatively narrowly spaced. During phase III ($\pm60 - \pm120$ msec), a V-shaped activation

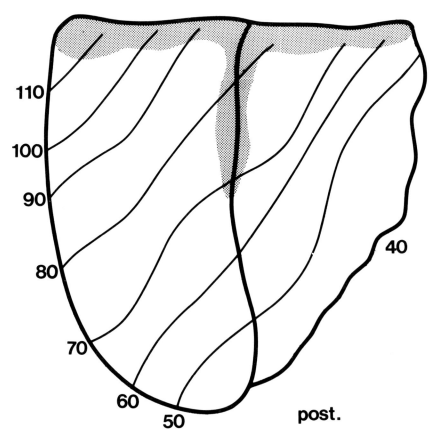

Fig. 9. Epicardial activation sequence on the posterior surface of the same human heart with CLBBB as illustrated in figure 8. Same legends as in figure 8.

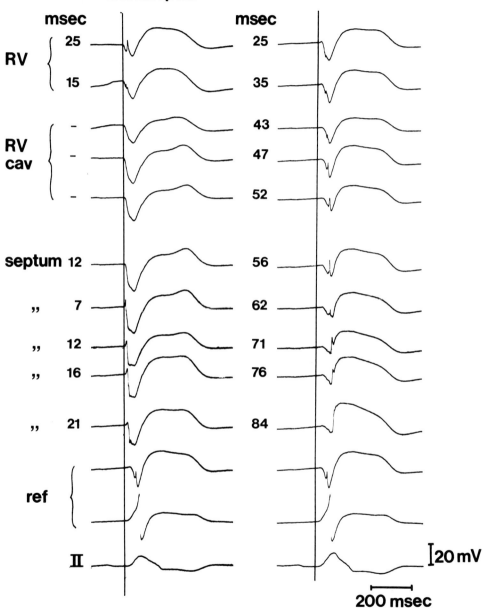

Fig. 10. Unipolar complexes recorded from a 20-terminal needle-electrode inserted by the right ventricle into the interventricular septum in the same case of human CLBBB. These data served in the construction of figure 12. Lower 3 channels: reference leads. Upper 10 channels: unipolar complexes from the intramural terminals 1–10 (right column) and 11–20 (left column).

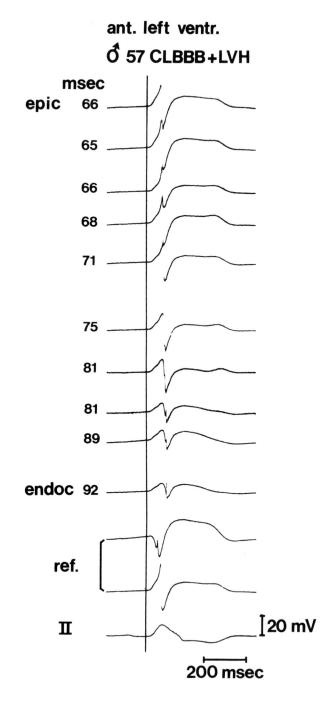

Fig. 11. The intramural unipolar complexes recorded from a needle-electrode inserted into the paraseptal anterior left ventricular wall, of a human heart with CLBBB. These data were used for the construction of figure 12.

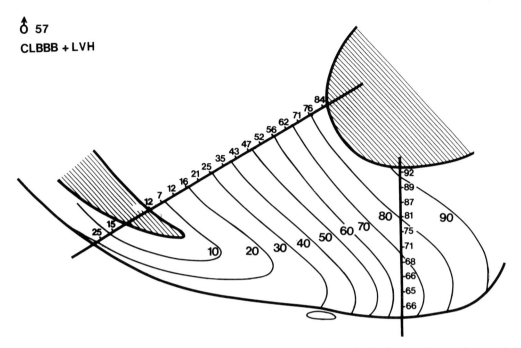

♂ 57

CLBBB + LVH

Fig. 12. Intramural activation sequence as studied with 2 needle-electrodes in the same human heart with CLBBB as illustrated in figures 8, 9, 10 and 11. Discussion in text.

front moves to the basolateral corner of the left ventricle. Because of the presence of excessive fat deposits, the latest activation, occurring at about 120 msec according to the standard electrocardiogram, has not been found during epicardial exploration.

2. *Intramural activation* (fig. 10, 11 and 12)

The unipolar complexes, recorded from the two needle-electrodes are shown in figures 10 and 11. The transseptal needle carried 20 terminals, was inserted into the lower half of the interventricular septum via the right ventricle and initially just reached into the left ventricular cavity. Activation times were measured from the onset of the right ventricular cavity potential, that preceded by ±20 msec the first discernable ventricular deflection in lead II. The advancing wave front induces a slight positivity in the unipolar complexes recorded from the left half of the interventricular septum. Apart from a local spreading back to the lining of the right ventricular cavity, there is a continuous conduction from right to left in the septum.

The left sided endocardium is reached at 84 msec in this part of the septum. The unipolar complexes recorded from the needle-electrode inserted in the paraseptal part of the left ventricular wall, and carrying 10 terminals at an interelectrodedistance of 2 mm. all display a well developed positivity appearing before the local intrinsic deflection. In this area, the activation front is curved and in the subepicardial layers approximately 25 msec advanced as compared to the middle and subendocardial layers. The intramural data from this heart are summarized in figure 12, in which also the hypothetical isochrones are indicated. The main features of epicardial and intramural activation correspond rather closely to the activation-sequence observed in the canine heart with CLBBB, given the larger diameter of the human hypertrophic left ventricle.

DISCUSSION

The main purpose of the present study has been the analysis of the ventricular activation-sequence in chronic bundle branch block, both in the canine and in the human heart.

The results in the canine heart are in general agreement with the earlier findings mainly in acute experiments, of Becker et al. (54) and Erickson et al. (256) and also of Moore et al. (565) who studied epicardial activation in chronic canine CRBBB. In the dog heart, at least two types of CRBBB seem to occur. Our fig. 1 illustrates the type, in which the latest activation occurs in the pulmonary conus and the same pattern has been described by Erickson et al. (256); some secondary involvement of the right ventricular subendocardial Purkinjeplexus is probably occurring in this type, accelerating conduction along the posterior half of the right ventricle. In the other type, a more lateral localization of the latest activation is present.

This type has been described by Moore et al. (565) and has been observed several years ago in our laboratory in a 12 year old dog with a 'spontaneous' CRBBB. The human case studied by us corresponds to this latter type of canine CRBBB. The equal spacing of iso-chrones at both sides at the right ventricle, and the relatively slow conduction suggest little or no participation of the conduction system in right ventricular activation in this type of CRBBB, however our recordings do not offer a definite proof for this hypothesis.

The same applies to our results on CLBBB, in which the intramural recordings did not display any electrical activity that could with certainty be attributed to the left ventricular Purkinje-system.

In chronic CLBBB in the human and in the canine heart, left ventricular and septal activation appear to occur exclusively by myocardial conduction during the first two phases of activation, as witnessed by the neat and parallel arrangement of the isochrones. In the interventricular septum, we have not found evidence of a local delay at the junction between right and left ventricular components of the septum. Most probably, the findings of Sodi Pallares et al, suggesting a local 'barrier' between both ventricles, are related to acute injury to the myocardium during the experiments.

The crescent-shaped activation waves present in the anterior and posterior left ventri-cular wall during phase II strongly suggest pure myocardial conduction. Our studies on Paired Stimulation (172) have demonstrated that activation conducted by the myocardium in the ventricular wall in a direction tangential to the epicardial surface, will result in such crescent-shaped activation waves, whereas secondary invasion of the subendocardial Purkinje plexus and its involvement in further propagation will result in a faster and preferential conduction in the subendocardial layers. This latter type occurs during phase III in canine CLBBB and suggests participation of the Purkinje-system in the distribution of activation.

Also, the more wide spacing and irregular arrangement of the isochrones during phase III, and the appearance of sudden 'jumps' in the activation sequence, that cannot be accounted for on the basis of continuous myocardial conduction, strongly support the hypo-thesis of secondary participation of the Purkinjeplexus in left ventricular activation during CLBBB. It has been shown by Venerose et al. (857) that the Purkinje-system in CLBBB in invaded, at least in acute experiments, as soon as the activation-wave progressing from the right ventricle has reached the left side of the interventricular septum. In previous studies we, and also Myerburg, have shown that impulses entering the Purkinje-system from the myocardium are distributed by this system to more distant parts of the myo-cardium. However, since a myocardial activation wave already is in progress, this secondary Purkinje-excitation sometimes has to travel over a relatively large distance before it is able to enter excitable myocardium, because of the transitional time-delays and detours involved.

As judged from the epicardial activation sequence and the samples of intramural excita-tion derived from the two needle electrodes in our human case, human CLBBB demon-strates the same basic activation-pattern as observed in the canine heart. During phase III, the wider spacing of epicardial isochrones suggests a more rapid spread of activation that possibly is due to participation of the Purkinje system. As pointed out by Kulbertus in this workshop, most degenerative lesions of the conduction system leading to left ventri-cular conduction-block tend to be localised in the proximal fascicles, although also the peripheral parts may be affected. In contrast, in our patient with CLBBB, the organic disease-process localized in the region of the aortic valve may have caused a purely local-ized interruption of the main stem of the left bundle branch, leaving the peripheral parts of the conduction system able to participate in the distribution of activation.

SUMMARY

The sequence of ventricular activation during chronic complete right and left bundle branch block (CRBBB and CLBBB) has been studied in two human cases and in chronic experimental bundle branch block in canine hearts by means of epicardial mapping pro-cedures and recordings from intramural terminals.

In chronic canine CRBBB, activation starts in the left ventricle according to the normal initial left ventricular activation pattern, it traverses the interventricular septum and enters the free right ventricular wall anteriorly and posteriorly by continuous myocardial conduc-tion. In the right ventricular wall, the anterior and posterior waves merge near the apex, forming a V-shaped activation front that moves towards the pulmonary conus which is activated as the latest part, by tangential conduction in the right ventricular wall and by an activation front conducted from the top of the interventricular septum along the crista supraventricularis. In a human case of CRBBB, approximately the same epicardial activa-tion sequence was found, with a more lateral localization to the area of late activation. The possibility of the occurrence of two types of CRBBB, with a different degree of secondary participation of the subendocardial Purkinjeplexus is discussed.

In chronic canine CLBBB, activation begins in the right ventricle according to the normal initial right ventricular activation-pattern and invades the left ventricle by con-duction in the myocardium across the interventricular septum and in the anterior and posterior left ventricular wall. The fronts meet at the lateral apical region and merge into an activation-front that is V-shaped on the epicardial surface and recedes into the latest area of left ventricular activation, the basolateral corner of the left ventricle. The acceleration and irregularities occuring during the later part of ventricular activation, probably are caused by secondary participation of the Purkinjeplexus in the distribution of activation. In a case of human CLBBB, associated with severe aortic stenosis and left ventricular hypertrophy essentially the same activation pattern as in the canine heart was observed.

ACKNOWLEDGEMENTS

Sincere thanks are due to the cardiac surgeons Prof. G. Brom, M.D. and Prof. N. G. Meyne, M.D. for their cooperation in the human cases, to Prof. D. Durrer, M.D. and L. Rossi, M.D. for their helpful suggestions and encouragement, and to Prof. J. P. Roos, M. J. Janse, M.D., F. J. L. van Capelle, Ph.D. and Mrs. Carla Mater for their participation in the experiments.

22

DEPRESSED CONDUCTION AND UNIDIRECTIONAL BLOCK IN PURKINJE FIBRES[1]

EUGENE DOWNAR, M.D., AND MENASHE B. WAXMAN, M.D.

INTRODUCTION

Re-entry is a mechanism basic to many of the rhythm disturbances that are clinically encountered. An understanding of such disturbances occurring at the ventricular level is perhaps all the more urgent in view of the potentially lethal consequence of ventricular arrythmias. In order to gain some further insight into conditions necessary for re-entry to occur within the Purkinje system we examined the character of depressed conduction produced within the system by a method of focal cooling. Others have used techniques such as 'blocking current' (921), graded pressure (546) and local hyperkalemia (160). Focal cooling had the advantages of allowing fine control of the degree of depressed conduction and could be rapidly and completely reversed to allow repeated observations in the same preparation. Furthermore many of the effects produced were qualitatively similar to those reported using other techniques, suggesting that depressed conduction has certain basic characteristics no matter how it arises.

METHOD

Sheep Purkinje fibres were obtained from freshly killed animals in an abbatoir and instantly placed in cooled oxygenated Tyrode's solution. Canine preparations were obtained by rapid excision after induction of anaesthesia using 30 mg/kg of intravenous sodium pentobarbitol. Similar results were obtained in both kinds of preparations. These were pinned out across a U-shaped 16G steel tube (fig. 1) through which CO_2 could be passed from a standard CO_2 cylinder source. Cooling was achieved by the Joule-Thompson effect which occured at points of pressure reduction when CO_2 was allowed to pass through the system. The degree of cooling was monitored by a miniature thermistor on the steel tube (close to the point of contact between the tube and the Purkinje fibre) and controlled by regulating gaseous flow by a needle valve.

Expelled CO_2 was exhausted away from the tissue bath by a polyethylene tube to prevent disturbances at the surface of the bath. In order to localise the cooling to the portion of Purkinje fibre immediately adjacent to the steel tube, the circulation of superfusant solution was arranged to proceed as shown in figure 2. Freshly heated Tyrode's solution

1. This work was supported by grants from the Ontario Heart Foundation and Medical Research Council of Canada.

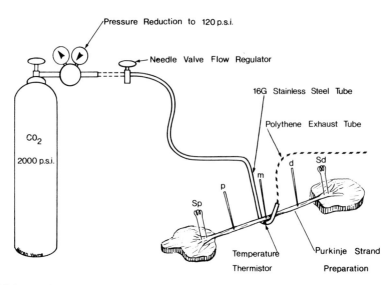

Fig. 1. Purkinje stand preparations. Stimulating electrodes on septal side-Sp. Stimulating electrodes on papillary muscle side-Sd. Intracellular electrodes-p, m and d recording from proximal, middle and distal sites along the strand. Electrode m records from the cooled zone, while p and d record from normothermic regions.

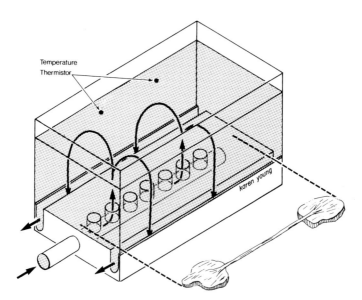

Fig. 2. Special tissue bath. Arrows denote direction of incoming and outgoing Tyrode's solution.

(K^+ 4.0 meg/1) aerated with 95% O_2 5% CO_2 entered the bath at points closest to the Purkinje fibre and rose to the surface. On being cooled by coming into contact with the steel tube, the cool solution left by sinking laterally into grutters which drained into a sump. Scavenging spent solution exclusively from the sump ensured that the coolest solution was always the first to be removed before it could influence remote portions of the Purkinje fibre. In this way it was possible to limit the cooled zone of the Purkinje fibre to a region within a few millimetres of the steel tube. Elsewhere within the tissue bath the temperature was maintained at $37 \pm 0.25°$ C.

Intra-cellular action potentials (APs) were recorded from the Purkinje fibres in the standard way using KCl filled glass microelectrodes. The preparations were paced by bipolar silver electrodes placed proximal and distal to the site of cooling. In certain situations intracellular stimulation and recording was performed through the same glass microelectrode by means of a switching circuit (569).

RESULTS

The initial effect of the cooling was to increase principally the duration of phase 2 of action potentials recorded from within the cooled zone (fig. 3). Subsequently the major changes noted were a decrease in resting membrane potential, slowing of phase 0 and a reduction in maximal amplitude of the AP (fig. 4). The final sequence of changes leading up to the failure in conduction across the cool region included firstly the emergence of a break in phase 0 which with further cooling became more distinct as a prepotential preceding a second more typical AP. Further cooling increased the separation between the two responses until finally conduction failed and only the prepotential remained in response to each stimulus (fig. 4, panels E and F).

With suitable adjustment in the flow rate of CO_2 it was possible to maintain for prolonged periods of time, stable incomplete block with a simple arithmetic relationship between blocked and conducted responses. Most frequently a 2:1 pattern of conduction

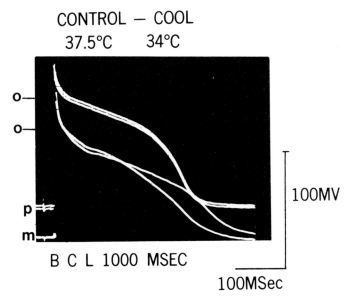

Fig. 3. Localisation of cooling effect. Two superimposed sweeps from electrodes p and m (separated by 5 mm) during control and regional cooling to a temperature of 34°C. Selective prolongation in action potential (AP) duration of m is seen. Preparation driven at a basic cycle length (BCL) of 1000 msec.

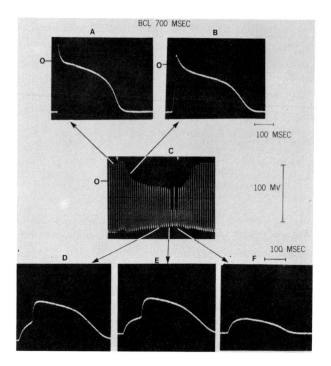

Fig. 4. Configurational changes in AP recorded from electrode m during focal cooling to the point of block. Panel C shows the uninterrupted sequence at slow sweep. White arrows indicate onset and offset of cooling. Resting membrane potential (RMP) and AP amplitude are reduced during cooling but rapidly restored when cooling stops. Panels A, B, D, E and F are fast sweep displays at different stages indicated by the black arrows. A and B show the AP at control temperature and on initial cooling respectively. Panels D and E show the gradual emergence of a prepotential which alone persists when block supervenes (panel F). Normal configuration as well as amplitude and RMP returns rapidly when cooling stops.

was produced. Conduction disturbances often displayed unidirectional characteristics by simultaneously maintaining 1:1 conduction in one direction in the face of complete block in conduction in the opposite direction (fig. 5, panel 4). Further degrees of cooling produced complete block in both directions (fig. 5 panel 5). It was always possible to rapidly restore normal bidirectional conduction by cessation of cooling.

THE MECHANISM OF BLOCK BY FOCAL COOLING

In contrast to the effects of generalized hypothermia, focal cooling produced a characteristic break in phase 0, even at an early stage when little slowing in conduction velocity has occurred (fig. 5, panel 2). As the degree of cooling is increased, the AP resolves in to two definite components—an early prepotential and after an increasing delay, a second response superimposed on that prepotential. The delay between these components parallels precisely the conduction delay across the cooled zone. Finally when conduction fails only the prepotential remains.

Close scrutiny of the prepotential reveals that there is a small but definite reduction

BCL 600 MSEC

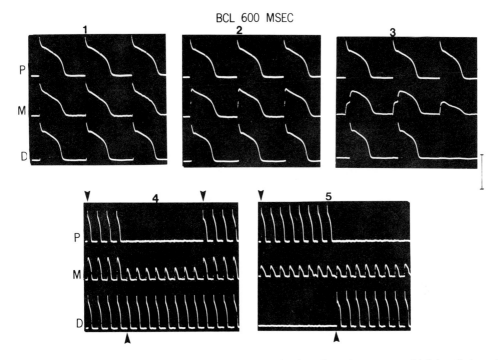

Fig. 5. Sequence of conduction disturbances produced by focal cooling of a segment of left bundle branch tissue. All panels show AP's from electrodes p, m and d. Panels 1, 2 and 3 are recorded during antegrade stimulation. Panel 1 is taken under control conditions (37 °C.) Panel 2 is taken during early cooling and shows a break in phase 0 of signal m associated with only a slight delay in antegrade conduction. Panel 3 shows a well-developed prepotential associated with second degree block with a 3:2 conduction ratio. Panel 4 shows while antegrade stimulation (upper arrows) still resulted in 1:1 conduction switching to retrograde stimulation (lower arrow) exposed already a coexistant retrograde block. Panel 5 recorded after further cooling, shows complete block with both antegrade and retrograde stimulation. Cessation of cooling at this point could rapidly restore normal bidirectional conduction.

in its amplitude prior to the onset of block (fig. 6). The prepotential not only loses amplitude with distance travelled (fig. 7). It represents a process of decremental conduction and/or electrotonic decay through refractory cells in the cooled region. The process represented by the prepotential is doomed to extinction unless it can penetrate, with sufficient amplitude, through to responsive cells at the distal end of the cooled region.

The manner in which the threshold of excitability is raised in the cooled region is illustrated in figure 8. It shows a strength-interval curve obtained (during a stable period of cooling) by intracellular stimulation. Compared with the control situation the curve is shifted up and to the right and becomes smoothly curvilinear. In addition to showing a raised threshold and a prolongation of the absolute refractory period, it shows a marked prolongation of the relative refractory period during which partial responses may be elicited.

From the foregoing it is apparent that conduction across the cooled zone is blocked when the diminishing amplitude of the excitation front fails to meet the rising threshold of exciteability.

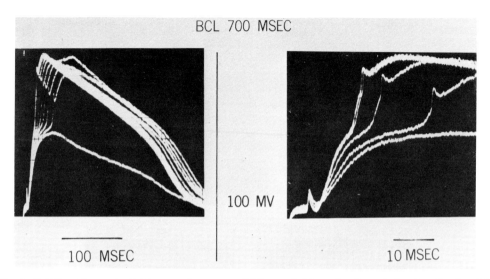

Fig. 6. Relation of prepotential to second response of AP recorded from focally cooled region. Panel on left shows sequential changes in AP recorded during onset of cooling and displayed as a series of superimposed sweeps. Right panel shows same sequence at a faster sweep. The initial break in phase 0 develops into a distinct prepotential and a superimposed increasingly delayed second response. This delay is related to a falling rate of rise and maximal amplitude of the prepotential. The second response coincides precisely with the timing of the upstroke of the AP immediately distal to the cooled region and parallels the delay in conduction. As soon as conduction fails, the second response disappears and only the prepotential remains.

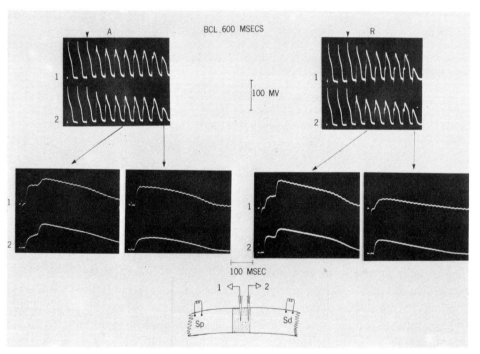

Fig. 7. Decremental nature of the prepotential. Electrodes 1 and 2 are both situated in the cooled region, in the same longitudinal axis, separated by 3 mm. Sequential changes leading to block are shown in the top two panels during antegrade (left panels) and retrograde stimulation (right panels). In each instance the amplitude of the prepotential is greatest in the electrode closest to the stimulated side. The prepotential loses significant amplitude even over the 3 mm between the two electrodes. By contrast the second response is greatest in the electrode further away from the stimulated side.

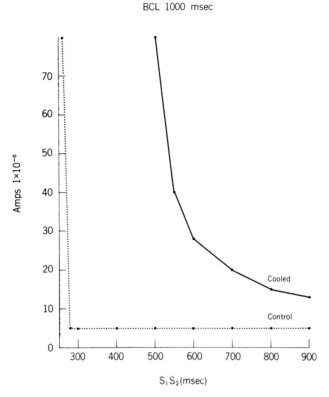

Fig. 8. Intracellular strength-interval curves obtained in the same cell under control and stable cooled conditions (see text).

RELATIONSHIP OF THE PREPOTENTIAL TO THE SECOND RESPONSE

As mentioned earlier the second response of the AP recorded within the cooled region, is intimately related to the response beyond the region. It precisely parallels the degree of conduction delay and in fact depends entirely on successful conduction in order to be seen. Furthermore, in contrast to the prepotential, the amplitude of the second response is greater the closer it is to the exit from the cooled region (fig. 7). These observations strongly suggest that, whereas the prepotential represents electrotonic decay of decremental conduction in to the cooled region, the second response is an electrotonic reflection back into the cooled region from a successful regenerative wavefront elicited beyond the cooled region.

Further evidence for this view is shown in figure 9. Two microelectrodes were situated in the proximal (A) and distal (B) sites in the cooled region. Extracellular pacing from the proximal end of the fibre produced a typical complex with prepotential and secondary response in both electrodes. Intracellular stimulation and recording was then initiated through electrode A. Complexes 1, 2 and 3 were recorded when conduction succeeded in penetrating to the distal side and produced a regenerative response. Complexes 4, 5

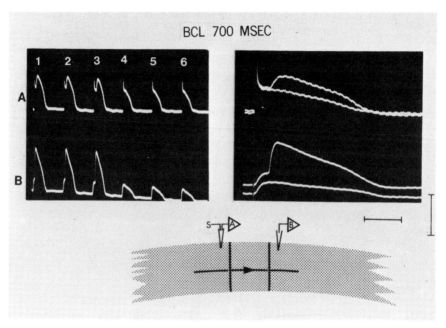

Fig. 9. Intracellular stimulation during onset of block (see text).

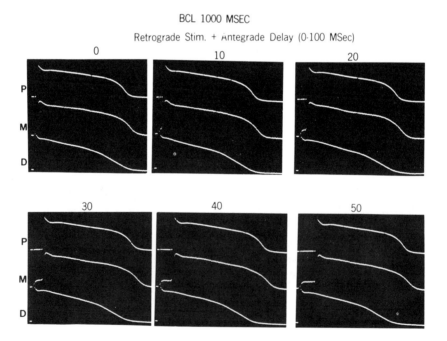

Fig. 10. Dependence of second response on activity beyond site of block. During a period of retrograde block when only a prepotential was recorded from electrode m, a second response at m could be produced by delayed stimulation of the antegrade end. The delay between retrograde and antegrade stimulation was increased by 10 msec increments to 50 msec. As is clearly shown the timing of the second response was determined by antegrade activation. This models precisely the behaviour of the second response prior to the onset of block.

and 6 show the configuration of the response of the stimulated cell when antegrade conduction failed to penetrate the cooled zone but retrograde conduction to the proximal
end of the fibre still occurred. The moment conduction failed to penetrate to the distal
side, the second response disappeared even in the intracellularly stimulated cell. This
suggests that the second response is not an intrinsic component of the stimulated cell's
AP since the cell is responsive and allows conduction to occur retrogradely in a normal
fashion. Furthermore in a situation where block across the cooled region had occurred and
the only response to a retrograde impulse was a prepotential in the cooled region, a typical
second response superimposed on the prepotential could be produced by stimulation of
the proximal end of the fibre (fig. 10). The timing of the second response was determined
entirely by the timing of stimulation of the proximal end of the fibre.

BCL 700 msec

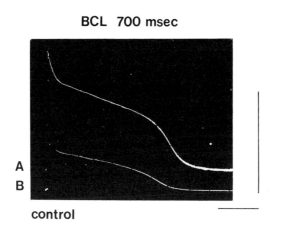

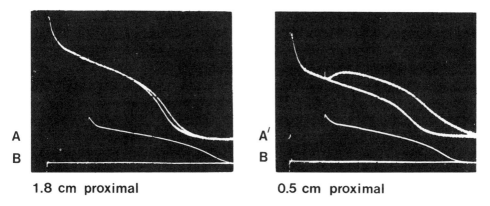

Fig. 11. Action potential shortening proximal to site of block. Signals A and B (reduced sensitivity) are
recorded proximal and distal to site of 2:1 block (top panel under control conditions with normal 1:1 conduction). Two superimposed sweeps are shown—one conducted and one blocked impulse. Slight shortening of
AP duration with each blocked impulse is seen 1.8 cm proximal to site of block (lower left panel). This
shortening is greatly magnified closer to site of block. (lower right panel).

THE NATURE OF ELECTROTONIC INTERACTION ACROSS THE
COOLED REGION

The effect of such electrotonic interactions as described above, reaches outside of the cooled zone to influence both the AP configuration and the duration of the refractory period of normothermic cells. As has been reported in instances of block produced by other techniques (160, 545, 719) focal cooling also causes shortening of AP duration (APD) refractory period of cells proximal to the block. Figure 11 illustrates the shortening in APD seen in a typical experiment. A stable 2:1 block had been set up and even though the recording site A was 1.8 cm from the cooled zone, some shortening in APD is seen with each blocked impulse. The recording electrode was then moved closer to site A, only 0.5 cm from the site of block. Marked shortening of the APD by about 100 msec is now seen with each blocked impulse.

The extent to which APD could be influenced by the timing of activity distal to the block was investigated in the following way: in a stable 2:1 block, the distal end of the fibre was excited after a varying delay following each blocked proximal impulse (fig. 12). It was found that delays up to 150 msec restored the duration of the proximal AP to what it was with each conducted impulse. Delays of more than 150 msec produced some prolongation of the late part of phase 3 while still precisely restoring phase 2 and early phase 3. The striking feature was the limited way in which the proximal cell responded, always trying to assume the configuration of the conducted AP regardless of the delay.

These changes in configuration in the proximal AP were accompanied by parallel changes in the refractory period. It was shortened in blocked impulses but could be lengthened by activation of the distal end to stimulate conduction.

UNIDIRECTIONAL BLOCK

As already stated unidirectional block (U.B.) was frequently observed in focally cooled Purkinje fibres. In fact UB almost invariably occurred prior to the development of complete block provided conduction was allowed to deteriorate gradually. Since the conduction disturbances produced by such cooling were completely reversible many observations were made on the effect of repeated cooling in the same preparation, without any apparent change in the conditions. In such repeated observations it was not uncommon to find a given preparation would manifest UB in one direction one time and in the opposite direction next time it was cooled. Our suspicion was that the cooled region was not a symmetrical band but rather changed its contour according to changes in microcurrents of the heated superfusant as it passed around the cooling probe. We thought that accurate definition of the shape of the cooled zone might predict the direction of UB. Efforts directed toward mapping the precise shape of the cooled zone were unsuccessful. We consequently contrived to produce deliberately asymmetric cooled regions by making the surface of contact between the fibre and the cooling probe, triangular shaped. The apex of such a triangular metal form by projecting into the heated Tyrode's solution was warmer than the base of the triangle which was flush with the probe. Encouraged by our

BCL 500 msec

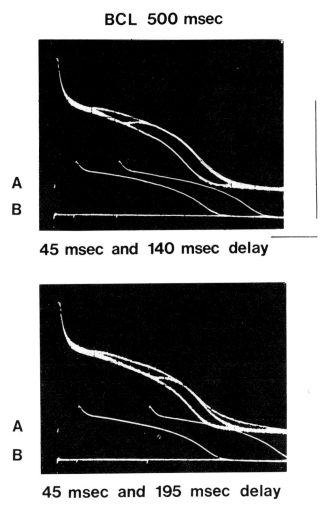

45 msec and 140 msec delay

45 msec and 195 msec delay

Fig. 12. Effect of conduction delay on proximal action potential duration. Same preparation as in figure 11 in a state of 2:1 antegrade block. Each panel shows three superimposed sweeps taken during blocked impulses *only*. One sweep shows the proximal action potential (A) with no distal activity (straight line on B). The other sweeps show the change in A when the distal end is also stimulated 45, 140 and 195 msec after proximal stimulation. The result is prolongation of the proximal action potential to what it would have been had antegrade conduction been successful (see text).

observations with this technique, we went on to examine the effect of an asymmetric pressure lesion. To produce this, a bevelled crushing probe was applied to the Purkinje fibre with carefully graded pressure. Maximal pressure on the fibre occurred under the apex of the bevelled probe with a region of diminishing pressure under the bevel.

The results of both techniques were the same and are shown in figure 13. UB almost invariably occurred in the direction of a wave front of excitation moving from the region of minimal injury to that of maximal.

Since the normal bidirectional conduction could be restored immediately on stopping the cooling, it was possible to examine the effect of repeatedly reversing the cooling

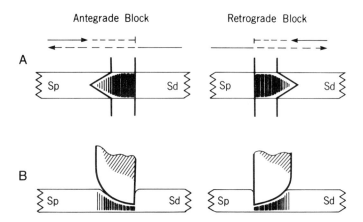

Fig. 13. Unidirectional Block. Schematic representation of direction of block. The *top panels* represent the triangular cooling probe while the *bottom panels* describe the crushing probe. The heavier shading indicates the region of greatest cooling or compression. The preparation is stimulated antegradely or retrogradely from a proximal (Sp) or distal (Sd) site respectively. The direction of block corresponds with the wave front which meets the least depressed zones first. On the other hand, successful conduction occurs in the direction in which the wave front encounters the most depressed zone first. Thus, antegrade block occurs when the least depressed zone faces the proximal stimulating site, while retrograde block occurs when the least depressed zone faces the distal stimulating site.

triangle in the same preparation (fig. 14). Each reversal of the cooling triangle was accompanied by a reversal of the direction of UB once it was re-established. By contrast, in the crush experiments the reversibility of UB could not be demonstrated because of residual injury from the first crush.

Whereas orientation of the lesion produced was the determinant of the direction of UB, the anatomic orientation of the preparation was not i.e. the direction of the block did not preferentially occur toward the periphery (papillary muscle end) nor centrally toward the ventricular septal end. Moreover, pre-existing functional differences as expressed by differences in conduction velocity in the two directions, did not predict the direction of UB (fig. 15) and could be overridden.

UB is not an infrequent occurrence whenever conduction disturbances occur in myocardial tissue. In special circumstances the direction of block can be predicted. Conduction across Purkinje-muscle (P-M) junctions fails in the P-M direction when M-P conduction remains still intact (547). In atrial muscle, UB occurs across an isthmus linking a large mass of muscle with a smaller mass (187). Conduction across the isthmus fails when it proceeds from the small mass to the large mass while conduction in the reverse direction is maintained. Such observations have been explained by considerations of a falling space constant as one proceeds from a small mass of tissue to a larger. The term 'impedance mismatch' (187) has been applied to such circumstances. The eccentric lesion we produced in Purkinje fibres may be viewed as a junction between a large and a smaller mass of cells. There may well be a falling space constant on moving from the region of least injury to the region of maximal injury since the latter has an abrupt interface with uninjured Purkinje cells across the full diameter of the fibre.

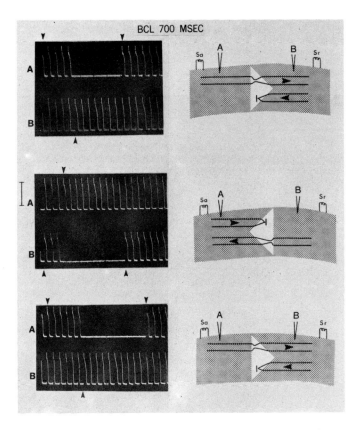

Fig. 14. Asymmetric focal cooling. A proximal cell (A) and distal cell (B) are impaled across a zone of cooling. The fibre crosses over a triangular platform as indicated. By rotating the entire cooling probe, the direction of the triangle could be reversed. The arrows over the action potentials indicate the direction of stimulation i.e. downward arrows denote antegrade, while upward arrows denote retrograde stimulation. The *top panel* shows unidirectional block in a retrograde direction. This corresponds to the triangular platform being directed so that the zone of least cooling pointed toward the distal portion of the fibre. In the *middle panel* the triangular probe has been rotated so it is directed in the opposite direction. This produces antegrade unidirectional block; restoration of the direction to its original position causes a reversion to unidirectional retrograde block (see bottom panel).

Figure 16 summarizes a proposed mechanism by which UB may have arisen in the circumstances that we saw it. We have assumed that the cooling or crushing raises the exciteability threshold of cells in the depressed zone. The region of greatest injury shows a very sharp rise in threshold and the region of lesser injury shows a more gradual rise. An impulse coming in retrogradely encounters a zone of inexciteable cells abruptly and decays electrotonically according to the space constant. Depending on the gap of inexciteable tissue and the threshold of cells on the opposite end of the lesion this electrotonic input may be just sufficient to initiate a regenerative response at point 'X' and thus complete retrograde conduction. By contrast an impulse coming in antegradely encounters a gradually rising threshold which results in decrement of the active wavefront. At point 'X' this decremental conduction ceases active propagation and decays electrotonically according to the space constant. In attempting to bridge the zone of inexcitable cells

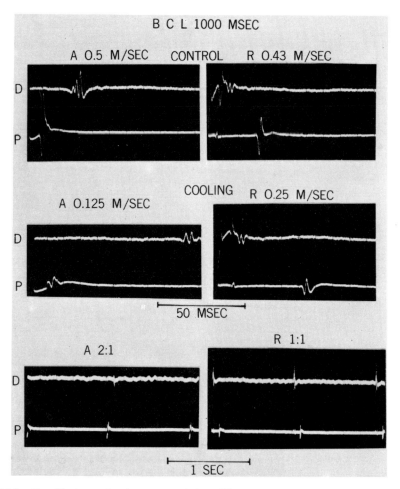

Fig. 15. Unidirection block unrelated to pre-excisting differences in conduction velocity. Two external electrograms are recorded proximal (P) and distal (D) to a zone which is being cooled. Control antegrade conduction velocity is faster (0.5 m/sec) than retrograde conduction (0.43 m/sec). Despite the faster antegrade conduction velocity, the greatest slowing and block during cooling occur in an antegrade direction.

electrotonically the antegrade input fails while the retrograde input succeeds because of two factors. Firstly, it starts of from a lower voltage at point 'X' instead of the full 120 mV. Secondly it contends with a shortening space constant instead of the lengthening space constant that operates retrogradely.

A possible third determinant of UB may well be the nature of active conduction within the partially depressed zone. Conduction through this region retrogradely, being augmental, may be more self-sustaining than antegrade conduction, which is decremental.

DISCUSSION

The observations described were produced by focal cooling. They differ markedly in many respects from the effects seen when generalised cooling of an entire Purkinje fibre occurs

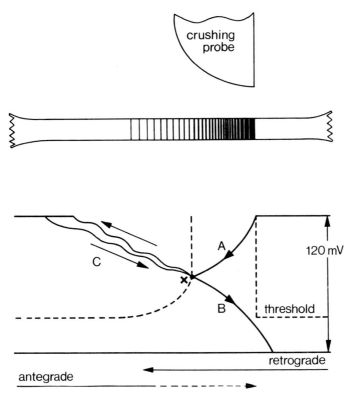

Fig. 16. Proposed schema by which unidirectional block may arise. The top figure illustrates a Purkinje fibre with asymmetric injury produced by crush. The lower figure illustrates influence of the injury on excitability threshold and contrasts the amplitude of antegrade (C-X-B) and retrograde (A-X-C) wavefronts at corresponding points. C represents decremental or augmental conduction depending on direction, through region of partial injury. X represents point of transition between partially excitable cells and refractory cells in zone of maximal injury. A and B represent electrotonic conduction through refractory cells. The retrograde wavefront succeeds in conducting across while an antegrade wavefront fails. (see text for discussion)

(366). Among the more striking points of difference are the relatively small amount of AP prolongation and the relatively marked effects on the upstroke and amplitude of the AP when focally cooled. The differences are due in part to decremental conduction within the cooled zone and in part to electrotonic interaction of the cooled zone with adjacent normothermic cells.

In contrast to these differences, configuration of the complexes recorded in the cooled zone bore marked similarities to complexes recorded from regions of depressed conduction brought about by other techniques such as hyperkalemia, compression and depolarising currents. They were also reminiscent of complexes recorded from N-cells of the rabbit atrio-ventricular (AV) junction, especially when AV conduction is stressed (366, 408, 545). There is increasing evidence that such complexes are due to slow Na^+ current or Ca^{++} current and are manifest when the fast Na^+ current is inhibited (166, 527, 705, 855). Such inhibition may be due to a reduced resting membrane potential (brought about by an elevated external (K^+), depolarising current, injury to the cell membrane or as an intrinsic property of certain normal cells (958) or due to hypothermia (215). If applicable the latter process was probably more important in producing the complexes we saw since there was only a minor degree of resting depolarisation in our preparations.

The character of such depressed AP's produced by hyperkalemia has been described (162) and differs from normal in some important respects. They behave paradoxically in being capable of responding to a second stimulus during inscription of the complex and then are refractory for some time after repolarisation. In consequence, depending on the timing of collision of two such depressed AP's the result may be summation of two decremental wavefronts to produce a regenerative wavefront, or inhibition with resultant extinction of decremental conduction (187). We have observed similar summation and inhibition properties of decremental conduction in focal cooling. We also saw marked disparity between the voltage time course and the time course for recovery of exciteability similar to that described in focal hyperkalemia and in normal N-cell of the AV junction (162, 548). Such a disparity suggests that the depressed action potentials seen in decremental conduction are dependent on a slow activation current whose carrier is more time-dependent for recovery than voltage-dependent. The double responses observed in focal areas of depressed conduction which ultimately succeeds, emphasize the extent to which the AP configuration of a particular cell is determined by surrounding conduction. Although especially true for cells within a depressed region it also applies to normal adjacent cells which manifest shortening of APD proximal to the site of block. In the case of focal cooling this shortening even affects normal cells a considerable distance from the

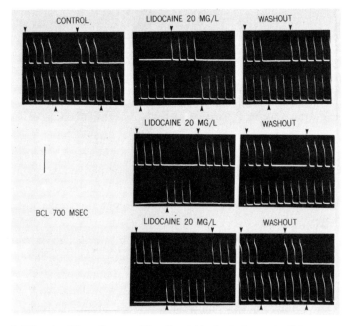

Fig. 17. Effects of Lidocaine 20 mg/L on unidirectional block. Action potentials are recorded from a cell proximal and distal to a zone of crushing. The downward arrows denote antegrade stimulation, while the upward ones signify retrograde conduction. In the *control panel*, unidirectional retrograde block has already been produced. Lidocaine converts this zone into bidirectional block. Washout of the drug restores unidirectional block, *without* a stage of bidirectional conduction. Here we show 3 consecutive administrations and washouts of Lidocaine. The results are always the same. Note how Lidocaine reduces action potential duration.

site of block. Such shortening of APD is accompanied by a parallel shortening of the refractory period. The frequent occurrence of unidirectional block in depressed Purkinje fibres together with slow conduction and shortening of refractory periods sets the scene for re-entrant phenomena via a classic circuit pathway. Re-entry by reflection (930) without a circuit may also occur if antegrade conduction is successful but slow enough to produce proximal shortening of recovery times and a sufficient retrograde wavefront arises from the distal regenerative activity.

Our observations on unidirectional block indicate that the prime requisite for its occurrence is a zone of depressed conduction which is asymmetric, with the zone of maximal depression interfacing with an underpressed region. Conduction fails when a wavefront approaches this interface from the region of minimal depression before it fails in the opposite direction. Recently, van Capelle, using an analogue model of asymmetric depressed conduction has obtained identical results with block first arising in the predicted direction. (See chapter 18 by van Capelle.) Directional differences in electrotonic space constant (187,547) would appear to play a key role but the role of directional differences in decremental conduction may be important and remain to be clarified. The *in vitro* model of unidirectional block produced with pressure on the fibre is stable enough to allow observation on antiarrhythmic drug actions and we have been able to observe the action of xylocaine in this context (fig. 17). Contrary to its proposed action of unidirectional block (70) we did not see the facilitation of conduction in low doses but in high doses did see the development of bidirectional block. The effects of other drugs await examination.

23
NEWER ASPECTS OF
CONCEALED CONDUCTION OF THE CARDIAC IMPULSE

RICHARD LANGENDORF, M.D.

This article will not give an exhaustive presentation of the subject of concealed conduction (c.c.) of the cardiac impulse; but will review newer aspects of this phenomenon. Actually, no new material will be shown. The figures obtained from our own material were selected to demonstrate the more recently recognized manifestations of c.c., mainly localized in the A-V junction, but examples will also be shown of its occurrence in the ventricles and atria. The emphasis will be on the effects of concealed re-entry and on enhancing effects of c.c. on subsequent conduction. In addition to electrocardiographic records a number of tables will be given to present a more complete analysis of the manifestations of c.c. The overlap of the tables, unavoidable because of the different criteria used to classify the effects of c.c., may prove useful from a didactic standpoint.

In our appreciation of c.c. progress was mainly due to microelectrode studies of the electrophysiologists with recordings of action potentials from the various portions of the conduction system and the study of His bundle recordings in man in conjunction with artificial pacing of the atria or ventricles.

Table 1 presents a listing of the manifestations of c.c. in general terms. Subsequent tables will enumerate the specific effects of c.c. of the impulse.

In 1925 Lewis and Master (498, their fig. 25) did the classical dog experiment demonstrating the first and indirect evidence of concealed A-V conduction, the effect of blocked impulses on subsequent conduction. When, in the middle portion of their figure, the rapid rate

Table 1. Manifestations of concealed conduction I (without presence of accesory A-V pathway).

A. *Effect on subsequent impulse conduction*

1. Delay
2. Block
3. Concealment ('repetitive concealed conduction')
4. Enhancement
5. Re-entry (manifest or concealed)

B. *Effect on subsequent impulse formation*

1. Premature discharge ('Resetting') of dominant pacemaker

C. *Combined effects* on subsequent impulse conduction and impulse formation (A & B)

of atrial stimulation, associated with 2:1 ventricular response, is reduced to one half, the ventricular rate remains the same (1:1 response), however, the P-R interval shortens. In 1965, forty years later, we repeated the same experiment in man (461), stimulating the right atrium via a transvenous catheter electrode. In 1968 Damato and co-workers (471) showed with His bundle recordings that the A-V conduction delay during 2:1 A-V response was due to delay of transnodal transmission, caused by penetration of the 'blocked' impulses into the A-V node.

Figure 1 shows in the bottom strip an instance of atrial flutter with *2 :1 A-V response and alternation of ventricular cycle length.* The mechanism, as indicated in the diagram, concealed penetration of alternate 'blocked' impulses, was the first explanation in clinical electrocardiography of the effect of blocked impulses on subsequent conduction, given by Kaufmann and Rothberger in 1927 (427). The top portion of the figure shows the same phenomenon of alternation of ventricular cycle length during sinus rhythm and 2:1 A-V block with more obvious alternation of the P-R interval of the conducted beats. Here, the interpretation is substantiated by the occurrence of 3:2 conduction in the center of the middle strip.

In 1972 Watanabe and Dreifus (888, fig. 1) examined the phenomenon in the rabbit heart, recording action potentials from the lower portion of an NH fiber in addition to surface records from an area close to the S-A node and from the ventricle. Record B shows

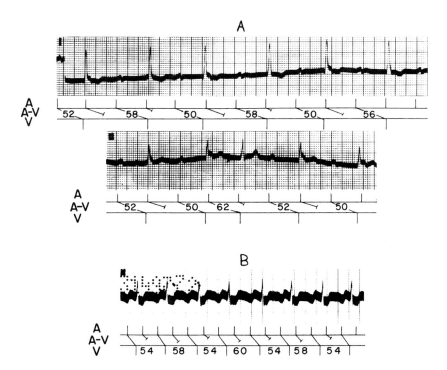

Fig. 1. 2:1 A-V response with alternation of ventricular cycle length. In the top and middle record the numbers indicate A-V conduction times in hundredths of a second, in the lower record R-R intervals. Discussed in text. From R. Langendorf: Entstehungsprinzipien seltener in der Klinik beobachteter Herzrhythmusstörungen. *Verh. dtsch. Ges. Kreisl. Forsch.* 35: 69, 1969, figure 1. By permission.

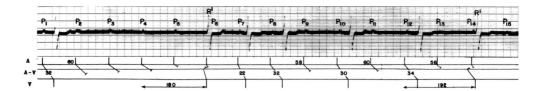

Fig. 2. A-V block, Type I, with repetitive concealed conduction and repetitive concealed discharge of the subsidiary pacemaker (R′). Discussed in text. From R. Langendorf and A. Pick, ref. 459, figure 6. By permission.

2:1 block with alternation of ventricular cycle length and reveals the intricate mechanism of the disturbance, namely, a 4:3 Type I block in an upper region of the A-V junction and a second region of block below the site of inscription of the NH action potential.

Consecutive blockage of several atrial impulses is common in so-called Type II A-V block, but may also occur in Type I block (464). In patients with evidence of Type I block we called a resulting 3:1 block 'abortive 3:2 block' (459) long before the introduction of His bundle recordings. Dhingra et al. (199) (fig. 19.3) showed the occurrence of a 3:1 A-V response during rapid atrial pacing. The deeper penetration of the first blocked impulse, responsible for H of the blocked atrial impulse (with lengthening of the A-H time) demonstrates the mechanism. That does not mean that in all such cases of 3:1 block the deeper penetration has to reach past the A-V node.

Figure 2 shows a rare case of Type I A-V block with *repetitive concealed conduction* (459, 558) and repetitive concealed discharge of the subsidiary pacemaker, a Wenckebach period of concealed conduction (459).

Now, I wish to demonstrate the simplest type of the *gap phenomenon of A-V conduction* (927, fig. 2), a subject that will be discussed in detail by Dr. Damato. During premature atrial stimulation (A_2) with progressive shortening of A_1-A_2, conduction to the ventriciles ceases in the two middle strips. Inscription of an H_2 following the blocked A_2 indicates concealed penetration. In the bottom record, when the shortest A_1-A_2 is associated with the longest H_1-H_2, impulse A_2 reaches the ventricles and imitates a supernormal phase of A-V conduction in the surface ECG.

In 1973 Damato and co-workers (177, fig. 2) described that in certain individuals rapid atrial stimulation may induce 1:1 A-V conduction if started early in the cycle, or 2:1 response with block below H when started later in the cycle, representing a functional subnodal A-V block.

In 1970 Rosen and co-workers (669, fig. 2) showed that premature His bundle depolarizations can cause *pseudo A-V block* as we and Mehlman (456) postulated in 1947. The top strip of their fig. 2 imitates Type II A-V block, the middle strip, Type I block, and the bottom strip first degree A-V block. The third beat in the bottom strip, with the longest H-H′, becomes manifest as junctional premature systole.

Puech and Grolleau (642, fig. 31) published a beautiful example of a His bundle parasystole in a case of complete subnodal A-V block and demonstrated the *effect of concealed conduction upon concealed conduction*, revealed by His bundle recordings. In the upper tracing the prolongation of A-H proves concealed retrograde conduction of H′.

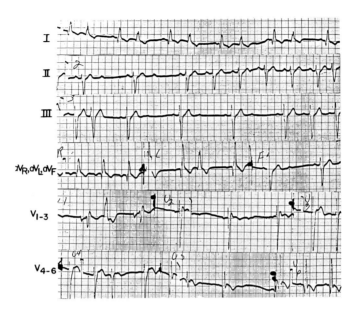

Fig. 3. Pseudo A-V block in a patient with right bundle branch block and left anterior fascicular block. Intermittent parasystole orginating in the posterior fascicle of the left bundle branch. Discussed in text. From R. Langendorf and A. Pick, ref. 467, figure 3. By permission.

At the end of the lower tracing H'-A is so short that the concealed retrograde conduction of H' prevents the inscription of H after the subsequent A.

In 1973, in a study of intermittent parasystole from our laboratory (134) we showed that pseudo A-V block can also be the result of concealed depolarization in a proximal portion of a fascicle of the ventricular conduction system. In the 12 lead ECG of fig. 3 the bigeminy seen in lead I was due to parasystole (as discussed by Pick in chapter 8), and the 2:1 block in II and III were pseudo-blocks due to concealed depolarization in the posterior fascicle of the left bundle branch. Figure 4, with the help of His bundle electrograms shows that the H-Q interval of the parasystolic beats (35 msec) is shorter than that of the sinus beat (65 msec), ruling out a His bundle site of the premature beats with aberrant conduction. A similar case was reported by Castellanos et al. (114). The occurrence of other effects of concealed impulse formation can be postulated (table 2), notably such occurring late in

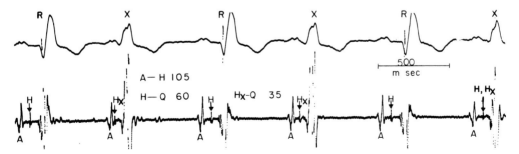

Fig. 4. His bundle recording of the patient of figure 3, indicating fascicular origin of the parasystolic pacemaker (X). Discussed in text. From H. Cohen, R. Langendorf and A. Pick, ref. 134, figure 6. By permission.

Table 2. Manifestations of concealed conduction II.

A. Re-entry (manifest or concealed) after slow concealed conduction

1. Single echo (ventricular, atrial, sino-atrial)
2. Initiation, perpetuation, termination of reciprocating A-V junctional, ventricular, atrial tachycardia

B. Effects of concealed re-entry ('abortive echo') (effects of concealed conduction of *reflected* re-entrant impulse) after slow conduction or slow concealed conduction

1. Wenckebach period of A-V and V-A conduction (intermittence due to abortive atrial or ventricular echo)
2. Atypical Wenckebach period (atypical lengthening of last cycle)
3. Pseudo supernormal phase of A-V conduction (ventricular echo following abortive atrial echo)
4. Pseudo A-V block (bidirectional block of re-entrant impulse)
5. Resetting of junctional pacemaker by abortive ventricular or atrial echo in A-V dissociation
6. Resetting of parasystolic pacemaker by its own impulse

the cycle, particularly in instances of infranodal, unidirectional A-V block, initiating concealed retrograde conduction. However, to our knowledge, they have not been demonstrated yet with His bundle recordings. They may occur in paroxysmal A-V block and subsequent conduction in the opposite direction.

In 1971 Moore and Spear (570, fig. 3) investigated the enhancing effect of concealed

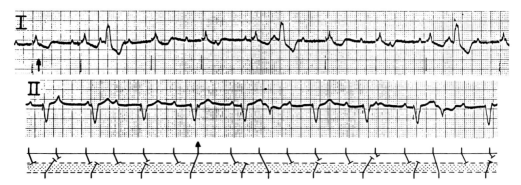

Fig. 5. Facilitation of A-V conduction (due to supernormal phase in the wake of concealed retrograde conduction) in 'complete A-V block' with evidence of unidirectional block, during ventricular pacing. Discussed in text. From R. Langendorf: Entstehungsprinzipien seltener in der Klinik beobachteter Herzrhythmusstörungen. *Verh. dtsch. Ges. Kreisl. Forsch.* 35: 69, 1969, figure 3. By permission.

retrograde conduction of a premature ventricular systole on A-V conduction of a subsequent atrial premature systole, the so-called 'pealing back' phenomenon of a refractory
barrier by pre-excitation, as described by Moe, Abildskov and Mendez (558) in their experimental study of c.c. in 1964, also assumed before by others (943, 512). This type of facilitating effect of pre-excitation of the ventricle or atrium, due to concealed penetration of the
premature impulse resulting in pre-excitation of the A-V junction, is certainly not the
same that can be observed so frequently in patients with chronic A-V block of Type II,
intraventricular block and preserved retrograde conduction, as seen in figure 5. Here,
during ventricular pacing the atrial impulses falling shortly after the T wave tend to be the
only ones to elicit a ventricular response. A supernormal phase of conduction in the His-
Purkinje system may be the underlying mechanism (628) or the phenomenon may be
related to the newly described summation phenomenon (161). An enhancing effect of
concealed retrograde conduction of a different, yet somewhat similar type, is seen in
bradycardia-dependent bundle branch block due to accelerated phase-4 depolarization
giving rise to paroxysmal A-V block. As Coumel (147, fig. 8) indicates in his diagram, concealed retrograde conduction of an escape beat reestablishes A-V conduction of an
appropriately timed atrial impulse.

Figure 6 is reminiscent of the enhancing effect of transseptal and retrograde conduction
assumed by Cohen et al. (136) in 1969, and later confirmed experimentally (48), to account
for the alternate patterns of premature ventricular excitation during induced atrial
bigeminy. Figure 6 shows the phenomenon recently observed in our Laboratory (185),
the mechanism of electrical alternans in bradycardia dependent bundle branch block.
Transseptal and retrograde conduction shortens the cycle in the vulnerable bundle branch.
In the upper strip of the figure the alternans is initiated by the atrial pause following a

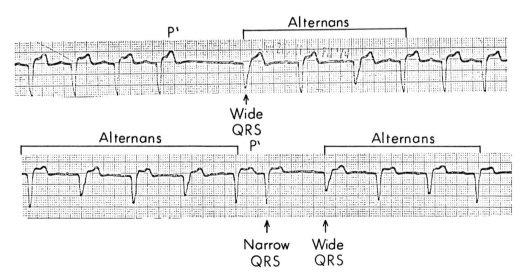

Fig. 6. Intermittent electrical alternans due to accelerated phase-4 depolarization. Initiated (top strip)
by a non-conducted atrial premature systole, terminated and re-initiated (bottom strip) by a conducted atrial
premature systole. Transseptal and retrograde concealed conduction. Discussed in text. From I. A. D'Cruz,
H. Cohen, A. Pick and R. Langendorf, ref. 185. By permission.

Table 3. Manifestations of concealed conduction III. *Effects of concealed impulse formation* with partial propagation (in the A-V junction, in the bundle branch system or in the atria)

A. Concealed *premature* impulse

    1. on subsequent impulse conduction: Delay or block (pseudo A-V block, pseudo i.v. block)
    2. on subsequent impulse formation: Resetting of dominant pacemaker

B. 1. Concealed *escape*

    a. Facilitation ('supernormal conduction') in Type II A-V block with unidirectional block (following concealed retrograde conduction)
    b. Resumption of A-V conduction in paroxysmal, bradycardia-dependent A-V block (prevention of phase IV depolarization)

Table 4. Manifestations of concealed conduction IV.

Enhancing effects on subsequent impulse conduction

A. On conduction in *opposite direction*

1. Following *premature* concealed retrograde depolarization of the A-V junction or a bundle branch (by a ventricular premature systole)
   a. 'Peeling back' of the refractory period
      Change from 2:1 to 1:1 A-V conduction
   b. Termination of aberrant ventricular conduction in paroxysmal supraventricular tachycardia
2. Following concealed retrograde depolarization of the A-V junction or a bundle branch by a ventricular *escape*
   a. Facilitation of A-V conduction (supernormal A-V conduction in Type II A-V block following concealed retrograde conduction across area of unidirectional block)
   b. Prevention of Phase 4 diastolic depolarization of His-Purkinje system in bradycardia dependent paroxysmal A-V block (resumption of A-V conduction)
3. Normalization of intraventricular conduction in bradycardia dependent bundle branch block by prevention of Phase 4 diastolic depolarization in a bundle branch with acceleration of atrial rate (concealed transseptal and retrograde conduction)
4. Alternation of aberrant ventricular conduction in supraventricular bigeminy (shortening of the refractory period by shortening of the cycle in the affected bundle branch consequent to its concealed transseptal penetration)
5. Electrical alternans due to bradycardia dependent BBB and normalization of intraventricular conduction in alternate beats

B. On conduction in the *same direction*

Prevention of expected aberrant ventricular conduction of a supraventricular impulse terminating a short ventricular cycle that follows a long cycle (by concealed A-V conduction into vulnerable bundle branch during long ventricular cycle) non-conducted atrial premature systole, in the lower strip it is terminated and re-initiated by a conducted atrial premature systole.

Table 3 lists a few additional examples of the *enhancing effect* of c.c. We just want to call attention to the one listed as A,1,b: Termination of aberrant ventricular conduction in paroxysmal supra-ventricular tachycardia as described by Wellens and Durrer in 1968 (901).

Further manifestations of c.c. to be discussed are *re-entry or concealed re-entry*, and those of *concealed conduction of the reflected re-entrant impulse* (465) (table 4).

Figure 7 is taken from a paper with Dr. Pick, published in 1950 (625). The lower strip shows an A-V junctional rhythm (the retrograde P wave is upright in lead CF1) with alternation of ventricular cycle length and also alternation of the R-P interval. The lengthening of the ventricular cycle following the longer R-P interval (0.28 sec.) is explained by concealed re-entry with discharge of the junctional pacemaker by the re-entrant impulse that is blocked below the site of the pacemaker. This interpretation is confirmed by the upper strip, where in the middle portion the re-entrant impulse elicits a ventricular response (ventricular echo) with aberrant ventricular conduction. As expected, the long cycles with concealed re-entry resetting the junctional pacemaker are about equal to the cycles bridging an echo.

In figure 8 the dominant rhythm is again junctional with progressive lengthening of the retrograde conduction time. However, here, at the time of the long ventricular cycle a concealed ('abortive') ventricular echo with concealed discharge of the junctional pacemaker occurs after concealed retrograde conduction, since there is no retrograde P wave superimposed on the T wave of the re-entrant beat. This illustrates that in man the atrium is not a necessary link in the re-entry pathway (465).

In 1973, Cranefield, Wit and Hoffman (163, their fig. 11) showed concealed re-entry in the depressed loop of a canine Purkinje fiber. Whereas, the action potentials on the left side of A indicate that the impulse did not travel around the loop (no potential is recorded from site C), those on the right side of A indicate that the impulse travelled around the loop, re-exciting site 2, but without returning to site 1, concealed re-entry.

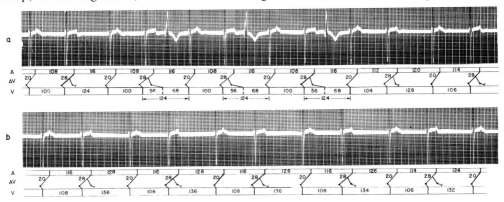

Fig. 7. A-V junctional rhythm with progressive lengthening of V-A conduction and (middle portion of top record) manifest, or (bottom record) concealed re-entry. The abortive ventricular echo is responsible for resetting the junctional pacemaker (lengthening of the ventricular cycle). Discussed in text. From A. Pick and R. Langendorf, ref. 625, figure 2. By permission.

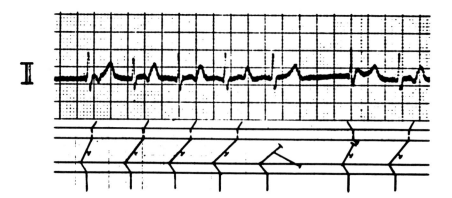

Fig. 8. A-V junctional rhythm with progressive lengthening of V-A conduction. Long ventricular cycle due to concealed discharge of junctional pacemaker after concealed retrograde conduction (abortive ventricular echo after abortive atrial echo). Discussed in text. From R. Langendorf and A. Pick, ref. 465, figure 4. By permission.

Figure 9 we owe to the Veterans Administration Hospital of Indianapolis. The short groups of sinus rhythm show at the end d. a 3:2 A-V Wenckebach period; at the beginning a., the second P wave is followed by an atrial echo following concealed antegrade conduction, and in the following group b. the same mechanism initiates a miniature circus movement.

Such reflection to the ventricles of the re-entrant atrial impulse may also occur after an abortive atrial echo, as seen in figure 10. In the first portion of the record a Wenckebach period is terminated by an atrial echo (premature retrograde P after the longest P-R), in the following portion—as indicated in the lower diagram—the retrograde re-entrant atrial impulse fails to give rise to a premature retrograde P wave; the sinus P wave appeared on time, however, the abortive atrial echo gave rise to a premature ventricular complex, a ventricular echo. This mechanism may a. imitate a supernormal phase of A-V conduction, b. initiate a reciprocating supraventricular tachycardia. Damato and his co-workers (176) have investigated in beautiful experiments and later in man (290, their fig. 3, 4) the mechan-

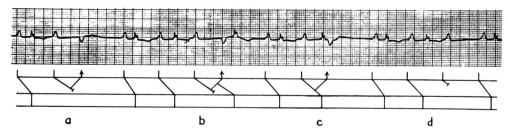

a   b   c   d

Fig. 9. Second degree A-V block, Type I; 3:2 block in (d), atrial echo after concealed antegrade conduction in (a), ventricular echo after such an atrial echo (miniature circus movement) in (b). From A. Pick and R. Langendorf: Approaches to the Diagnosis of Complex A-V Junctional Mechanisms. Mechanisms and Therapy of Cardiac Arrhythmias, edited by L. S. Dreifus and W. Likoff, Grune & Stratton, New York, figure 11, 1966. By permission.

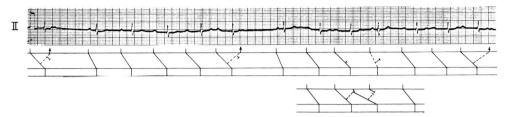

Fig. 10. Second degree A-V block, Type I, with atrial echoes after longest R-P intervals. On one occasion ventricular reciprocation followed *abortive* atrial echo (indicated in lower diagram). Discussed in text.

ism of A-V nodal Wenckebach periods by ventricular pacing and His bundle recordings of the re-entrant beat. Collision of the concealed re-entrant impulse that followed a long R-P interval with the next ventricular pacer impulse was clearly responsible for the absence of the retrograde P wave, the intermittence of the retrograde Wenckebach period. Cessation of ventricular pacing permits manifestation of the ventricular echo (with aberrant conduction), that would have prevented a retrograde P wave if a third pacer impulse had been delivered at the time of the two arrows.

How often the analogous mechanism is responsible for Wenckebach periods of ante-

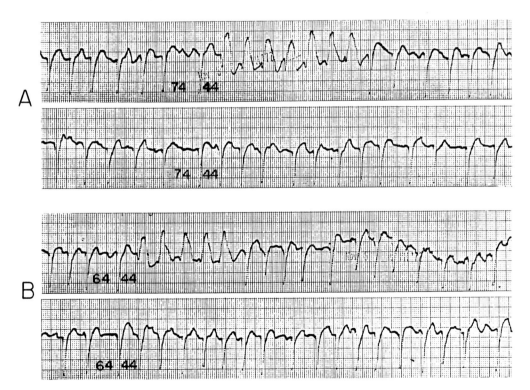

Fig. 11. Atrial fibrillation with runs of repetitive aberrant ventricular conduction in top strip of A and B, perpetuated by transseptal and retrograde conduction into vulnerable bundle branch. Failure of initiation of aberrant conduction in lower strips of A and B probably due to concealed conduction of atrial fibrillatory impulse into the vulnerable bundle branch during long cycle (74 and 64 msec) preceding the short one (44 msec). From R. Langendorf and A. Pick, ref. 467, figure 1. By permission.

grade conduction, i.e. blockage of the sinus P wave by an abortive atrial echo of the preceding beat has not been ascertained.

Table 2 summarizes the manifestations of re-entry or concealed re-entry following c.c., and in addition lists the effects of concealed conduction of the reflected re-entrant impulse. The last point (B,6) refers to a recent observation of concealed re-entry during parasystole, described by Singer et al. (762).

So far we dealt primarily with the effects of c.c. taking place in the A-V junction, mostly in the A-V node, less frequently in the bundle of His. In addition, partial penetration of impulses from above or from below into the bundle branch system can give rise to further manifestations of *intraventricular c.c.* (367,467).

Figure 11 shows in the top record of both A and B perpetuation of aberrant ventricular conduction initiated by functional bundle branch block of a beat that terminates a short cycle that follows a long cycle. The continuation of this well known type of aberration is explained by concealed transseptal conduction and retrograde penetration into the vulnerable bundle branch (318). In the lower record of both A and B with the same timing, aberrant ventricular conduction does not develop. This might be due to c.c. of an atrial fibrillatory impulse into the vulnerable bundle branch, thus shortening the measurable manifest long ventricular cycle (467,531).

Figure 12 shows in A, at the end, a similar phenomenon, absence of aberration of a beat

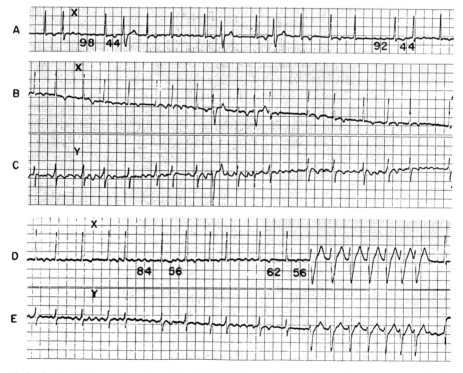

Fig. 12. In the two bottom strips, D and E, atrial fibrillation with runs of repetitive aberrant ventricular conduction starting rather late in the ventricular cycle—possibly initiated by preceding concealed antegrade conduction into the vulnerable bundle branch. Discussed in text.

with a short coupling (44 msec) that follows a long manifest ventricular cycle, and, in contrast in D and E, repetitive aberrant conduction starting rather late in the ventricular cycle. Here, the unexpected initiation of aberrant conduction could be explained by concealed penetration of an atrial fibrillatory impulse into the vulnerable bundle branch during the rather long coupling of the first aberrant beat, making the ventricular cycle appear longer than it is (531). The assumptions made to explain both the lack of aberration of an early beat and initiation of aberration by a rather late beat are still waiting for verification by the demonstration of a His bundle depolarization at the time of the postulated concealed antegrade penetration into the bundle branch system.

Guérot and co-workers (328, their fig. 5) observed during atrial pacing functional bundle branch block and initiation of a reciprocating tachycardia involving both bundle branches, which can be terminated by c.c. of ventricular stimuli.

Termination of a re-entrant ventricular tachycardia by appropriately timed ventricular stimuli can be best explained by concealed penetration of the impulse into the re-entry pathway (100, 781, 903, 904).

Wellens et al. (906, their fig. 3) gave an example of termination of a ventricular par-

Table 5. Manifestations of concealed intraventricular conduction (CIVC).

A. *Transseptal Retrograde* CIVC

  1. Perpetuation of functional BBB initiated by a premature supraventricular impulse
  2. Alternation of aberrant ventricular conduction in supraventricular bigeminy
  3. Normalization of intraventricular conduction of alternate beats in electrical alternans with bradycardia-dependent BBB
  4. Normalization of intraventricular conduction with acceleration of rate in bradycardia-dependent BBB
  5. Prevention of manifest Wenckebach periods of conduction in a BB or fascicle

B. *Antegrade* CIVC

  1. Prevention of expected aberrant ventricular conduction
  2. Exceptions of the 'rule of bigeminy'
  3. Aberrant ventricular conduction late in the ventricular cycle
  4. Initiation and termination of reciprocating ventricular tachycardia

C. *Retrograde CIVC of a Ventricular Escape in Association with Unidirectional BB or Fascicular Block*

  1. Resumption of the A-V conduction in paroxysmal A-V block with BBB
  2. Facilitation of the A-V conduction in type II A-V block due to bilateral BBB

D. *Retrograde CIVC of a Premature Ventricular Impulse*

  1. Initiation or termination of a reentrant ventricular tachycardia
  2. Resetting of an idioventricular pacemaker
  3. Pseudo-intraventricular and pseudo-A-V block
  4. Termination of aberrant ventricular conduction in paroxysmal supraventricular tachycardia

oxysmal tachycardia by concealed conduction of a critically timed atrial premature beat.

Table 5 summarizes the manifestations of concealed intraventricular conduction. I want to call attention to point B,2 exceptions to the 'rule of bigeminy'. The postulated antegrade concealed conduction during the long ventricular cycle will have to be proved by a His bundle recording.

Finally (fig. 13), we want to discuss a few examples of concealed conduction at the atrial level. In 1962, in a case of atrial parasystole observed in Miami Beach (460) we attributed shortening of the returning sinus cycle to concealed conduction of the premature atrial impulse into the region of the S-A node with prolongation of the subsequent S-A conduction time and 'pseudo-interpolation' (460) of the parasystolic beat., reminiscent of the 'postponed compensatory pause' (457). Similar observations were published by Fleischmann (274) and by Louvros et al. (506). Today we are not entirely sure of that interpretation because of the difficulty to rule out sino-atrial reciprocation.

Panlay et al. (620, their fig. 6) showed initiation (in A) and termination (in B) of a *reciprocating atrial rhythm involving the S-A node*, due to c.c. of an appropriately timed premature atrial impulse.

Klein et al. (445, their fig. 5) described the phenomenon of *concealed atrial impulse formation* proved by conduction of the concealed impulse to the sinus node and re-setting of the latter. In their record on the left, in C and D the strength of atrial stimulation varies. In C the use of threshold stimulation permits the atrial impulse to reach end reset the sinus, but fails to be propagated to the atrial recording site (no P'), whereas in D a suprathreshold stimulus results in a stimulus which reaches both the atrial and S-A nodal recording sites.

To summarize, we have shown that c.c. a. has its specific effects on subsequent impulse conduction and/or impulse formation, mainly in the A-V junction, but also in the ventricles and atria; b. in addition to inhibitory it may exert important enhancing effects; c. it may

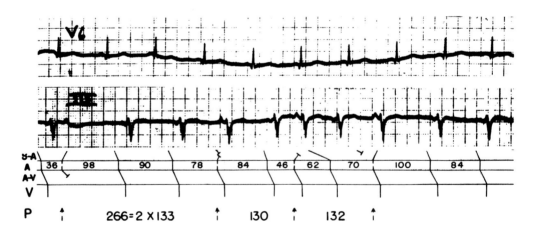

Fig. 13. Top strip shows regular sinus rhythm, lower strip reveals atrial parasystole (P) with varying duration of the returning atrial cycle. On one occasion it becomes shorter than the sinus cycle. This is attributed to *concealed A-S conduction* of the parasystolic impulse (see diagram) giving rise to the lengthening of the S-A conduction time and 'pseudointerpolation' of the parasystolic beat. Discussed in text. From R. Langendorf, M. E. Lesser, P. Plotkin and B. D. Levin, ref. 460, Figures 3 and 4. By permission.

initiate re-entry or concealed re-entry and perpetuate or terminate reciprocating tachy-cardias. Finally, we illustrated specific effects of c.c. of the reflected re-entrant impulse.

In our incomplete presentation we omitted to consider the role of c.c. in the presence of accessory pathways and we have not examined its role in conjunction with summation, inhibition, disinhibition or its relation to the conduction with the 'slow response' (Crane-field 168).

24
THE ROLE OF THE CONDUCTION SYSTEM IN SUPRAVENTRICULAR TACHYCARDIAS

PHILIPPE COUMEL, M.D., PATRICK ATTUEL, M.D., AND
DANIEL FLAMMANG, M.D.

INTRODUCTION

Unequivocal proof of the reciprocating mechanism of ectopic tachycardias is difficult to obtain if the criteria of initiation and termination by appropriate electrical stimulations are not considered as perfectly reliable. Localizing precisely the pathways of conduction which are involved by the re-entrant impulse, or at least the macroscopic size of the re-entry circuit is the best way to rule out both automatic focus and micro-re-entry. The methods used are exemplified in ten cases of supraventricular tachycardia. In two cases the circus movement is intra-atrial, and in one of them it is possible to evidence the macroscopic size of a sinus node re-entry circuit. In A-V junctional tachycardias, localizing precisely the lower junction of the circuit shows that strictly intra-nodal longitudinal dissociation is rarer than usually admitted. Either longitudinal dissociation of the His bundle itself, or the presence of latent accessory pathways (James fibers, Kent bundle and Mahaim fibers) might be more frequent than realized. An exceptional case is reported, where the A-V nodal-His axis does not participate in the re-entry circuit, but two Kent bundles exist, one of them being latent.

Since the experimental work of Mendez and Moe (544), many experimental (409) and clinical studies have been devoted to re-entry phenomena. Various criteria have been proposed to differentiate them from the activity of automatic foci. These criteria are based on the modes of initiation and termination of tachycardias by programmed stimulations. Their value has been challenged by some electrophysiologists, and recent experiments (165) have pointed out the possibility of meeting these criteria in actual automatic foci. In fact, the problem is that initiating and terminating a tachycardia by appropriately-timed stimulations might not suffice in some cases to differentiate an automatic focus from a *micro*-re-entry. (13) In other words, for the physician, the best way to prove the actual existence of a re-entry is not only to fulfill the preceding criteria, but also to evaluate as precisely as possible both location and size of the circuit. Once its macroscopic size has been proven, the re-entry is challenged no more. But the difficulty may vary with the location of the phenomenon. For example it is rather easy to evaluate precisely the pathways of conduction involved by the reciprocating impulse in a Wolff-Parkinson-White syndrome (W.P.W.) (154). It becomes more difficult when the re-entry is located within the nodal-His axis, though in such cases studying the re-entry phenomenon from both atrium, ventricle and even His bundle provides useful arguments. It may be very difficult or almost impossible when the circuit is confined within the atrium or the ventricle.

We shall try to point out the various possible locations of circus movements in the different forms of supraventricular tachycardias (S.V.T.), i.e. atrial tachycardias and overall tachycardias arising from the atrio-ventricular (A-V) junction, including the W.P.W. syndrome. We should underline that most of the 10 cases taken as demonstrative examples would necessitate many figures and extensive discussions: we shall try to give the most important positive arguments supporting the proposed hypothesis. We know that in some cases they may not be considered as perfectly convincing or unquestionable. They often make the hypothesis just highly probable. On the other hand, it should be noted that this is the case among some other publications. In this field it is rather rare to gather arguments which can be considered as pathognomonic.

Another preliminary remark is necessary concerning the conditions required for the creation of a circus movement (152). These conditions are: 1. a potential circuit pathway, 2. a unidirectional block in this circuit and 3. a slowed conduction, as the time needed for the impulse to traverse the whole circuit must exceed the duration of the refractory period of the involved pathways. Condition 2 can be obvious, for example by the disappearance of a delta wave at the beginning of the tachycardia in a W.P.W. syndrome, but it can well be latent and its apparent absence cannot be taken as an argument against re-entry. Along the same vein, we have shown (146, 152) that condition 3 can be latent, and the absence of prolongation of the conduction times at the beginning of a tachycardia is perfectly compatible with the diagnosis of re-entry: it means only that the conduction speed in the circuit is already slow enough to permit re-entry. In conclusion, proving that condition 1 is present, i.e. providing evidence concerning the *macroscopic* size of the circuit pathway, is in our opinion, the best way to prove the re-entry phenomenon. Our goal is to discuss this point in the following examples.

The following topics will be discussed.

I. Intra-atrial re-entry.
    1. Sinus node re-entry (case 1, fig. 1–4)
    2. Intra-atrial, but not sinus node re-entry (case 2, fig. 5–6)
II. Junctional re-entry.
    1. Junctional re-entry *without* overt or latent pre-excitation.
        a. Re-entry involving only a part of the A-V node (case 3, fig. 8–9)
        b. Re-entry involving both A-V node and His bundle (case 4, fig. 10–11)
    2. Junctional re-entry with overt or latent accessory pathways.
        a. Re-entry involving James fibers (case 5, fig. 12)
        b. Re-entry involving Kent bundle:
            — latent accessory pathway proved by ventricular stimulation (case 6, fig. 13)
            — latent accessory pathway proved by BBB-dependent rate of tachycardia (case 7, fig. 14)
            — re-entry involving *two* Kent bundles, one of them being latent (case 8, fig. 15–18)
        c. Re-entry involving Mahaim fibers:
            — with overt pre-excitation (case 9, fig. 19–20).
            — with latent pre-excitation (case 10, fig. 21–22).

I – INTRA-ATRIAL RE-ENTRY

Experimental (334,621) and clinical (10) studies have shown the reality of sinus node re-entry, and more generally-speaking of intra-atrial re-entry. Two kinds of criteria are given by the authors: 1. initiation and termination of a more or less sustained S.V.T. by programmed pacing without any relationship with the mode of A-V conduction; and 2. an atrial mode of depolarization originating from the sinus node area or at least not from the A-V junction. The two following examples will show the value but also the limits of this concept.

1. Sino-atrial re-entry (case 1)

Basic tracings are presented in figure 1. In strip A[a] 2/1 sino-atrial block is intermittent. In strip B episodes of atrial bradycardia alternate with attacks of atrial tachycardia: the P waves have about the same morphology as during sinus rhythm. The initiation of the episodes of tachycardia is not related to the A-V conduction, as they can occur (strip C) when an A-V dissociation is present.

Tracings of figures 2 through 4 were recorded a few days later. The atrial tachycardia is then permanent, and a complete right bundle branch block (B.B.B.) is present. Figure 2 shows that the tachycardia can be stopped if the atrial stimulation is early enough. A His bundle escape beat then occurs. As there is no retrograde atrial activation, it is followed by an atrial escape beat. Its pattern differs clearly from that of a sino-atrial P wave, suggesting a low atrial origin and this fact probably explains why the tachycardia does not recur. Along the same vein, atrial driving in this patient prevented the recurrence of the

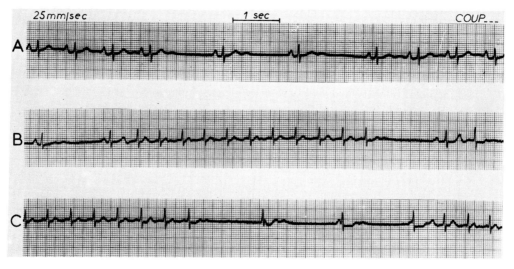

Fig. 1. (case 1) Sinus node re-entry. Basic tracings. A. Intermittent 2/1 sino-atrial block. B. Spontaneous onset and termination of the atrial tachycardia. C. Spontaneous termination of the tachycardia, followed by an A-V dissociation, which does not prevent the tachycardia to start again. Tracings A to C are not continuous. They are recorded in lead II.

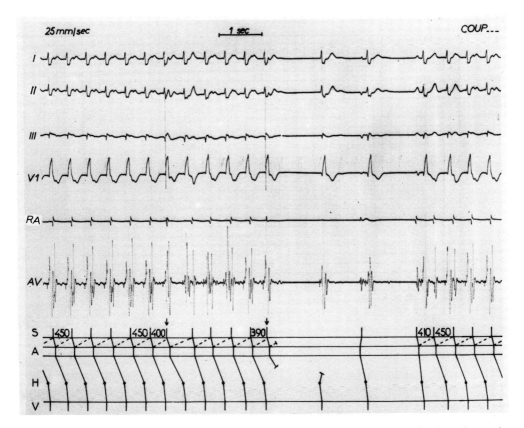

Fig. 2. (case 1) Sinus node re-entry. Atrial stimulation. A single premature atrial stimulation (arrow) stops the tachycardia if it is appropriately timed. The recurrence of the tachycardia is possible neither after a His bundle escape beat nor an atrial escape beat, but only after the first sino-atrial P wave. R.A. = right atrial electrogram, A-V = His bundle electrogram. In the diagram, S is supposed to be the sinus node area, A is the low right atrium, H the His bundle and V the ventricle. (See the text for discussion.)

S.V.T. as long as it continued. Sino-atrial P waves only could start again the tachycardia, as in the right part of figure 2.

The intra-atrial mapping (fig. 3) demonstrates clearly that the P waves of the S.V.T. (upper strip) originate from the high right atrium. Furthermore, the lower tracing shows the perfect similarity of the atrial depolarization for the first (sinus P wave) and the second P wave of the tachycardia.

The preceding facts meet the criteria for a sinus node re-entry. Such phenomenon is supposed to be a microscopic re-entry, or at least a re-entry strictly limited to the sinus node area. As the size of the re-entrant circuit is not known, strictly speaking one can keep wondering as to whether a true re-entry or an automatic focus is in cause. However, figure 4 does prove the re-entry mechanism, as it demonstrates that the circuit is indeed macroscopic.

In the upper and lower tracings of figure 4, a stimulation is given in two different points of the right atrium. In the upper strip, the sinus node area is stimulated 390 msec after the preceding P wave. The atrial depolarization of the electrically-induced beat is

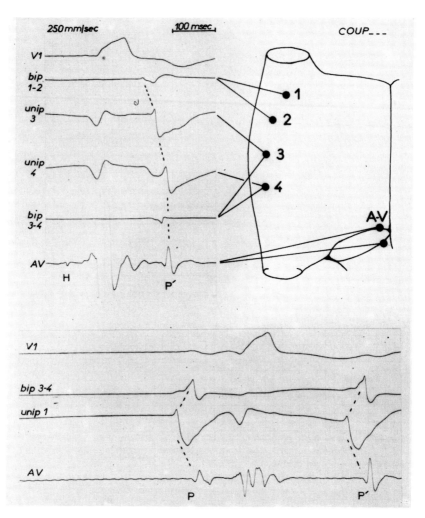

Fig. 3. (case 1) Sinus node re-entry. Intra-atrial mapping. *Upper panel*: a P wave of the tachycardia is recorded in various areas of the right atrium (1 to 4) in either unipolar (unip) or bipolar (bip) leads. The atrial activation spreads in a cranio-caudal direction. *Lower panel*: the comparison between the first P wave (of sino-atrial origin) and the second of the tachycardia shows that the spread of activation is quite identical. (See the text for discussion.)

the same as during the tachycardia, the course of which is influenced: a more than compensatory pause (600 msec) is followed by cycles alternatively shorter (440 msec) and longer (480 msec) than the basic one of 460 msec. In the lower strip, the stimulus is given far from the sinus node area, in the lateral wall of the right atrium (point labelled '3–4'). The timing of the induced beat in this area is the same (390 msec) as in the upper strip. However, this time the tachycardia is interrupted. Moreover, the induced beat has *not* captured the sinus node area (labelled '1–2') where the cycle remains 460 msec. This phenomenon proves undoubtly that the reciprocating impulse has been blocked somewhere in the circuit far away from the sinus node area: thus the circus movement is ensured by the fact that the circuit is macroscopic.

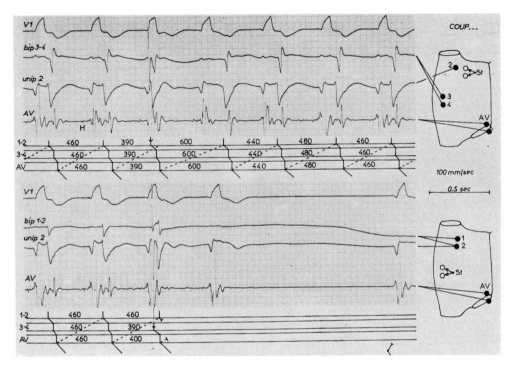

Fig. 4. (case 1) Sinus node re-entry. Atrial stimulation in various areas. *Upper panel*: the stimulation of the high right atrium influences the course of the tachycardia. *Lower panel*: the stimulation given in points labelled '3–4' with the same timing as in the upper panel does not depolarize the sinus node area but it stops the tachycardia, thus proving the macroscopic size of the re-entry circuit. (See the text for details and discussion.)

2. Intra-atrial but not sinus node re-entry (case 2)

Figure 5 shows an S.V.T. with a type I second-degree A-V block not influencing the course of the tachycardia. Nevertheless, a re-entry phenomenon is highly suggested by the possibility of modifying (upper strip) or interrupting readily (lower strip) the tachycardia thanks to an appropriately-timed paired atrial stimulation. The initiation of the tachycardia is made possible by either a stimulus test or a progressively accelerated atrial driving, and figure 6 shows that the re-entry is situated far away from the sinus node area. The stimulation is given in the high right atrium. The intra-atrial conduction is impaired, as shown by the P wave lasting about 300 msec, and the stimulus—'A' (low right atrium) of about 200 msec. The atrial activation of the echo beat (the last P wave in the tracing) is far different from that of either stimulated or spontaneous P waves. This indicates that the echo beat cannot originate from the high right atrium. On the other hand, the low right atrial depolarization preceeds the high right atrial one by about 20 msec. Thus the echo beat cannot be supposed either to arise from the A-V junction but from somewhere else, probably in the left atrium as this patient had twice undergone mitral commissurotomy. However, an intra-atrial mapping which included stimulation in various areas, particularly the left atrium, could not be carried out in the present case. It would have been of great interest, as in case 1. In its absence the diagnosis between macro and micro-re-entry (13) is still uncertain.

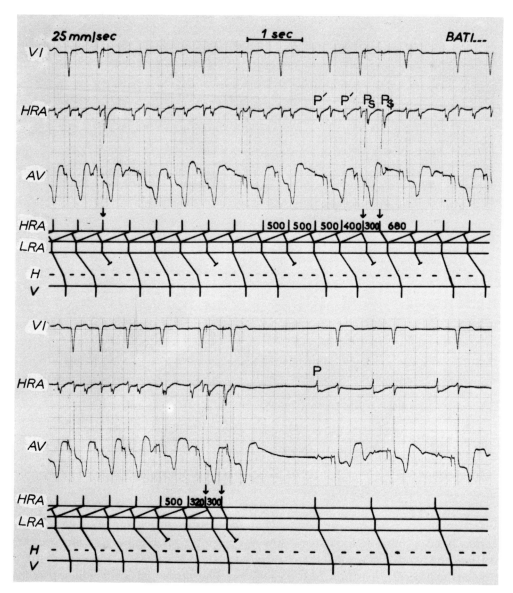

Fig. 5. (case 2) Intra-atrial re-entry. Termination of the tachycardia. *Upper panel:* a paired atrial stimulation (Ps waves) influences the course of the tachycardia, but it does not stop it. *Lower panel:* the atrial tachycardia is stopped if the timing of the first stimulation is reduced from 400 to 320 msec. HRA = high right atrium. LRA = low right atrial electrogram recorded in the A-V lead ('A' waves).

II JUNCTIONAL RE-ENTRY

In most publications, two types of reciprocating S.V.T. are usually distinguished depending on whether a ventricular pre-excitation pattern is present or not during sinus rhythm. The re-entry circuit is supposed to be intra-nodal whenever there is no evidence of pre-excita-

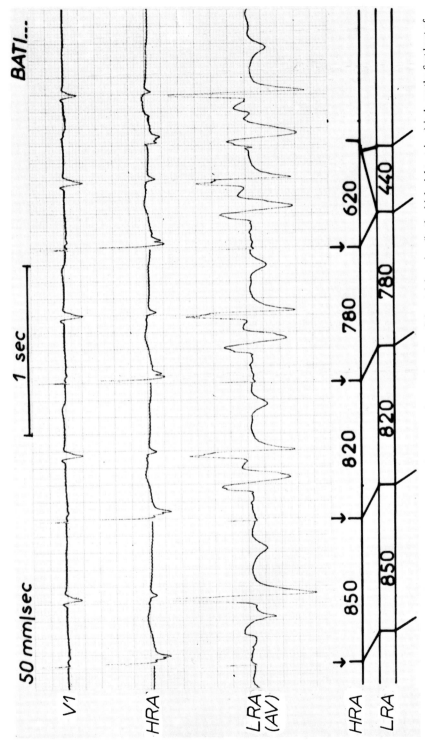

Fig. 6. (case 2) Intra-atrial re-entry. Atrial echo beat. The progressive acceleration of the atrial pacing (in the high right atrium) induces the first beat of the tachycardia (the last P wave on the tracing). The timing of the intrinsic deflection in both HRA and LRA is about the same, indicating that this 'atrial echo beat' arises from neither HRA nor LRA but from somewhere else. (See the text for discussion.)

tion. Reversely, the re-entrant impulse is thought to involve the accessory pathway every time its presence is known. In fact, the problem is in knowing precisely that no accessory pathway is operating during the tachycardia even in cases where there is no visible pre-excitation during sinus rhythm (150,159,598). Using the methods exposed below, it is very frequent in those cases to uncover unsuspected accessory pathways. In contrast, one should be sure that a known by-pass is actually involved by the re-entrant impulse, though we have no example of an intra-nodal reciprocating tachycardia coexisting with a ventricular pre-excitation known with certainty not to be responsible for the re-entry. Experimental data (187) as well as human studies (593,911) give more and more support to these possibilities. In a recent series of 65 consecutive cases of A-V junctional reciprocating tachycardia (155) we observed, aside from 30 cases of W.P.W. syndrome, 13 cases of latent pre-excitation with an unidirectional anterograde block in the accessory pathway (fig. 7).

Thus we shall distinguish cases without an either overt or latent pre-exciting pathway from those in which its presence is undoubted.

1. Junctional re-entry without latent for or overt pre-excitation

This label means only that the presence of an accessory pathway has not been evidenced, whatever the method used. In other words, it is probable that in some of our cases a latent accessory pathway might be present, but that the study has not been precise enough. Anyway, even if we considered our methods as perfectly reliable, such label would not mean that the re-entry circuit is thought to be actually intra-nodal. As a matter of fact, even in these cases, a precise evaluation of the level of the lower junction with respect to the point of recording of the His bundle activity and the bifurcation, leads to the conclusion that the re-entry circuit is not limited to the A-V node. In the preceding series (155) the lower junction was situated within the His bundle in 12 cases, and at the point of recording of the H wave in 5 cases (fig. 7). In 5 cases only (out of 65) the re-entry was thought to be strictly

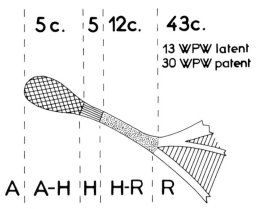

Fig. 7. A-V junctional reciprocating tachycardias. The level of the lower junction of the re-entry circuit in 65 consecutive cases. In 43 cases out of 65, the lower junction of the circuit was found below the His bundle bifurcation, i.e. within the ventricle: in 30 cases the W.P.W. syndrome was present during sinus rhythm, but in 13 cases it was latent. In the 22 remaining cases, the lower junction was located 12 times within the His bundle, 5 times at the level of the H wave. In 5 cases only, the circus movement was found to be probably intra-nodal. (See the text for discussion.)

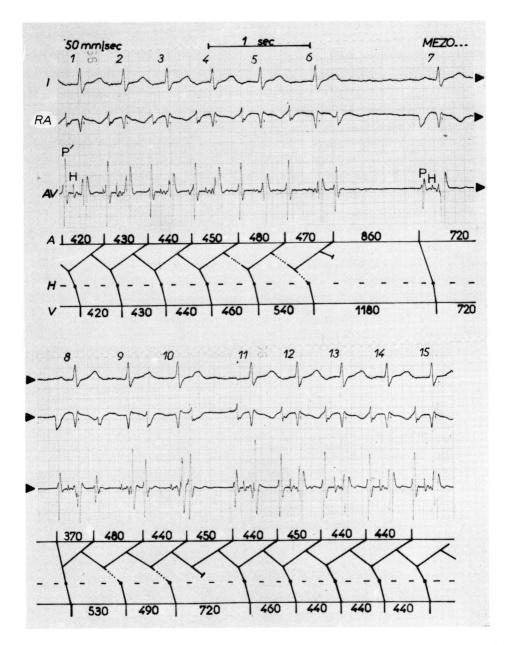

Fig. 8. (case 3) Re-entry involving the upper part of the A-V node. The two tracings are continuous. In the upper one, a Wenckebach phenomenon explains clearly the spontaneous termination of the tachycardia, indicating that the circus movement is located within the A-V node. The tachycardia starts again in the lower tracing and this time, a Wenckebach phenomenon (from beat 9 to beat 11) does not influence the course of the tachycardia, indicating that the lower part of the A-V node is probably not involved by the re-entry circuit. (See the text for discussion.)

intra-nodal, or at least the proof could not be yielded that it was not. In short, we consider that the diagnosis of functional longitudinal dissociation of the A-V node, as described experimentally (409, 544) should be made in humans only after having eliminated a wider re-entry circuit. We shall give two examples in which the A-V node is most probably concerned by the dissociation.

a. Re-entry involving only the upper part of A-V node (case 3)
In figure 8 the S.V.T. resembles that of cases 1 and 2: the onset of the tachycardia is not related to a prolongation of P-R (beat 8), and the occurrence of a type I second-degree A-V block (beats 9 to 11) apparently does not influence its course. In addition, stopping the tachycardia is easy by a premature atrial stimulation, but impossible by a ventricular one. All these phenomena suggest an intra-atrial re-entry, while in fact the upper part of the A-V node is certainly involved. As a matter of fact, in the upper tracing the spontaneous termination of the episodes is announced by a Wenckebach phenomenon starting at beat 2 and becoming evident at beat 5: the prolongation of P'5–R5 makes longer the P'5–P'6 interval, and the prolongation of R5–R6 explains the blocked P' following R6 which ends the tachycardia. The absence of prolongation of P-R in beat 8 which preceeds the next episode is not inconsistent with the diagnosis of A-V nodal reciprocating tachycardia (309) as it is well-known in the 'permanent' form of such tachycardia (146, 151, 152). Finally, the endocavitary atrial mapping (fig. 9) confirms that the activation of P' waves originates from the A-V junction and differs clearly from that of sino-atrial P waves.

   In short, in this case, the Wenckebach phenomenon in the upper tracing proves the A-V nodal location of the re-entry, while in the lower tracing another Wenckebach phenomenon strongly supports the hypothesis that the lower part of the A-V node is *not* involved by the re-entry.

b. Re-entry involving not only the A-V nodal but also the distal conducting system: a longitudinal dissociation of the His bundle? (case 4)
Even though the A-V nodal location of the re-entry circuit is highly suggested by the characters of the tachycardia, this does not mean that the longitudinal dissociation of the conducting system is confined in the A-V node. Figure 10 (as fig. 8 in case 3) proves that both anterograde and retrograde pathways of the circuit involve the A-V node: the spontaneous termination of the S.V.T. is preceeded by a Wenckebach phenomenon concerning both A-V (P'-H progressively increasing from 85 to 110 msec) and V-A conduction (R-P' progressively increasing from 315 to 350 msec). Though the strict intra-nodal location of the circus movement is highly suggested by these facts, as in case 3, figure 11 permits more precise localization of the lower junction of the circuit.

   A ventricular stimulation is given during the tachycardia at the very upper part of the ventricular septum, in a point (strip A) normally depolarized 20 msec after the onset of R. A stimulation in this area is delivered 370 msec after the preceding R wave (strip B) and the induced impulse is assumed to reach the bifurcation of the His bundle 20 msec after the spike, i.e. 390 msec after the preceding R. Thus the induced impulse is premature by 60 msec ($450 - 390 = 60$ msec) if we consider only what happens at the very upper part of the ventricular septum, viz. at the His bundle bifurcation. This impulse

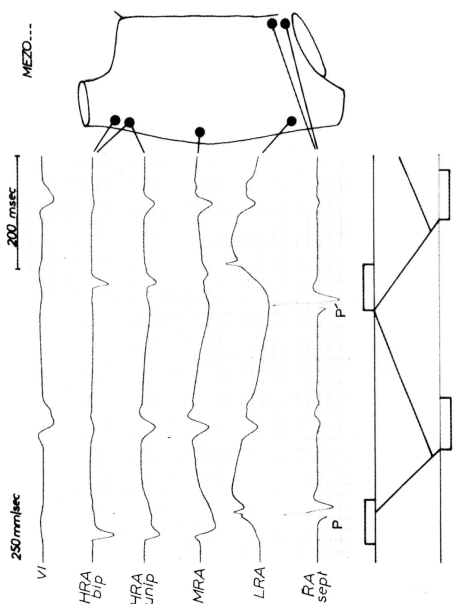

Fig. 9. (case 3) Intra-atrial mapping in A-V nodal tachycardia. The first P wave is of sino-atrial origin: the impulse spreads in a cranio-caudal direction. The second P wave (P') is the first atrial echo beat, and the atrial activation originates clearly from the A-V junction (MRA = mean right atrium. RA sept = low septal right atrium.) (See text for discussion, and compare with fig. 3.)

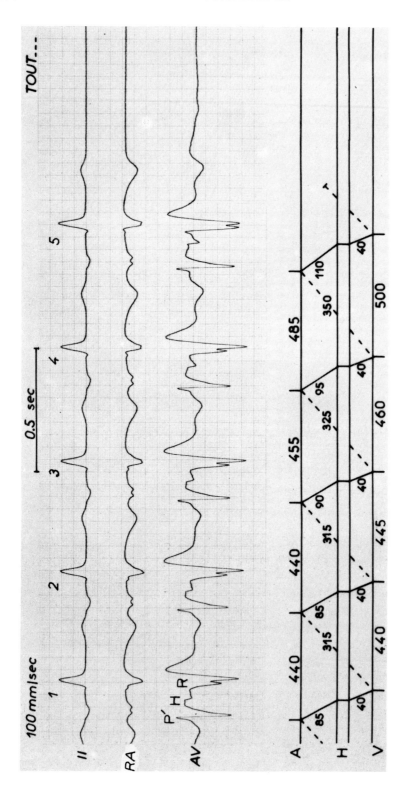

Fig. 10. (case 4) A-V nodal-His bundle longitudinal dissociation. Spontaneous termination of the tachycardia. A Wenckebach phenomenon occurs in both anterograde and retrograde pathways, as shown by the progressive prolongation of P'-H and R-P' intervals. The retrograde V-A block is directly responsible for the end of the tachycardia. These facts highly suggest that both anterograde and retrograde impulses of the tachycardia traverse the A-V node.

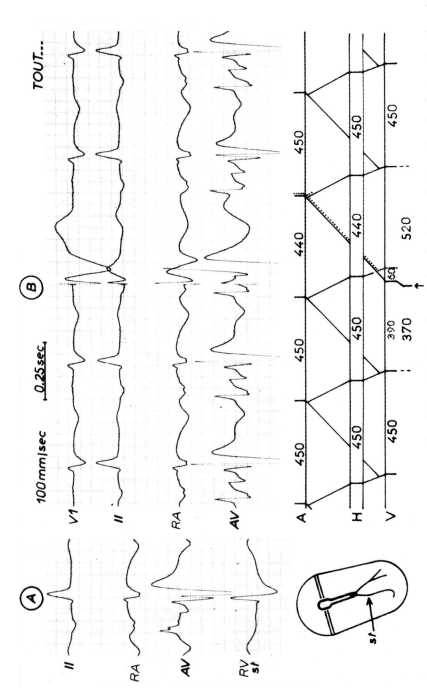

Fig. 11. (case 4) A-V nodal-His bundle longitudinal dissociation. The effect of ventricular stimulation, allowing to localize the lower junction of the circuit. *Left panel:* the intrinsic deflection is recorded in the pacing electrode (bipolar) located at the upper part of the inter-ventricular septum. It occurs 20 msec after the onset of QRS in lead labelled RVst. *Right panel:* the stimulated impulse given in the preceding point is supposed to reach the His bundle bifurcation 20 msec later, then premature by 60 msec (dotted numbers) with respect to the next expected R wave. As it captures the following P' wave, the induced ventricular impulse cannot be supposed to have reached the atrium by involving the entire His bundle in the retrograde direction. This assumption is made sure by recording the anterograde His bundle potential in the A-V lead. (See the text for discussion.)

does capture the atrium, which appears premature by 10 msec: it is impossible to conclude that the stimulated impulse has reached the supposed intra-nodal re-entry circuit by traversing the His bundle in the retrograde direction. In addition, the direct proof of such an assumption is given by the His bundle electrogram ('A-V' lead) showing clearly a normally-timed anterograde H wave.

The longitudinal dissociation of the His bundle, suggested by experimental studies (46) is proved in this case, unless one invokes the possibility of Mahaim fibers (see below) operating only retrogradely: this is a matter of semantics.

2. *Junctional re-entry* with *overt or latent accessory pathways*

Classically, three types of accessory pathways are described as the entire normal A-V nodal-His axis, or its upper part, or its lower part only are by-passed. As the 'Kent bundle', the 'James fibers' or the 'Mahaim fibers' are alone or associated, as they are right or left-sided or even septal, one can imagine an infinity of possible re-entry circuit (225), and they do probably exist.

The most frequent situation is that of an overt pre-excitation with a direct A-V by-pass (bundle of Kent) forming the retrograde pathway for the reciprocating impulse. As this situation has been extensively studied in many publications (225, 227, 325, 589), we shall give no example of it. We shall study some particular problems arising in this kind of pre-excitation. On the other hand, reciprocating tachycardias involving Mahaim fibers seem to be much rarer. As far as James fibers are concerned, their role in participating to re-entrant circuits may be considered as frequent as well as very rare. It depends upon the criteria admitted for their diagnosis.

a. *Re-entry circuit involving James fibers (case 5)*

Theoretically, the following conditions enable an atrio-His by-pass to be considered as participating in a re-entry circuit. 1. Either the anterograde or the retrograde conduction time during the tachycardia should be less or equal to 120 msec. 2. Anterograde or retrograde conduction should respect the all-or-none law. 3. The lower junction of the circuit should be localized distal to the His bundle, but on the other hand its ventricular situation (i.e. W.P.W. syndrome) should be accurately ruled out, for instance by the presence of a second-degree A-V block, even though transient, an occurrence rather rare (150, 151). 4. The upper junction of the circuit should be localized within the atrium, and this absence of an initial common pathway is very difficult to be proved. Conceivably, all these conditions are hardly met, though the role of A-V nodal by-passes is probably more frequent than realized. Figure 12 shows by which methods one can approach the localization of the upper and lower junctions of the circuit, by determining as precisely as possible the distance between the atrial and ventricular areas of stimulation and the circuit itself.

In the left panel (fig. 12) the various points which will be taken into account in the discussion are recorded. 1. The very beginning of the retrograde P' waves during the tachycardia, and 2. The intrinsic deflection recorded by a bipolar catheter located at the lower atrial septum: the interval between these two points is 20 msec, and the atrial stimulation will be delivered in the high inter-atrial septum. 3. The H wave and 4. The very beginning of

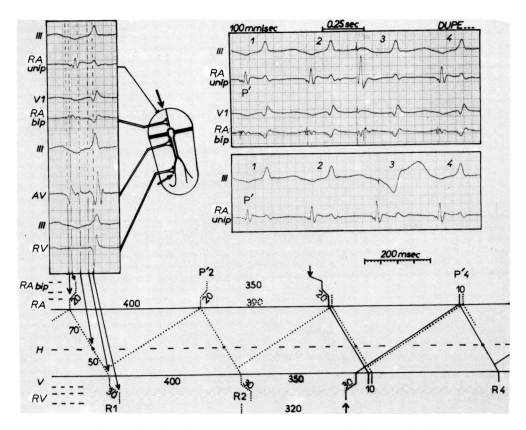

Fig. 12. (case 5) Re-entry circuit involving James fibers in the anterograde direction. The left panel where are recorded the different leads necessary for the discussion, as indicated in the diagram. Arrows in the diagram indicate where the stimulations will be given in the right panel: in the high right atrial septum (above the bipolar electrogram labelled RAbip) and in the bipolar ventricular electrode labelled RV. The effects of the atrial and ventricular stimulations are shown in the right upper and lower panels respectively, and represented in the lower diagram where P' and R waves of both panels are numbered 1 to 4. Both stimulations capture the alternate chamber which is premature by 10 msec in both cases, so that both impulses can be superimposed in the diagram (solid lines) with respect to the expected impulses. Assuming that both anterograde and retrograde conduction speeds remain constant in either pathways, one can conclude that there is no initial common pathway between the atrium and the re-entry circuit, and that the lower junction is situated in the lower part of the His bundle. This highly suggest the presence of James fibers operating antegradely, with an A-V conduction time of 120 msec. (See the text for discussion and further details.)

R: the H-R interval in this case is 50 msec. 5. The intrinsic deflection (RVst) recorded on the bipolar pacing electrode located at the upper part of the ventricular septum: this R-RVst interval is 30 msec. In the right upper and lower panels, two strips of four beats of the S.V.T. are compared, in which an either atrial (upper panel) or ventricular (lower panel) stimulation is delivered. Either stimulus captures the alternate chamber then premature by 10 msec with respect to the next expected R or P' wave. The results are drawn in the diagram, and comparing them allows the determination of the respective levels of the upper and lower junctions of the circuit. The diagram suggests that there is no initial common pathway in this case. Thus the short P'-R interval of 120 msec should be considered as the actual A-V conduction time, and not only an apparent one as is seen in intra-nodal reciprocating tachycardias. On the other hand, the lower junction is found distal to the H wave, a situation suggesting the existence of an atrio-His accessory pathway.

However, it should be emphasized that these conclusions rely on the following assumptions. 1. The anterograde conduction time of the induced atrial impulse between points 2 and 1 is presumed to be equal to the basic retrograde time between 1 and 2, i.e. 20 msec. 2. In a similar fashion, the retrograde conduction time of the induced ventricular impulse between points 5 and 4 is presumed to be the same as the basic anterograde conduction time, i.e. 30 msec. 3. Finally, the conduction speed of the capturing impulses within the anterograde and the retrograde pathways of the circuit is not presumed to be slowed though they are premature: that is why the stimulations should be as late as possible in the cardiac cycle. Anyway, it should be underlined that the eventual slowering of either impulse in either pathway would make either stimulation point 'closer' to the circuit depicted in the diagram, so that the hypothesis of an extra-nodal by-pass in this case would be reinforced.

b. Re-entry circuit involving a latent bundle of Kent

1. Latent accessory pathway as proved by ventricular stimulation (case 6)

The preceding method may lead to the conclusion that a pre-exciting pathway is indeed present, whether or not a delta wave is seen during sinus rhythm. This is the case in figure 13, where two similarly-timed ventricular stimulations are delivered in two different areas of the right ventricle. In the upper tracing, the pacing catheter is positioned at the upper part of the septum: the stimulus premature by 70 msec ($340 - 270 = 70$) is followed by an atrial capture premature by only 50 msec ($340 - 290 = 50$). This difference of 20 msec ($70 - 50 = 20$) indicates that the stimulus has been given in an area situated 20 msec 'distant' from the re-entry circuit. If the lower junction were presumed to be proximal to the point of stimulation, i.e. within the His bundle, putting the pacing catheter at the right ventricular apex should increase the preceding difference. On the contrary, this manoeuvre makes the prematurity of the captured P' equal to that of the stimulation (lower tracing): this kind of result ('exact' atrial capture) does prove (151, 154, 155) that the stimulation has been delivered within the re-entry circuit itself, which involves the ventricle and hence is related to an accessory pathway. The pathway was completely latent in the present case.

2. B.B.B.–dependent rate of reciprocating tachycardia (case 7)

This phenomenon is not a rarity, as we have observed it 17 times out of a total of about 120 cases of reciprocating tachycardia studied. It can be considered as pathognomonic (150, 598, 782) of a ventricular preexcitation, localizing the accessory pathway on the side of the 'slowed' B.B.B. It is rather easy to recognize, on the condition that account is taken not only of the changing rate of the tachycardia, but also the changing R-P' interval: in some cases the B.B.B.–dependent rate of the tachycardia may be cancelled by a more or less 'compensatory' prolongation of the P'-R interval (150).

A particular pattern of this phenomenon is seen in figure 14, in a case of latent left-sided

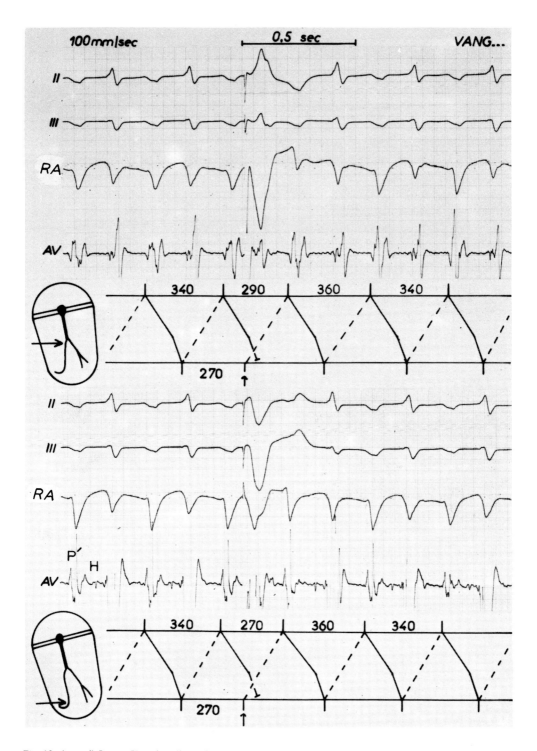

Fig. 13. (case 6) Latent Kent bundle as the retrograde pathway in a reciprocating tachycardia. The ventricular stimulation has the same timing in both tracings, and is followed by a captured P'. Paradoxically, the atrial capture is earlier when the stimulation is given farther in the ventricle, i.e. at the apex (lower strip) instead of the septum. The presence of an accessory pathway taking off from the ventricle is the only possible explanation. (See the text for discussion.)

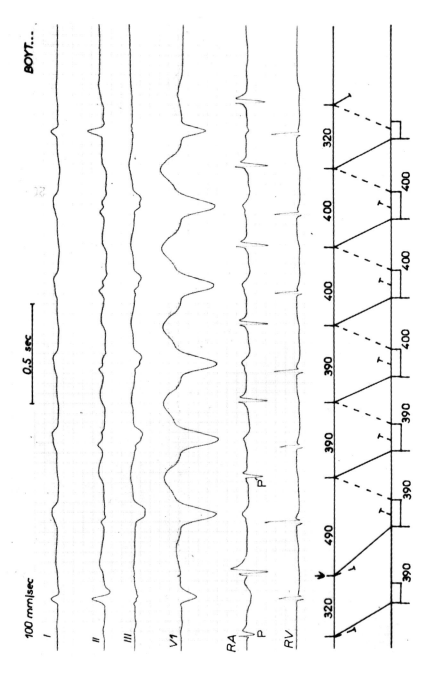

Fig. 14. (case 7) Left B.B.B.-dependent retrograde conduction time, evidencing a latent left-sided Kent bundle. The first beat of the tracing is of sino-atrial origin, and there is no pre-excitation pattern. A premature atrial stimulation initiates the reciprocating tachycardia, with a left B.B.B. pattern. After 5 beats, the disappearance of the functional left B.B.B. makes the atrial cycle shorter than the preceding one by 80 msec. This proves that the intraventricular conduction time of the reciprocating impulse has been shortened, and that an accessory pathway taking off from the left ventricle constitutes the retrograde pathway of the circuit. Otherwise, the blocked premature P' terminates the tachycardia.

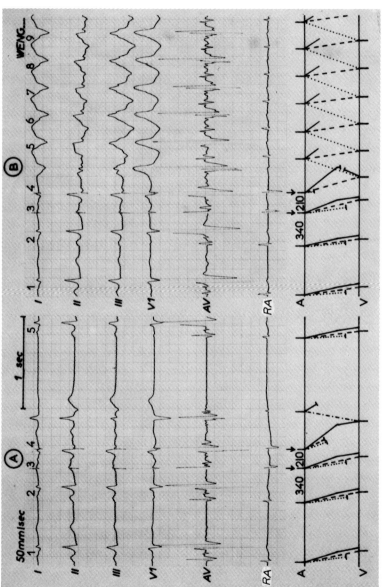

Fig. 15. (case 8) Re-entry involving two Kent bundles, one of them being latent. In both tracings a left ventricular pre-excitation is present during sinus rhythm (beats 1 and 2). The W.P.W. deformity is increased by the first atrial stimulation (beat 3). The effect of the second atrial stimulation (beat 4) differs in either tracings. In panel A the W.P.W. deformity is followed by a long P-R and a normalized QRS with an isolated atrial echo beat: the retrograde conduction has occurred by either right or left accessory pathway (see below). In panel B, though the timing of stimulation 4 is the same as in panel A, the left Kent bundle is not refractory: the reciprocating tachycardia starts, with a maximal W.P.W. deformity. Though the H wave of beat 4 is not visible in the tracing, in the diagram its timing is assumed to be the same as in panel A. If such an assumption is correct, the retrograde impulse cannot involve the His bundle with must be refractory. The presence of a latent accessory pathway has to be assumed in the diagram. Solid lines represent the A-V nodal-His conducting system, dashed lines represent the left Kent bundle, and dotted lines represent the supposed latent accessory path. (See the text and figures 16 to 18 for further details and discussion.)

ventricular pre-excitation. A reciprocating tachycardia is initiated by a premature atrial stimulation. The first five beats of the tachycardia are enlarged by a left B.B.B., and the cardiac cycle is 400 msec. The functional left B.B.B. disappears for the sixth beat, and the atrial cycle is lessened by 80 msec, according to the shortening of the intraventricular part of the re-entry circuit. As a consequence, the last P′ is blocked, and the tachycardia stopped in this patient every time the R wave is narrowed. This value of 80 msec is the biggest we have ever observed in studying this phenomenon. The shortening of the retrograde conduction time ranges from 20 to 80 msec, with a mean value of about 40 msec.

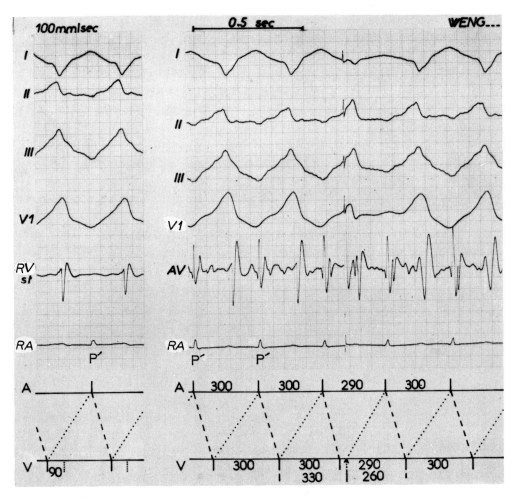

Fig. 16. (case 8) Re-entry involving two Kent bundles. Paradoxically-premature atrial capture. *Left Panel:* the intrinsic deflection is recorded at the right ventricular apex in the bipolar pacing electrode during the tachycardia. It occurs about 90 msec after the onset of QRS. *Right panel:* a stimulation is given in this point 30 msec *after* the onset of QRS, and does capture the following P′ wave, indicating that the re-entry circuit involves the ventricle itself. (See the text for discussion.)

3. Overt left-sided and latent right-sided Kent bundles: reciprocating tachycardia
involving two accessory pathways (case 8)

The circuit of a re-entrant tachycardia should be precisely studied before it is formally accepted. In the tracings of figure 15, a left ventricular pre-excitation is clearly visible. In this patient, a premature atrial stimulation can produce either a normalized R wave followed by a single atrial echo beat (fig. 15A) or a sustained reciprocating S.V.T. involving anterogradely the left Kent bundle with a maximal W.P.W. deformity. In such published cases, the retrograde pathway is always supposed to be the normal nodal-His axis, a fact proved only in some cases (227) by demonstrating the position of the retrograde H′ wave just after R. In most cases, as in the present one, the retrograde H′ is hardly recorded and difficult to authenticate as it is buried within the wide R wave.

However, figure 16 proves that the re-entry circuit involves the ventricle itself. The pacing catheter is placed at the right ventricular apex and, during the tachycardia, the intrinsic deflection in this point occurs 90 msec after the onset of R (left panel). Stimulating this point produces a 'paradoxically-premature' atrial capture (154, 155). As a matter of fact, the stimulation is delivered 30 msec *after* the onset of QRS, when the anterograde impulse has already invaded the left ventricle. Nevertheless, an atrial capture does occur, as the P′ following the stimulation is premature by 10 msec. This kind of phenomenon is not unusual in the W.P.W. syndrome, and it proves that the pacing catheter is located within the re-entry circuit.

Moreover, in figures 17 and 18, the effects of His bundle stimulation lead to the conclusion that the A-V nodal-His axis is *not* the retrograde pathway in this case. In figure 17A the His bundle deflection is recorded at the end of an atrial tachycardia with block and normalized QRS. A short time later, while the catheter has been left in the same position, it does not permit identification of the required retrograde H′ wave during an episode of reciprocating tachycardia. There is no H wave *after* QRS, and a His bundle deflection might be present before, labelled 'H?'. A stimulation is delivered thrice in this electrode-catheter in panel C, and captures the R wave: stimulations 1 and 3 are followed by a normalized QRS, while after stimulation 2 QRS is enlarged by a functional right B.B.B. In figure 18, the effects of stimulations 1 and 2 are studied at a faster paper speed. The fact that the His bundle can be activated at this time of the cardiac cycle proves that an eventual retrograde activation has not occured *after* QRS, as one should suppose a very short refractory period. The most important conclusion concerns the atrial captures. Stimulation 1 is followed by a P′ wave premature by 10 msec, while after stimulation 2 the P′ wave is *delayed* by 15 msec with respect to the basic cycle length. The difference of 25 msec between these atrial captures is certainly not related to the timing of the stimulations, since it is exactly the same in both situations. The only possible explanation is that the difference is accounted for by the presence of the right B.B.B. following stimulation 2: the induced His bundle impulse has penetrated the circuit before the reentrant impulse, as in stimulation 1, but the impaired intraventricular conduction has delayed the atrial capture. Obviously, the stimulated impulse has reached the atrium traversing neither the A-V nodal-His axis, nor the left accessory path, but the ventricular myocardium and a latent right-sided accessory pathway.

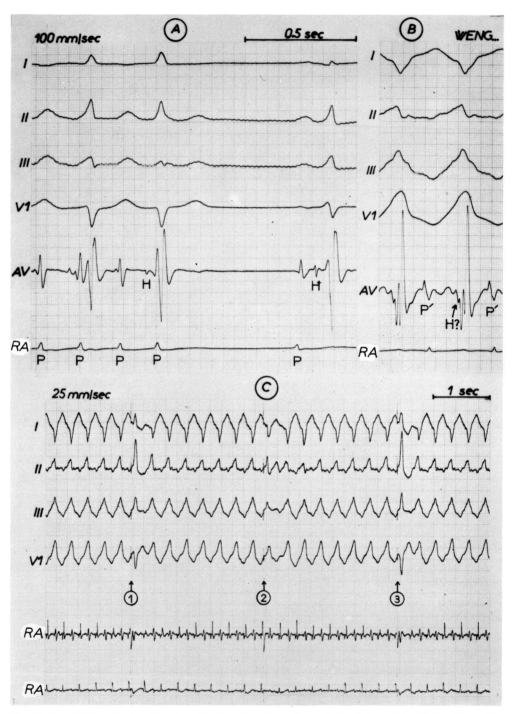

Fig. 17. (case 8) Re-entry involving two Kent bundles. Recording and stimulation of the His bundle. A. The His bundle potential is recorded at the end of an atrial tachycardia with normalized QRSs: the H-R interval is 40 msec, and it decreases as the pre-excitation pattern is resumed, in the last beat of the tracing. B. During the reciprocating tachycardia with a maximal W.P.W. deformity, the H wave is not visible after QRS, and might be present before it ('H?') C. Stimulation of the His bundle during the tachycardia: stimulations n° 1 and 3 are followed after 40 msec by a normalized QRS, while after stimulation 2 a right B.B.B. is present. The effect of these stimulations is more precisely studied in figure 18. (See the text and figure 18 for discussion.)

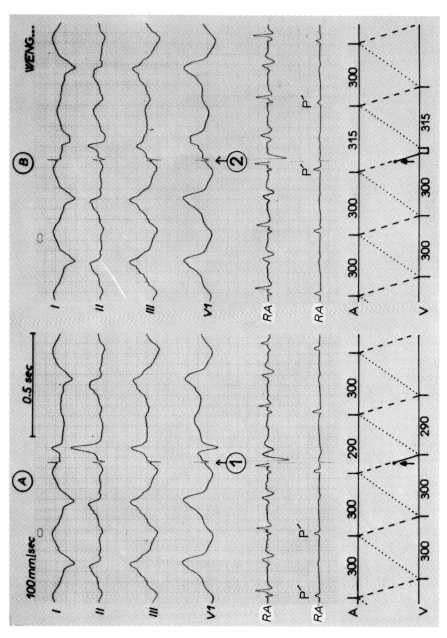

Fig. 18. (case 8) Re-entry involving two Kent bundles. Stimulation of the His bundle during the tachycardia. Stimulations n° 1 and 2 of figure 17 are recorded at a faster paper speed. Their timing is the same, and both are followed 40 msec later by an R wave activated via the normal conducting system. The only difference is the presence of a functional right B.B.B. after stimulation 2. This is the only apparent explanation for the fact that the atrial capture following the His bundle stimulation is premature in tracing A (10 msec) and delayed in tracing B (15 msec), thus proving that the retrograde impulse has involved a latent right-sided accessory pathway. (See the text for discussion.)

c. Re-entry circuit involving Mahaim fibers

In a similar fashion as for James fibers, it is difficult to determine whether this situation is frequent or rare. Mahaim fibers are frequently encountered anatomically, which does not mean that they are frequently functioning, at least anterogradely: a very few cases only have been published (148). If a oneway retrograde conduction is supposed to be frequent in these fibers, a re-entry circuit involving the His bundle and its branches as the anterograde pathway is conceivable, on the condition that impaired conduction facilitates a sustained re-entry.

Theoretically, the following conditions enable a His bundle or an A-V nodal—ventricular by-pass to be considered as participating in a re-entry circuit. 1. The presence of an initial common pathway between the atrium and the circuit should be proved. 2. A ventricular portion of the circuit should be demonstrable. 3. A true ventricular tachycardia, including a re-entry involving only the branches of the His bundle should be ruled out. In practice, all these conditions are rarely met.

1. Re-entry circuit involving Mahaim fibers, with an overt pre-excitation (case 9)

In figure 19, a left ventricular pre-excitation is present, albeit intermittent. It was not possible to modify either the amplitude or duration of the delta wave, a strong argument against the presence of a Kent bundle. In figure 20, a reciprocating S.V.T. has been

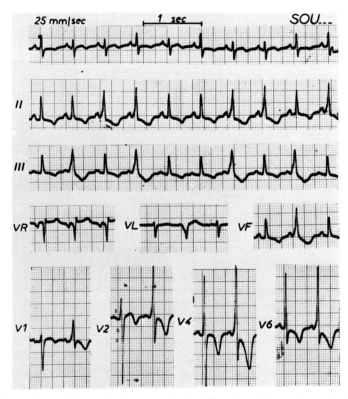

Fig. 19. (case 9) Intermittent left ventricular pre-excitation. The sino-atrial rate is constant, and there is no apparent reason for the intermittent W.P.W. pattern.

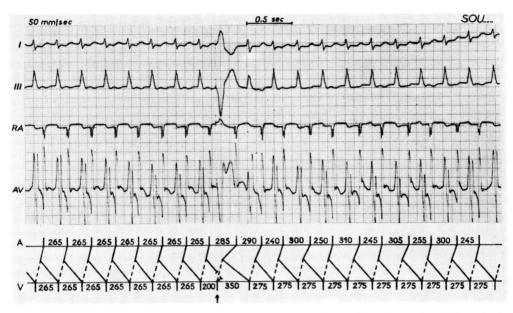

Fig. 20. (case 9) Particular effect of a premature ventricular stimulation. The A-V relationship is perfectly constant before the premature stimulation of the right ventricle, and the rate of the reciprocating tachycardia is regular at 226/min. An atrial capture with delay follows the induced ventricular premature beat. The course of the tachycardia is then modified, as the atrial cycle length becomes alternating, while the ventricular rate becomes slower (218/min). These facts suggest a changing re-entry circuit, and the presence of an initial common pathway between the atrium and the circuit. (See the text for discussion.)

produced with a regular cardiac cycle of 265 msec. A single ventricular stimulation provokes a quite unusual change in the course of the tachycardia. The following atrial capture occurs with delay (cycle length of 285 msec), a phenomenon presuming a first-degree block in the retrograde pathway. Then a more than compensatory pause occurs, and the A-V relationship is completely changed. The atrial cycle not only becomes alternating, with long-short cycles differing by up to 50 msec, but also the ventricular cycle remains regular but increased by 10 msec (275 msec). Thus, in this case, the re-entry circuit is clearly separated from the atrium, but proof is not afforded that the ventricle itself is a part of the circuit. If fact, the lower junction of the circuit was certainly distal to the H wave, i.e. within the His bundle, but neither exact nor paradoxically-premature atrial capture by ventricular stimulation could be demonstrated, which would have proved that the lower junction was actually intraventricular.

2. Re-entry involving probably unidirectionally-blocked Mahaim fibers: the differential diagnosis with His bundle branches re-entry (case 10)

The re-entry circuit in this case is certainly supraventricular, though located below the atrium. In basic tracings (fig. 21), a right B.B.B. is present during sinus rhythm in this 25 year-old and healthy patient. Two kinds of tachycardia were recorded spontaneously, with either a cardiac rate of 240/min and a right B.B.B. pattern, or a rate of 200/min and a left B.B.B. pattern. During the study, only the first variety was observed (fig. 22A). The tachycardia is started by a single atrial premature stimulation with a prolonged P-R

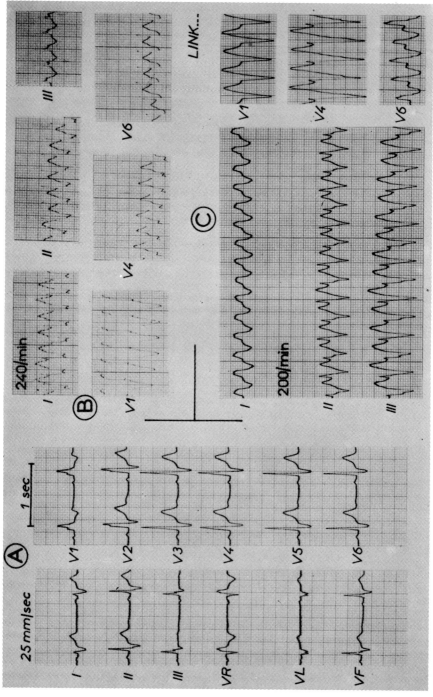

Fig. 21. (case 10) Ventricular or supra-ventricular tachycardia? A. Basic tracings showing a permanent right B.B.B. B. Regular tachycardia at 240/min: QRSs have the same pattern as in basic tracings, but the atrial activity is not visible. C. Regular tachycardia at 200/min: this time a left B.B.B. pattern is present, and 2/1 retrograde P' waves are clearly visible in standard II and III. Theoretically, the diagnosis of ventricular tachycardia should be made by comparing tracings A and C. (See the text and figure 22 for further details and discussion.)

interval, and the QRS pattern is identical to that observed during sinus rhythm. In addition, the initiation of the tachycardia does not coincide with a further impaired intraventricular conduction, a strong argument against the hypothesis of an intraventricular re-entry. A 2/1 retrograde V-A block (fig. 22A) or an A-V dissociation (panels B and D) are present during the tachycardia which is interrupted readily by a paired ventricular stimulation (in B). Before this stimulation, a single right ventricular stimulation coinciding with the very beginning of the spontaneous QRS not only makes it narrow, but also shortens

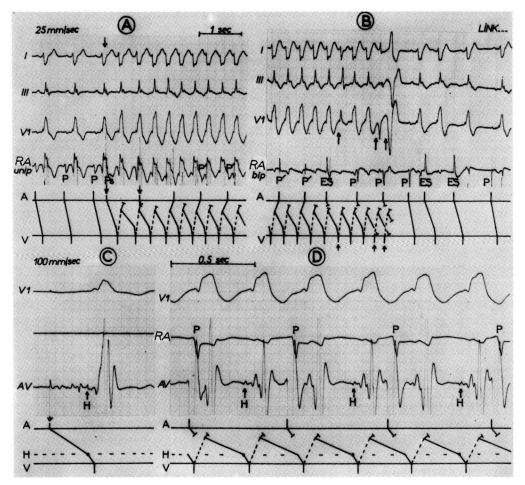

Fig. 22. (case 10) Supraventricular tachycardia with A-V dissociation. A. A premature atrial stimulation (Ps wave) is followed by a prolonged P-R interval which initiates the tachycardia. The QRS pattern is unchanged, suggesting the supra-ventricular origin of the tachycardia, though a 2/1 V-A block is present. B. A single and a paired right ventricular stimulations (arrows) are successively given. The first one coincides with the very beginning or QRS and is responsible for a narrow fusion beat which does capture the tachycardia, as the following beat occurs earlier than expected. The paired stimulation terminates the tachycardia. The atrial activity is either of retrograde (two first P' waves) or extrasystolic (third P wave labelled 'ES') or sino-atrial origin. Tracings C and D compare the His bundle activity during atrial driving and during the tachycardia with A-V dissociation: it is unchanged, confirming the supra-ventricular origin of the tachycardia. As tracing B proves the existence of a ventricular segment of the re-entry circuit, the presence of latent Mahaim fibers is highly suggested in this case. (See the text of discussion.)

the following cycle length, thus indicating that the re-entry circuit involves the ventricular myocardium. Finally, comparing tracings C (during atrial driving) and D shows that the H-R interval is normal and unchanged during the tachycardia.

The existence of attacks of tachycardia with a left B.B.B. pattern is not inconsistent with the diagnosis of S.V.T. in this case, as the right B.B.B. was in fact a first degree block: appropriately-timed atrial stimulations could be followed by either a left B.B.B. with a prolonged H-R interval or even a normalized QRS with a prolonged H-R. Contrarywise, the slower rate of the tachycardia with a left B.B.B. pattern does suggest the existence of a B.B.B.-dependent rate of the tachycardia, and the supposed Mahaim fibers might be left-sided.

CONCLUSION

The concept of re-entry has gained wide acceptance, to the point where now it is virtually impossible to rule out this mechanism in most cases of ectopic tachycardia. Usually admitted criteria of initiation and termination by appropriate electrical stimulation might not be perfectly reliable, as recent experiments suggest that some automatic foci could follow the same rules. On the other hand, it is never possible to eliminate in humans the hypothesis of micro-re-entry. It is why, in our opinion, very precise investigations should be carried out each time the re-entry mechanism is suspected, in order to localize as exactly as possible which circuit is involved.

The three above-mentioned conditions for re-entry are highly favoured in the A-V junction by its anatomic and electro-physiological properties. Various kinds of accessory pathways by-passing more or less completely the normal conducting system are frequent anatomically, and constitute potential circuits (condition 1). These pathways are frequently unidirectionally-blocked, fulfilling condition 2. Finally, the decremental conduction within the A-V node allows a sustained re-entry to occur (condition 3). Thus, if the A-V node undoubtly participates in most re-entrant tachycardias, the more precise the evaluation of the involved pathways, the less frequent the strictly intra-nodal location of the circus movement.

On the other hand, there is no doubt that strictly intra-atrial, and strictly intra-ventricular re-entry circuits do exist. But the problem remains in these cases that participation of the A-V junction must be unequivocally excluded. However, care must be taken in separating atrial and ventricular from A-V junctional re-entry, as cases 3 and 10 suggest that the limits of such forms are not clear-cut.

25

ELECTROPHYSIOLOGICAL DIAGNOSIS AND MANIFESTATION OF DUAL A-V NODAL PATHWAYS

KENNETH M. ROSEN, M.D., PABLO DENES, M.D.,
DELON WU, M.D., AND RAMESH C. DHINGRA, M.D.

Animal studies by Rosenbleuth and Moe et al. suggested that the A-V node could undergo longitudinal dissociation into two pathways (555,698). The presence of two pathways was implied by the development of echo phenomenon following varying patterns of coupled stimulation. The occurrence of echo beats implied the existence of longitudinal dissociation of the A-V node. Subsequently, Mendez et al. provided more direct evidence by demonstration of sudden prolongations of retrograde A-V nodal conduction times (from His bundle to low atrium), utilizing coupled His bundle stimulation (543). Sudden prolongations were noted at critical coupling intervals, suggesting block in a fast A-V nodal pathway, with conduction from the His bundle to the atria occurring via a slow A-V nodal pathway. Subsequent microelectrode studies in rabbit hearts by Mendez and Moe suggested that functional dissociation into dual pathways occurred in the proximal portion of the A-V node (544). Schuilenburg and Durrer provided experimental demonstration of a similar phenomenon in man (742). They demonstrated sudden prolongations of retrograde conduction time (ventricle to atrium) with simultaneous occurrence of ventricular echoes at critical coupling intervals. These observations were made prior to the utilization of catheter His bundle recording techniques, so that exact sites of retrograde conduction delay could not be identified in their patients.

Recently, Goldreyer and co-workers provided strong evidence that A-V nodal reentry was responsible for many cases of paroxysmal supraventricular tachycardia (PSVT) in man (309,310). They were able to induce atrial echoes and PSVT utilizing critically timed atrial stimulation, with demonstration of echo zones. They suggested that induction of atrial echoes depended upon achieving a critical A-V nodal delay (A-H interval), which could be induced by both coupled atrial stimulation and during pacing induced A-V nodal Wenckebach periods. The presence of A-V nodal reentry in patients with PSVT implied but did not prove the existance of dual A-V nodal pathways.

Our laboratory, utilizing His bundle recording and atrial extra-stimulus technique, described sudden prolongation of A-H intervals upon achievement of critical coupling intervals in a patient with two P-R intervals, and in several patients with A-V nodal reentrant PSVT (190,674). Plotting of A_1-A_2, H_1-H_2 curves in these patients, revealed discontinuities, suggestive of dual A-V nodal pathways. Subsequent studies suggested that dual A-V nodal pathway were common, and often directly related to the occurrence of PSVT. In addition, a number of other observations were made regarding the electrophysiological manifestations of dual A-V nodal pathways.

In this presentation, we will attempt to summarize our findings regarding dual A-V nodal pathways and their significance.

ELECTROPHYSIOLOGICAL DIAGNOSIS OF DUAL PATHWAYS

The normal A-V nodal conduction curve generated with atrial extra-stimulus technique (H_1-H_2 responses plotted against A_1-A_2 coupling intervals) is smooth (266, 268, 369, 806, 925). Smooth curves generated by atrial extra-stimulus technique can be described as 'Type I', Type II or truncated. Type I curves show relatively constant intervals between paced and premature responses as the interval between paced and premature stimuli applied to the atrium is shortened. Type II curves demonstrate exponential increases in H_1-H_2 at close coupling intervals. Curves are truncated, when atrial refractoriness limits A-V conduction, so that the portions of the curve at close coupling intervals are never visualized.

A discontinuous conduction curve is suggestive of dual A-V nodal pathways (190, 195, 674, 947). Such a curve is characterized by a sudden increase in H_1-H_2 (and of necessity A_2-H_2) upon achievement of critical coupling intervals (fig. 1). The portion of the curve to the right of the discontinuity, can be described as the fast pathway curve, and the portion to the left, the slow pathway curve. The slope of the slow pathway curve can be positive (decrease in H_1-H_2 with decreasing A_1-A_1 coupling intervals), flat (no change in H_1-H_2 with decreasing A_1-A_2) or negative (increase in H_1-H_2 with decreasing A_1-A_2) (fig. 1). Overlaps of fast and slow pathway curves are frequent, so that at a given coupling interval, either fast or slow responses may be noted. It is important to note that intermediate responses are not demonstrated in the zone of overlap.

For a given discontinuous A_1-A_2, H_1-H_2 conduction curve, a number of definitions can be provided. The fast pathway effective refractory period (ERP) is defined as the longest A_1-A_2 coupling interval, in which conduction does not occur via the fast pathway. The fast pathway functional refractory period (FRP) may be defined as the shortest attainable H_1-H_2 interval on the fast pathway curve. The slow pathway effective refractory period

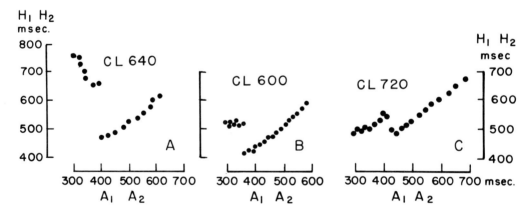

Fig. 1. Three types of dual A-V nodal curves (from Denes et al. (925). In each panel, A_1-A_2 coupling intervals are plotted on the abscissa and H_1-H_2 response on the ordinate. CL = cycle length. Numbers are expressed in msec. Note a sudden jump in H_1-H_2 at a critical A_1-A_2 coupling interval. The portion of the curve to the right of the jump represents the fast pathway, and to the left, the slow pathway. Panel A shows a slow pathway curve with negative slope. Panel B, a slow pathway curve with flat slope, and panel C, a slow pathway curve with positive slope (from Denes et al. (195).

can be defined as the longest A_1-A_2 coupling interval at which conduction does not occur via the slow pathway. In those patients in whom conduction is atrial limited, the slow pathway ERP is less than the shortest achievable A_1-A_2 coupling interval. The slow pathway FRP is defined as the shortest attainable H_1-H_2 interval on the slow pathway curve. In those patients with positive slope slow pathway curves in whom conduction is atrial limited, the slow pathway FRP is shorter than the shortest H_1-H_2 on the slow pathway curve. The definitions of slow pathway properties given above are somewhat arbitrary, since these are determined with an extra-stimulus during sinus or a driven rhythm which is conducted via the fast pathway. A truer assessment of slow pathway properties would be provided if sinus or driven beats were conducted via the slow pathway. This latter condition is rarely fulfilled in human studies.

The electrophysiological diagnosis of dual A-V nodal pathways as described above, is derived totally from data generated with atrial extra-stimulus technique. In a small percentage of patients, dual pathways may be apparent by examination of A-H intervals during sinus rhythm or at constant atrial driving rates (674,951). In this small group of patients, the diagnosis of dual pathways is made by observing the presence of two non-overlapping ranges of A-V nodal conduction times (A-H intervals) at equivalent cycle lengths. Extra-stimulus studies in this group of patients may not allow a diagnosis of dual pathways since all extra-stimuli may be conducted only via the slow pathway. Thus, only one curve is generated, this being the slow pathway curve.

The presence of an extra-nodal accessory pathway between atria and His bundle (James Tract) must be excluded if one is to diagnose dual intra-nodal pathways utilizing extra-stimulus technique (193). This determination is provided by examination of fast pathway properties. An extra-nodal fast pathway should be characterized by a short A-H (less than 54 msec during sinus rhythm), lack of significant A-H prolongation with constant atrial pacing, and a fixed A_2-H_2 with coupled atrial stimulation (prior to the jump in curve). An intra-nodal fast pathway should be characterized by normal or prolonged A-H interval, increase in A-H with atrial pacing at increased rates, and increase in A_2-H_2 with decreasing coupling intervals (prior to the jump in curve).

FREQUENCY OF DUAL PATHWAYS

Atrial extra-stimulus studies were performed in 397 patients without pre-excitation in our laboratory between July 1971 and July 1974. Forty-one of these patients had discontinuous conduction curves suggestive of dual A-V nodal pathways (195).

In 27 of the 41 patients, discontinuous curves were demonstrable with atrial extra-stimulus technique during sinus rhythm. In the remaining 14 patients, conduction curves were smooth during sinus rhythm, and discontinuous only at cycle lengths that were significantly shorter than those of sinus rhythm. The inability to detect dual pathways in these 14 patients during sinus rhythm could have reflected the presence of a fast pathway with a shorter ERP than that of the slow pathway. Shortening of cycle length could have prolonged fast pathway ERP relative to slow pathway ERP, unmasking the presence of dual pathways. The shortening of atrial FRP with decrease in cycle length might also contribute to the unmasking of a slow pathway, allowing delivery of atrial impulses at close coupling intervals. It is also possible that dual pathways were not present during sinus rhythm, and that inhomogeneity of A-V nodal conduction related to shortening of cycle length was a necessary prerequisite for the development of functional dissociation of the A-V node. Additional abnormalities of the A-V node were suspected in many of the patients with discontinuous conduction curves (195). Twenty-two (54%) of the 41 patients with dual A-V nodal pathways studied in our laboratory, had either an etiologic factor strongly associated with A-V nodal dysfunction (previous diaphragmatic myocardial infarction, previous intracardiac surgery, myxedema) and/or one or more abnormalities suggestive of A-V nodal dysfunction (prolonged A-H during sinus rhythm, prolonged A-V nodal ERP or slow pathway ERP during sinus rhythm, prolonged A-V nodal FRP or fast pathway FRP during sinus rhythm, or development of A-V nodal Wenckebach periods at pacing rates of 110/minute or less). It is our impression, that dual pathways relate to the presence of anatomic A-V nodal disease in some patients. Actual anatomic septation of the node due to scar may relate to some discontinuous conduction curves.

The presence of discontinuous conduction curves also related to the occurrence of paroxysmal supraventricular tachycardia (195) (fig. 2). Of the 41 patients studied who had discontinuous curves, 17 of the patients had known documented paroxysmal supraventri-

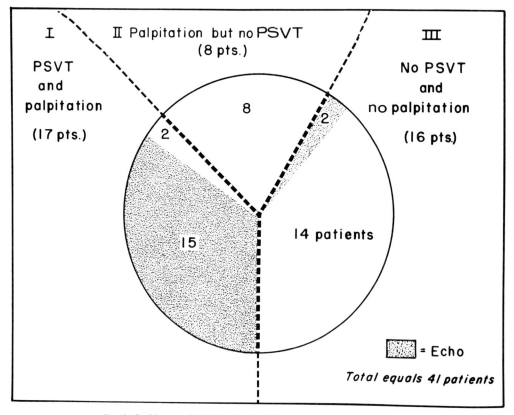

Fig. 2. Incidence of PSVT and palpitations in dual pathway patients.

cular tachycardia (group 1) and 8 of the patients had recurrent paroxysmal palpitation without documentation of paroxysmal tachycardia (group 2). Only 16 of the patients had neither palpitation or documented paroxysmal tachycardia (group 3). Echo zones were demonstrable in most of the patients in group 1. Approximately 50% of the patients studied in our laboratory with known recurrent paroxysmal supraventricular tachycardia, have discontinuous conduction curves demonstrable during extra-stimulus studies.

ELECTROPHYSIOLOGICAL MANIFESTATIONS OF DUAL A-V NODAL PATHWAYS

Paroxysmal tachycardia and the echo phenomenon
At the present, the most important electrophysiological manifestation of dual A-V nodal pathways relates to the presence of echo phenomenon and paroxysmal supra-ventricular tachycardia (190,195,674,950,974). In most patients with intra A-V nodal reentrant PSVT, extra-stimulus studies demonstrate discontinuous conduction curves

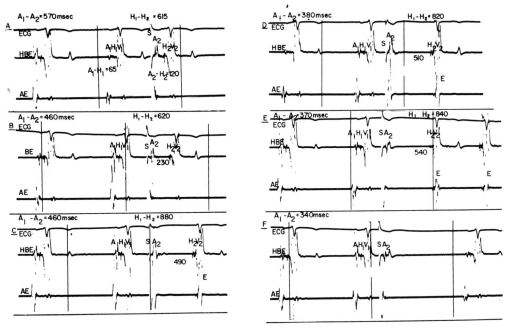

Fig. 3. Demonstration of dual pathways in a patient with PSVT utilizing extrastimuli technique (from Denes et al. (190). The effect of shortening of the A_1-A_2 coupling interval on the A-V conduction of the premature heat (A_2-H_2) and the H_1-H_2 responses. Electrocardiographic lead V_1 (ECG), His bundle electrogram (HBE) and atrial electrogram (AE) are shown in each panel. A_1, H_1, V_1, and A_2, H_2, V_2, represent the atrial, His bundle and ventricular electrograms of the basic sinus and the premature atrial beats, respectively. S represents the pacing stimulus and E echo beats. The A_1-A_2, H_1-H_2, A_2-H_2 intervals are listed in milliseconds. Shortening of A_1-A_2 interval results in lengthening of the A_2-H_2 (A and B). At an A_1-A_2 interval of 460 msec, a sudden increase A_2-H_2 and H_1-H_2 is seen (B and C). When propagation occurs through the slow pathway echo beats are present (C to E). In panel E induction of reentrant PSVT is seen. The cycle length of the tachycardia varied between 550 and 500 msec. At an A_1-A_2 of 340 msec the premature atrial impulse is blocked above H (F). Time lines are at one second.

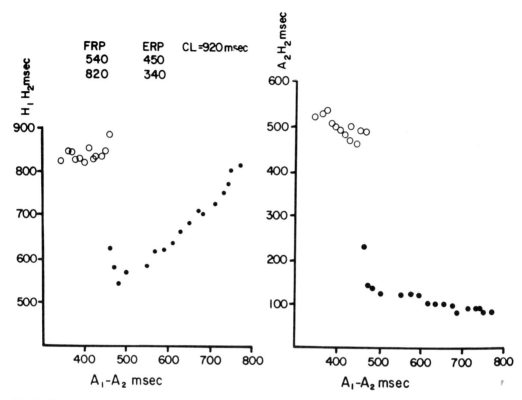

Fig. 4. Conduction curves from patient with PSVT and dual pathways (from Denes et al. (190). Premature atrial coupling to the patient's sinus rate. A_1-A_2 in the abscissa is plotted as a function of the H_1-H_2 responses in the ordinate (left panel). Numerical values on the top indicate the effective and functional refractory periods (ERP and FRP) of the fast and slow pathways expressed in msec. CL indicates basic drive cycle length. Filled circles (●) indicate responses to atrial premature beats introduced at varying prematurity during the basic cycle length, empty circles (○) indicate atrial premature beats that resulted in echo beats. At a coupling interval of 460 msec two H_1-H_2 responses (left panel) and A-V nodal conduction times (right panel) can be observed. Further decrease in prematurity results in a second curve.

suggestive of dual A-V nodal pathways. Examples are presented in figures 3 and 4. At critical A_1-A_2 coupling intervals, there are sudden increases in H_1-H_2 (secondary to sudden increase in A_2-H_2). Coincident with the sudden increase in H_1-H_2 are the occurrence of A-V nodal reentrant atrial echoes. Single echoes, and/or sustained episodes of PSVT (A-V nodal reentrant) may be induced. Echo zones frequently coincide with the total slow pathway curve.

The proposed explanation for the electrophysiological events in such a case are as follows (fig. 5). At achievement of a critical coupling interval, failure of the fast A-V nodal pathway occurs. This results in an impulse being conducted via the slow pathway (which has a shorter refractory period than the fast pathway) resulting in the increase in A_2-H_2 and jump in the A_1-A_2, H_1-H_2 curve. Conduction via the slow pathway is slow enough, so that the failed fast pathway is available for retrograde conduction. The atrial echo occurs because of retrograde conduction in the fast pathway. If appropriate critical relationships between antegrade slow pathway properties (conduction time and refractori-

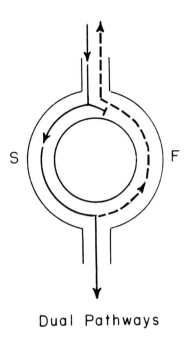

Dual Pathways

Fig. 5. Schematic demonstration of relationship of dual A-V nodal pathways to A-V nodal reentrant circus movement.

ness) and retrograde fast pathway properties (conduction time and refractoriness) are present, sustained reentrance results due to circus movement located within the A-V node. Proximal and distal common pathways must connect the fast and slow pathways so that circus movements may exist. Neither the atria or ventricles appear to be necessary for sustaining of this reentrant circuit.

Determinants of fast and slow pathway conduction
Patients who manifest two non-overlapping ranges of A-H intervals (P-R intervals) at identical cycle lengths, provide a unique opportunity for study of the determinants of fast and slow pathway conduction. These patients are equivalent to patients with pre-excitation, where the presence of short P-R and delta wave graphically reflects the presence of anomalous pathway conduction. In the dual A-V nodal pathway patients with dual conduction times, examination of A-H intervals allow an immediate diagnosis of whether the fast or slow A-V nodal pathway is being utilized (951).

The occurrence of two P-R or A-H intervals depends upon a long fast pathway ERP relative to cycle length (951). At critical heart rates, a premature impulse may encounter the effective refractory period of the fast pathway and conduct via the slow pathway (fig. 6). Subsequent repetitive retrograde concealed conduction (and possible antegrade concealed conduction) to the fast pathway can keep the fast pathway refractory for subsequent antegrade conduction and maintain persistant slow pathway conduction (fig. 6C). With slow rates, the fast pathway can recover for subsequent antegrade conduction, despite concealed conduction (fig. 6A). Thus, the shift to persistant slow pathway conduction may be induced by a critically timed premature atrial beat only at critical heart rates.

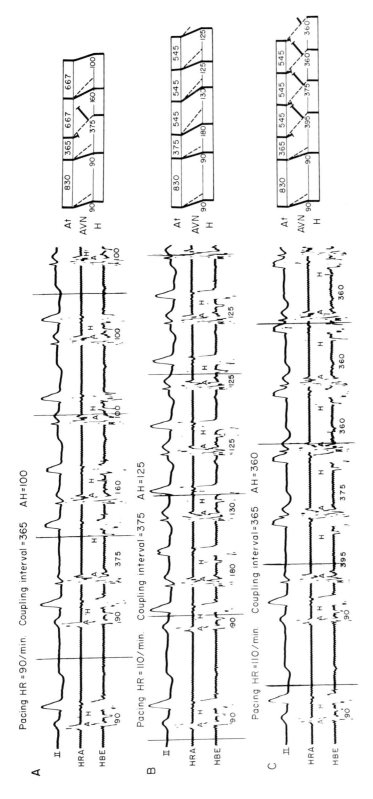

Fig. 6. Determinants of fast and slow pathway conduction (from Wu et al. (951). Shown are ECG lead II. high right atrial electrogram (HRA) and His bundle electrogram (HBE). In each panel, the first two beats are sinus with a cycle length of 830 msec and an A-H of 90 msec. The third and subsequent beats are paced beats. In panel A, a pacing rate (HR) was 90/min. The first paced beat had a coupling interval of 365 msec (equal to fast pathway ERP) and was conducted via the slow pathway with an A-H of 375 msec. The second and subsequent paced beats were conducted via the fast pathway with an A-H of 100 msec. Panels B and C show pacing rates of 110/min. In panel B, the coupling interval of the initial paced beat was 375 msec (> fast pathway ERP) and was conducted via the fast pathway with an A-H of 180 msec. The subsequent beats were also conducted via the fast pathway with an A-H of 125 msec. In panel C, the coupling interval of the first paced beat was 365 msec (equal to fast pathway ERP) and was conducted via the slow pathway with an A-H of 360 msec. Proposed mechanisms are presented in the ladder diagrams on the right, which depict atrium (AT), A-V node (AVN), and His bundle (H). Solid lines reflect fast pathway conduction, and broken lines reflect slow pathway conduction.

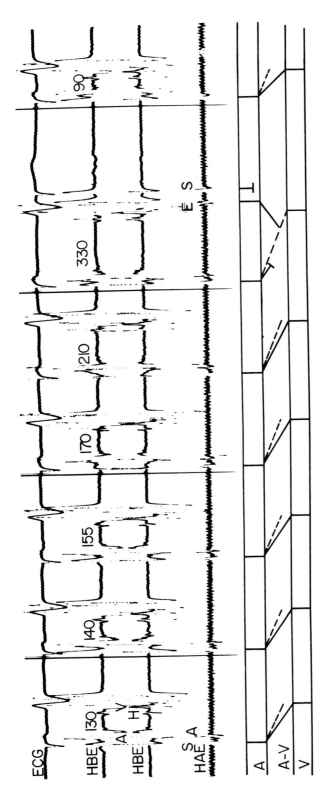

Fig. 7. Atypical Wenckbach periods with echo phenomenon in a patient with dual A-V nodal pathways. The sixth paced P shows sudden A-H prolongation and is followed by an atrial echo.

Shift of conduction to the slow pathway can occur at heart rates which induce Type I block in the fast pathway. Shift of conduction from slow to fast pathway occurs when the premature atrial impulse is blocked in both pathways, allowing recovery of the fast pathway for subsequent antegrade conduction.

Atypical Wenckebach periodicity

In our experience, virtually all patients with discontinuous A-V nodal conduction curves manifest a somewhat characteristic from of atypical Wenckebach periodicity with atrial pacing. These patients develop sudden increases in A-H in the middle or terminal portions of pacing induced Wenckebach periods (fig. 7). The sudden increase in A-H may be accompanied by the simultaneous appearance of an atrial echo, if the pacing rate is such that the echo phenomenon is not concealed by the subsequent pacing stimulus and atrial capture.

Another remarkable manifestation of dual pathways is the demonstration of a double QRS response to one paced P wave in the course of pacing induced Wenckebach periods (951). Pacing induced Type I block involving both pathways, may put these pathways out of phase so that the distal conduction system and ventricles are able to respond to both fast and slow antegrade impulse. Sudden cessation of pacing can allow demonstration of these double responses.

Supernormal conduction and demonstration of dual pathways with additional extra-stimuli

Although the evidence provided strongly supports the existence of longitudinal dissociation of the A-V node into fast and slow pathways, it is possible to fashion explanations for the discontinuous curves, by suggesting inhomogeneous conduction in a single pathway.

The presence of dual A-V nodal pathways can be further substantiated by examining the responses to additional extra-stimuli (atrial or ventricular). In a patient recently reported with discontinuous conduction curves, a third impulse (A_3) often occurred spontaneously following A_2 conducted via the slow pathway (196). During slow pathway conduction of A_2 critical timing of A_3 allowed fast pathway conduction, resulting in an earlier than expected QRS (a form of supernormal conduction) (fig. 8). This was interpreted as reflecting fast pathway conduction during slow pathway conduction, and thus provided strong additional evidence for the existence of dual A-V nodal pathways.

In a recent series of studies, we have been introducing a ventricular extra-stimulus (V_s) in patients with discontinuous conduction curves (948). V_s is introduced at varying coupling intervals relative to A_2, while A_1-A_2 is fixed at a coupling interval which reliably produces an A-V nodal reentrant atrial echo (E) with constant A_2-E interval. At a critical range of A_2-V_s intervals, V_s conducts to the atrium, shortening the apparent A_2-E interval. The ability of V_s to preempt control of the atria, strongly suggests the presence of dual A-V nodal pathways in these patients. If only a single pathway were present, V_s would of necessity collide with the antegrade impulse and would not reach the atria.

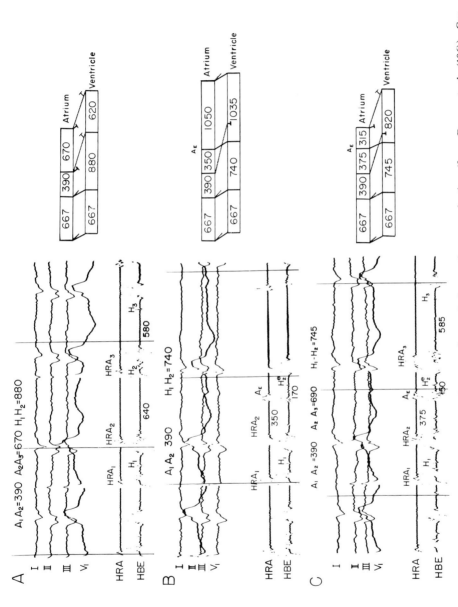

Fig. 8. Supernormal conduction due to simultaneous fast and slow pathway conduction (from Denes et al. (196)). Conventions are similar to previous illustrations. A_2 in panel A is conducted via the slow pathway. In panel B, an atrial premature beat (atrial reentry) (A_e) results in an earlier than expected QRS. A similar phenomenon is shown in panel C. The proposed mechanisms are shown in the ladder diagrams on the right.

DRUGS AND DUAL PATHWAYS

The acute effects of propranolol were studied in seven patients with dual pathways and recurrent PSVT (947). In one of these patients, conduction curves were smooth prior to propranolol administration, and discontinuous after the drug. In the other six patients, discontinuous curves were noted prior to and following the drug. Propranolol tended to increase fast pathway ERP and FRP, as well as slow pathway ERP and FRP (fig. 9). In most patients, the total duration of the slow pathway curve increased, reflecting a greater increase in the outer limit of this curve (fast pathway ERP) than of the innter limit (slow pathway ERP or atrial FRP) following propranolol administration (fig. 9). Echo zones coincided with either part or all of the slow pathway curve. In two of the patients, echo zones were abolished after propranolol administration suggesting that this drug increased retrograde fast pathway refractoriness (fig. 9). In four of the patients, echo zones were unchanged in total duration after propranolol. In two of these four, echo zones were shifted to the right. In one of the patients, there was a marked increase in echo zone following propranolol administration. In this patient, echo zone coincided with the total slow pathway curve. Two patients lost the ability to sustain PSVT after propranolol administration. In those patients with sustained PSVT before and after propranolol, rates

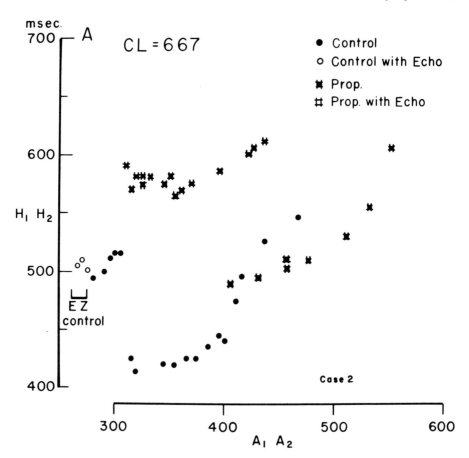

of induced PSVT were slightly but significantly decreased following propranolol administration.

In summary, propranolol shifted both fast and slow pathway curves upwards and to the
right with increase in both fast and slow pathway refractory periods. This presumably
reflected the effects of beta blockade on two pathways, both located within the A-V node.
The results on echo zones were variable. The slowing of PSVT rate following this drug,
presumably reflected slowing of conduction time in one or both pathways.

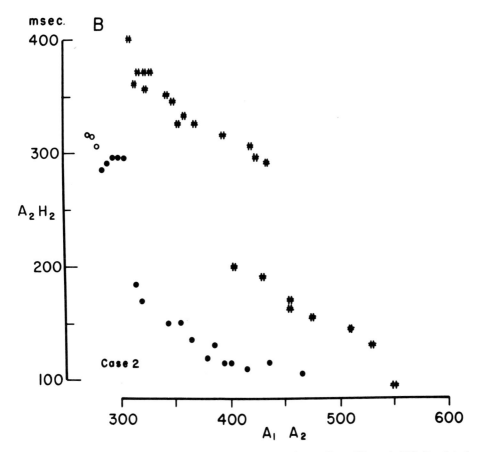

Fig. 9. Effect of propranolol in a patient with PSVT and dual pathways (from Wu et al. 947). Panel A shows
H_1-H_2 responses plotted against A_1-A_2 coupling intervals. Panel B shows A_2-H_2 responses plotted against
A_1-A_2 coupling intervals. Control responses are shown as circles and post propranolol responses as squares.
Open circles and squares reflect responses followed by echo beats. Echo zones are designated in the A panel.
The basic driving cycle length (CL) was 667 msec. A: Before propranolol, the ERP of the fast pathway was
305 msec, which coincided with the onset of the slow pathway curve. The echo zone was noted on the inner side
of the slow pathway curve at A_1-A_2 between 275 to 265 msec. The atrial FRP of 265 msec limited slow pathway
conduction. After propranolol, both the slow and the fast pathway curves shifted rightward and upward
indicating increase of the ERP and FRP of both pathways. The echo zone was abolished. Overlaps of the fast
and slow pathway curves were also noted. B: Before propranolol, the critical A-H interval was 305 msec. After
propranolol, the critical A-H interval was 305 msec. After propranolol, there was no critical A-H interval
even at the longest attainable A_2-H_2 of 400 msec, suggesting increased refractoriness of the fast pathway for
retrograde conduction. A_2-H_2 lengthened at any given A1-A_2 intervals.

We recently reported a similar study regarding the effects of Ouabain in patients with recurrent PSVT and dual pathways (950). The results following Ouabain administration were generally similar to those described above in regard to propranolol. Ouabain shifted both fast and slow pathway curves rightwards and upwards. The effect of Ouabain on echo zones were variable (echo zone abolished in one patient, decreased in duration in three patients, and increased in one patient). The ability to sustain PSVT was lost in two of the patients. In contrast to propranolol, rates of induced PSVT were similar before and after Ouabain administration.

The clinical management of dual pathway A-V nodal reentrant PSVT has not been well defined. Reported drug studies have been limited to Ouabain and propranolol, both of which were studied acutely in the catheterization laboratory. There is no reported information concerning the effects of quinidine on induction of dual pathway A-V nodal reentrant PSVT. It is our current impression, that digitalis is the drug of choice for prevention of PSVT in patients with dual pathway reentrant PSVT.

This is in contrast to our experience in patients with recurrent PSVT and smooth conduction curves (947,950). It is our impression, that drugs which depress A-V nodal conduction (Ouabain and propranolol) frequently potentiate PSVT induction in such patients. This may reflect the fact that many smooth curve cases reflect the occurrence of concealed extra-nodal bypass pathways. Drugs which depress the A-V node, allow additional time for concealed extra-nodal pathways to recover (following antegrade concealed penetration from premature stimuli) potentiating the echo phenomenon (197).

CONCLUSIONS

About three and a half years ago, we studied a patient with two P-R intervals, in whom extra-stimulus studies revealed discontinuous conduction curves suggestive of dual pathways. At that time, we felt the case studied to represent an electro-physiological curiosity. Over the next two years, we learned that discontinuous conduction curves were present in the majority of patients with A-V nodal reentrant PSVT, and in some patients without PSVT.

We presently suspect a direct relationship between the presence of dual pathway curves and PSVT. However, the basis for the presence of these curves in patients with and without underlying organic heart disease is unknown. It is possible that with appropriate conditions, all patients are capable of manifesting discontinuous conduction curves. These curves could possibly be potentiated by a number of interventions that produce inhomogeneity of A-V nodal conduction. Examples of such interventions might include shortening of cycle length, depression of A-V nodal conduction with drugs, and development of A-V nodal ischemia. The presence of dual pathway curves and recurrent PSVT in young patients without organic heart disease could reflect congenital development abnormalities of the A-V node (or perhaps lack of appropriate maturation of the A-V node).

26
INCIDENCE OF DIFFERENT TYPES OF A-V BLOCK
AND THEIR LOCALIZATION BY HIS BUNDLE RECORDINGS

PAUL PUECH, M.D., ROBERT GROLLEAU, M.D., AND CLAUDE GUIMOND, M.D.

The recordings of the His bundle electrogram in cases of atrioventricular block has demonstrated the inability of the surface electrocardiogram to localize exactly the site of the conduction disturbance, especially when the QRS complexes, of either conducted or escape beats, are widened.

Only His bundle recordings enable us to diagnose conduction disturbances not discernable in the standard leads, and to localize conduction block in the subdivisions of the conducting system. Moreover, when His bundle recordings combined with certain interventions such as vagal reflexes, endocavitary stimulation and pharmacological tests, facilitate the diagnosis of paroxysmal atrioventricular block.

MATERIAL

656 patients with different types of AV blocks were studied, and the conduction disturbance localized by means of His bundle recordings (table 1). First degree, second degree, and third degree spontaneous AV block, with the atria in sinus rhythm, occurred in 118, 141 and 222 patients respectively. In 41 patients, high degree, or complete block occurred in the presence of atrial flutter or fibrillation. Four patients had paroxymal AV block with narrow QRS complexes and normal PR intervals. Complete unilateral, or bifascicular block was present in 130 patients. In these patients, the HV interval was measured, in most cases also during stress-tests, in order to evaluate whether conduction in the other parts of the conducting system was normal or not.

The criteria for the topographic diagnosis of AV block using His bundle recording have been given in detail by several authors (173, 585, 672, 747) and in previous publications from our department (641, 642, 645).

Table 1. Material.

First-degree AV block (S-A R)	118
Second-degree AV block (S-A R)	141
Third-degree AV block (S-A R)	222
High-degree AV block + atrial flutter or fibrillation	41
Normal PR and narrow QRS (paroxysmal AV block)	4
Normal PR and wide QRS	130
TOTAL	656

Table 2. First-degree spontaneous AV blocks (118 cases).

QRS	No of cases 118	Supra His 55(47%)	Intra His 15(13%)	Infra His 24(20%)	Mixed 24(20%)
Narrow	45	39(87%)	6(13%)	—	—
Wide	73	16(22%)	9(12%)	24(33%)	24(33%)

Intra-atrial blocks are not included in the present study. They do in fact rarely result in 1 degree AV block, whereas 2nd degree intraatrial block has only been documented during atrial stimulation (112,436,588,644).

CORRELATION BETWEEN SURFACE ECG AND HIS BUNDLE RECORDING

First degree AV block

In this group of patients, defined by a PR interval longer than 0.20 second (table 2), the conduction disturbance is localized in 47% proximal to the site where the His potential is recorded, in 13% in the common bundle itself, and in 20% distal to the recording site. In 20% the conduction time is prolonged both above and below the recording site.

When QRS morphology is considered, it appears that a prolonged PR interval with narrow QRS complexes corresponds most often to a first degree AV block localized in the proximal part of the conducting system (87%), but also in a not insignificant number of cases in the common bundle of His (13%). When QRS complexes are widened (longer than 0.12 sec), the conduction disturbance is proximal to the His bundle in 22%, distal to the His bundle in 33%, localized within the His bundle in 12%, and mixed (both supra- and infra His) in 33%.

Second degree AV block

In their totality, second degree blocks are localized in about an equal percentage above and below the His bundle (table 3). *Important differences* come to light when the type of conduction disorder and the morphology of the conducted QRS complexes are considered. In type I second degree AV block (Wenckebach phenomenon) the conduction

Table 3. Second-degree spontaneous AV blocks (141 cases).

Type of block and QRS pattern	No of cases 141	Supra His 58(41%)	Intra His 24(17%)	Infra His 59(42%)
Type I	53	38(72%)	5(9%)	10(19%)
Type II	15	—	3(20%)	12(80%)
2:1 or 3:1	73	20(27%)	16(22%)	37(51%)
Narrow QRS	65	43(66%)	18(28%)	4(6%)
Wide QRS	76	15(20%)	6(8%)	55(72%)

disturbance is predominantly localized in the AV node (72%), only in 9% within the His bundle, and in 19% distal to the His bundle. The data of Narula (595) are nearly identical.

In our experience, a type II second degree AV block (Möbitz II) is never localized proximal to the His bundle, but always represents a lesion of the common bundle (20%) or the bundle branches (80%).

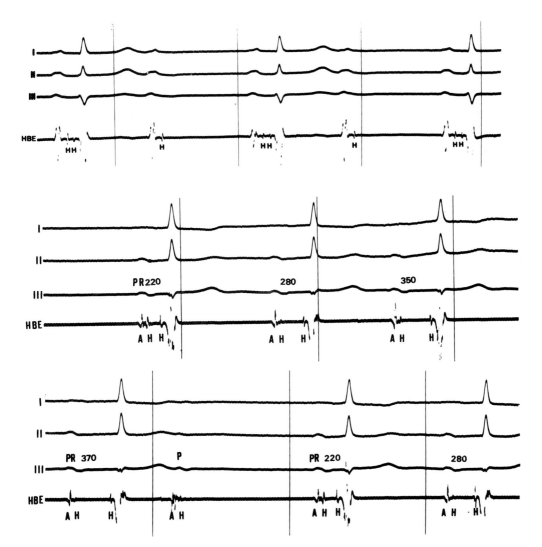

Fig. 1. Second degree block in the common His bundle. *Upper panel* 2:1 AV block with conducted QRS complexes of normal morphology. In the conducted beats, the His potential is split. The blocked P waves are followed by a single His complex, corresponding to depolarization of the proximal His bundle above the very circumscribed lesion in the common bundle. *Middle and lower panel* (continuous tracing). 5:4 type I (Wenckebach) block with normal QRS complexes. The prolongation of AV conduction time takes place between the proximal His potential (fixed to atrial activity) and the distal His potential (fixed to ventricular activity), while the P wave is blocked after the proximal His potential, proving that the site of block is the common bundle. Note the reduction in amplitude of the proximal His potential in successive beats, when conduction time increases progressively.

Absence of type II block in the node of Tawara, is considered the rule (594). Blocks of the 2:1 (or 3:1) variety can be localized both in and below the AV node, but occur predominantly in the His-Purkinje system.

Second degree AV block associated with narrow QRS complexes occurs most often in the node of Tawara (66%). In a third of the cases, a lesion in the His bundle is responsible, as shown by the presence of a split His potential (fig. 1). In the absence of a split His potential, stimulation of the His bundle resulting in 1:1 conduction to the ventricles without a change in QRS morphology, which remain narrow, argues in favour of an origin of the block in the common bundle, distal to recording site (fig. 2).

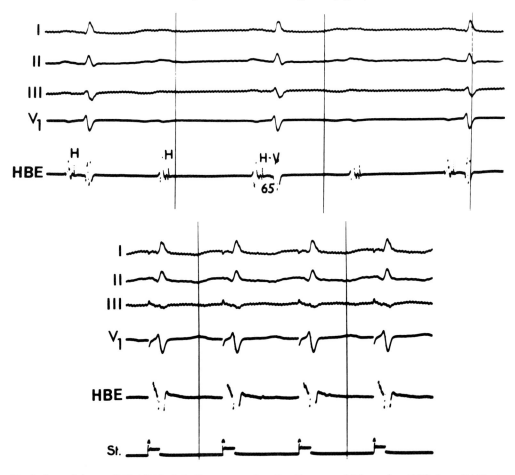

Fig. 2. Second degree (2:1) AV block in the common bundle. *Upper panel.* The surface ECG shows 2:1 block with narrow QRS complexes. The His bundle electrogram shows that the AH interval is normal (intact AV nodal conduction) and that block is localized below the site where the His potential is recorded. In the conducted beats the HV interval is prolonged (65 msec), and only every second beat is conducted to the ventricles. The narrow QRS complexes are an argument in favor of a localisation of the block in the common bundle, but block distal to the bifurcation, with equal prolongation of conduction time in both bundle branches cannot be ruled out. *Lower panel.* His bundle stimulation (arrows) at 110/min results in 1:1 conduction to the ventricles; QRS complexes remain narrow. The ability to overcome the block while stimulating an intact part of the common bundle, below the site of block and above the bifurcation, is an argument in favour of a localized block in the common bundle.

Table 4. Third-degree spontaneous AV blocks (222 cases).

QRS	No of cases 222	Supra His 47(21%)	Intra His 40(18%)	Infra His 135(61%)
Narrow	53	28(53%)	25(47%)	—
Variable	8	2(25%)	6(75%)	—
Wide	161	17(11%)	9(5%)	135(84%)

Second degree block with widened QRS complexes due to bundle branch block (unilateral or bifascicular) is in two thirds of the cases caused by lesions below the His bundle.

Very long PR intervals of the conducted beats correspond as a rule to a localization above the bifurcation (the common bundle or the node of Tawara), whereas normal or slightly prolonged PR intervals are mostly associated with infra-His blocks.

Third degree AV block

In these patients (table 4), block is usually infranodal (18% in the common bundle, 61% in the bundle branches).

The frequent occurrence of complete block localized in the common bundle has been noted in other large series (Narula 14% (594), Rosen et al. 17% (673).

When QRS complexes are constantly narrow, the localisation of block is divided equally between the AV node (53%) and the common bundle (47%). Escape beats having both wide and narrow QRS complexes are associated three times more often with block in the common bundle than with intra nodal block. Third degree block with permanently widened QRS complexes most often corresponds to complete bilateral bundle branch block (84%). It is probable that certain cases of complete AV block with narrow QRS complexes are due to lesions high in the His bundle and not in the AV node. These occur in elderly women, the escape rhythm has a rate below 40/min, and the QRS complexes are permanently narrow. Intravenous injection of atropine, which clearly accelerates AV nodal pacemakers, and has little or no influence on His bundle pacemakers, may be of help in the diagnosis (594,645).

When block is localized in the common bundle and a split His potential is present, atrial stimulation at increasing rates permits recognition of the proximal His potential when it is superimposed on the terminal part of the P-wave at basic rates, as it becomes separated from the atrial electrogram at faster rates (fig. 3).

In our series of 222 cases of complete antegrade AV block, retrograde conduction frequently occurred, thus making the block unidirectional. When both manifest retrograde conduction, apparent in the surface ECG, and concealed retrograde conduction were considered, unidirectional block occurred in 15% of the cases (table 5).

The occurrence of retrograde conduction depends on the site of block. Thus, third degree block due to bilateral bundle branch block was most often associated with intact retrograde conduction, both manifest and concealed (137,330).

The diagnosis of unidirectional block in the intraventricular part of the conducting system is based on the presence of a His potential occurring after the QRS complex, when the preceding A and H potentials occur at a certain time prior to that His potential, and on

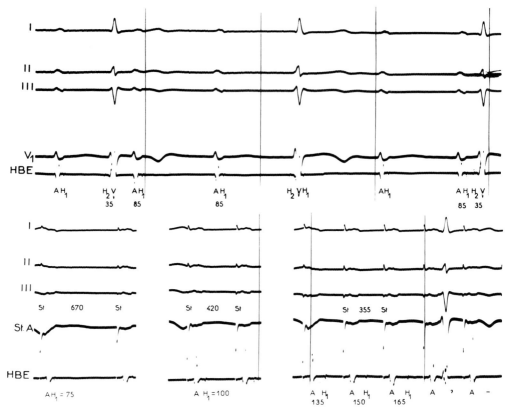

Fig. 3. Complete intra His block. *Upper panel* 3rd degree AV block. Atrial rate 87/min, ventricular rate 37/min. The His bundle electrogram shows 2 His potentials which are completely dissociated, H_1 being linked to atrial activity (AH_1 being normal at 85 msec) and H2 being linked to ventricular depolarization, H_2V being normal at 35 msec. The QRS complexes are narrow. *Lower panels.* Atrial stimulation at increasing rates to validate the proximal His potential which might be confused with late atrial activity due to widening of the P wave. AH_1 prolongs progressively on increasing rate (left to right). At 170/min an intranodal Wenckebach phenomenon occurs, separating clearly the proximal His potential from atrial activity.

Table 5. Third-degree spontaneous AV blocks (222 cases).

Site of block	No of cases 222	Bidirectional 188(85%)	Unidirectional 34(15%)
Supra His	47	45(96%)	2(4%)
Intra His	40	36(90%)	4(10%)
Infra His	135	107(79%)	28 Retrograde atrial cond. 18(13%) Concealed cond. 10(7%)

the prolongation of the AH interval (or the absence of a His potential) following the next P wave (sinus or retrograde). This is shown in figure 4. Following these criteria, it can be shown that the specific conducting system is in fact involved in the retrograde conduction, and that in the case of manifest retrograde conduction, the atria are not activated retrogradely by way of an accessory pathway. Moreover, the fixed time relationship between the ventricular escape beat and the retrograde His potential makes the differentiation possible

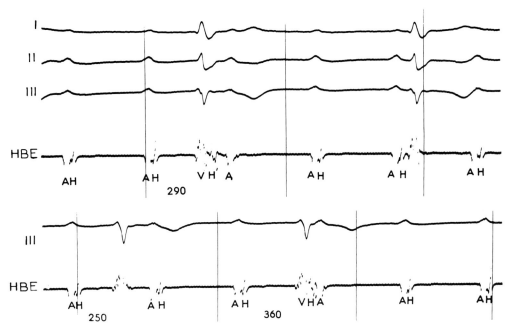

Fig. 4. Unidirectional infra His block with concealed retrograde conduction. The ECG shows complete AV block with widened QRS complexes and a ventricular rate of 38/min. The His bundle electrogram demonstrates the intra His localization of the block (coupled A-H potential with no ventricular response). Retrograde conduction from the ventricular escape focus is shown in the endocavitary recording by: a. retrograde His potentials (H') when the preceding A-H interval occurs sufficiently before the QRS complex to permit recovery of excitability of the His bundle; b. absence of the antegrade His potential (H) after the succeeding sinus P wave indicating that the specific conducting system was depolarized by the retrograde wavefront. In the surface leads, the retrograde conduction is concealed, the atria being activated by sinus impulses. Thus, the retrograde impulse is blocked in the node of Tawara.

between unidirectional block and His bundle extrasystole (or parasystole) with retrograde atrial capture (fig. 5).

When unidirectional block is located in the common bundle, the absence of a proximal His potential after the retrograde P wave shows that the part of the common bundle above the site of antegrade block is in fact involved in retrograde conduction of an escape beat originating in the lower part of the His bundle (fig. 6).

As for the infrequent (4%) occurrence of unidirectional block in the node of Tawara, it is impossible to confirm by His bundle recording alone that the AV node is involved in retrograde conduction and to exclude conduction via an accessory pathway only functioning during retrograde conduction. However, the effect of ventricular stimulation at increasing rates, and the effect of vagal reflexes and drugs on retrograde conduction time are of help to distinguish between retrograde conduction via the AV node or Kent bundle, because these structures behave differently during these interventions (640, 802).

High degree, or complete AV block, and atrial flutter or fibrillation
In the present series (table 6), block above the His bundle predominates (75%). This is partly explained by the fact that the block is frequently caused by digitalis, and partly because concealed intranodal conduction augments the degree of functional intranodal

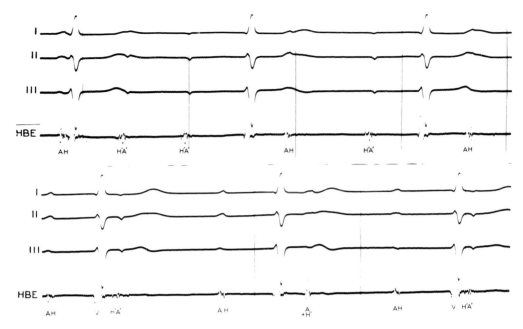

Fig. 5. Complete bidirectional infra His block. His bundle extrasystoles with retrograde conduction. In the surface ECG atrial activity is completely dissociated from ventricular activity. His bundle electrogram shows infra His location of block. Two types of P waves exist: positive P waves of sinus origin, negative P waves occurring after variable intervals following ventricular depolarization. The His bundle electrogram shows that the negative P waves are caused by His bundle extrasystoles (H′). The variable interval between H′ and QRS (sometimes quite long) permits the differentiation between His bundle extrasystoles with retrograde conduction and unidirectional AV block. Note the difference in polarity of the His potential during sinus rhythm and His bundle extrasystoles.

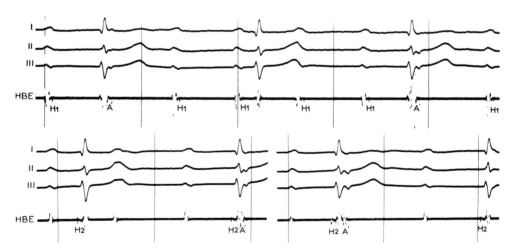

Fig. 6. Unidirectional intra His block with retrograde conduction to the atria. Complete antegrade AV block with narrow QRS complexes with LAH configuration. The ventricular rate is 40/min. The His bundle electrogram shows that block is located in the common bundle, with H_1 being linked to the atrial activity (upper panel) and the distal H_2 complex preceding ventricular depolarization (lower panel), the AH_1 and H_2V intervals being completely dissociated. Retrograde conduction from the focus low in the His bundle is preserved (unidirectional block), and is discernable in the surface ECG by the negative P waves in leads II and III. Retrograde conduction along the common bundle is demonstrated by the absence of the proximal His potential following the retrograde P waves, showing that the upper His bundle and node of Tawara are retrogradely activated.

Table 6. High-degree AV blocks in atrial fibrillation and flutter (41 cases).

QRS	No of cases 41	Supra His 31(76%)	Intra His 4(10%)	Infra His 6(15%)
Narrow or Variable	23	19(83%)	4(17%)	—
Wide	18	12(67%)	—	6(33%)

block. From a practical point of view, it is of interest to note that even in the presence of widened QRS complexes, of conducted or escape beats, block above the His bundle predominates. Both for prognosis, which is better than for block in or below the His bundle, and indication for an artificial pacemaker, this is of importance. Figure 7 shows an example of complete block at the level of the His bundle in the presence of atrial flutter. Figure 8 illustrates complete infra-His block with atrial fibrillation.

It is often difficult to demonstrate the presence of a His potential, when atrial flutter, and particularly when atrial fibrillation is present, because the proximal His deflection may be taken for atrial activity. Searching for activity in the distal part of the His bundle with

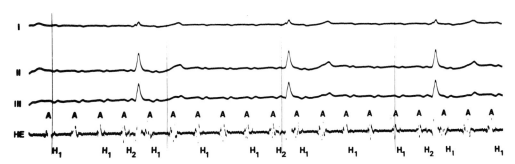

Fig. 7. Atrial flutter and complete block in the His bundle. The ectopic atrial rhythm has a rate of 275/min, the ventricular rate is regular at 45/min with normal QRS complexes. There is a physiological 2:1 AV nodal block caused by the high atrial rate, shown by the 2:1 relationship between atrial deflections and proximal His potential (H_1). A complete (pathological) block is present distal to the proximal part of the common bundle. The ventricular escape rhythm originates in the common bundle, below the zone of block (the distal H_2 potential precedes the ventricular complex at a normal interval).

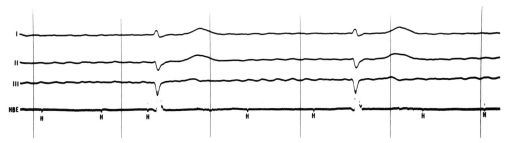

Fig. 8. Atrial fibrillation and complete infra His block. The activity of the fibrillating atria is discernable in the surface ECG but not in the endocavitary lead, recorded close to the distal end of the His bundle. The His bundle potentials occur irregularly at an average rate of 85/min, and conduction fails completely below the His bundle. The ventricular escape rhythm has a rate of 25/min, and the QRS complexes are widened and not preceded by a His potential, indicating the intraventricular origin of the escape rhythm.

a bipolar catheter (interelectrode distance of 0.5 to 1 mm) may facilitate the localization of block.

Bundle branch block and His bundle recording
AV conduction was studied in patients whose QRS complexes showed complete mono- or bifascicular bundle branch block (QRS ≥ 0.12 sec) with normal P̊R intervals, as well as with 1° and 2nd degree AV block.

Complete right bundle branch block
The findings differ according to whether isolated RBBB without marked axis deviation is present (table 7), or RBBB with either left anterior hemiblock (LAH, table 8) or left posterior hemiblock (LPH, table 9).

Table 7. Right BBB without marked axial deviation (conducted beats) (64 cases).

AV Conduction	No of cases	Supra His block	Subnodal block	Mixed block
Normal PR	26	—	5 HV ≥ 55(19%)	—
First-degree AV block	10	5	2 HV ≥ 55 (50%)	3
Second-degree AV block	28	5	23 (82%)	

Table 8. Right BBB and LAD (conducted beats) (107 cases).

AV Conduction	No of cases	Supra His block	Subnodal block	Mixed block
Normal PR	48	—	18 HV ≥ 55(37, 5%)	—
First-degree AV block	33	8	13 HV ≥ 55(76%)	12
Second-degree AV block	26	4	22 (85%)	—

Table 9. Right BBB and RAD (conducted beats) (30 cases).

AV conduction	No of cases	Supra His block	Subnodal block
Normal PR	23	—	17 HV ≥ 55 (74%)
First-degree AV block	1	—	1
Second-degree AV block	6	—	6

When the PR interval is *normal*, an infranodal conduction disturbance can be present, not diagnosable on the surface ECG, as shown by the finding of a prolonged HV interval (≥ 55 msec) in 19% of cases with isolated RBBB. When RBBB is associated with LAH, this conduction disturbance is present in 37, 5% and in 74% of RBBB + LPH.

When *1° degree AV block* is present, prolongation of the HV interval (partly or completely responsible for the prolonged PR interval) is observed in half of the cases of isolated RBBB, and in 76% of the cases of RBBB + LAH.

In 2nd degree AV block, block is infranodal in 82% when the conducted beats have an isolated RBBB configuration, in 85% when RBBB is associated with LAH, and in all cases of RBBB + LPH.

Left bundle branch block (Table 10)

In complete left bundle branch block, absence or presence of left axis deviation did not significantly influence the HV interval, as was found also in other series (595).

When PR is *normal*, infranodal conduction is often abnormal (67%) with HV prolongation in some instances related to a conduction disturbance in the common bundle (fig. 9). Narula (595) has also emphasized the frequent occurence of prolonged conduction time in the common bundle associated with left bundle branch block.

Table 10. Left **BBB** (conducted beats) (78 cases).

AV conduction	No of cases	Supra His block	Subnodal block	Mixed block
Normal PR	33	—	22 HV $\geq$ 55 (67%)	—
First-degree AV block	29	3	17 HV $\geq$ 55 (90%)	9
Second-degree AV block	16	6	10 (62%)	

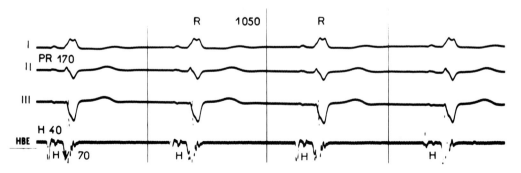

Fig. 9. First degree block in the His bundle associated with complete left bundle branch block. In the surface ECG the PR interval is normal (170 msec) and the QRS complexes have a complete left bundle branch block configuration. The His potential is deformed, wide (40 msec) and slowly rising. The HV interval, if measured from the beginning of the His complex, is prolonged to 70 msec, due to slow conduction in the common bundle.

In *1° degree AV block*, the HV interval is prolonged in 90% accounting partly or completely for the prolongation of the PR interval. In other series this figure is lower (489).

When no split His potential is found signs of conduction disturbances in the common bundle have to be looked for systematically, by placing the catheter end successively at the proximal end of the His bundle (juxta-atrial position) and the distal end (juxta-ventricular position) (fig. 10).

In *2nd degree AV block*, LBBB is in 62% associated with an infranodal lesion (common bundle or right bundle branch), which is less often than in RBBB with 2nd degree block.

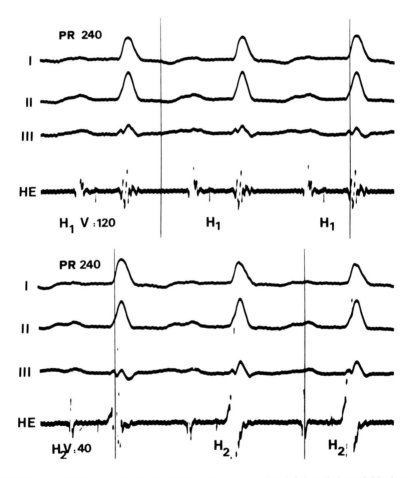

Fig. 10. First degree AV block located in the His bundle and complete left bundle branch block *Upper panel*: His bundle electrogram showing prolonged conduction time from proximal His potential (H_1) to ventricle (H_1V being 120 msec) accounting for prolonged AV conduction (240 msec). When the investigation would have been limited to this recording, the diagnosis of bilateral bundle branch block (complete LBBB and 1st degree block in the right bundle) would erroneously have been made. *Lower panel*. Recording of a distal His potential (H_2) preceding a QRS complex at a normal interval ($H_2V = 40$ msec), showing that the 1° degree AV block is located in the common bundle, and that conduction in the right bundle branch is normal. When only this recording would have been available, the erroneous diagnosis of left bundle branch block associated with a supra-His conduction disturbance would have been made. Conduction time in the common bundle is prolonged by 80 msec.

Paroxysmal AV block

Diagnostic problems often arise and the diagnosis is especially difficult when no episodes of bradycardia are documented. Most often, paroxyxmal block is located below the His bundle. Recordings made between attacks, when sinus rhythm is present and PR is normal or slightly prolonged, show evidence of alterations in intraventricular conduction such as complete mono- or bifascicular bundle branch block. More rarely, the ventricular asystole responsible for the syncope is due to paroxysmal block at the level of the His bundle. In these cases the diagnosis is most difficult because recordings made between attacks may be completely normal, or show only insignificant abnormalities such as a slightly prolonged PR interval, or isolated LAH.

Figure 11 is an example of spontaneously occurring periods of asystole due to block of sinus impulses at the level of the His bundle. The proximal His complex has a large amplitude during the conducted beats and gradually becomes smaller until it disappears during the period of asystole. This change in the His bundle electrogram seems independent of catheter movement, and should be compared to identical observations made during experimental His bundle block due to ischemia in the dog heart (245).

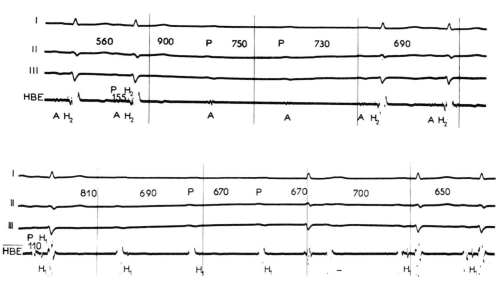

Fig. 11. Paroxysmal AV block located in the common bundle. *Upper panel:* Recordings made at the distal part of the His bundle. The first two beats are of sinus origin and have normal PR intervals (190 msec), narrow QRS complexes and an AH$_2$ interval of 155 msec. The blocked sinus P waves are not followed by a His potential suggesting intra nodal block. This is disproved by recording at a more proximal site. *Lower panel:* Recording at the proximal part of the His bundle (note higher amplitude of atrial complexes), AH of the conducted beat is 110 msec, showing 1st degree intra His block with a conduction delay of 45 msec at basic rates. During ventricular asystole, conduction is blocked distal to H, demonstrating that the paroxysmal AV block is located in the common bundle. Note the progressive reduction in amplitude of the proximal His complex, until it disappears altogether during the period of asystole, and the large amplitude of the His complex before and after the pause. Voltage and morphology of the atrial complexes remain unaltered, suggesting that the change in amplitude of the His potential is related to the conduction disturbance and not to catheter displacement. It should be noted that the sinus rate varies spontaneously and that the paroxysms of block are initiated by the longest sinus intervals, suggesting 'phase 4 block' (diastolic block induced by relative bradycardia) in the common bundle.

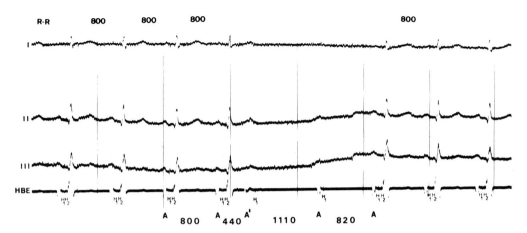

Fig. 12. Paroxysmal block in the common bundle initiated by an atrial extrasystole. During the basic rate, the PR interval is normal (190 msec), and the QRS complexes are normal. A 1st degree block exists in the common bundle, as shown by the presence of a split His potential, both components being separated by 40 msec. An atrial premature beat (coupling interval 440 msec) is followed by block distal to the proximal His potential ('phase 3 block', or systolic block following a short cycle). The next sinus P wave is also blocked in the common bundle, which may be interpreted on 'phase 4 block' (diastolic) caused by the long post-extrasystolic pause.

Some paroxysmal blocks are initiated by extrasystoles (atrial or ventricular) and can be evoked by programmed endocavitary stimulation. Figure 12 is an example of paroxysmal intra His block initiated by atrial premature beats. Conduction block in the common bundle (after the first complex of a split His potential) occurs not only after the

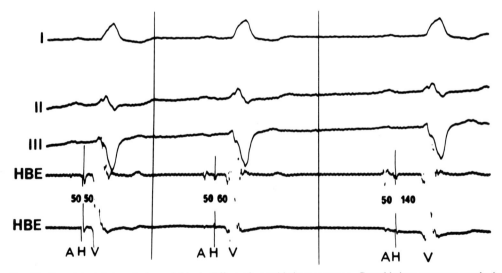

Fig. 13. Complete left bundle branch block. Effect of carotid sinus massage. Carotid sinus massage results in slowing of the sinus rate which does not affect AV nodal conduction (AH interval remains 50 msec) but prolongs the HV interval which changes from 50 to 140 msec. This prolongation of conduction time in the subnodal part of the conducting system (distal part of common bundle or right bundle branch) is probably due to the bradycardia itself ('phase 4 block' or 'diastolic block') rather than to a direct vagal effect on the specific conducting system.

premature atrial beat but also after the succeeding sinus impulse. The sequence may be regarded as 'phase 3 block' followed by 'phase 4 block' (caused by the post extrasystolic pause) in the common bundle.

Vagal reflexes, in practice carotid sinus massage, are of value in demonstrating slowing or block in conduction in the specific conducting system *below* the AV node, as shown in figure 13. Infra-His conduction disturbances which are revealed or aggravated, during sinus bradycardia following carotid sinus message (155,416) can be considered as 'phase 4 blocks' (diastolic blocks). They indicate latent pathology at the cellular level, such as a low membrane potential, diastolic depolarization and/or elevated threshold potential (144, 147, 244, 313, 694). However, proof that these blocks are dependent only on the bradycardia itself, and not on a direct vagal effect on the infranodal conducting system, can only be obtained by comparing the results of carotid sinus massage during sinus rhythm and during atrial stimulation at a fixed rate.

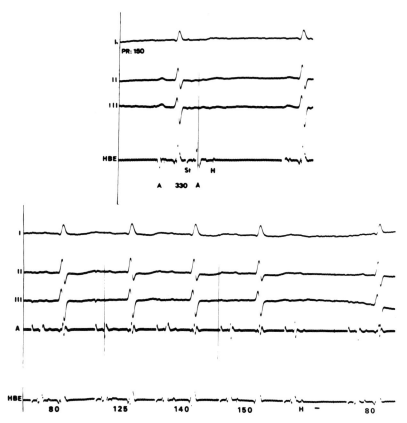

Fig. 14. Paroxysmal block in the common bundle. Effects of atrial stimulation. During the *basic rate* the PR interval is normal (150 msec), QRS complexes are narrow with isolated LAH configuration. The HV interval is long (80 msec) suggesting 1st degree block in the distal part of the common bundle. *Premature atrial stimulation* (coupling interval 330 msec), as shown in the upper panel, results in a prolongation of conduction through the node and block below the His potential. *Atrial stimulation at a fixed rate* at 110/min (lower panel) gives rise to type I second degree block (Wenckebach phenomenon) between H and V, located in the distal part of the common bundle, intranodal conduction time remaining constant at an AH interval of 110 msec. QRS complexes remain narrow.

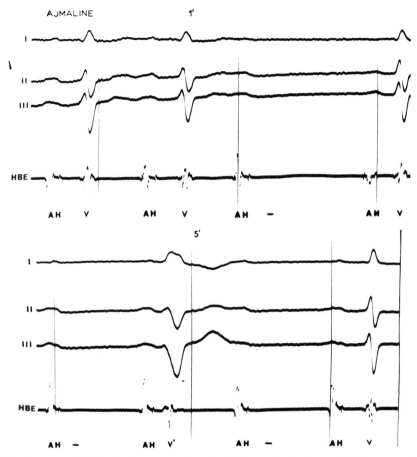

Fig. 14 bis. Paroxysmal block in the common bundle. Effects of Ajmaline. Administration of Ajmaline (1 mg/kg) results within one minute in type II 2nd degree block below the His bundle (upper panel). After 5 minutes, complete block occurs with a ventricular escape (widened QRS complex, lower panel).

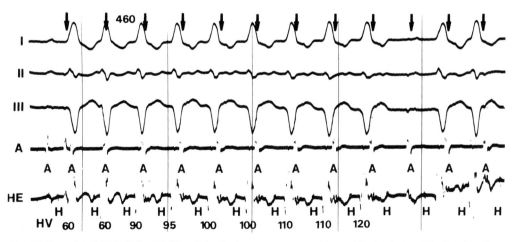

Fig. 15. Complete LBBB. Infra His Wenckebach phenomenon caused by atrial stimulation. The first beat is a sinus beat; PR interval is normal (190 msec), HV interval is prolonged (60 msec). Atrial stimulation (arrows) at 130/min results in 1:1 conduction to the His bundle and a Wenckebach phenomenon below the His bundle. HV progressively increases from 60 to 120 msec until block occurs.

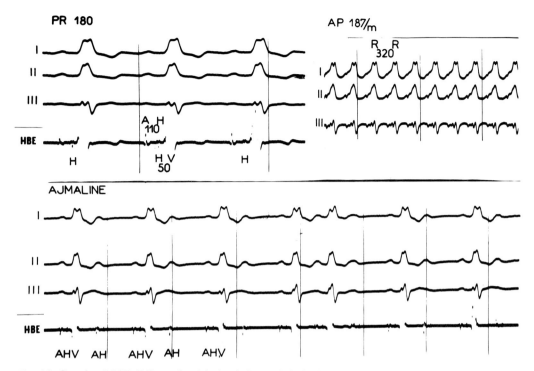

Fig. 16. Complete LBBB. Effects of atrial stimulation and of Ajmaline. Left upper panel: sinus rhythm. Normal PR interval (180 msec) and complete LBBB. HV is normal (50 msec). Right upper panel: Atrial stimulation at 187/min results in 1:1 AV conduction (negative result). Lower panel: Intravenous injection of 50 mg Ajmaline results in 2nd degree block (2:1 or 3:2) below the site where the His potential is recorded, indicating that a latent conduction disturbance exists at the most distal part of the common bundle or the right bundle branch. Conduction through the AV node remains normal.

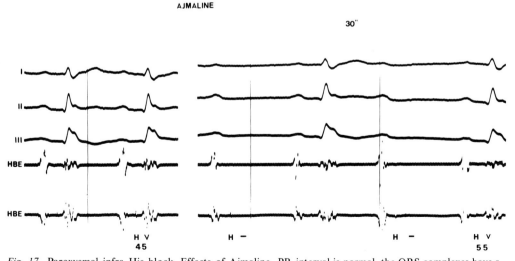

Fig. 17. Paroxysmal infra His block. Effects of Ajmaline. PR interval is normal, the QRS complexes have a RBBB + LPH configuration, the HV interval is normal at 45 msec. 30 msec after the injection of *Ajmaline* (1 mg/1kg), a 2:1 infra His block occurs, revealing the instability of conduction in the intraventricular part of the conduction system.

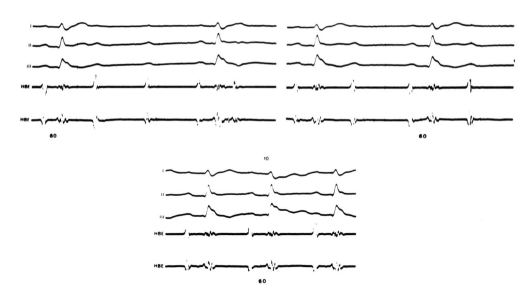

Fig. 17 bis. Two minutes after injection of Ajmaline 3:1 infra His block exists. Progressively, AV conduction ameliorates: 2:1 block after 5 minutes, and 1:1 conduction after 10 minutes with a slightly prolonged HV interval of 60 msec.

Intravenous injection of Ajmaline (1mg/kg body weight injected in 30 sec) is a sensitive method to explore conduction (101, 327, 538). Examples of paroxysmal AV block brought to light by Ajmaline are illustrated in figure 14 (block in common bundle) and figure 16 and 17 (infra His block). It is true, both for atrial stimulation (fig 14–16) and pharmacological tests that they are only of value in demonstrating conduction disturbances, when the response is positive. More experience is needed to determine the significance of these tests as far as indication for pacemaker implantation is concerned.

27

PATTERNS OF V-A CONDUCTION IN THE HUMAN HEART IN THE PRESENCE OF NORMAL AND ABNORMAL A-V CONDUCTION

REINIER M. SCHUILENBURG, M.D.

The combined technique of intracardiac electrocardiography and stimulation has proven to be a valuable method in the study of atrioventricular conduction in man. As compared to the vast literature on the subject of A-V conduction in antegrade direction, accumulated in recent years, the number of papers reporting studies on retrograde conduction is relatively small (8, 9, 11, 116, 117, 308, 593, 677, 742, 743, 905). With the exception of a few recent reports (11,593) most studies concerned a relatively limited number of patients and antegrade and retrograde conduction were not compared systematically.

A definition of the characteristics of ventriculo-atrial conduction in patients with normal and abnormal antegrade conduction might also be of interest in the further clasification of some rhythm disturbances, especially of those in which a reentry mechanism seems to be involved.

This paper reports a study on 200 consecutive patients, in whom antegrade and retrograde conduction were compared. The antegrade conduction was tested with the atrial incremental pacing and single test stimulus methods. The stimulation and recording techniques and the characteristics of a normal response to these tests have been described earlier (744). After completion of the study of antegrade conduction the right ventricular apex was stimulated at a rate just above the sinus rate. One hundred patients proved to have retrograde conduction, no V-A conduction was found in the other 100 patients. Table 1 shows that 50 of the 200 cases had a normal antegrade conduction (that is, they had normal A-H and H-V intervals, a normal A-V nodal Wenckebach rate, normal functional and effective refractory periods of the A-V node and no conduction disturbances in the His bundle or bundle branches). Of these 50 patients 34 (68%) had V-A conduction, while it was present in 44% of the patients with any kind of antegrade conduction disturbance. ($p < 0.001$).

Table 2 represents the distribution of the patients according to the existing principal abnormality of the antegrade conduction. From this table it appears that the percentage of successful retrograde conduction did not differ much from the 68% found in patients with normal antegrade conduction in the patients with first degree block in the His bundle (71%)

Table 1. V-A conduction in 200 patients.

A-V conduction	N	V-A +		V-A −	
		n	%	n	%
Normal	50	34	68%	16	32%
Abnormal	150	66	44%	84	56%

Table 2. V-A conduction in 150 patients with impaired A-V conduction.

A-V conduction	N	V-A +		V-A −	
		n	%	n	%
A-V nodal block					
1°	34	13	38%	21	62%
2°	5	1	20%	4	80%
3°	6	0	0%	6	100%
His bundle block					
1°	7	5	71%	2	29%
2°	14	5	36%	9	64%
3°	6	0	0%	6	100%
Bundle branch block					
CLBBB	15	8	53%	7	47%
CRBBB	23	15	65%	8	35%
CRBBB + LAH	19	12	63%	7	37%
CRBBB + LPH	2	2	100%	0	0%
2° HV block	6	3	50%	3	50%
3° HV block	13	2	15%	11	85%

or (partial bilateral) bundle branch block with 1:1 A-V conduction (37 out of 59 cases, 63%).

There was, however, a much lower incidence of V-A conduction in the whole group of patients with conduction impairment in the A-V node and in those with second or third degree His bundle or H-V block. Remarkable is, that as compared with the groups of second and third degree block in A-V node and His bundle the percentage of successful retrograde conduction was higher in those with second and third degree H-V block (even 15% in the last category).

These results indicate, that the absence or presence of V-A conduction cannot be deduced with certainty from the characteristics of the antegrade conduction.

V-A CONDUCTION ABSENT

In the group of patients without retrograde conduction we tried to localize the site of the retrograde block. A handicap in the study of retrograde conduction is that the retrograde His potential is visible in only a few patients, in most cases it is hidden within the broad ventricular complex. The site of the retrograde block, therefore, could not be easily identified by the presence or absence of retrograde His potentials, and indirect methods had to be used. This was accomplished in three ways.

In the *first method* utilized, we looked at the influence of the ventricular activations of a regularly driven rhythm upon the antegrade conduction of the atrial activations originating from the independent activity of the sinus node. In the patient of figure 1 the P-H conduction was slowed down or even blocked when the atrial activation followed a ventri-

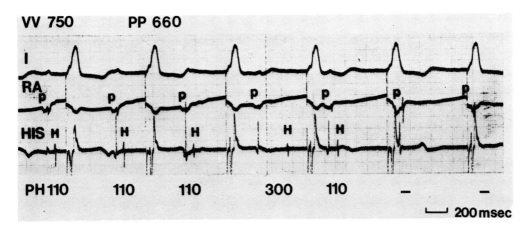

Fig. 1. Complete antegrade bilateral bundle branch block. Ventricular pacing (cycle length 750 msec). The ventricular complexes influence the antegrade conduction through the A-V node when the atrial activations follow the ventricular complexes closely (fourth, sixth and seventh P-wave). This indicates that retrograde concealed conduction into the A-V node took place. The P-H interval of the fifth P-wave is normal although the V-P interval is short, because the short H-V interval of the preceding cycle prohibits retrograde activation of the His bundle and thereby of the A-V node.

cular activation closely. Therefore, in this patient with complete bilateral bundle branch block, concealed retrograde conduction of the ventricular activations into the A-V node hand to be assumed and by consequence the retrograde block had to be localized within the A-V node. If the antegrade conduction of the atrial beats appeared to be independent on the time relation with the preceding ventricular beat a subnodal localization of the retrograde block had to be postulated. The phenomenon of concealed retrograde conduction into the A-V node has also been observed and described recently by others (137,644) in patients with complete antegrade A-V block.

Our experience indicates that this phenomenon can also be used as a test to localize the site of the retrograde block in patients with less advanced disturbances of antegrade conduction or even normal A-V conduction.

The *second method* was also based on concealment of retrograde conduction, but allowed a more systematic approach.

Figure 2 shows an example of this test. During a basic rhythm in which the atria were stimulated synchronously with the ventricles in order to obviate interferences with the sinus nodal activity, a stimulus V_2 was applied to the ventricles after an interval equal to the cycle length of the basic rhythm. An atrial test impulse A_3 was given after V_2 and the influence of gradual shortening of the V_2-A_3 interval upon the antegrade A-V conduction of A_3 was noted. In the patient of figure 2, who had a rate-dependent complete left bundle branch block, A_3 was blocked at the A-V nodal level at a critical V_1-A_3 interval of 910 msec (middle panel). When V_2 was omitted A-V nodal conduction of A_3 was successful (lower panel) with an A-H interval, which was shorter than at a 10 msec longer V_1-A_3 interval in the presence of V_2 (upper strip). From this sequence it can be concluded that the retrograde conduction of the V_2 impulse was blocked within the A-V node. If on the other hand the A_3-H_3 interval was independent of the time relation between V_2 and A_3, it had to

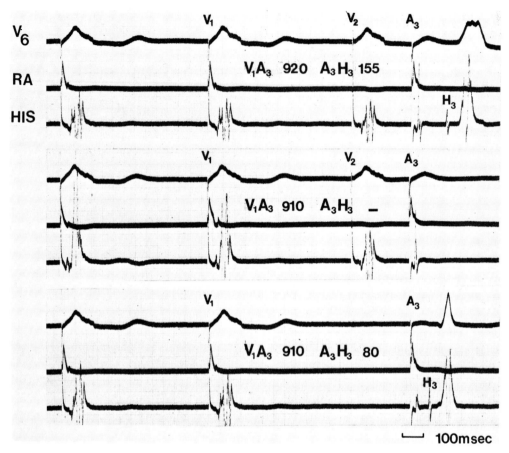

Fig. 2. Synchronous pacing of right ventricle and atrium (cycle length 670 msec). Test stimulus V_2 applied to the ventricle with V_1-V_2 650 msec shows concealed retrograde conduction into the A-V node, as is evident from its influence upon the antegrade A-H conduction of a test stimulus A_3 which is delayed at a V_1-A_3 interval of 920 msec and even blocked at a 10 msec shorter V_1-A_3 interval. If V_2 is omitted at that V_1-A_3 interval, A_3-H_3 conduction is normal. This patient had a rate-dependent left bundle branch block.

be assumed, that the retrograde block of the V_2 impulse was localized at a subnodal level.

It is obvious that successful application of the two fore-mentioned methods is only possible if the antegrade conduction through the A-V node is normal or only slightly depressed. They are useless in the presence of a second or third degree antegrade A-V nodal block.

The *third method* utilized partly overcomes this problem. It is based upon direct visualization of retrograde His bundle activations by premature ventricular stimulation. If, like is demonstrated in figure 3, a retrograde His potential (H_2) becomes visible after a ventricular test activation V_2 due to delayed retrograde conduction at the bundle branch-Purkinje level when the coupling interval (V_1-V_2) of this test stimulus is shortened, one may assume, that V_2-H_2 conduction is also intact at longer coupling intervals approaching the cycle length of the stimulated rhythm and therefore, that

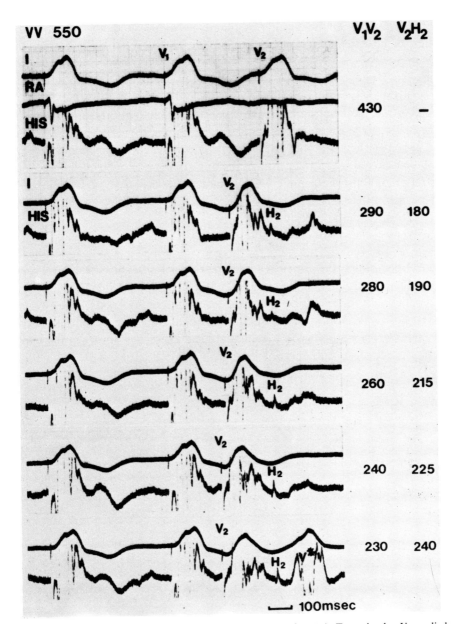

Fig. 3. Synchronous ventricular and atrial pacing (cycle length 550 msec). Test stimulus V_2 applied to the ventricle. The coupling interval V_1-V_2 is gradually shortened. At V_1-V_2 290 msec a retrograde His potential with a V-H interval of 180 msec can be discerned. Further shortening of V_1-V_2 results in widening of V_2-H_2, until at a critical V_2-H_2 interval of 240 msec ventricular re-entry occurs. The retrograde V-A block in this patient is located at a level higher than the His bundle recording site, that is, in the A-V node (or in the very proximal part of the His bundle).

the retrograde block is located in the A-V node, although a localization in the proximal part of the His bundle is not excluded completely.

Conclusions from this test may only be drawn if retrograde His potentials are visualized, since we have evidence that in some patients retrograde block of ventricular premature beats in the bundle branch system may occur suddenly without preceding retardation to an extent large enough to let the H_2 potential emerge from the ventricular complex V_2.

In this figure one can also see the relatively frequent phenomenon of ventricular reentry occurring at a critical lengthening of the V_2-H_2 interval.

Absence of V-A conduction does not necessarily mean that the conduction system is always incapable to retrograde conduction.

In the patient of figure 4, who had a sinus bradycardia and normal antegrade conduction, V-A conduction was absent even at the low driving rate of 50 per minute. After the administration of 1 mg of atropin 1:1 V-A conduction was present up to a rate of 100 per minute, at which rate a V-A Wenckebach phenomenon was found. The V-A block before atropin was located in the A-V node.

Table 3 shows the localization of the retrograde block in the 100 patients with V-A block as it was assessed with the use of the three just described methods. Again the material was split up according to the principal antegrade conduction disturbance. In all 16 patients with normal antegrade conduction and in 30 of the 31 cases with impaired antegrade A-V nodal conduction, the retrograde block was located in the A-V node. The A-V node was also the weakest link in most cases with bundle branch block even if it was bilateral of if the H-V interval was prolonged. A subnodal localization was found in the majority of patients with second or third degree antegrade block in the His bundle or bundle branch system.

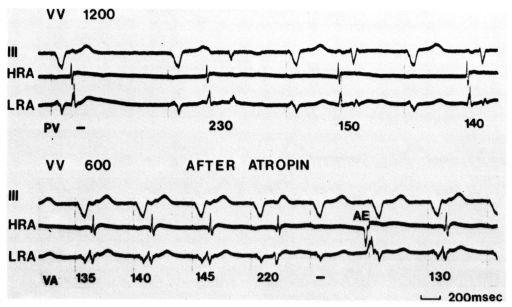

Fig. 4. Sinus bradycardia with normal antegrade A-V conduction. On ventricular pacing even with a low rate (50, cycle length 1200 msec, upper panel) there is no A-V conduction. The dependence of the antegrade conduction time of the sinus impulses on the interval to the preceding ventricular beat suggests retrograde concealed conduction into and therefore block within the A-V node. After administration of atropin 1:1 V-A conduction was present up to a ventricular rate of 100 (cycle length 600, lower panel), at which rate a V-A Wenckebach phenomenon occurred. AE is an atrial escape beat.

Table 3. Localization of retrograde block in 100 patients with V-A block.

		Localization of V-A block			
A-V conduction	N	In A-V node		Subnodal	
		n	%	n	%
Normal	16	16	100%	0	0%
A-V nodal block					
1°	21	21(11″)	100%	0	0%
2°	4	3(1″)	75%	1(1″)	25%
3°	6	6	100%	0	0%
His bundle block					
1°	2	2	100%	0	0%
2°	9	1	11%	8(3″)	89%
3°	6	0	0%	6	100%
Bundle branch block					
CLBBB	7	7(3′)	100%	0	0%
CRBBB	8	7(1′)	88%	1	12%
CRBBB+LAH	7	5(3′)	71%	2	29%
2° HV block	3	1	33%	2	67%
3° HV block	11	4	36%	7	64%

″with BBB
′HV prolonged

V-A CONDUCTION PRESENT

In this group of 100 patients the V-A conduction was stressed by increasing ventricular driving rate and with the single test stimulus method.

1. Response to increasing ventricular pacing rate
The usual response was a lengthening of the V-A interval as rate went up (88%) until a second degree V-A block occurred. In a minority (11%) 1:1 V-A conduction remained intact at the highest rates studied (180–200 per minute).

Presumably most of the conduction delay at higher rates took place in the A-V node as is demonstrated in figure 5 of a patient with complete right bundle branch block and left anterior hemiblock, in whom retrograde His potentials could be recorded. The increase of the V-A interval at the higher rate was exclusively due to a lengthening of the H-A interval (40 to 90 msec), the V-H interval remaining constant (95 msec). In some patients the V-A interval remained constant at incremental pacing. An example is given in figure 6. This patient had a 2:1 H-V block, and a complete right bundle branch block and posterior hemiblock of the conducted beats. V-A conduction remained present up to rate 190. At this rate the V-A interval was identical to that at rate 110 (165 msec). The V-A interval was found to be independent of the driving rate

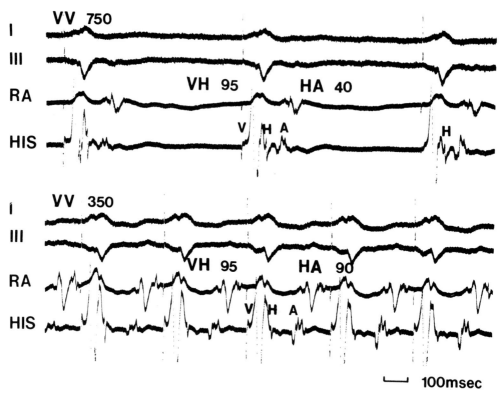

Fig. 5. Complete right bundle branch block and left anterior hemiblock. On ventricular pacing retrograde His potentials are visible, with a V-H interval of 95 msec and an H-A interval of 40 msec at a cycle length of 750 msec (upper panel). Increasing pacing rate (cycle length 350, lower panel) results in lengthening of H-A. The V-H interval, however, remains constant.

in 12% of our material. This figure corresponds with the 15% incidence reported recently by Narula (593). A maximum increment of less than 20 msec was found in an additional 31%. Retrograde conduction through anomalous bypass fibers has been advanced as an explanation for this phenomenon (593). None of our patients with no or only slight increase of the V-A interval, constituting 43% of the group with V-A conduction, had had any signs of antegrade pre-excitation or a history of paroxysmal tachycardias. No re-entrant tachycardias could be elicited by atrial or ventricular premature stimulation. In all patients there was a marked lengthening of the A-H interval when atrial driving rate was increased. We are aware that the absence of antegrade pre-excitation or re-entry phenomena does not rule out the possibility of the existence of bypass fibers with exclusive conduction in retrograde direction. However, the high incidence of a constant or nearly constant V-A interval (43% of our material), as compared to the general occurrence of antegrade pre-excitation, suggests, that other explanations have to be contemplated as well. In the absence of direct recordings from the A-V nodal area these explanations can only be tentative, but one might speculate that in some human hearts the retrograde wave front originating from the His bundle may be and remain more homogeneous on rate increases than the antegrade wave front approaching from the atrium, or that in retrograde direction a different, perhaps shorter pathway is followed through the A-V node than in antegrade

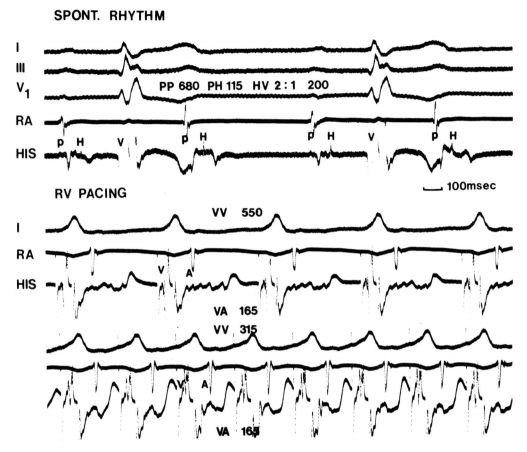

Fig. 6. Complete right bundle branch block with left posterior hemiblock and 2:1 H-V block (upper panel). Note that the H-V interval of the conducted beats is markedly prolonged: 200 msec. There is, however, 1:1 V-A conduction with a relatively short V-A interval of 165 msec, which appeared to be independent of the ventricular pacing rates (middle and lower panels).

direction. Both possibilities might result in a smaller rate-dependency of the retrograde A-V nodal conduction time.

The rate at which a second degree V-A block occurred varied considerably and showed no relation with the atrial rate at which a second degree A-V block was found.

As in antegrade conduction, retrograde second degree V-A blocks may be of the Wenckebach or Mobitz II variety. In the patients in whom retrograde His potentials could be discerned, it could be demonstrated that the Wenckebach type may be localized in the A-V node or in the bundle branch system (fig. 7). A Mobitz II type of block was located predominantley in the bundle branches, but in a few patients the Mobitz II sequence occurred apparently in the A-V node. This is shown in figure 8. This patient with a complete right bundle branch block developed an A-H Wenckebach at an atrial cycle length of 400 msec. and an H-A Mobitz II block at a ventricular cycle length of 700 msec. Although a localization in the proximal part of the His bundle cannot be excluded completely, the Mobitz II block seems to occur in the A-V node.

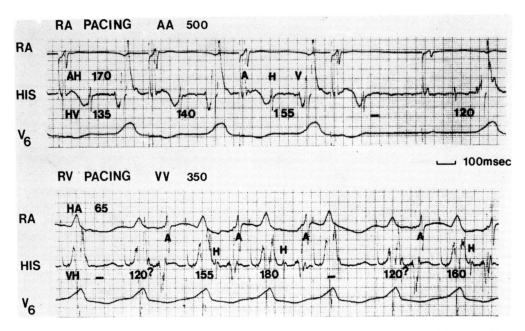

Fig. 7. Complete left bundle branch block. *Upper panel*: H-V Wenckebach occurring at atrial pacing with a cycle length of 400 msec. *Lower panel:* V-H Wenckebach at ventricular pacing with cycle length 350 msec.

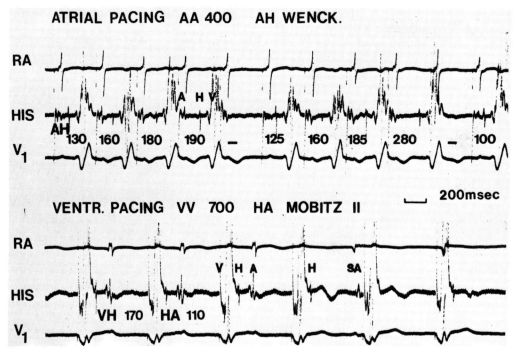

Fig. 8. Complete right bundle branch block. *Upper panel*: A-H Wenckebach occurring at atrial pacing with a cycle length of 400 msec. *Lower panel*: H-A Mobitz II type of block on ventricular pacing with cycle length 700 msec. SA is an atrial complex of sinus nodal origin.

A V-A Mobitz II block was found in 26% of all cases with V-A conduction. Its occurrence was associated with a small increment of the V-A interval on increasing ventricular driving rate. It occurred in 8 of the 12 patients with a constant V-A interval (in 3 of the 12 1:1 V-A conduction remained present up to the highest rate studied) and in 14 of the 31 patients with a maximum V-A increment of less than 20 msec (in 3 patients 1:1 V-A conduction was intact at rates of 190 and higher). On the other hand it was observed in only 4 patients of the 57 cases with a V-A increment of 20 msec or more.

In 34 of the 100 patients it was found that V-A conduction remained intact up to higher rates than A-V conduction did during atrial pacing. A differentiation according to the properties of antegrade conduction is given in table 4.

V-A conduction was better than A-V conduction as far as the response to incremental pacing was concerned in 9% of the group with normal antegrade conduction, while this was the case in an overall 36% of the patients with a conduction disturbance at any level, but 1:1 A-V conduction. Of course V-A conduction had to be considered better than A-V conduction in all 11 patients with second or third degree A-V block, who had 1:1 V-A conduction.

In comparing V-A conduction with A-V conduction it has to be kept in mind, that ventricular pacing in itself may influence the functional properties of the V-A conduction system, possibly by a neurogenic feed-back mechanism, activated by the altered hemodynamic state, which goes along with the change in the temporal relation of atrial and ventricular contractions. This is demonstrated in figure 9 of a patient with a slightly

Table 4. Incidence of better V-A conduction than A-V conduction in 100 patients.

A-V conduction	N	V-A better than A-V	
		n	%
Normal	34	3	9%
A-V nodal block			
1°	13(7″)	7(5″)	54%
2°	1	1	100%
His bundle block			
1°	5(1″)	2	40%
2°	5	5	100%
Bundle branch block			
CLBBB	8(4′)	5(2′)	63%
CRBBB	15(4′)	4	27%
CRBBB+LAH	12(4′)	2(1′)	17%
CRBBB+LPH	2(2′)	0	0%
2° HV block	3	3	100%
3° HV block	2	2	100%

″ with BBB
′ HV prolonged

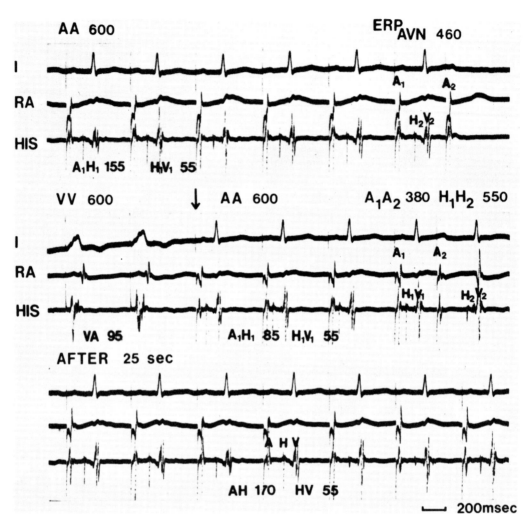

Fig. 9. Influence of ventricular pacing upon A-V nodal conduction properties. In the upper panel the A-H and H-V intervals (resp. 155 and 55 msec) and the effective refractory period of the A-V node (ERP$_{AVN}$: 480 msec), at atrial pacing with a cycle length of 600 msec during the control period are shown. The middle panel shows the transition of ventricular pacing of a few minutes duration at the same driving rate into atrial pacing. The A-H interval is now 85 msec, the H-V interval is unchanged. An atrial test stimulus A$_2$ with an 80 msec shorter coupling interval than the ERP$_{AVN}$ during the control period is now conducted successfully through the A-V node. After 25 sec the A-H interval has increased to 170 msec (lower panel).

depressed A-V nodal conduction. The upper panel shows the A-H interval (155 msec) and the effective refractory period of the A-V node (460 msec) at atrial pacing with a cycle length of 600 msec. In the middle strip the transition from ventricular pacing of a few minutes duration into atrial pacing with the same cycle length of 600 msec is shown. The A-H interval after ventricular pacing is 70 msec shorter than before (resp. 85 and 155 msec). It is also shown, that an atrial premature beat A$_2$ with a A$_1$-A$_2$ interval which is 80 msec shorter than that of the effective refractory period of the A-V node during the control period is now conducted succesfully through the A-V node. Twenty-five seconds after

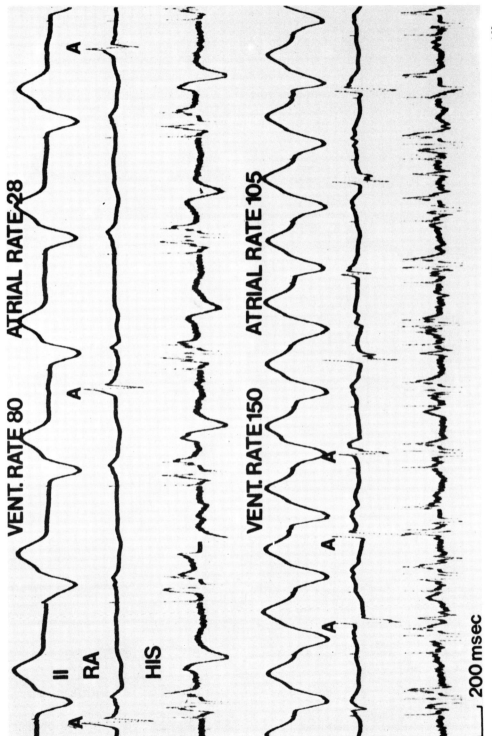

Fig. 10. Sinus bradycardia. No V-A conduction. Atrial rate at ventricular pacing rate 80:28. On increasing the ventricular rate to 150 the atrial rate rises to 105.

498 R. M. SCHUILENBURG

ventricular pacing the A-H interval has again a duration comparable to that before ventricular pacing. Similar results were obtained in the three other patients studied in this way. These findings indicate that ventricular pacing may alter the functional state of the A-V node prevailing during atrial pacing at the same rate in a positive sense. In the same way rapid ventricular pacing may influence sinus nodal function. This is shown in figure 10 of a patient with sinus bradycardia and no V-A conduction. On increasing the ventricular rate from 80 to 150 the atrial rats rose from 28 to 105.

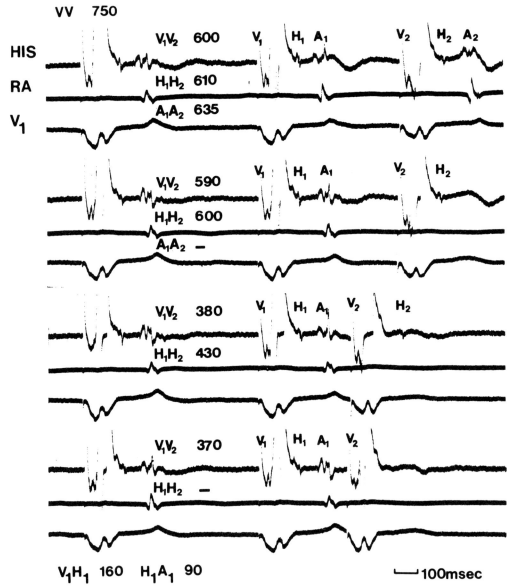

Fig. 11. Complete right bundle branch block. Ventricular pacing with cycle length 750 msec. The V_2-A_2 conduction delay of a premature ventricular beat V_2 with coupling interval 600 msec (upper panel) is partly due to a lengthening of H_2-A_2, partly to a lengthening of V_2-H_2. The retrograde effective refractory period of the A-V node is reached at V_1-V_2 590 (second panel). Further shortening of V_1-V_2 results in widening of V_2-H_2 until V_2-H_2 block occurs at V_1-V_2 370 (third and fourth panel).

2. Response to the single test stimulus method

In this test a single stimulus (V_2) was applied to the ventricle after each eighth beat (V_1) of a regularly driven ventricular rhythm. The coupling interval V_1-V_2 was gradually diminished. The usual response in this test is, that the V_2-A_2 interval lengthens as the V_1-V_2 interval shortens. This lengthening of the V_2-A_2 interval may be due to an increase of the conduction times through the A-V node as well as through the bundle branch-Purkinje system. An example is given in figure 11 of a patient with a complete right bundle branch

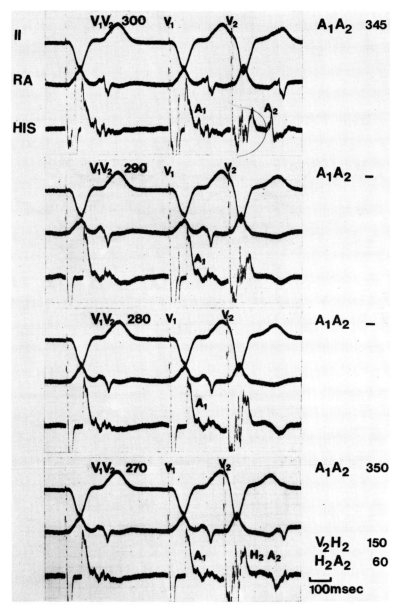

Fig. 12. Retrograde gap phenomenon. No V_2-A_2 conduction takes place at V_1-V_2 coupling intervals 290 and 280. Resumption of V_2-A_2 conduction occurs at V_1-V_2 270, due to lengthening of the V_2-H_2 conduction time.

block in whom retrograde His potentials could be identified in the basic rhythm. In the upper panel the widening of the A_1-A_2 interval as compared to the V_1-V_2 interval can be seen to be caused partly by a widening of the H_1-H_2 interval. At a critical H_1-H_2 interval V_2-A_2 conduction is blocked in the A-V node (second panel). Further shortening of V_1-V_2 results in a further increase of the V_2-H_2 interval, until ultimately the V_2 impulse is blocked at a level below the His bundle (lower panel).

This conduction delay below the His bundle at short coupling intervals may, if it is pronounced, lead to resumption of previously blocked conduction through the A-V node, like is shown in figure 12. This so-called *gap phenomenon*, which has been described earlier by Damato's group (8), can be observed relatively frequently. We have found it in 20% of our patients with V-A conduction. It occurred in 17% of the cases with normal antegrade conduction.

In a few patients (5%) the V_2-A_2 interval was found to remain constant. In all of them the

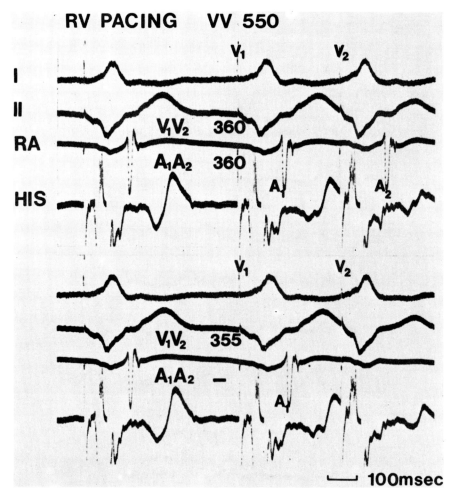

Fig. 13. No V-A conduction delay of ventricular premature beats with coupling intervals down to that at which the V_2-A_2 conduction is blocked.

V-A interval was also constant during incremental ventricular pacing. In the patient of figure 13, who had an antegrade 2:1 H-V block and complete right bundle branch block and left posterior hemiblock of the conducted beats, the V_2-A_2 interval remained constant until the retrograde effective refractory period was reached. The V_2-A_2 block was localized

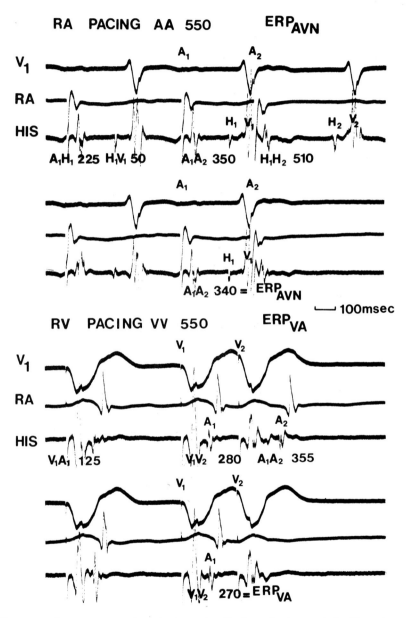

Fig. 14. Discrepancy between antegrade and retrograde effective refractory periods. Upper two panels: effective refractory period of A-V node at atrial pacing with cycle length 550: 340 msec. Antegrade block takes place in the A-V node. Lower two panels: effective refractory period of retrograde conduction at ventricular pacing with the same rate: 270 msec. Note that on atrial pacing the A-V interval is 275 msec and on ventricular pacing the V-A interval 125 msec.

below the level of the A-V node, as could be demonstrated with an atrial test stimulus A_3 as described above.

Comparison in 89 patients with 1:1 A-V conduction of the effective refractory period of the conduction system in retrograde direction (ERP_{VA}) with that of the weakest link in antegrade direction (ERP_{AV}) at the same stimulation rate yielded a percentage of 43% in which the ERP_{VA} was shorter than the ERP_{AV}, while the outcome was reversed in 42%. In 15% both values were equal. Further studies are in progress to identify the weakest link in the retrograde conduction of premature ventricular beats and to compare it with that in the antegrade conduction of premature atrial beats.

Figure 14 gives an example of a patient, in whom the ERP_{VA} was 70 msec shorter than

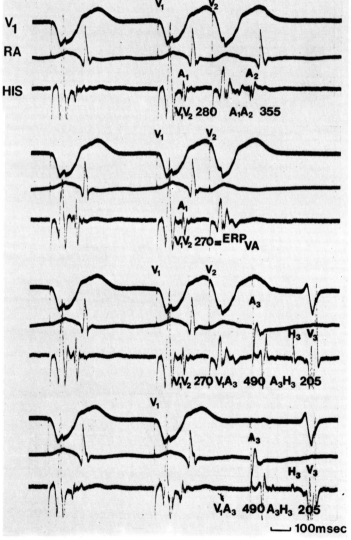

Fig. 15. Same patient as in figure 14. Test stimulus A_3 is used to eludicate location of V_2-A_2 block at the ERP_{VA} (third and fourth panel). Since the presence of V_2 has no influence upon the A_3-H_3 conduction time, the V_2-A_2 block occurred in the bundle branch system or the distal part of the His bundle.

the ERP_{AV}. Note the difference of 150 msec between the A-V and V-A intervals of the beats of the basic rhythm. While the A-V node proved to be the weakest link in the antegrade conduction, it could be demonstrated with an atrial test stimulus A_3 that the V_2-A_2 block took place at a subnodal level (fig. 15).

A few remarks on two phenomena, which may be observed during ventricular premature stimulation.

The first is the *ventricular echo phenomenon* in which re-excitation of the ventricle takes place presumably due to longitudinal dissociation in the upper part of the A-V node (742, 743). This was found in 20% of our material. The second phenomenon is that of the *ventricular re-entry* occurring in the His-Purkinje system (9). This type of ventricular re-excitation takes place at shorter coupling intervals than the fore-mentioned ventricular echo beats, it is related to a critical lengthening of the V_2-H_2 interval in 90% and the re-entrant beat has a QRS configuration which resembles that of the stimulated beats. In 10% there was no His potential interposed between V_2 and the re-entry beat. In the total material of 182 patients studied with the single test stimulus method, we observed this phenomenon in 25% regardless whether V-A conduction was present or absent.

In conclusion, the findings of this study indicate that the characteristics of ventriculo-atrial conduction are often markedly different from those of atrio-ventricular conduction. The functional properties of the conduction system during retrograde conduction can not be predicted with certainty from the results of a study of antegrade conduction. This holds especially in patients with normal A-V conduction or conduction disturbances at the His bundle-bundle branch level. Further work has to be done to clarify the underlying mechanism of these differences.

28
GAP PHENOMENA: ANTEGRADE AND RETROGRADE[1]

ANTHONY N. DAMATO, M.D., MASOOD AKHTAR, M.D., JEREMY RUSKIN, M.D.,
ANTONIO CARACTA, M.D., AND SUN H. LAU, M.D.

The phenomenon of 'Gap in A-V Conduction' was originally described by Moe and associates (559). During experiments designed to evaluate conduction characteristics with the canine heart, it was noted that premature atrial beats evoked progressively earlier in the cardiac cycle conducted to the ventricles with prolonged P-R intervals. With decreasing prematurity a zone within the cardiac cycle was reached where in premature atrial responses no longer conducted to the ventricles. However, as the atrial responses were made even more premature, conduction resumed. Within this context, the term 'gap in A-V conduction' as originally used, defined a zone within the cardiac cycle where in premature atrial impulses failed to evoke ventricular responses while atrial beats of greater and lesser prematurity did.

The application of His bundle recordings has aided significantly in the understanding of the mechanisms responsible for antegrade and retrograde gap phenomena.

To date, a total of six types of gaps have been described for antegrade conduction and two for retrograde conduction (5,7,8,10,102,222,289,927,946).

METHODS

The techniques used to study gap phenomena in the human heart have been previously described (927). Essentially, it involves recording bundle of His activity from an electrode catheter positioned in the region of the tricuspid valve. For the study of gaps during antegrade conduction, the atria are driven at a basic cycle length (A_1-A_1) and premature atrial beats (A_2) are elicited at progressively decreasing A_1-A_2 intervals up to the point of atrial refractoriness. For the study of gaps in V-A conduction, the right ventricle is driven at a basic cycle length (V_1-V_1) and premature ventricular beats elicited at progressively decreasing V_1-V_2 intervals up to the point of ventricular muscle refractoriness.

DEFINITIONS

A_1, H_1, V_1: The atrial, His bundle, and ventricular depolarizations during the basic atrial drive.

A_2, H_2, V_2: The atrial, His bundle, and ventricular depolarizations resulting from coupled premature atrial stimulation.

1. This work was supported in part by Bureau of Medical Services Grant Py76–1 and National Heart and Lung Institute Grant No. HL-12536-05.

Effective refractory period (ERP) of the atrioventricular (A-V) conduction system
The longest $A_1 A_2$ interval at which A_2 fails to evoke a ventricular response.

ERP of the atrium
The longest $S_1 S_2$ interval at which S_2 does not cause an atrial depolarization.

ERP of the A-V node
The longest $A_1 A_2$ interval at which A_2 does not conduct to the bundle of His.

ERP of the His-Purkinje system (HPS)
The longest $H_1 H_2$ interval at which A_2 blocks within the HPS.

Functional refractory period (FRP) of the atrioventricular (A-V) conduction system
The shortest $V_1 V_2$ interval in response to a given range of $A_1 A_2$ intervals.

FRP of the A-V node
The shortest $H_1 H_2$ interval in response to two successive atrial impulses both propagated through the A-V node.

FRP of the His-Purkinje system
The shortest $V_1 V_2$ interval in response to two successive atrial impulses, both propagated through the bundle of His.

Relative refractory period (RRP) of the HPS
The longest $H_1 H_2$ interval at which H_2 conducts to the ventricles with a longer H-V time than the basic drive beat or with a QRS of aberrant configuration.

Retrograde conduction
The onset of induced ventricular depolarization was measured from the corresponding stimulus artifact. Ventriculo-atrial intervals were measured from the corresponding stimulus artifact to the onset of low atrial electrogram.

Retrograde refractory period measurements
The retrograde His deflection for the basic drive beats during 1:1 V-A conduction was obscured by the ventricular electrogram and could not be identified. Data from experimental studies indicate that for the basic ventricular drive beats the interval between the stimulus artifact and the retrograde His deflection is constant. Thus, H_1, was taken from the onset of ventricular activation of the last beat of the basic drive (V_1). During ventricular premature stimulation, the retrograde His deflection emerged from the ventricular electrogram and was identified by its morphology and expected physiologic behavior. For purposes of comparison, $V_1 H_2$ can be used interchangeably with $H_1 H_2$ intervals, since the former interval always exceeds the latter by a constant amount. The following definition of terms during retrograde refractory period studies applies to conduction through the normal pathways in the absence of functional bypass tracts.

Effective refractory period (ERP) of the ventriculo-atrial (V-A) conduction system
The longest $V_1 V_2$ interval at which V_2 fails to propagate the atria.

ERP of the A-V node
The longest $V_1 H_2$ interval at which the retrograde His bundle deflection of the premature beat (H_2) is not followed by atrial depolarization.

ERP of the HPS
The longest $V_1 V_2$ interval at which the premature impulse blocks within the HPS. This can be determined only if the retrograde His bundle deflection of the premature beat is clearly identifiable prior to the blocked beats.

ERP of the ventricular myocardium
Longest $S_1 S_2$ interval at which S_2 does not evoke a ventricular response.

Functional refractory period (FRP) of the V-A conduction system
The minimum interval between two successive atrial responses $(A_1 A_2)$, both propagated from the ventricle.

FRP of the A-V node
The shortest $A_1 A_2$ interval in response to two successive retrograde impulses, both propagated from the His bundle.

FRP of the HPS
The shortest $V_1 H_2$ interval in response to any $V_1 V_2$ intervals.

RESULTS

For the purposes of this presentation, the various gaps occurring during antegrade and retrograde conduction will be arbitrarily designated numerically.

Type 1 gap in A-V conduction
Figure 1 is an example of a so-called Type I gap in A-V conduction (327). At an $A_1 A_2$ coupling interval of 445 msec (panel B), A_2 initially blocks within the HPS. The ERP of the HPS is encountered at an $H_1 H_2$ interval of 510 msec. At shorter coupling intervals $(A_1 A_2$ 400-360) A-V conduction resumes because A_2 encounters sufficient A-V nodal delay that the resultant H_1-H_2 intervals (545 and 515) are now outside the ERP of the HPS. Very often, though not always, the QRS complex during resumed A-V conduction is normal because the degree of A-V nodal delay is of such magnitude that the resultant H_1-H_2 interval is greater than the relative refractory period of the HPS (panel C).

Demonstration of a Type I gap requires that the ERP of the HPS exceed the ERP of both the atrium and A-V and the FRP of the A-V node. These requirements also apply to Types 2 and 3 gap phenomena. Figure 2 is a plot of a Type I gap depicting the relationships between $A_1 A_2$ intervals and corresponding $H_1 H_2$ and V_1-V_2 intervals.

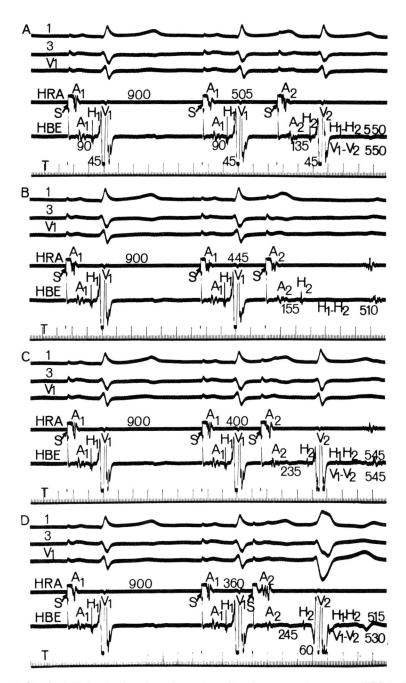

Fig. 1. Type 1 Gap in A-V Conduction. In each panel, tracings from top to bottom are: ECG leads 1, 3 and V_1, a high right atrial electrogram (HRA), His bundle electrogram tracing (HBE) and time lines at 10 and 100 msec. A_1, H_1, V_1 are the atrial His bundle and ventricular electrograms of the basic drive beats. A_2, H_2, V_2 are the atrial, His bundle and ventricular electrograms of the premature beats. S denotes stimulus artifact. Similar abbreviations will be used for subsequent figures. The basic drive rate (A_1A_1) is 900 msec and premature atrial depolarizations (A_2) are elicited progressively earlier (505–360 msec). In Panel B, A_2 blocks within the His-Purkinje system. The ERP of the HPS is encountered at an H_1H_2 interval of 510 msec. In Panels C and D, A-V conduction resumes at shorter A_1A_2 intervals (400 and 360). Note the increase in A-V nodal delay (235 and 245 msec). The resultant H_1H_2 intervals (545 and 515) are now outside the ERP of the HPS. Note that during resumption of A-V conduction, the QRS complexes may be normal (Panel C) or abnormal (Panel D). (From Akhtar et al., *Circulation* 44, 624, 1974).

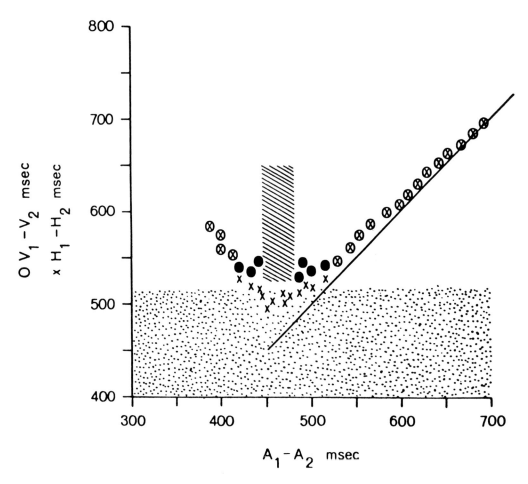

Fig. 2. Plot of a Type 1 gap in A-V conduction (not the same patient as shown in figure 1) at a basic cycle length of 900 msec. A_1A_2 intervals are plotted on the abscissa and the H_1H_2 intervals (X) and V_1V_2 (O) plotted on the ordinate. Conduction delay of premature atrial impulses occurred only in the A-V node at A_1-A_2 intervals of 650 to 525 msec, as indicated by deviation of the descending limb of the curve from the line of no A-V conduction delay (H_1-H_2 and V_1-V_2 intervals were identical). At an A_1-A_2 interval of 525 msec, conduction delay of A_2 also began to occur in the ventricular specialized conduction system (VSCS), as indicated by the differences in the V_1-V_2 and H_1-H_2 intervals. An aberrant QRS complex on the ECG is indicated by the solid circles. At A_1-A_2 intervals of 480 to 440 msec, A_2 was not conducted to the ventricles and the gap in A-V conduction occurred (diagonal lines). During the gap, A_2 still conducted to the bundle of His as indicated by the Xs. The gap occurred at H_1-H_2 intervals of less than 513 msec which is within the effective refractory period of the VSCS (stippled area). At the end of the gap, H_1-H_2 intervals increased to values greater than 513 msec and conduction to the ventricles resumed. (From Wit et al. *Circulat. Res.* 27: 679, 1970).

Type 2 gap in A-V conduction

Figure 3 is an example of a Type 2 gap in A-V conduction. In this form of gap, the ERP of the HPS also exceeds both the ERP and FRP of the A-V node and consequently A_2 initially blocks within the HPS. However, unlike Type I gap, A-V conduction resumes at shorter and not longer H_1-H_2 intervals. Thus, the A-V node is eliminated as the site of proximal delay accounting for resumption of conduction. Resumption of conduction at shorter

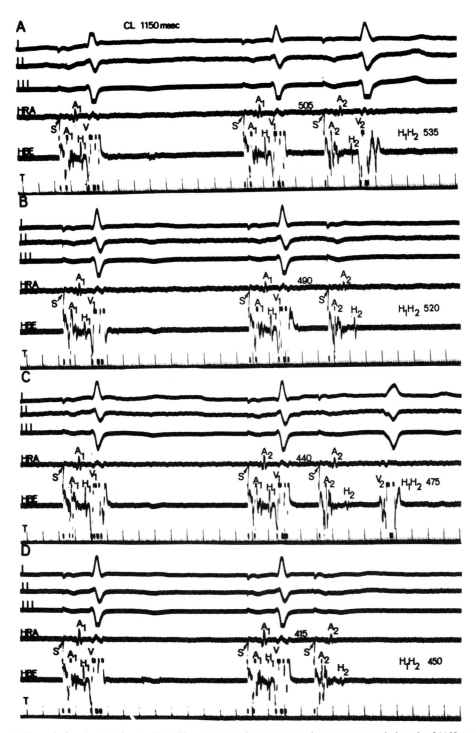

Fig. 3. Type 2 Gap in A-V Conduction. The coronary sinus was paced at constant cycle length of 1150 msec. Note the low to high sequence of atrial activation and inverted P waves in leads 2 and 3. The ERP of some portion of His-Purkinje system is encountered at an H_1 H_2 interval of 520 msec (panel B). At closer A_1 A_2 intervals (panel C) resumption of A-V conduction occurs at a shorter H_1 H_2 interval (475 msec) and is associated with a prolonged H_2 V_2 interval. It is postulated that because A_2 arrives earlier within the HPS it encounters proximal delay thereby allowing the more distal area (i.e. the initial site of block) time to recover. In panel D, the ERP of a more proximal region of the HPS is encountered at an H_1H_2 interval of 450 msec.

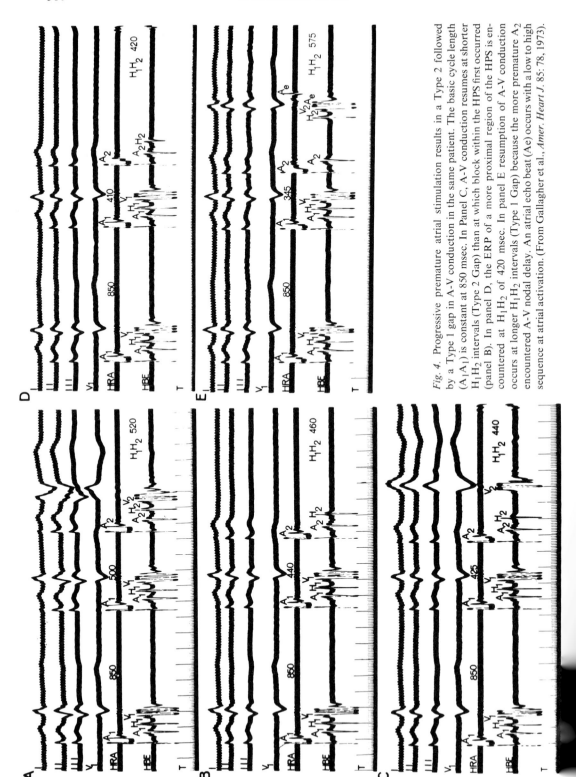

Fig. 4. Progressive premature atrial stimulation results in a Type 2 followed by a Type 1 gap in A–V conduction in the same patient. The basic cycle length (A_1A_1) is constant at 850 msec. In Panel C, A–V conduction resumes at shorter H_1H_2 intervals (Type 2 Gap) than at which block within the HPS first occurred (panel B). In panel D, the ERP of a more proximal region of the HPS is encountered at H_1H_2 of 420 msec. In panel E resumption of A–V conduction occurs at longer H_1H_2 intervals (Type 1 Gap) because the more premature A_2 encountered A–V nodal delay. An atrial echo beat (Ae) occurs with a low to high sequence at atrial activation. (From Gallagher et al., *Amer. Heart J.* 85: 78, 1973).

H_1-H_2 intervals in association with long H_2-V_2 intervals suggests that some portion of the distal His-Purkinje system was the site of initial block and that the requisite delay occurred at a more proximal site within the HPS. The site of proximal delay is probably within the bundle branches rather than the bundle of His itself because the latter (as will be shown below) usually results in so-called split His bundle deflections (H-H′). Almost without exception, the QRS complexes during the period of resumed conduction in Type 2 A-V gap are aberrant.

Figure 4 illustrates both a type 2 and Type 1 gap in A-V conduction occurring consecutively in the same patient during progressive premature atrial stimulation (289).

Type 3 gap in A-V conduction
In type 3 gap, the site of initial block is within the His-Purkinje system and the site of proximal delay which accounts for resumption of conduction is within the bundle of His itself (946). This is reflected in so-called split His bundle deflections ($H_2 H_2'$) an example of which is illustrated in figure 5. During resumed A-V conduction, the $H_1 H_2$ interval exceeds the $H_1 H_2$ interval at which A_2 initially blocked within the HPS. If, for one of several possible reasons, the second of the split His bundle deflections (H_2') is not recorded, the electrophysiological findings in Type 3 gap would be identical to those in Type 2 gap.

Type 4 gap in A-V conduction
Infrequently we have observed a possible fourth type of gap in A-V conduction (fig. 6) characterized by the following: (a) During the gap zone, non-conducted atrial premature beats are not followed by His bundle deflections implying that block occurred because the ERP of some portion of the A-V node was encountered. (b) During the period of resumed A-V conduction, the more closely coupled premature atrial beats are conducted with prolonged A-H intervals and the QRS complexes are similar to those of the basic drive beat. It is possible that this form of gap results because the site of initial block is within a distal portion of the A-V node and at closer coupling intervals conduction delay occurred within a more proximal region of the A-V node thereby allowing the more distal area time to recover.

Alternative explanations for the phenomenon illustrated in figure 6 include the following: 1. During the gap zone, block is occurring within the proximal portion of the bundle of His, the electrical activity of which is insufficient to generate a recordable electrogram. Resumption of conduction occurs because of proximal delay occurring within the A-V node. Thus, this would be a subtle form of Type 1 gap. 2. What appears to be a conducted beat is in reality a junctional escape beat and therefore resumption of conduction is spurious. However, the alternative of a spurious gap is a less attractive possibility when it is observed that longer post-extrasystolic intervals are always terminated by sinus escape beats, never by junctional escape beats and the gap phenomenon is reproducible upon repeat atrial scanning. 3. Dual A-V nodal pathways, as originally proposed by Moe and associates (559), and as illustrated in figure 7, offers a third possible explanation of this phenomenon. During the gap zone, atrial premature beats conduct along a fast pathway and block within an A-V nodal final common pathway. Impulses conducting simultaneously along the slow pathway, encounter refractory tissue. During the period of resumed

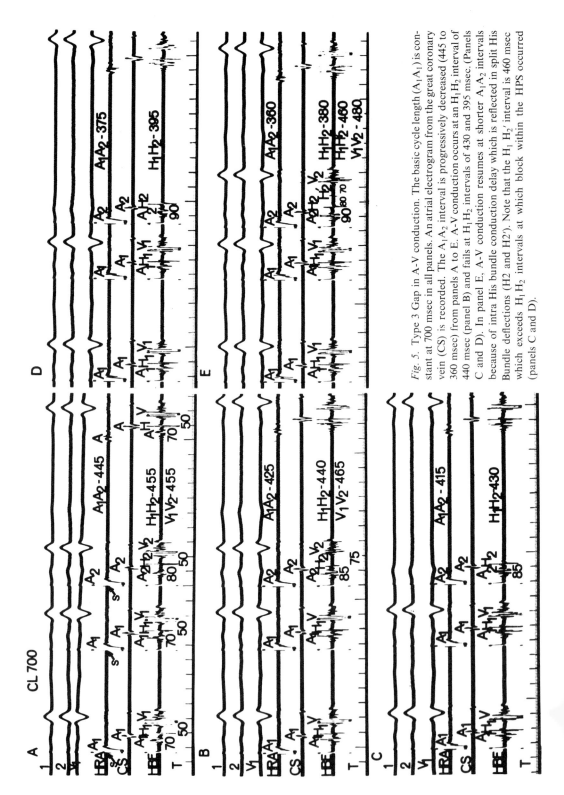

Fig. 5. Type 3 Gap in A–V conduction. The basic cycle length (A_1A_1) is constant at 700 msec in all panels. An atrial electrogram from the great coronary vein (CS) is recorded. The A_1A_2 interval is progressively decreased (445 to 360 msec) from panels A to E. A–V conduction occurs at an H_1H_2 interval of 440 msec (panel B) and fails at H_1H_2 intervals of 430 and 395 msec. (Panels C and D). In panel E, A–V conduction resumes at shorter A_1A_2 intervals because of intra His bundle conduction delay which is reflected in split His Bundle deflections (H2 and H2'). Note that the H_1 H_2' interval is 460 msec which exceeds H_1 H_2 intervals at which block within the HPS occurred (panels C and D).

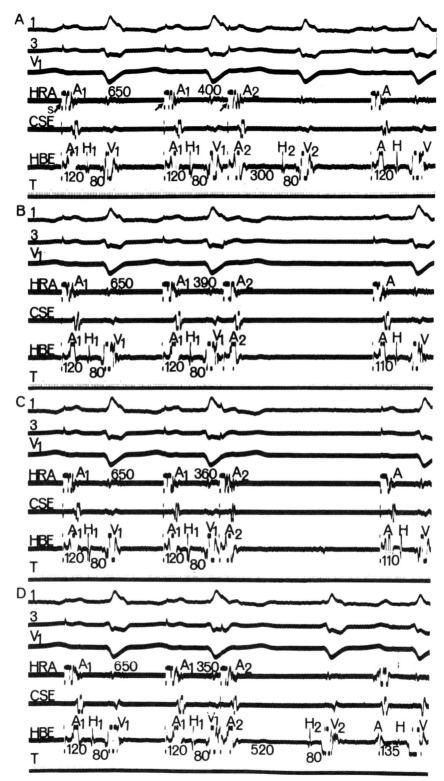

Fig. 6. Type 4 gap in A-V conduction. In panels B and C A_2 presumably blocks in the Distal A-V node and in panel D, resumption of conduction occurs presumably because of delay occurring within a more proximal region of the A-V node. See text for discussion.

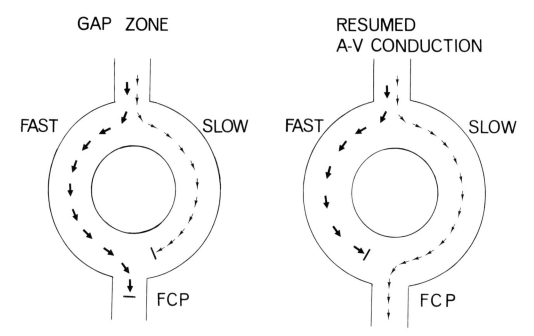

Fig. 7. Schematic representation of an alternative theoretical explanation for Type 4 gap in A-V conduction involving fast, slow and final common pathways (FCP), all within the A-V node. During the gap zone, A_2 blocks within the FCP of the A-V node, after reaching it by the fast pathway. The impulse traveling the slow pathway finds the FCP refractory. During resumed A-V conduction the earlier A_2 blocks proximal to the FCP leaving the latter available to conduct an impulse traveling the slow pathway.

A-V conduction, the more premature atrial impulses block within the fast pathway leaving the final common pathway available for the impulse traversing the slow pathway to activate the ventricles.

Type 5 gap in A-V conduction
A fifth type of gap has been described by Wu and associates (946). During the zone of no A-V conduction, atrial premature beats may block within the A-V node or HPS. Resumption of conduction occurs because intra-atrial delay (i.e. from the high right atrium, which is the site of stimulation, to the low right atrium) permits later arrival of the impulse at the site of initial block. A pseudo form of this type of gap is illustrated in figure 8. It is to be noted that during resumed A-V conduction, latency exists between the stimulus artifact and the atrial responses which causes the $A_1 A_2$ interval to equal values to the right of the gap zone (see fig. 2). Strictly speaking, therefore, it is questionable whether the findings in figure 8 qualify as a gap phenomenon since atrial responses of less prematurity were not achieved.

Type 6 gap in A-V conduction
Castellanos and Associates (5) described in patients with Mobitz Type II A-V block a form of gap in which the duration of the periods of A-V and no A-V conduction were reversed; the gap zone extended for several hundred milliseconds whereas the period of A-V conduc-

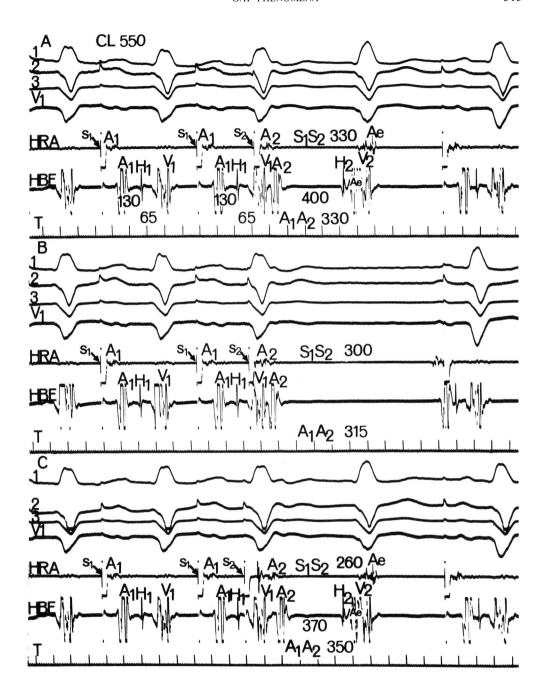

Fig. 8. Pseudo Type 5 gap in A-V conduction. The atrium is prematurely stimulated (S₂) at progressively decreasing S₁S₂ intervals. In Panel A, S₁ S₂ and the resultant A₁ A₂ intervals are the same (330 msec). A-V conduction occurs followed by an atrial echo beat (Ae). In panel B, a 15 msec latency exists between S₂ and the A₂ response which blocks in the A-V node. In panel C, a 90 msec latency exists between S₂ and the A₂ response. This results in an A₁ A₂ response of 350 msec which explains why A-V conduction resumed.

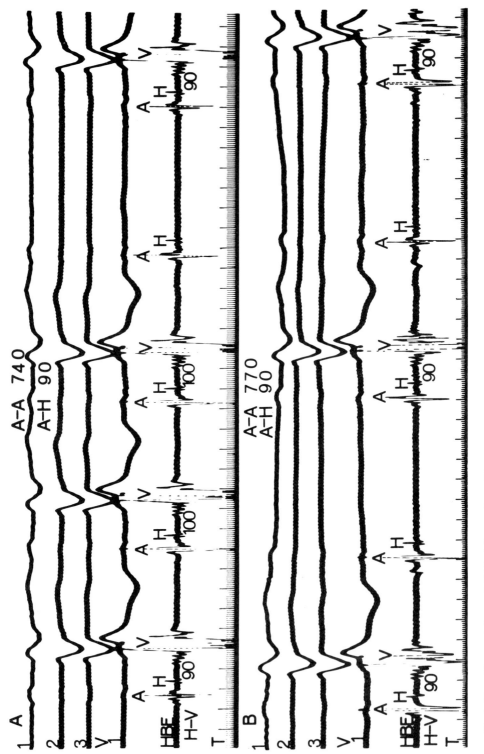

Fig. 9. Type II second degree A-V block in a patient with RBBB-LAH. Panel A shows that at a sinus cycle length of 740 msec the fourth P wave blocks within the His-Purkinje system. The H-V interval of conducted beats is variably prolonged between 90–100 msec. In panel B 2:1 block within the His-Purkinje system is present.

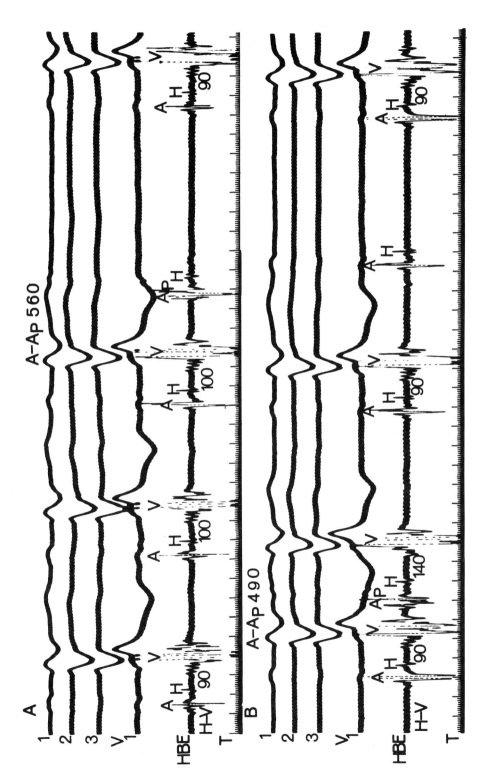

Fig. 10. (same patient as in figure 9). In panel A, a premature atrial beat (Ap) occurring 560 msec after the third sinus beat fails to conduct to the ventricles. In panel B, a more premature atrial beat (A-Ap 490) conducts to the ventricles with a prolonged H-V interval (140 msec).

tion at very close A_1-A_2 intervals was extremely narrow (fig. 9 and 10). Although A-V conduction always occurred at H_1-H_2 intervals which were significantly less than those at which block occurred, it is obvious that proximal delay allowing distal recovery is not the mechanism for this type of gap. Resumption of A-V conduction is more in keeping with the phenomenon of supernormality.

Demonstration of gap phenomena is not possible in every patient in whom the ERP of the HPS is greater than the ERP of the A-V node. Gap phenomena may not be demonstrated because: 1. atrial refractoriness occurs before a sufficient delay in a proximal region can be achieved; or 2. the ERP of the A-V node is only slightly less than the ERP of the HPS and decreasing the A_1-A_2 interval results in block in the A-V node. Figure 11 is an example in which atrial refractoriness precluded demonstration of an A-V gap after the ERP of the HPS had been reached.

Masking of gap phenomena
Since the more commonly encountered gaps in A-V conduction, namely Types 1, 2 and 3, are dependent upon the ERP of the HPS exceeding the FRP of the A-V node, it is apparent that alterations in the relationship between refractoriness of various part of the A-V conducting system can significantly modify demonstration of gaps.

Decreases in the basic cycle length invariably lead to abolishment of gap phenomena primarily because the ERP of the HPS decreases to a value less than the FRP of the A-V node. The effect of cycle length is demonstrated in figures 12 and 13.

Alternatively, if the FRP of the A-V node is increased to a value greater than the ERP of the HPS, as may occur following administration of beta adrenergic blocking agents or digitalis, gap phenomena are abolished (927).

The abolishment of gaps by interventions which either shorten the ERP of the HPS or prolong the FRP of the A-V node point to the functional nature of this phenomenon. Generally speaking, long basic cycle lengths favor demonstration of gap phenomena whereas shorter cycle lengths do not.

Unmasking of gap phenomena
The unmasking of gap phenomena and the conversion of one type to another type by atropine provides further evidence in support of its functional nature (7).

Akhtar and associates studied in 9 patients the effects of small doses of atropine on gap phenomena (7). Atropine in doses of 0.2 to 0.5 mg produced a Type 1 gap in six patients in whom no gap in A-V conduction was present in control studies at comparable cycle lengths. Representative findings are illustrated in figures 14 and 15. The unmasking of gaps in A-V conduction results because atropine enhances A-V nodal conduction and decreases both the functional and effective refractory periods of the A-V node. These changes enhance the likelihood of premature atrial depolarizations being delivered to the HPS during its ERP and in addition cause very early premature atrial beats to encounter sufficient A-V nodal delay that A-V conduction resumes.

In three subjects no gap in A-V conduction was present prior to administration of atropine whereas after drug administration a Type 2 gap occurred at comparable cycle lengths.

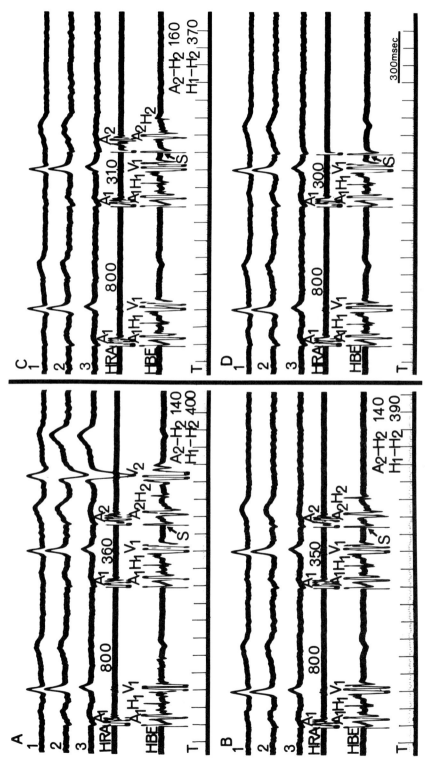

Fig. 11. Failure to demonstrate a gap phenomenon due to atrial refractoriness. Panels B and C demonstrate that the HPS has the longest ERP, which is requisite for demonstration of Types 1, 2 and 3 gaps. However, atrial refractoriness as shown in panel D (no atrial response to stimulation) precludes demonstration of any proximal delay which would allow resumption of conduction.

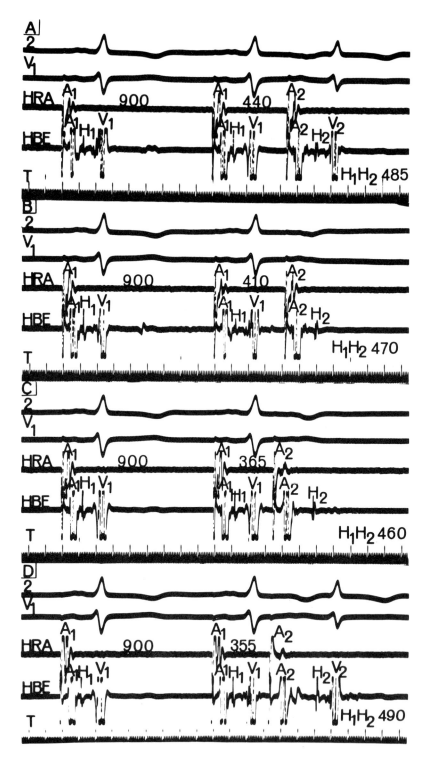

Fig. 12. A Type 1 gap in A-V conduction occurred at a basic drive rate of 900 msec. The ERP of the HPS was encountered at an $H_1 H_2$ interval of 470 msec. (panel B).

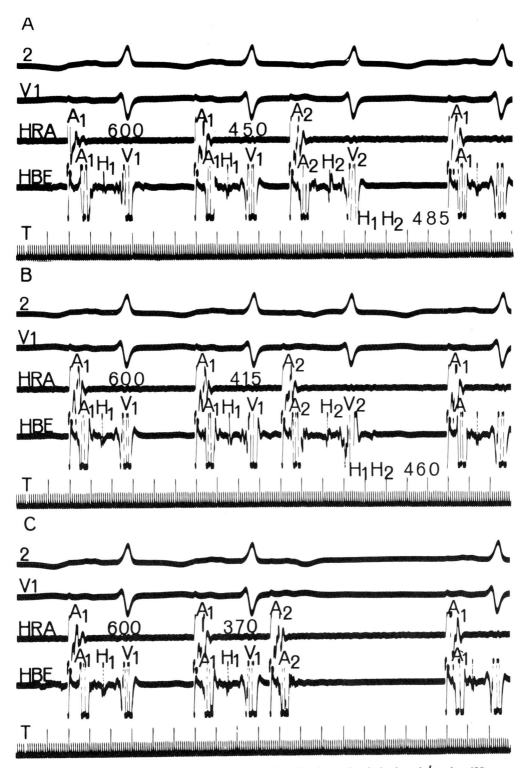

Fig. 13. (same patient as in figure 11). Type 1 gap is abolished by decreasing the basic cycle length to 600 msec. At the shorter cycle length the ERP of the HPS is decreased. Note that in panel B, A-V conduction occurs at an $H_1 H_2$ interval of 460 msec. In panel C, A_2 encountered the ERP of the A-V node.

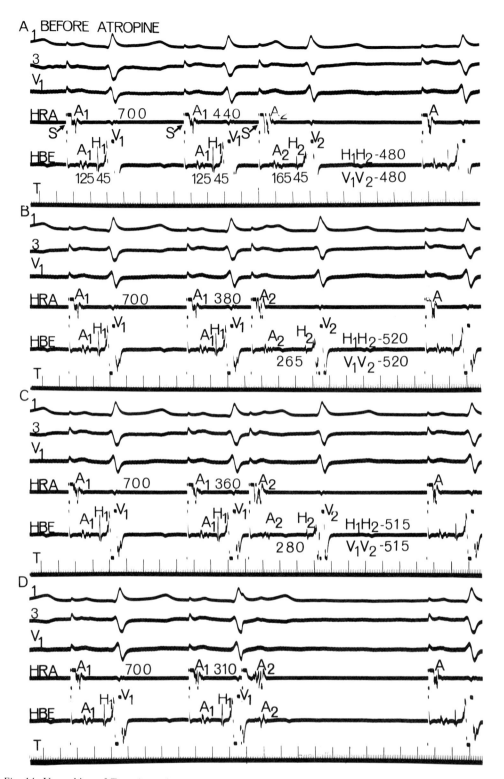

Fig. 14. Unmasking of Type 1 gap in A-V conduction. At a cycle length of 700 msec progressive premature atrial stimulation before administration of atropine fails to uncover any gap phenomena. The FRP of the A-V node (measured as the shortest $H_1 H_2$ interval) is 480 msec (panel A). The ERP of the A-V node is encountered at an $A_1 A_2$ interval of 310 msec (panel D). (From Akhtar et al., 49: 624, 1974).

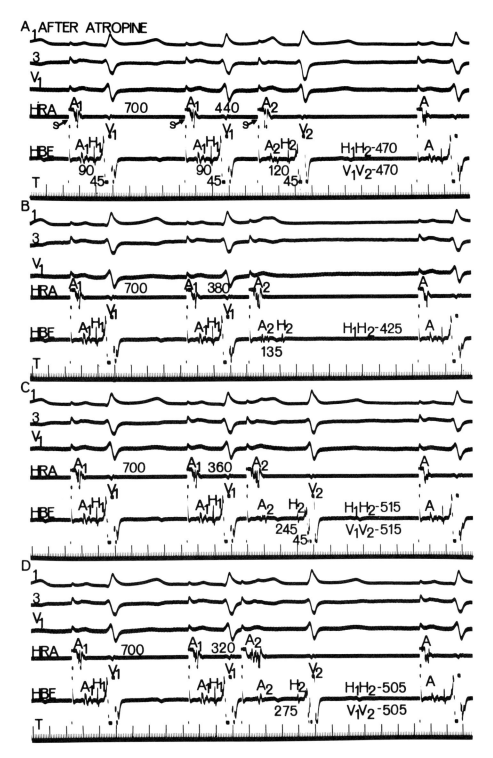

Fig. 15. Unmasking of Type 1 gap in A-V conduction. Same patient as in figure 14 after administration of atropine. Atropine shortens the FRP of the A-V node thereby permitting the A_2 impulse to encounter the ERP of the HPS (panel B) which was measured at an $H_1 H_2$ interval of 425 msec. As the $A_1 A_2$ interval was decreased (panels C and D), A_2 encountered A-V nodal delay and A-V conduction resumed because the resultant $H_1 H_2$ intervals were greater than the ERP of the HPS. (From Akhtar et al., 49: 624, 1974).

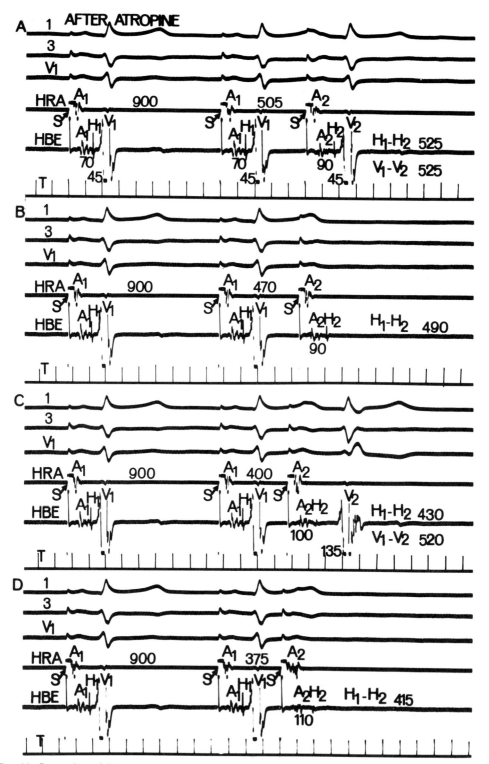

Fig. 16. Conversion of Type 1 into a Type 2 gap in A-V conduction, (same patient as in figure 1 which shows a Type 1 gap). Atropine, by virtue of decreasing the FRP of the A-V node permits the attainment of shorter $H_1 H_2$ intervals. Conduction delay within the proximal HPS (panel C) permits resumption of conduction at shorter $H_1 H_2$ intervals (430 msec). (From Akhtar et al., *Circulation* 49: 624, 1974).

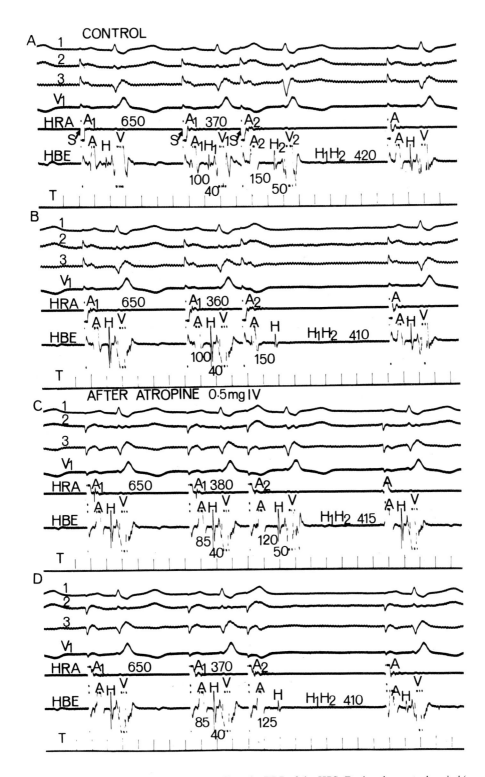

Fig. 17. Demonstration that atropine does not effect the ERP of the HPS. During the control period (panels A and B), the ERP of the HPS is encountered at an H_1 H_2 interval of 410 msec. Following 0.5 mg of atropine (panels C and D), the ERP of the HPS is the same, 410 msec (panel D). Note that atropine shortened the A-H intervals but did not alter H-V intervals.

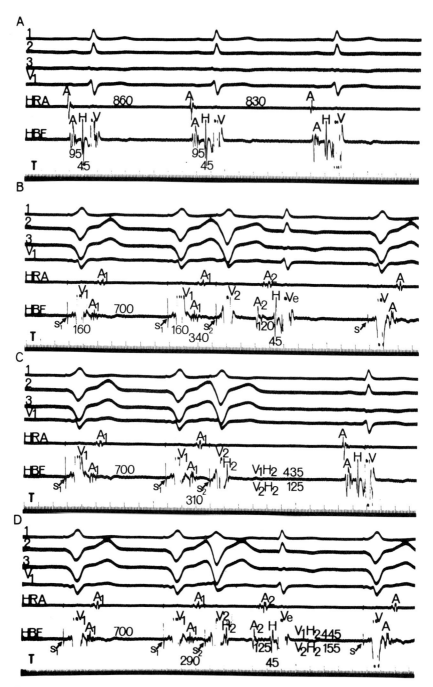

Fig. 18. The 1 gap in V-A conduction. Panel A shows sinus rhythm with normal high to low sequence of atrial activation. In panels B to D the ventricles are driven at a constant cycle length of 700 msec and prematurely stimulated (V_2) at progressively decreasing coupling intervals (V_1 V_2 340 to 290 msec). In panel B, V_2 retrogradely conducts to the atria and is followed by a ventricular echo beat (Ve) of normal QRS morphology. Note the low to high sequence of retrograde atrial activation for both the basic drive and premature beats. In panel C, V_2 is retrogradely delayed within the His Purkinje system (V_1 H_2 125 msec). The H_2 electrogram emerges from the ventricular electrogram and block occurs within the A-V node. In panel D, a closer premature ventricular beat (V_1 V_2 290 msec) encounters greater delay within the His-Purkinje system (V_2 H_2 155 msec). The later arrival of the V_2 impulse at the A-V node permits retrograde conduction to the atria followed by an echo beat (Ve).

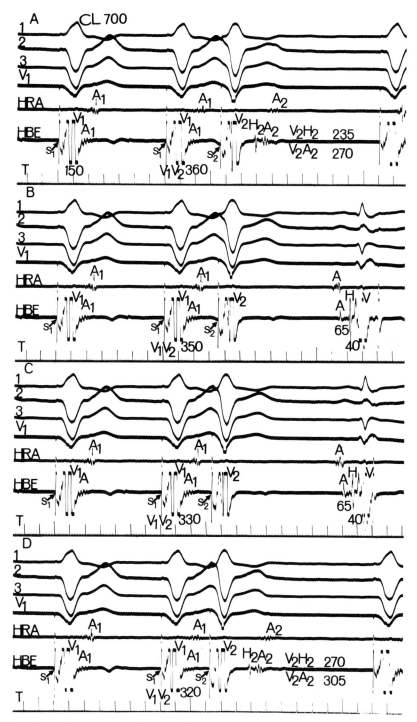

Fig. 19. Type 2 gap in V-A conduction. Ventricular drive rate is constant at 700 msec. Note low to high sequence of atrial activation. In Panel A, V_2 encounters retrograde conduction delay below the bundle of His. The $V_2 H_2$ interval is 235 msec, and retrograde activation of the atria occurs. At closer $V_1 V_2$ intervals (panels B and C), V_2 blocks within the His-Purkinje system and retrograde conduction to the atria does not occur. At a $V_1 V_2$ interval of 320 msec (panel D), V_2 encounters delay proximal to the initial site of block which allows the latter time to recover. Consequently, V-A conduction resumed. (From Akhtar et al., Circ. 49: 811, 1974).

Atropine can cause a Type 1 gap to be converted into a Type 2 gap. The patient who tracing is depicted in figure 1 (Type 1 gap) was given atropine after which a Type 2 gap resulted (fig. 16).

Since atropine has no direct effect on refractoriness of the HPS (see fig. 17) both the unmasking and conversion of gaps are the result of altering refractoriness within the A-V node (10).

Gap phenomena during retrograde conduction
Gap phenomena also occur during retrograde conduction (8). In fact, gaps during retrograde conduction occur more frequently than during antegrade conduction. Using the ventricular extrastimulus method, Akhtar and associates demonstrated two types of retrograde gaps in 6 of 12 unselected patients. In only one of these 12 patients was a gap during antegrade conduction demonstrated. The initial site of retrograde block was the A-V node in 2 patients and in the HPS in 4 patients. In both groups of patients, resumption of V-A conduction at shorter V_1-V_2 intervals occurred because of retrograde delay within the HPS.

Figure 18 illustrates an example of a retrograde gap in V-A conduction in which the initial site of block was the A-V node and resumption of conduction occurred because of retrograde delay in the HPS. A long ERP of the A-V node favors the demonstration of retrograde gaps but limits demonstration antegrade gaps.

Figure 19 illustrates an example of a retrograde gap in which the site of retrograde block was the HPS and at closer V_1-V_2 intervals, delay within the HPS resulted in resumption of conduction.

Table 1 summarizes the six types of antegrade and the two types of retrograde gaps which have thus far been observed or reported.

Table 1. Gap phenomena during A-V conduction.

Type	Site of initial block	Site of proximal delay
1	HPS	A-V node
2	HPS (distal)	HPS (proximal)
3	HPS	bundle of His
4	HPS or A-V node	atrium
5	distal A-V node	proximal A-V node
6	HPS	none (supernormality)

	Gap phenomena during V-A conduction	
Type	Site of initial block	Site of proximal delay
1	A-V node	HPS
2	HPS	HPS

29

ACCOMMODATION OF A-V NODAL CONDUCTION AND FATIGUE PHENOMENON IN THE HIS-PURKINJE SYSTEM

ONKAR S. NARULA, M.D. AND MANFRED RUNGE, M.D.

INTRODUCTION

To understand the mechanisms responsible for disturbances in cardiac rhythm and conduction, it is useful to have a working knowledge of electrophysiologic events underlying normal and abnormal impulse propagation through different segments of the A-V conducting tissue. The ability to study these events in man has been facilitated by the development of the catheter technique for recording His bundle (BH) electrograms. Artificial pacing of the human heart, by permitting variations in site, rate and duration of stimulation, when used in conjunction with BH recordings have contributed significantly to the understanding of disturbances in impulse formation and conduction.

Various characteristics of impulse transmission through the normal or abnormal A-V node and His Purkinje System (HPS) have been previously elucidated to a large extent by animal experiments and studies in man (304, 362, 364, 407, 422, 541, 548). However, certain aspects of conduction have not been systematically analyzed. The purpose of this presentation is to explicate the following two characteristics: a. the phenomenon of accommodation in the normal A-V node; and b. the "Fatigue" phenomenon in the diseased HPS.

I. ACCOMMODATION OF A-V NODAL CONDUCTION

The changes in A-V nodal conduction time associated with sustaining of an increased but constant rate have been defined as A-V nodal accommodation. These changes in A-V nodal conduction time are over and above the expected rate related increase in conduction time, since the A-V nodal conduction velocity during its relative refractory period is frequency dependent. The latter is noted in the first beat at the establishment of the new cycle length. However, the phenomenon of accommodation pertains to changes in A-V nodal conduction noted in the subsequent beats of the new cycle length. A-V nodal accommodation is related to the magnitude of increase in rate and the duration for which the increase is sustained. Except for a preliminary report from this laboratory this phenomenon has not been defined previously in man (707).

Patients with normal sinus rhythm and a normal P-R interval were studied during diagnostic right heart catheterization. Patients were studied in the postabsorptive state and were premedicated with 100 mg of Nembutal administered intramuscularly 30 minutes prior to the study. His bundle electrograms were obtained by the standard technique and A-H interval was normal in all. The recordings were made at a paper speed of 100 mm/sec.

The right atrium was stimulated at 100 and 120/min for periods of two and five minutes at each level. Continuous BH recordings were obtained before atrial pacing (AP), during AP and on termination of AP. The A-H time was measured during normal sinus rhythm, during AP in the first 10 or more paced beats and thereafter at intervals of one minute through the duration of pacing. A-H time was also measured in the sinus beats immediately following the cessation of AP.

Two types of A-V nodal conduction responses were observed as follows:

Type I: This type of response was exhibited by a majority (80%) of the cases. During AP, the first beat at the established new cycle length showed a lengthening of A-H time as compared to that of sinus beats and is a rate related phenomenon. The subsequent ten paced beats showed a gradual lengthening of A-H time despite the maintenance of a constant pacing rate and is due to A-V nodal accommodation. This increase in A-H time in the first ten paced beats was usually 15–30 msec (range 0–55 msec). Additional A-H increments of a lesser magnitude were usually observed in the subsequent beats with stabilization and occurrence of a plateau by one minute in most of the cases (fig. 1 and 2). In a few patients further A-H lengthening (range 5–65 msec) was seen between one and five minutes of pacing levels. The magnitude of total A-H lengthening was greater at higher pacing rates. For example, figure 2 shows a total increase of 35 msec in A-H time during AP at 120/min as compared to an increase of 20 msec during AP at 100/min

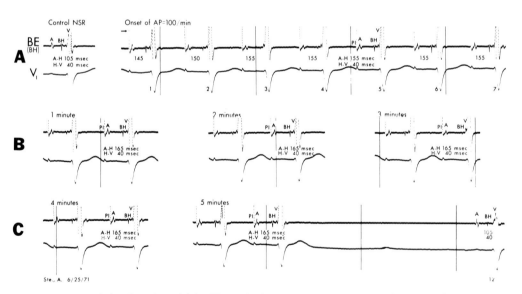

Fig. 1. Accommodation in A-V nodal (A-H) conduction and type I response during onset of atrial pacing (AP) at 100/min. *A.* First beat shows control A-H (105 msec) time during normal sinus rhythm (NSR). The beat numbered one, is not the very first paced beat but is the first paced beat after the establishment of the new atrial rate (100/min) and shows an A-H time of 145 msec. A gradual increase in A-H time (145–155 msec) is noted in the first three beats and is due to A-V nodal accommodation. *B & C.* Further increase in A-H time (155 to 165 msec) is noted after one minute of AP as compared to the seventh paced beat in panel A, despite a constant rate. This suggests additional accommodation in A-V nodal conduction reaching a plateau after one minute with a constant A-H time up to five minutes of AP (panel C). Cessation of AP is immediately followed by a return to control A-H (105 msec) time in the first sinus beat. The H-V time (40 msec) remained constant throughout.

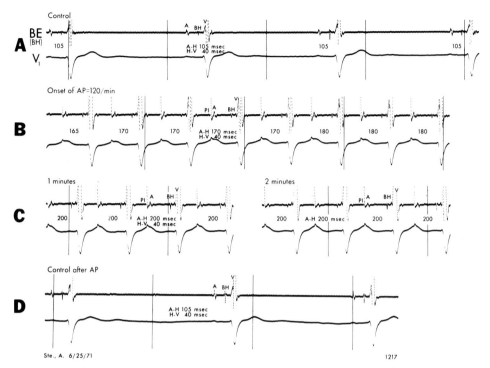

Fig. 2. Accommodation in A-H conduction with type I response during AP at 120/min. (Same patient as in fig. 1) *A*. Control recordings during sinus rhythm. *B*. A gradual lengthening of A-H time (165 to 180 msec) is noted in the first eight paced beats after the onset of AP. *C* Additional increase in A-H (180 to 200 msec) time occurs up to a level of one minute with subsequent stabilization. The total increment in A-H time (35 msec) due to A-V nodal accommodation during AP at 120/min is proportionally higher as compared to the 20 msec increase during AP at 100/min (fig. 1). This suggests that the degree of A-V nodal accommodation is to some extent rate related. *D*. The A-H conduction time after cessation of AP is similar to that of control (panel A).

seen in figure 1. In a few patients with a control normal A-H time, during continuous AP at 120/min after one or two minutes of 1:1 A-V conduction, a progression to second degree Wenckebach type I A-V block was noted despite a constant atrial rate. On the other hand, an occasional patient exhibited second degree type I A-V block initially with the onset of AP which subsequently, with continuation of pacing at a constant rate, manifested stable and persistent 1:1 A-V conduction. An example of this type of response is shown in figure 3. In a rare case the increments in A-H time subsequent to the first paced beat were absent suggesting the absence of any accommodation in A-V nodal conduction.

Type II: This type of response was seen in a small number of cases (20%). In these patients: a. subsequent to the first paced beat the A-H increments were of great proportion, and b. a wide range of wild beat to beat fluctuations in A-H time, especially during the first 30 seconds (occasionally up to two minutes) were noted prior to stabilization and occurrence of plateau at the new level (fig. 4). These fluctuations were without any cyclic or phasic pattern and were noted at more than one pacing rate. These variations in A-H time ranged from 150–225 msec in some cases. Somewhat similar observations have been

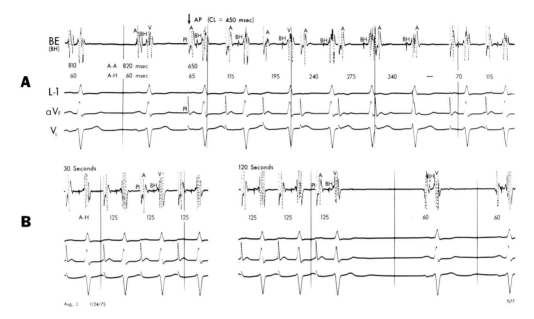

Fig. 3. An unusual response seen during accommodation in A-H conduction. *A.* First two beats show NSR with an A-H time of 60 msec. The onset of AP at a cycle length (CL) of 450 msec initially resulted in second degree type A-H block. *B.* Continuation of AP at the same cycle length after 30 seconds shows disappearance of second degree A-V block and conversion to 1:1 conduction which persisted up to two minutes. The initial development of second degree A-V block probably indicates an overshoot of the processes participating in A-V nodal accommodation which after 30 seconds stabilized to an appropriate level. This may be an intermediate response between types I and II.

reported in a brief communication by others (324). However, the latter report did not delineate the total duration of AP and the duration for which fluctuations persisted in their studies. In the studies by others, although BH recordings were not obtained and the site of fluctuations in A-V conduction time (P-R interval) cannot be localized with certainty, it may be reasonably assumed that these changes occurred in the A-V node (324).

In cases with both type I and type II responses A-H time immediately returned to control levels upon cessation of AP. In all of these patients, the H-V time remained constant throughout the study, i.e. sinus rhythm or AP.

Effect of atropine on A-V nodal accommodation

In some of the cases with type II responses subsequent to intravenous administration of atropine (1.5–2 mg) the wide fluctuations and marked increments in A-H time were abolished. Figure 5 shows a typical type II response in a patient with A-H time varying between 120 and 270 msec, whereas figure 6 shows the absence of fluctuations in A-H after atropine. In addition, only a minimal increment of 10 msec in A-H time is noted after atropine despite AP at a higher rate (120/min versus 100/min) and for a longer duration (fig. 5 and 6). The abolition of type II response and variations in A-H time suggests a major role of neurogenic mechanisms in the production of type II responses.

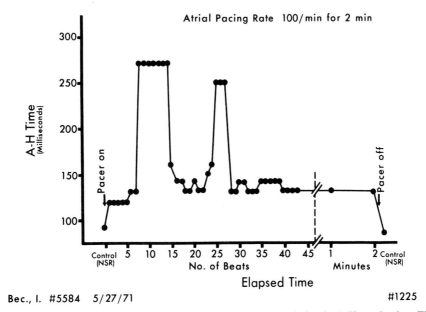

Atrial Pacing Rate 100/min for 2 min

Bec., I. #5584   5/27/71   #1225

Fig. 4. Graphic representation of a type II response during accommodation in A-H conduction. The A-H time is plotted on the vertical axis. Horizontal axis shows the first 45 paced beats (the left half) followed by the duration of AP in minutes (the right half). The control A-H time (80 msec) during NSR is normal. Onset of AP at 100/min is followed by wide swings and fluctuations of A-H time during the first 40 paced beats. Subsequently the A-H time stabilized at a level only slightly higher than the very first five paced beats.

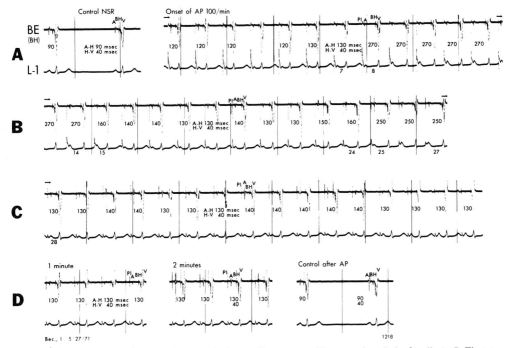

Fig. 5. His bundle recordings during a typical type II response. (Same patient is in fig. 4) *A–C.* First two beats show a control A-H time (90 msec) during NSR. Onset of AP at 100/min is followed by sudden and marked variations in A-H time (ranging between 120 and 270 msec) during the first 40 paced beats. Panels A to C show continuous recordings during atrial pacing. *D.* Subsequent recordings at one and two minute levels show stabilization of A-H time to 130 msec.

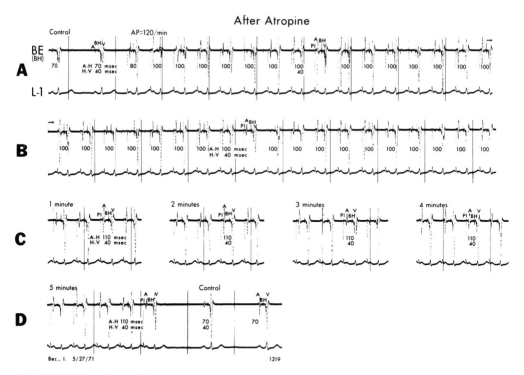

Fig. 6. Abolition of type II response or wide and sudden fluctuations in A-H time subsequent to intravenous administration of 2 mg of atropine. (Same patient as in fig. 5.) *A & B.* Continuous recordings show a stable and constant A-H time (100 msec) in the first 34 beats. following onset of AP at 120/min. *C & D.* After one minute of pacing a minimal increase (100 to 110 msec) in A-H time is seen which subsequently remained constant up to five minutes.

During type I responses the initial and gradual lengthening of A-H time prior to the occurrence of a plateau is an adaptive response in A-V nodal conduction, during alterations in atrial rate, resulting from different mechanisms. These adaptive mechanisms in all probability are comprised of a neurohumoral component and also of independent or primary A-V nodal accommodation to the changes in rate. The degree to which reflex mechanisms are mediated through the sympathetic and parasympathetic system and their precise role in the type I A-V nodal adaptive mechanisms cannot be determined from the present data as atropine was not administered to most of the cases. However, the available limited data do suggest that the A-H increments are not entirely due to vagotonia. This is supported by the demonstration of A-H lengthening (although of a smaller magnitude in some cases) despite atropine administration (fig. 7 and 8).

Clinical significance of A-V nodal accommodation
The phenomenon of A-V nodal accommodation is clinically significant under the following settings:
a. Several investigators have indicated that the manifestation of second degree type I A-H block at AP rates $\leq$ 130/min is suggestive of abnormal A-V nodal conduction (594,672). Therefore, the consideration of A-V nodal accommodation is important

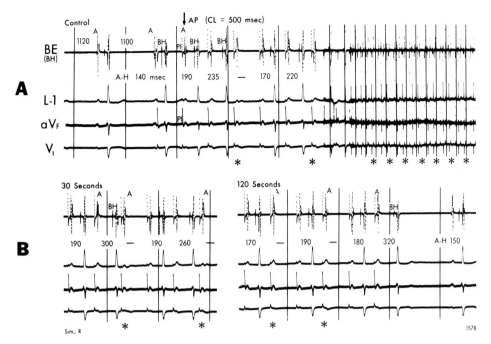

Fig. 7. During control state atrial pacing at a cycle length (CL) of 500 msec resulted in second degree type I A-H block. During the initial 30 seconds, conduction ratios were predominantly 3:2 whereas after two minutes of AP then were mostly 2:1.

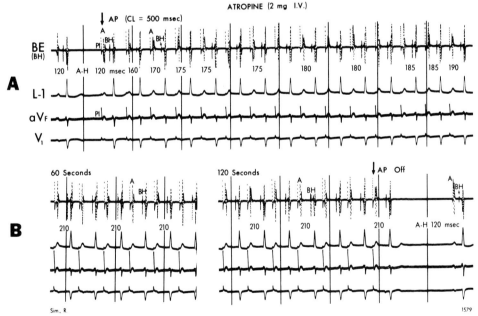

Fig. 8. Demonstration of accommodation in A-V nodal conduction following vagal block with intravenous (IV) administration of 2 mg of atropine. (Same patient as in fig. 7). A. Following onset of AP (CL = 500 msec) a gradual lengthening in A-H interval from 160 to 190 msec is noted in the initial 14 paced beats at the new cycle length. B. Additional lengthening of A-H time (from 190 to 210 msec) is manifested until the one minute level at which time a plateau effect is reached. The occurrence of A-V nodal accommodation under these settings suggests the participation of an adaptive mechanism localized with the A-V node itself.

during clinical evaluation of the A-V node by determining the AP rate at which second
degree type I A-V block is exhibited. The rate at which second degree block develops
may be modified by the magnitude of increments in the AP rate and the duration of
pacing at each level preceding a change to the next level.

b. The phenomenon of accommodation should be considered during studies evaluating
the effect of various degrees on A-V nodal conduction by utilizing the following
criteria: 1. the atrial rate at which second degree type I block occurs; 2. the A-H time
at different paced cycle lengths; and 3. the refractory periods.

c. A-V nodal accommodation may explain atypical Wenckebach periods showing a lack
of progressive or sustained lengthening of A-H or P-R intervals. (590, 591).

d. The type II responses with beat to beat fluctuations in A-H are important in clinical
interpretations of the standard ECG and may explain some of the cases reported by
others as examples of type II block in the A-V node (671). An example of such a

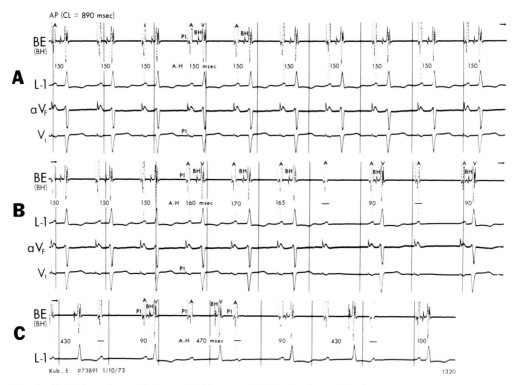

Fig. 9. Simulation of second degree Mobitz type II A-H block possibly due to accommodation in A-V
nodal conduction with a type II response. Continuous recordings from top to bottom. *A–C.* During AP
(CL = 890 msec) 1:1 A-V conduction is present for the first half of the recordings with a constant
A-H time (150 msec). A minimal increase (160, 170, 165 msec) is noted in the beats preceding a dropped beat
and simulates Mobitz type II block (panel B). This is not a type II block as the A-H time in the next conducted
beat is markedly shorter (90 msec). The second degree A-H block in all probability is due to a type II response
in A-V nodal accommodation associated with a marked and sudden retardation in conduction leading to a
dropped beat which simulates Mobitz type II block. This mechanism is further supported by the subsequent
spontaneous manifestation of: a. classical type I A-H block; and b. by a disproportionate increment in A-H
time (from 90 to 470 msec) during 3:2 conduction ratios (panel C).

possibility is illustrated in figure 9 showing continuous recordings during AP at a cycle length of 890 msec. The A-H time remained constant at 150 msec for most of the period with 1:1 A-V conduction (fig. 9, panel A). Panel B of figure 9 shows a minimal increase in A-H time (160, 170, 165 msec) preceding a dropped beat proximal to the BH simulating type II block. The minimal increment may simply mark the beginning of wide fluctuations. The sudden and marked increase in A-V nodal delay is of such magnitude that it immediately results in complete block of the propagated impulse without manifesting intervening beats conducted with a marked lengthening of A-H time. Continuous recordings (fig. 9, panel C) demonstrate classical second degree type I periods and support the proposed reasoning. This is further supported by the sudden marked spontaneous increases in A-H time, associated with minimal sinus arrhythmia, leading to second degree type I A-V block in this patient (fig. 10).

e. These findings may provide another explanation for the sudden jump noted in A-V nodal refractory periods or conduction times attributed to dual A-V nodal pathways by others (197).

II. 'FATIGUE' PHENOMENON IN THE HIS PURKINJE SYSTEM

Depression of A-V conduction through the His Purkinje System following rapid driving has been defined as the 'Fatigue' phenomenon (708). The development of or an increase in A-V block subsequent to rapid pacing is probably secondary to repetitive penetration

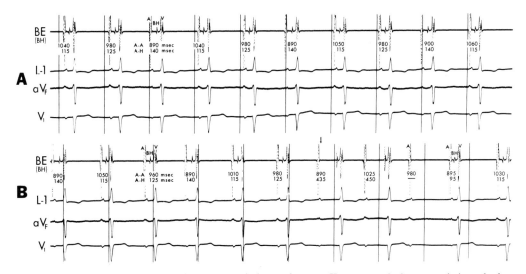

Fig. 10. The occurrence of A-V nodal accommodation and a type II response during normal sinus rhythm with minimal sinus arrhythmia. (Same patient as in fig. 9.) *A, B.* The sinus cycle length varies slightly (1040, 980, 890 msec) due to sinus arrhythmia and results in corresponding minimal changes in A-H time (115, 125, 140 msec). However, intermittently a sudden and disproportionate increase in A-H time (125 to 435 msec) is associated with a slight shortening of sinus cycles (panel B). The mechanism of this sudden jump in A-H time in all probability is a type II response in A-V nodal accommodation similar to that seen in figure 4.

and depolarization of the diseased HPS and transient exhaustion of its conduction capabilities. The resultant A-V block transiently prevents the penetration of the HPS, thereby providing the exhausted tissue with the necessary rest and recovery time.

The 'Fatigue' phenomenon has only been documented in patients with abnormal HPS as indicated by a prolonged H-V time or by spontaneous second degree A-V block localized distal to the BH deflection. This phenomenon has been documented in isolated bundle branch disease, partial bilateral bundle branch block, main His bundle and during 1:1

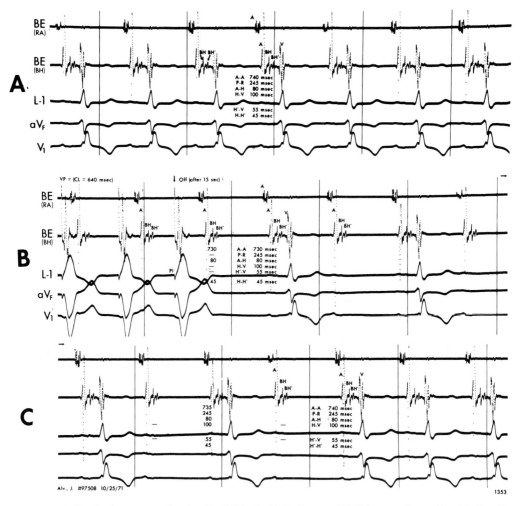

Fig. 11. 'Fatigue' phenomenon in the distal His Purkinje System (HPS) in a patient with right bundle branch block (RBBB) and left axis deviation (LAD). *A.* Simultaneous bipolar recordings (BE) from the high right atrium (RA), the area of the A-V junction (BH) and three surface ECG leads. During control NSR 1:1 A-V conduction is seen with a markedly prolonged H-V time (100 msec) and 'split' BH potentials are recorded indicating lesions at more than one site in the HPS. *B. C.* Termination of ventricular pacing (VP) at a CL of 640 msec after 15 seconds is followed by the development of second degree A-V block. In the non conducted beats the block is localized distal to the BH' deflection. The persistence of second degree A-V block for six seconds prior to the resumption of 1:1 A-V conduction demonstrates 'Fatigue' phenomenon in the distal HPS. The recordings in panels B and C are continuous.

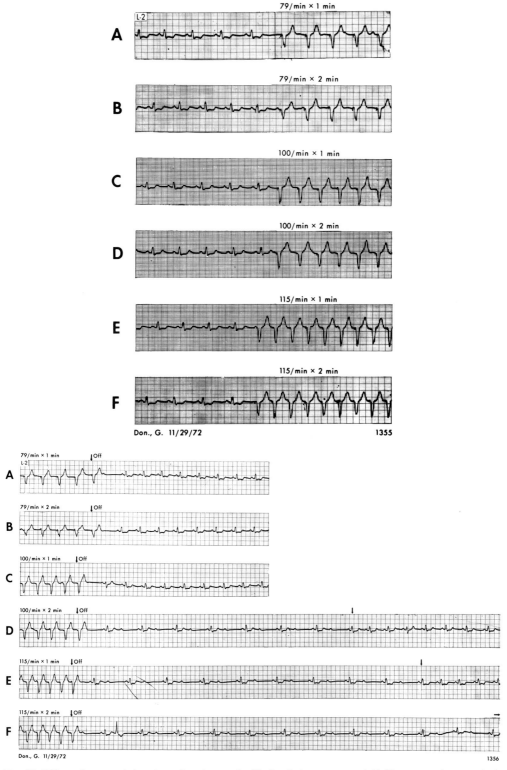

Fig. 12. Effect of rate and duration of pacing on the 'Fatigue' phenomenon. *A–F*. Upper part shows control NSR with 1:1 A-V conduction and onset of VP at different rates (79 to 115/min) for periods of one and two minutes at each level. Lower part shows termination of VP at different levels. 'Fatigue' phenomenon is manifested by the development of second degree A-V block (panels D-F) and is within limits related to the rate and duration of pacing. This phenomenon is absent at slower pacing rates (panels A to C).

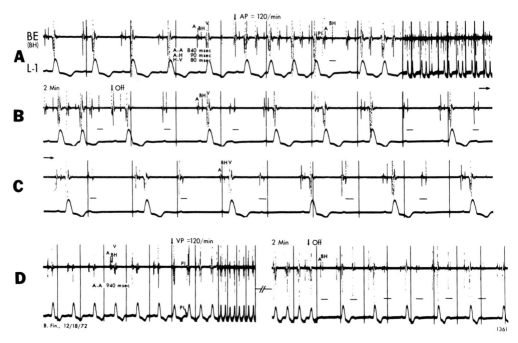

Fig. 13. Manifestation of 'Fatigue' phenomenon following both atrial or ventricular pacing. *A–C.* Control recordings during NSR show 1:1 A-V conduction with a prolonged H-V time (80 msec). Cessation of AP at a rate of 120/min (after 2 minutes) is followed by the development and transient persistence of second degree A-V block (2:1) distal to the BH. Recordings in Panels B and C are continuous. *D.* Shows control NSR with 1:1 A-V conduction, onset of VP at 120/min and manifestation of second degree A-V block (2:1) distal to the BH on termination of VP after two minutes.

A-V conduction or second degree A-V block. A typical example of 'Fatigue' phenomenon is illustrated by figure 11 showing recordings in a patient with right bundle branch block and left axis deviation. During normal sinus rhythm, 1:1 A-V conduction is seen with a severely prolonged H-V time and recordings of 'split' BH deflections (fig. 11, panel A). Termination of ventricular pacing after 15 seconds, at a rate slightly less than 100/min (cycle length = 640 msec), is followed by the manifestation of 2:1 A-V block lasting for 6 seconds prior to resumption of 1:1 A-V conduction. In the dropped P waves, the block is localized in the distal HPS or distal to the BH' (fig. 11, panels B and C).

The duration and degree of 'Fatigue' in the HPS, manifested as A-V block, are within limits directly related to the rate and duration of pacing. This is illustrated by figure 12, the upper part of which shows control sinus rhythm with 1:1 A-V conduction and onset of ventricular pacing (VP) at different rates (ranging from 79 to 115/min) for periods of one to two minutes at each level. The lower part (fig. 12) shows that cessation of VP at higher rates and/or after longer durations is followed by the development of second degree A-V block. In addition, the duration for which second degree A-V block persisted prior to resumption of 1:1 A-V conduction was directly proportional to the rate and duration of pacing (fig. 12, panels E to F).

This phenomenon may be observed following both atrial or ventricular pacing (fig. 13). The limited available data suggest that in a given patient VP results in a more pronounced

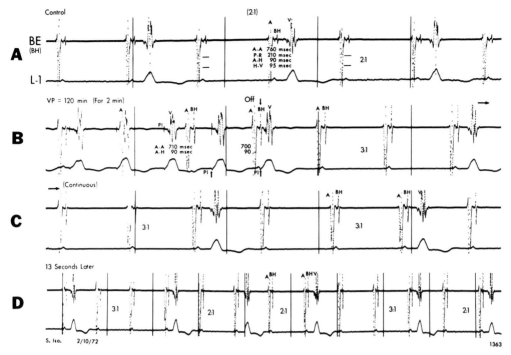

Fig. 14. 'Fatigue' phenomenon in a patient with second degree A-V block. *A.* Control recordings during NSR show 2:1 A-V conduction with block localized distal to the BH. *B–D.* Cessation of VP after two minutes of stimulation at a rate of 120/min exhibits an increase in the degree of second degree A-V block (from 2:1 to 3:1) (panel B). Continuous recordings show the persistence of 3:1 ratio for eight seconds prior to resumption of 2:1 A-V conduction.

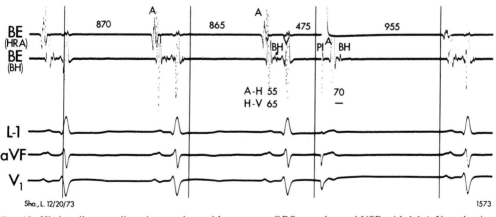

Fig. 15. His bundle recordings in a patient with a narrow QRS complex and NSR with 1:1 A-V conduction show a prolonged H-V time (65 msec) indicating intra-BH disease.

'Fatigue' effect as opposed to AP at comparable levels. This difference in response may be explained by the following: a. the diseased HPS is readily penetrated by ventricular pacing due to its proximity to and direct continuity with the ventricular myocardium; and b. a larger ventricular muscle mass may result in a greater input into the diseased HPS.

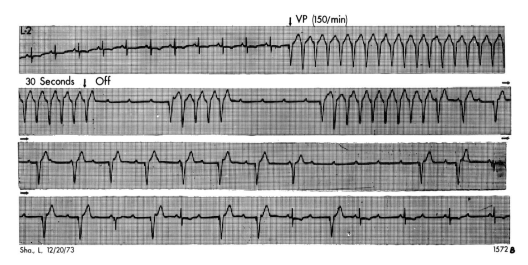

Fig. 16. 'Fatigue' phenomenon in a patient with a lesion in the main His bundle. (Same patient as in fig. 15). Top rhythm strip (lead L-2) shows NSR with 1:1 A-V conduction and onset of VP at 150/min. The next three strips show continuous recordings on cessation of VP after 30 seconds of stimulation. Transient manifestation of complete A-V block followed by 2:1 A-V conduction and eventual resumption of 1:1 A-V conduction after one minute demonstrate 'Fatigue' phenomenon in the His bundle.

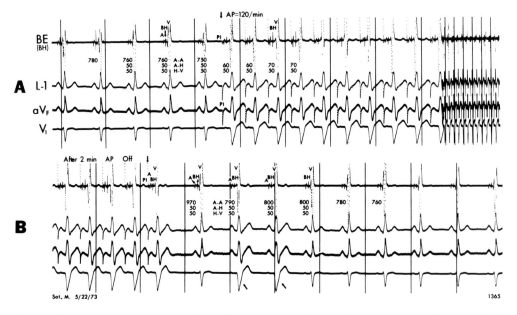

Fig. 17. 'Fatigue' phenomenon in the left bundle in a patient with rate dependent left bundle branch block (LBBB). *A.* Control recordings and onset of AP at 120/min. *B.* Cessation of AP after two minutes, exhibits a narrow QRS complex in the first spontaneous beat occurring at an R-R interval of 950 msec. This normalization is bradycardia dependent. However, the next two beats at regular and control R-R intervals (790, 800 msec) show LBBB. The first of these two beats with LBBB may be explained on the basis of Ashman's phenomenon but the second QRS with LBBB in all probability is secondary to 'Fatigue' phenomenon in the left branch.

'Fatigue' effect may be noted in a case with second degree A-V block by an increase in the degree of A-V block. Such an example is illustrated in figure 14 showing a transient increase in A-V block from 2:1 to 3:1 (for 13 seconds) on cessation of VP after two minutes of driving at a rate of 120/min. A possible example of this type has been previously reported by others in a case with bundle branch block and type II second degree A-V block (463). Despite the absence of His bundle recordings, type II second degree A-V block suggests that the block as well as the fatigue phenomenon were, in all probability, localized in the HPS (Ref. 463 fig. 2).

An example of 'Fatigue' effect in the diseased His bundle is illustrated by figures 15 and 16. During sinus rhythm, a normal P-R and QRS were seen with a prolonged H-V (65 msec) time indicating a diseased BH (fig. 15). Ventricular pacing at a rate of 150/min for 30 seconds only is followed by a period of transient complete A-V block. A decrease in VP rate and an effort to wean off the ventricular pacer is followed by an intermediate period of 2:1 A-V block prior to the resumption of 1:1 A-V conduction (fig. 16). The resultant A-V block was localized distal to the BH deflection during His bundle recordings indicating fatigue in the BH distal to the recorded deflection.

An interesting example of 'Fatigue' effect was seen in a patient with a rate dependent left bundle branch block (LBBB). During sinus rhythm the QRS complex was narrow and the sinus cycles ranged between 750–780 msec (fig. 17). AP at 120/min was associated with the development of LBBB. Termination of AP after two minutes showed a narrow QRS complex in the very first sinus beat appearing at a long R-R interval (950 msec). The long R-R interval, due to sinus node depression, provided a longer than normal

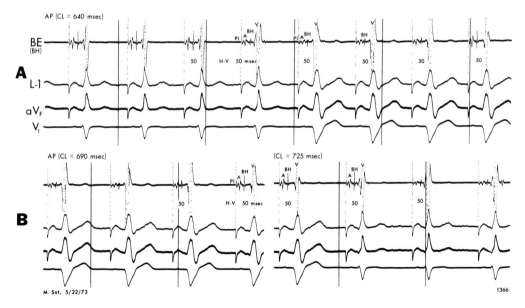

Fig. 18. 'On and off' effect in a patient with rate dependent LBBB. (Same case as in fig. 17). *A & B.* LBBB is manifested at a CL of 640 msec (panel A). However, the cycle length had to be decreased to 725 msec before the LBBB disappeared (panel B, right half). This shows development of LBBB at a faster rate and its disappearance at a comparatively slower rate. This on and off effect may be alternatively explained on the basis of 'fatigue' phenomenon in the left bundle branch.

recovery or resting period to the left bundle branch and thus a narrow QRS complex. However, the second and third spontaneous sinus beats (fig. 17 panel B and indicated by arrows) with cycle lengths almost equal to that of the control show LBBB. Ashman's phenomenon may be proposed to explain the LBBB in the second spontaneous QRS. However, the LBBB in the third spontaneous QRS complex cannot be explained by Ashman's phenomenon, and in all probability represents 'Fatigue' effect in the left bundle branch. Figure 18 shows that in this case LBBB is manifested at a higher pacing rate (CL = 640 msec) and once manifested it persists at a slower rate (CL = 690 msec). The LBBB disappears only after further slowing in pacing rate is achieved (CL = 725 msec). This type of response has been labeled as 'on and off' effect of rate dependent aberration. These data provide another explanation for the mechanism of 'on and off' effect on the basis of 'Fatigue' effect in the bundle branch conduction. A similar explanation has been offered in another report (272).

CLINICAL SIGNIFICANCE

1. Fatigue phenomenon provides possible mechanism to explain syncope associated with supraventricular or ventricular tachycardias in patients with diseased HPS.
2. In some patients rapid driving, preferably VP, may be used as a stress test for the diseased HPS. It is to be added that although a positive response is of diagnostic value, a negative response does not exclude disease in the HPS.

30

EPICARDIAL MAPPING AND SURGICAL TREATMENT IN SIX CASES OF RESISTANT VENTRICULAR TACHYCARDIA NOT RELATED TO CORONARY ARTERY DISEASE[1]

G. FONTAINE, M.D., G. GUIRAUDON, M.D., R. FRANK, M.D., R. COUTTE, M.D., AND C. DRAGODANNE, M.D.

INTRODUCTION

Surgical treatment of drug resistant ventricular tachycardia was first proposed by Cough in 1963 (145) when he excised a ventricular aneurysm which had developed following a myocardial infraction and which served as a source for arrhythmias. Similar reports were made by others (384,519,583,654,811). Recently, myocardial revascularization with or without resection of necrotic tissue, has been advocated (95,232,320). In these cases, the surgical intervention is guided by indirect data, obtained by angiography, or by macroscopic inspection of the anatomical lesions during operation. By contrast in the case of drug resistant ventricular tachycardia complicating cardiomyopathy or another non ischemic heart disease, radiological examinations are negative and inspection of the heart during surgery offers no particular clue to indicate where the tachycardia might originate. In such instances, two methods, based on the concept that the tachycardia is due to re-entrant mechanism make surgical interruption of the reentry circuit possible. Spurrell et al. (981) cut a branch of the specialized conducting system, and Fontaine et al. (277,278,329) performed a ventriculotomy at the epicardial breakthrough of the tachycardia.

In the present paper we report, in addition to two previously published cases, on our experience in 4 new cases of drug resistant ventricular tachycardia, not related to coronary artery disease.

CASE NO 1

Mr SIN . . . , a 33 year old man, was at the age of 30 when admitted to the hospital because of sudden pulmonary edema. After hemodynamic study in December 1969, the diagnosis of non-obstructive cardiomyopathy was made. After two years, during which the patient had only an occasional attack of retrosternal pain, he was suddenly taken to the hospital because of a sudden attack of ventricular tachycardia (VT) at a rate of 180/min. Electrical conversion was unsuccessfull, but the tachycardia disappeared finally following a drip of Procaïneamide. Several months later, the patient suffered from a new attack of VT, and in the following two months, 23 attacks of VT occurred. Numerous drugs were tried in an attempt either to interrupt a VT, or to prevent a new one. The effects appeared to be inconsistant. On radiological examination, the heart appeared moderately enlarged, with

1. This work was supported by la Caisse Régionale d'Assurance Maladie de la Région Parisienne (C.R.A.M.P.) and l'Association de Recherche et d'Entraide Cardiologique et Angéiologique (A.R.E.C.A.).

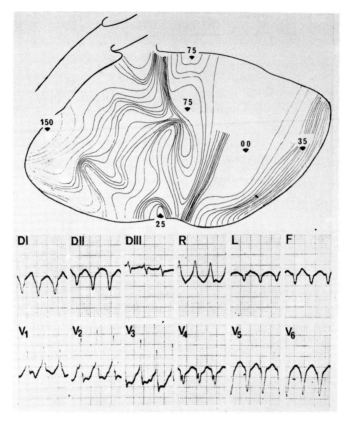

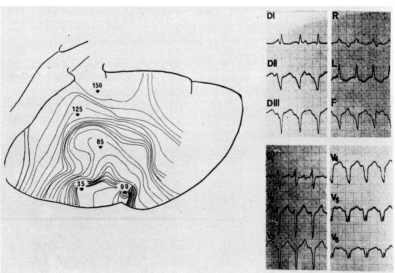

Fig. 1. Case No 1. Ventricular tachycardia with right bundle branch configuration and extreme right axis deviation. The epicardial map shows activation sequence during tachycardia. The isochrones are separated by 5 msec intervals. The total epicardial surface is depicted, the heart being folded out, after an imaginary cut was made along the posterior interventricular sulcus. During tachycardia, activation starts in the mid part of the lateral border of the left ventricle, while the posterior wall of the right ventricle is last to be activated at 150 msec. *b.* The second type of VT starts at the apex and progresses towards the base, which is the latest activated area, also at 150 msec.

diminished pulsations. The ECG during tachycardia showed two different QRS complexes (fig. 1). One showed right bundle branch block configuration with right axis deviation, the other showed left axis deviation. A ventricular angiogram revealed a slight mitral incompetence, and a slightly dilated left ventricle which was hypokinetic, especially at the apex. The coronary angiogram was normal. Because of the frequent attacks of VT, surgery was decided upon, and was performed on May 23rd, 1973.

Epicardial mapping during sinus rhythm showed a nearly normal pattern of activation (fig. 2) with late activation of the left lateral border of the left ventricle. Potentials recorded from that area showed a second component, occurring 70 msec after the first, at a time when no activity was seen on the surface ECG (278). The time interval between the two components increased during a premature beat. Epicardial mapping during VT (fig. 2a) permitted localization of the epicardial origin of both types of VT. One originated at the lateral aspect of the left ventricle (tachycardia with RBBB pattern), the other originated at the left ventricular apex (fig. 2b). A first ventriculotomy was performed at the apex, a second cut of 5 cm length was made, left of the interventricular sulcus towards the apex. The post-operative course was uncomplicated. The follow-up of this indisciplined patient

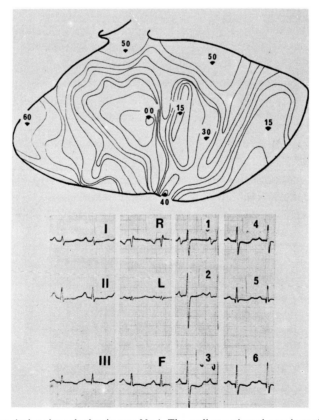

Fig. 2. Epicardial map during sinus rhythm in case No 1. The earliest activated area is on the right ventricular wall, in the anterior paraseptal region, marked 00. The lates activated parts are the basal area of the posterior wall of the right ventricle, the pulmonary infundibulum and the basal part of the anterior wall of the left ventricle.

was incomplete. Nine months after the operation, he suffered from acute heart failure, and died without having had an attack of VT. No autopsy was performed.

CASE NO 2

Mr CONA . . . , a man of 65 years, was admitted to the hospital because of repetitive attacks of VT, the first of which had occurred 20 years earlier. One of these attacks lasted for 11 days, and resulted in heart failure. For several years, the patient had only one attack per month, with an average duration of 24 to 48 hours, and with a rate of 180 to 200/min. During the last years, the attack became more frequent, until they occurred every week, despite the administration of different drugs, either alone or in combination. Physical examination was negative. On radiological examination the heart appeared normal; arterial blood pressure was 140/90 mm Hg. Only one type of VT existed, interrupted from time to time by a focal type of ventricular extrasystole. The ventricular angiogram suggested several slightly dyskinetic zones in the antero-superior part of the left ventricle. No coronary angiography was performed. Electrophysiological study revealed that VT could be initiated and terminated by a rapid burst of electrical stimuli.

On October 20th, 1973, surgery was performed. The epicardial map during sinus rhythm showed slightly delayed activation of the right ventricle (fig. 3). The zone of origin of the VT (fig. 4) was on the right lateral border, halfway between apex and base. A ventriculotomy was performed along the right lateral border extending from apex to base. The patient was regularly seen post-operatively, and has not suffered from arrhythmias since.

CASE NO 3

Mr TOU . . . , a 58 year old man, without known cardiac disease had his first attack of VT in 1970, for which he was admitted to the hospital, where cardioversion was performed. The ECG during sinus rhythm showed RBBB with an electrical axis of 30°.

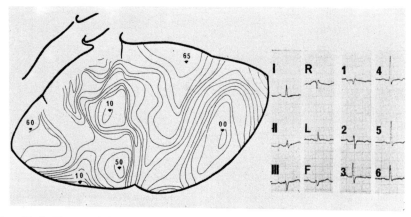

Fig. 3. Case No 2. The map during sinus rhythm shows earliest activation in the lower left paraseptal region; earliest right ventricular activation occurs 10 msec later, in the area normally activated early.

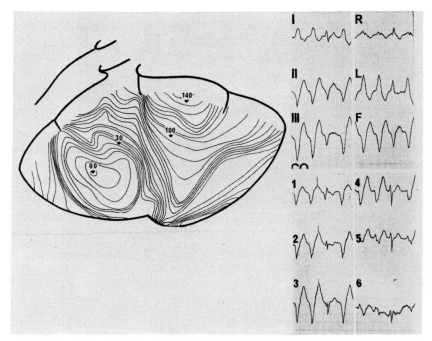

Fig. 4. Case No 2. During tachycardia, activation starts along the right lateral border, halfway between apex and base. The basal part of the left anterior wall is excited after 140 msec.

In 1973, auricular fibrillation was found to be present. A month later, a new attack of VT occurred with a LBBB configuration and left axis deviation. This attack was not well tolerated and had to be converted electrically. Thereafter, the attacks of VT became more frequent, until they occurred daily. During tachycardia, the QRS complexes always showed a LBBB configuration, however with a variable axis, either deviated to the left or to the right, in different attacks.

Angiography demonstrated hypokinesis of the left anterior wall, contractility elsewhere being normal. A coronary angiogram was made in December 1973. It showed a stenosis of 70% in the initial part of the left anterior descending artery, with a good artery distal to the narrowing.

Pre-operative electrophysiological study showed that the VT could be initiated and terminated by a single electrical stimulus, and also by rapid bursts of electrical stimuli.

A coronary bypass seemed to be indicated at the time, as well as epicardial mapping of the VT.

The patient was operated at the end of December 1973. Both atria and the left ventricle appeared normal on inspection. In the infundibular region, an area of several cm2 was found to be very thin-walled. The myocardium was yellowish, contracted little, and the area ballooned during systole as an aneurysm. During sinus rhythm epicardial mapping demonstrated late activation of the right ventricle (fig. 5). Earliest epicardial breakthrough occurred halfway between apex and base on the diaphragmatic aspect of the left ventricle. Late, polyphasic potentials were recorded from the infundibulum. During VT (fig. 6), mapping demonstrated an early wavefront, originating from

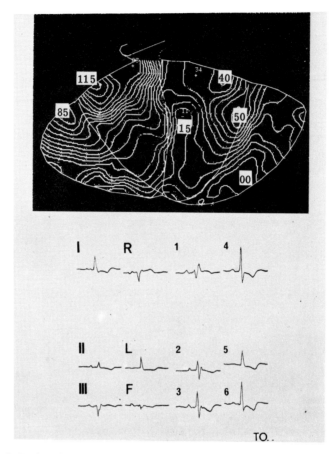

Fig. 5. Case No 3. During sinus rhythm, earliest epicardial breakthrough occurs in the left anterior and posterior paraseptal regions. The right precordial leads show a right bundle branch block configuration. The base of the right ventricular free wall is the last part to be activated.

the right border of the infundibulum. This wavefront propagated across diseased myocardium from the right to left towards normal myocardium. The latest part to be activated was the diaphragmatic aspect of the left ventricle.

The operation was performed in two stages: 1. a saphenous vein graft was made between aorta and left anterior descending artery; 2. a triangular piece of the infundibulum was resected with the apex of the triangle just below the pulmonary valves, and the base reaching the level of the papillary muscle of the tricuspid valve, extending towards the right border of the infundibulum. The suture ran transversally. The postoperative course was uneventful. No attacks of VT, nor signs of heart failure occurred. Only the auricular fibrillation persisted.

CASE NO 4

Mr GRI ..., a 29 year old man, suffered from attacks of VT since the age of 17. No known cardiac disease was present at that time. At the age of 24, a clinical examination revealed

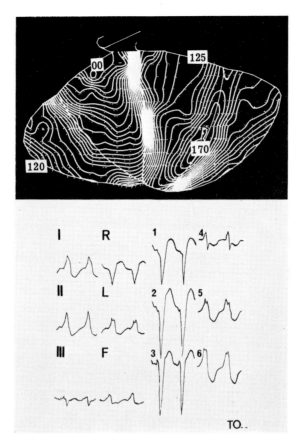

Fig. 6. Case No 3. The area to be activated latest during sinus rhythm is the site of origin of the ventricular tachycardia. The activation sequence during VT is the inverse of that during sinus rhythm (see fig. 5). The latest activated area is close to the apex at the left lateral aspect (170 msec.). The regular spacing of the isochrones suggests tangential activation through ordinary myocardium.

the existence of a protosystolic murmur in the 3rd and 4th left inter-costal space. The ECG showed sinus rhythm and LBBB. The VT had a rate of 150 to 160/min, and the QRS complexes had a configuration of RBBB + LAH.

Hemodynamic studies showed normal cardiac output and intra-ventricular pressures. Angiography showed a slightly enlarged left ventricle. The VT responded well to drug therapy. One year later, the VT became refractory to drugs. The combined administration of Digitaline (in discontinuous doses), Propanolol and Epanutin resulted in fewer attacks, and a better tolerance of the VT. Nevertheless, since the beginning of 1973, when the patient was 28 years old, the attacks of VT occurred every week and could not be suppressed by the administration of Amiodarone and Aprindine, either given alone or in combination. The administration of both drugs together succeeded in slowing the ventricular rhythm, but could not prevent the occurrence of the tachycardia. Electrocardiograms taken in 1974 showed 1st degree AV block. The possibility of surgery was considered after it was shown that the VT could temporarily be terminated by an appropriately timed electrical stimulus (fig. 13).

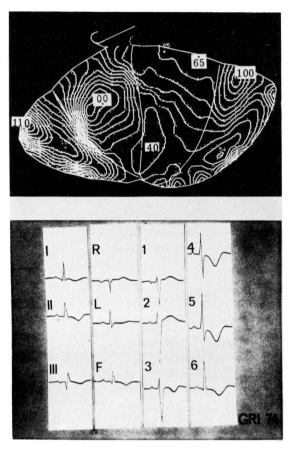

Fig. 7. Case No 4. Activation pattern during sinus rhythm, demonstrates a slight conduction delay in the right ventricle, and an irregular activation pattern in the anterior wall of the left ventricle.

On November 11th, 1974, surgery was performed. The heart especially the left ventricle, was considerably enlarged. Along the left lateral border, a fibrotic epicardial zone was present. The myocardium looked pale. No other abnormalities were seen. The coronary arteries were normal, as was already noted on coronary angiography. Mapping during sinus rhythm (fig. 7) showed an activation sequence which was nearly normal. During tachycardia, the earliest activated area was close to the apex (fig. 8) and close to the fibrotic epicardial zone. Late potentials were not found, neither during sinus rhythm, nor during VT. A 10 cm ventriculotomy was performed extending from the diaphragmatic aspect of the apex to the basal part of the anterior wall of the left ventricle. Wall thickness was relatively normal at 1 to 1.5 cm. After closure of the ventriculotomy, and defibrillation, sinus rhythm ensured, but when extra-corporeal circulation was stopped, ventricular tachycardia re-occurred, and was of the same type as pre-operatively. The ventriculotomy was therefore enlarged and a piece of myocardium (3 × 12 cm) was excised at the level of the apex, extending over anterior and diaphragmatic wall of the left ventricle. After defibrillation, again VT ensued at a frequency of 160 to 180/min. The arrhythmia could not be suppressed. A low output syndrome developed, and on the 18th postoperative day, the patient died.

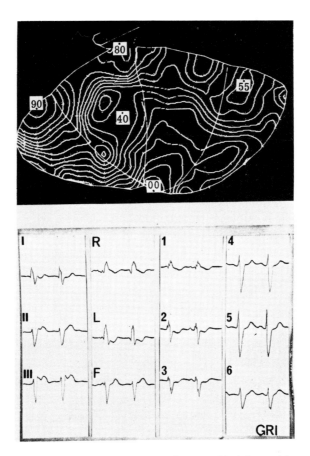

Fig. 8. Case No 4. During tachycardia, activation starts at the apex of the left ventricle, and progresses towards the base. In the mid portion of the free wall of the right ventricle, there is a relatively early activated zone suggesting participation of the right sided specialized conducting system, which might have been activated retrogradely by the tachycardia wavefront.

Histological examination of the excised fragments of myocardium revealed the presence of myocardium without evidence of fibrosis or recent necrosis. The endocardium was slightly fibrotic, but not significantly thickened.

CASE NO 5

Mr GON ... was 42 years old when admitted to the hospital. At the age of 38, abnormalities on his ECG were accidently discovered. The QRS complexes had a low voltage, there was late activation at the posterior division of the left bundle branch, and abnormal repolarization was present in the left precordial leads. He was asymptomatic until the age of 42. In December 1974, attacks of VT began which were not tolerated well, and which started with vaso-vagal phenomena. Almost immediately retrosternal pain occurred, vision disturbances followed and finally syncope ensued. During VT, the QRS complexes always had a RBBB configuration. Most often the VT had to be terminated by electroshock. Within one month more than 15 attacks of VT occurred. Their frequent occurrence, their ominous character, and failure to prevent them despite large doses of Procaïneamide, which initially was effective, resulted in the decision to perform surgery.

Pre-operative electrophysiological study showed that VT could be initiated and terminated after an artficial 'warming-up' period of several minutes. This tachycardia was different from the type occurring spontaneously, in that its QRS complexes showing different morphologies: LBBB configuration with right axis or left axis deviation.

On January 7th, 1975, surgery was performed. The heart was enlarged, due to involvement of the right ventricle which occupied the entire anterior aspect of the heart. The posterior aspect was pale. In the basal part of the infundibulum paradoxical pulsations were seen. The left ventricle appeared normal. The coronary arteries were not hardened, except for the middle portion of the left anterior descending artery. Epicardial mapping during sinus rhythm (fig. 9) demonstrated pathological potentials on the anterior paraseptal wall of the left ventricle, the pulmonary infundibulum and on the diaphragmatic wall of the right ventricle along the interventricular septum. Mapping during VT (fig. 10) showed early activation at the level of the enlarged infundibulum. Three incisions were made: a transverse incision over the infundibulum, a longitudinal incision in the diaphramatic

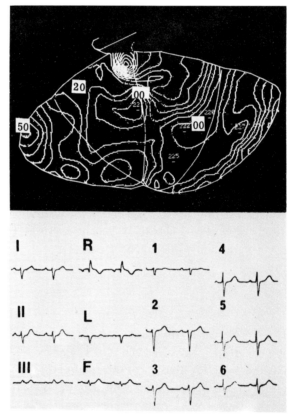

Fig. 9. Case No 5. Normal activation pattern during sinus rhythm. However, there is considerable slowing of conduction in the basal part of the pulmonary infundibulum.

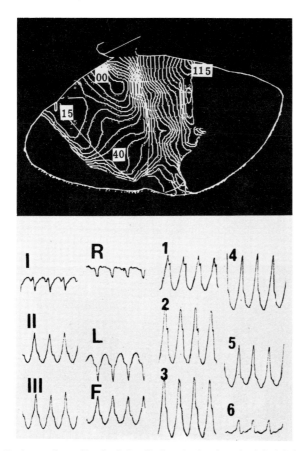

Fig. 10. Case No 5. During tachycardia, the infundibulum is the site of origin of the abnormal wavefront. The diaphragmatic aspects of the heart were not explored.

wall of the right ventricle from apex to base, and a small incision, 2 cm long, in the anterior paraseptal area of the left ventricle. After transient arrhythmias and conduction disturbances, occurring for 90 minutes after extra-corporal circulation had been stopped, sinus rhythm was restored and the hemodynamic situation became normal. The postoperative course was uneventful.

CASE NO 6

Mrs RAY ..., a 46 year old woman had a congenital heart disease, known since she was 11 year old. In the beginning of 1975, the diagnosis of Uhl's anomaly was made, following cardiac catheterisation and angiography. The findings were: Low pressures in the right ventricle (atrialization of the right ventricle), no pulmonary venous congestion, pulmonary plethora, an enormously dilated right ventricle, especially in the infundibular region, a normal left ventricle. Attacks of VT, which were tolerated well, and which first occurred 5 years previously, completed the picture of Uhl's anomaly. No symptoms of heart failure were present during sinus rhythm. The ECG showed sinus arrhythmia, associated with atrial extrasystoles, with an average rate of 50/min. There were signs of right atrial hypertrophy. The QRS complexes had a low voltage and showed extreme right axis deviation.

In the course of several weeks, the attack of VT became more frequent, being initiated by the slightest effort, and were resistant to drug therapy. Electrophysiologic study showed a ventricular refractory period of 310 msec, at a rate of 80/min, which was shortened to 280 msec at a rate of 120/min. A single extra stimulus induced VT, which was terminated by a train of 6 stimuli at a rate of 220/min.

On April 17th, 1975, surgery was performed. The pre-operative findings were confirmed. The right atrium and right ventricle were enormously enlarged. The left ventricle was hidden behind the right ventricle, which had a thin, pale-yellowish wall. The infundibulum was especially enlarged. The left ventricle was small and its myocardium seemed normal. The coronary arteries were normal. On epicardial mapping, the whole of the right ventricle

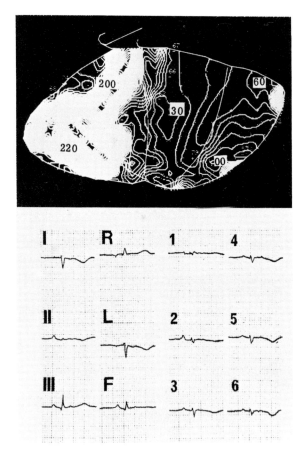

Fig. 11. Case No 6. The epicardial map during sinus rhythm is for a large part constructed by means of time measurements of late potentials, since at a number of sites no potentials were recorded which fell within the duration of the QRS complex of the surface ECG (see fig. 12). During tachycardia, recordings were made at too few sites to construct a complete activation map. Only the site of origin of tachycardia could be established, which was in the superior part of the anterior wall of the right ventricle.

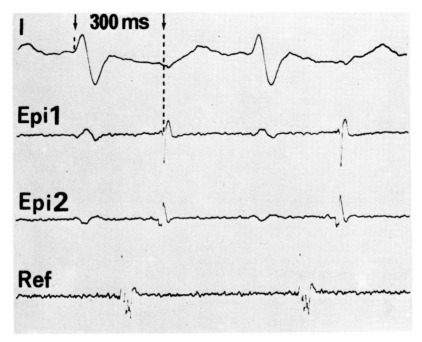

Fig. 12. Case No 6. Epicardial complexes recorded during sinus rhythm. Upper trace is standard lead I, the two middle traces are bipolar complexes recorded from a tripolar exploring electrode. The lower trace is a reference lead, recorded from the epicardial surface in a late activated area. Both the complex of the exploring electrode, and the reference complex occur after the QRS complex of the surface ECG, up till 300 msec after beginning of ventricular depolarization. During the QRS complex, no local activity is recorded by the exploring electrode.

was found to be abnormal (fig. 11), both its anterior and posterior aspects. Late potentials occurred after 300 msec (fig. 12). According to the poor hemodynamic condition, a fold maintained by sutures was made in the infundibulum, which seemed the most pathological area, and where tachycardia originated. Postoperatively no tachycardia occurred, despite large doses of Aramine and Isuprel. These drugs were given because of a persistent low output syndrome, which on the 7th postoperative day resulted in the death of the patient.

DISCUSSION

Clinical electrophysiological methods, such as the registration of endocardial potentials and electrical stimulation, established the concept of reentry as the basic mechanism underlying arrhythmias in the Wolff-Parkinson-White syndrome (81) and reciprocal junctional rhythm (146). Wellens (904,906) emphasized the important role played by intraventricular circus movements in the genesis of ventricular tachycardia. This concept opposes the generally accepted belief in which phenomena of hyperexcitability dominate (723). Basically, two major mechanisms have been proposed to explain the genesis of tachycardias:

1. An ectopic focus, in which fibers show an increase spontaneous activity. This mechanism

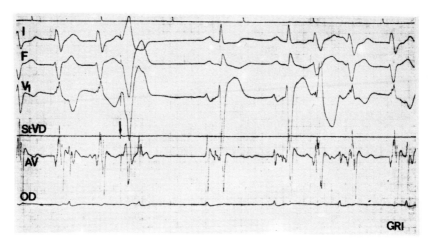

Fig. 13. Electrophysiological investigations in the 4th case. 1 = Standard lead I. F = AVF. V = Right precordial lead. AV = His bundle electrogram. OD = Lead from middle part of right atrium. A single well timed electrical stimulus (arrow) during tachycardia stops the arrhythmia for a few seconds, and sinus rhythm with normal AV conduction time is resumed. Tachycardia starts again, following a premature beat occuring just after the T wave of the last sinus beat. (See text for discussion.)

was demonstrated in the dog heart during Digitalis intoxication by Vasalle in 1962 (851) and Hoffman in 1964 (370). Kastor et al. in 1972 (423) explored the epicardial activation sequence during ventricular tachycardia by means of epicardial mapping techniques. They found that activation appeared to spread in concentric waves over the epicardium from an epicardial location (276,423).

2. Ventricular reentry, the concept of which was long ago suggested by McWilliams in 1887 (535) and experimental evidence for which was first published by Schmitt and Erlanger in 1928 (740). The same mechanism was proposed by Harris in 1947 (341) in his studies on experimental ischemia in the dog's heart. The same model was used in the experiments by Durrer et al. in 1961 (217) and 1964 (218), in which by means of bipolar electrodes late potentials were recorded, occurring 75 to 80 msec after the beginning of ventricular depolarization, at the time when the remainder of the myocardium was already depolarized (QRS duration being 50 msec). In a human heart in which considerable myocardial ischemia was present, the same author recorded multiphasic potentials (223) and with epicardial mapping during surgery of a large ventricular aneurysm, potentials were revealed which occurred 60 msec after the end of QRS in the surface ECG (223).

The physiological studies of Han in 1970 (370) on isolated fragments of tissue, showed that it was possible to elicit repetitive activity by a single premature stimulus applied during regular stimulation. The author suggested later that the circus movement could involve the specific ventricular conducting system (337,338). Due to its anatomical position, the conducting system is well suited to play a role in reentrant phenomena. In 1972, Wit, Hoffman and Cranefield (931) demonstrated for the first time experimentally a selfsustaining circus movement. This study emphasized the importance of slow conduction. A similar concept is found in the studies on experimental infarction of Boineau and Cox in 1973 (82).

These authors showed that in the intermediate zone between ischemic and healthy tissue late potentials could be recorded which occurred between 215 and 250 msec after the beginning of ventricular depolarization. The latest potentials occurred after the top of the T wave. Moreover, a premature ectopic ventricular beat occurred when the preceding interval of these late potentials increased sufficiently to result in a propagated wavefront, invading adjacent myocardium which had recovered its excitability. In contrast to studies in which repetitive activity is elicited by electrical stimulation at increasingly shorter coupling intervals, these data showed reentrant phenomena occurring spontaneously as a consequence of myocardial ischemia (82). With the aid of clinical electrophysiological techniques, Wellens in 1972 (904) showed for the first time that it was possible to initiate and to terminate a ventricular tachycardia by a single electrical stimulus, appropriately timed in the cardiac cycle. Two years later, in a larger series, he specified that ventricular tachycardias occurring after the acute phase of myocardial infarction (after the first 24 hours) behaved in nearly all cases as a reentrant tachycardia. One has therefore to substitute the classical concept of an ectopic focus due to hyperexcitability for a passive phenomenon associated with conduction disturbances.

The concept that the specific conducting system is involved in the reentry circuit is

Table 1. Main characteristics and results of surgery in 6 cases of drug resistant ventricular tachycardia, unrelated to coronary artery disease.

| No. of case | Diagnosis | Cavities reached during catheriza- tion | *Late potentials* | | Origin of VT | Survival M: months D: days | Cause of death |
			Present	Localisation			
1	N.O.C.	LV + RV	YES	LV	LV + Ap	9 M	Acute heart failure
2	I.V.T.	RV	YES	RV	RV	20 M	—
3	I.V.T.	RV	YES	RV	RV	18 M	—
4	N.O.C.	LV + RV	NO	—	Ap	18 D	VT + low output syndrome
5	N.O.C.	RV	YES	LV + RV	RV	5 M	—
6	UHL	RA + RV	YES	RV	RV	7 D	Low output syndrome

Abreviations:
N.O.C. = non obstructive cardiomyopathy
I.V.T. = idiopathic ventricular tachycardia
Uhl = Uhl's anomaly (paper-thin right ventricle)
LV = left ventricle.
RV = right ventricle.
RA = right atrium
Ap = apex

strongly supported in the literature, hence the attitude of Spurrell et al. (781), who thought
it is possible to prevent recurrent attacks of VT by cutting a branch of the specific conducting system. On the other hand, we have reported three cases in which a ventriculotomy was
performed at the site which seemed to us closest to the origin of the circus movement, that
is the site of earliest activity observed with an epicardial mapping technique during tachycardia (277). Table 1 summarizes aspects of our up-dated 6 consecutive cases of drug
resistant ventricular tachycardias. We have limited the cases to those in which the
arrhythmia was not related to myocardial ischemia. Although as already stated, reentrant
arrhythmias are associated with the chronic phase of myocardial infarction, we considered
it necessary to make this restriction for the following reasons: 1. Ventricular aneurysm, or
fibrotic scars are obvious targets for surgery, and we might argue that with the excision of
necotic tissue a possible ectopic focus might be removed as well (624). 2. In the course
of a myocardial infarction, the conduction disturbances seem more complicated and need
separate studies. 3. Chronic myocardial ischemia involves in general the myocardium and
subendocardium of the left ventricle, whereas in cardiomyopathy, or in idiopathic ventricular tachycardia, the involved areas are preferentially located in the epicardial layers of
the right ventricle (table 1).

Electrophysiological studies
In all cases except case No 4 (which will be discussed separately), it was possible to elicit
the tachycardia by electrical stimulation, using a single stimulus, or a pair of stimuli, or a
train of rapid stimuli. In cases 1, 2 and 5, an additional artificial 'warming-up' period was
necessary, during which the heart was stimulated for a period of 15 to 30 minutes at a rate
close to the tachycardia rate in order to elicit the arrhythmia by extra stimuli. The termination of VT could be effected by a single stimulus applied at the origin of the abnormal
wavefront during surgery in case No 1, and by endocardial stimulation of the right ventricle
in cases No 2 and 3, but only when the stimuli were applied at the *base* of the right ventricle,
and not when they were given in the *apical region*. This emphasizes the importance of the
site of stimulation relative to the reentrant circuit. A similar remark was made by Wellens
(903) concerning the termination of reentrant tachycardias in the Wolff-Parkinson-White
syndrome type A. In cases No 2, 5 and 6, a series of 3 to 4 stimuli, separated by short
intervals was needed to stop the arrhythmia.

The late potentials
At surgery, late potentials were recorded, similar to those observed with an intramural
electrode during myocardial ischemia by Boineau and Cox (82). The demonstration of
these late potentials is in our view of the utmost importance regarding the concept of
intraventricular reentry. They were consistently found in 5 of the 6 patients (not in case
No 4). The potentials showed two components: The first component was inscribed during
the QRS complex, had a low amplitude and a low frequency response; this one was used
to draw the maps; the second component was a high frequency response of a relatively
large amplitude, and occurred after the end of ventricular depolarization as observed on
the surface ECG. The coupling of both components varied from case to case, and within
one case from site to site. They were found on both right and left ventricle in cases No 2, 3

and 6, and occurred preferentially in those areas where the ventricular wall was estimated to be thin (Cases No 2, 5 and 6). They were found both during sinus rhythm and during ventricular tachycardia, in approximately the same areas. In case No 6, the late components were very late (about 300 msec after onset of ventricular depolarization) and were of low amplitude. The surrounding zones were electrically inactive. Moreover, in this case, no noticeable local activity was recorded during the QRS complex. Multiphase potentials were also observed with the latest component always occurring before the end of the ventricular refractory period (endocardial measurements were 310 msec at 80/min). It is conceivable that a premature impulse, resulting in a later occurrence of the late components were very late (about 300 msec after onset of ventricular depolarization) and were of results in reentry. The occurrence of reentry would be also facilitated by the shortening of the refractory period of the adjacent myocardium by the premature impulse, since refractory period decreases to 280 msec for 120/min. Both mechanisms could simultaneously be operative.

Site of origin of the ventricular tachycardia
In four cases, the site of origin of the ventricular tachycardia was in the right ventricle (sometimes at the level of the apex), in two cases in the left ventricle. In case No 1, there were two different zones of origin. In all cases, the area where the tachycardia originated coincided with the zone where the late potentials were recorded (this does not imply that all areas where late potentials were found acted as a source of tachycardia). Because in every case, mapping was performed during the sinus rhythm, the site of the origin of the tachycardia could be compared with the area where the main bundle branches contacted ventricular myocardium. Apart from two cases where the tachycardia originated at the apex, a region which normally can be activated early (224), it is clear, that the source of the tachycardia did not coincide with the areas of earliest epicardial activity during sinus rhythm (this does not exclude the possibility of a secondary penetration of the specific conduction system by the tachycardia wavefront).

Surgical aspects
The ventriculotomy was performed in the region, or regions, where the abnormal wavefront start. This region can be thought of as the site closest to the point where the circus movement started, all the more so because these regions coincided with the areas where late potentials were recorded from. The ventricular sectionswere made in case No 5, on the basis of this latter criterion, because one kind of VT had been mapped in a patient who had 3 different types of VT.

The fibrosis following the transmural section of the ventricular wall will constitute a barrier for conduction, and thus prevent the establishment of reentry circuits (906). In all cases, the conduction disturbances caused by the ventriculotomy, was not of such a degree as to be visible on the surface ECG, indicating that only a very limited part of the His-Purkinje system was involved in the section.

In case No 2, a temporary right bundle branch block appeared post-operative; two months later it had disappeared, and no tachycardias had occurred.

The length and the orientation of the ventriculotomy was determined by the anatomic conditions relative to the site of origin of the tachycardia. So the resection of a small piece of myocardium in case No 3, as well as revascularisation, might have been prevented.

The period during which extra-corporeal circulation was maintained, varied from 20 to 45 minutes. It would be desirable to reduce this time, or even to avoid it altogether. This was done in the 6th case, where the precarious condition of the myocardium led to the decision to make a single fold in the abnormal part of the ventricular wall, without extra-corporeal circulation. After the fold was made, electrical stimulation was unable to initiate VT, and despite large doses of Aramine and Isuprel, no tachycardia occurred post-operatively.

The fourth case
This case is discussed separately, because of its several special features. In the first place, the tachycardia was nearly continuous in this patient, and had the relatively slow rate of 110/min. As shown, the tachycardia originated in the apical region. During endocavitary stimulation of the right ventricle, the stimuli were delivered very close to the site of origin of the abnormal wavefront, and a properly timed single stimulus was able to stop the tachycardia only for 2 to 3 seconds and then the arrhythmia spontaneously started again.

Secondly during epicardial mapping, both during sinus rhythm and during ventricular tachycardia, only normal epicardial complexes were recorded, all of which fell within the QRS complex of the surface ECG. Finally, resection of the whole apical region failed to prevent the tachycardia.

If an intraventricular reentry was present, as suggested by the fact that tachycardia could be stopped by a single, properly timed stimulus, it must have possessed special character-istics since after its termination tachycardia started again immediately. On the other hand, the absence of late potentials can not exclude the presence of reentrant mechanism. The failure of the ventriculotomy, and the apical resection, lead to the conclusion that the surgical intervention, despite its size and despite the fact that it occurred at the correct site as indicated by the mapping during tachycardia, did not result in a conduction disturbance of sufficient magnitude to prevent reoccurrence of reentry. The results in this case are in sharp contrast to those in the other cases, notably in case No 1.

The concept of the ectopic focus seems better suited in this patient to explain the normal sequence of activation during both sinus rhythm and VT. Likewise, it offers a better explanation for the sequence of ventricular complexes which occurred when tachycardia was resumed after it had been temporarily stopped by electrical stimulation (446). Finally it could explain the failure of the surgical attempt, since the site and exact size of an active ectopic focus is unknown at the present time (624). The frequency of the VT (110/min) is is also compatible with activity of the type of 'accelerated idioventricular rhythm'. Because intracavity stimulation of the right ventricle was performed close to the site of origin of the tachycardia, one could think that what originally was interpreted as a criterion for reentry (termination of tachycardia by a single stimulus) might correspond to a pheno-menon of 'post stimulation inhibition', explaining the short period during which tachy-cardia was stopped before starting again.

The undeniable success of this treatment of resistant ventricular tachycardia should not conceal the fact that several questions remain unsolved. These questions are:

1. What are the precise mechanisms of intra-ventricular reentry in man and what is the mode of initiation.
2. What are the pre-operative electrophysiologic criterias which will distinguish between reentry and ectopic focus, for a better selection for surgery.
3. Which is the least aggressive surgical technique, so that it can be extended to the ventricular tachycardias associated with myocardial ischemia which concerns a much larger group of patients.
4. What is the future of those patients in whom zones of late potentials remain intact, and who theorically are susceptible to new attacks of VT. Thus far, no new attacks of VT have been observed in our series, the longest follow-up being 20 months.

SUMMARY

Electrophysiological studies in 6 patients with drug resistant ventricular tachycardia, not related to coronary artery disease, led to the conclusion that an intraventricular reentry might be the basic mechanism of the arrhythmias. Epicardial mapping with 110 test points was performed at surgery, both during sinus rhythm and during tachycardia elicited by electrical stimulation. The mapping during tachycardia permitted localization of the earliest excitation breakthrough, whereupon surgical intervention followed. In 5 of the 6 cases, the patients were free of ventricular tachycardia following surgery. This method apart from giving additional support to the concept of intraventricular reentry, opens new perspectives for the treatment of certain arrhythmias.

THE WOLFF-PARKINSON-WHITE SYNDROME

31

THE ELECTROPHYSIOLOGIC PROPERTIES OF THE ACCESSORY PATHWAY IN THE WOLFF-PARKINSON-WHITE SYNDROME

HEIN J. J. WELLENS, M. D.

Epicardial excitation mapping (99,220,278,281,873), stimulation studies (221,325,824, 902), His bundle recordings (110a) and results of surgery (132,203a,750,751, 874,908a) have demonstrated that in the Wolff-Parkinson-White syndrome two pathways are present between the atrium and ventricle.

Apart from a pattern of ventricular excitation which is different from that found in the presence of the A-V nodal—His pathway as the only atrio-ventricular connection, this may lead to arrhythmias specific for the syndrome and affect the significance and severity of other arrhythmias. This will depend upon the electrophysiologic properties of the accessory A-V pathway and A-V nodal—His pathway both in atrio-ventricular and ventriculoatrial direction. In this chapter data will be reported from 107 patients with the W.P.W. syndrome consecutively studied by electrical stimulation of the heart at the University Department of Cardiology, Wilhelmina Gasthuis, Amsterdam.

The outcome of these studies and a discussion of their relevance for our understanding of the role of the electrophysiologic properties of the two A-V connections in the genesis of arrhythmias and their treatment will be the subject of this chapter. Since most of our patients were referred because of recurrent tachyarrhythmias they represent a selected group from patients showing a W.P.W.-electrocardiogram. Our findings and their incidence can therefore not be transposed to all patients showing this electrocardiographic abnormality.

TECHNIQUE

Programmed electrical stimulation of the heart consisted of (903):
1. The study of the pattern of A-V and V-A conduction and of initiation of tachycardia by: a. regular pacing of the atrium and ventricle at increasing frequencies; and b. by using the single test stimulus method during atrial and ventricular pacing. During the latter procedure test stimuli were given with increasing prematurity right up to the effective refractory periods of atrium and ventricle.
2. The study of the effect of premature stimuli on the time relations during tachycardia and on termination of tachycardia. This was done by giving timed single or double atrial and ventricular stimuli during tachycardia. Atrial activation was registered by way of a unipolar or bipolar intracavitary high right atrial lead. In 38 patients a unipolar or bipolar electrogram from the left atrium was recorded by passing a catheter through a patent foramen ovale or by positioning the catheter in the coronary sinus.

An Elema EMT 12 was used for recording the electrical activity of the His bundle. Atrial leads and His bundle lead were recorded simultaneously with the ECG leads I, II, III, V_1 and V_6. All data were recorded on an Ampex FR 1300 tape recorder.

AGE, SEX AND CLASSIFICATION OF TYPE WPW

One hundred and seven patients with the electrocardiographic features of the W.P.W. syndrome were studied.

Patients showing evidence of A-V nodal bypass tracts, nodoventricular accessory connections, or fasciculo-ventricular accessory connections (34) were excluded from the study. Ages ranged from 8 to 76 years. Age distribution is given in table 1. Only 7 patients were over 60 years of age. There were 70 males and 37 females. This distribution is in agreement with other authors (455).

The QRS complex in W.P.W. is a fusion complex from ventricular activation over the A-V nodal pathway and the accessory pathway. When the contribution to ventricular excitation through the accessory pathway is small the ventricular complex may differ little from normal. A classification fitting the most likely site of the ventricular end of the accessory pathway should be based upon QRS configuration during maximal pre-excitation. When the single test stimulus method is used during atrial pacing, the contribution of conduction over the accessory pathway to ventricular activation increases as atrial stimulation is used progressively earlier in the cycle. The classification of our patients is therefore based upon the application of Rosenbaum's criteria (684a) to the QRS configuration in lead V_1 of the earliest atrial premature beat which is conducted to the ventricle over the accessory pathway.

As shown in table 1 thirty patients showed rS or QS complexes in lead V_1 and were classified as type B. Seventy-one patients had or developed high R-waves in lead V_1 and were classified as type A. In six patients the QRS complex in lead V_1 of the earliest atrial premature beat conducted over the accessory pathway showed wide notched R-waves measuring 0,08 sec or more, followed by S-waves of 0,06 sec or more. The refractory period of the accessory pathway was not long and thus contribution to ventricular activation over the accessory pathway was not minimal.

Table 1. Age, sex and type W.P.W. of the 107 patients studied.

Age (years)	Male	Female	A	B	Unclass
0–10	1	—	—	1	—
11–20	10	5	10	4	1
21–30	19	9	18	9	1
31–40	14	2	9	6	1
41–50	9	12	16	3	2
51–60	16	3	14	4	1
61–70	1	5	4	2	—
> 70	—	1	—	1	—
	70	37	71	30	6

These patients could not be classified as either type A or type B. It is of interest that the incidence of type A WPW which according to epicardial mapping and results of surgery is based upon an accessory pathway inserting into the left ventricle was more than twice as frequent as a right ventricular insertion (type B).

THE PROPERTIES OF THE ACCESSORY PATHWAY IN A-V DIRECTION

In all patients the properties of the accessory pathway were studied during atrial stimulation. Figure 1 shows the individual values for the effective refractory period of the accessory pathway obtained by the single test stimulus method. In most patients three basic pacing rates were used during atrial stimulation. In figure 1 the shortest value derived from these different pacing rates was chosen. Encircled points indicate those patients in whom A-V conduction over the AP occurred up to the effective refractory period of the right atrium. Values ranged from 180 to 700 msec. Table 2 gives the range and mean value of the effective refractory period of the AP in the different age groups. In 44 patients the ERP_{AP} was equal to or shorter than the ERP_{AVN}.

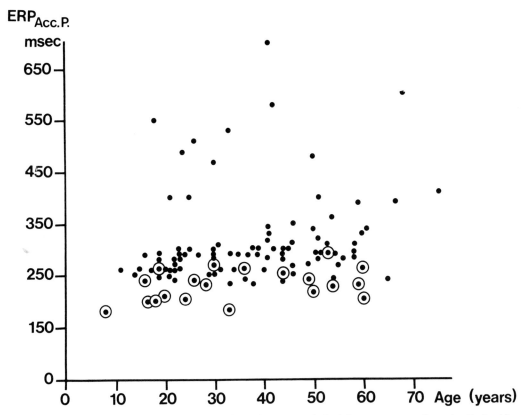

Fig. 1. Graph showing the length of the effective refractory period of the accessory pathway (vertical axis) and age (horizontal axis) of the 107 patients studied. The encircled points indicate those patients in whom A-V conduction over the accessory pathway was present up to the effective refractory period of the atrium.

Table 2.

Age (years)	No pts	Range ERP$_{AP}$(msec)	Mean ERP$_{AP}$(msec)
0–10	1		180
11–20	15	200–550	270
21–30	28	200–510	301
31–40	16	180–530	301
41–50	21	220–700	330
51–60	19	200–480	295
61–70	6	240–600	360
> 70	1		410

ERP = effective refractory period.
AP = accessory pathway.

In six patients the ERP$_{AP}$ was equal to or less than 200 msec. As shown in table 1 and 2 only seven patients were over 60 years of age. Studies on the natural history of the WPW syndrome (65,275,609) suggest that the electrocardiographic signs of pre-excitation disappear with time in a significant number of patients. Progressive lengthening of the ERP with ultimate block in the accessory pathway might explain a lower incidence of tachycardia in the older patient with the WPW syndrome (524). In our (selected group of) patients there was no significant difference in length of the ERP of the accessory pathway in the different age groups. This however does not give us insight into the natural history of the properties of the accessory pathway in the individual patient. Only follow up stimulation studies will answer that question. More data on the natural history of the WPW syndrome are also needed to exclude the possibility that patients suffering from this syndrome have a shorter life expectancy.

If conduction over the accessory pathway is stressed by pacing the atrium at increasing rates the pattern of sequential degrees of A-V block is different from that seen in the A-V node. While the A-V node shows: 1st degree block → Wenckebach type 2nd degree block → 2 to 1 block → complete block; the accessory pathway shows: Mobitz II block → 2 to 1 block → complete block (909). This can result in interesting combinations between different conduction disturbances in the two A-V pathways (fig. 2). Occasionally it is possible to observe Wenckebach type conduction delay in the accessory pathway (904b). One has to exclude however intra-atrial conduction delay, which might mimic this phenomenon (112,588).

The rarity of the Wenckebach type conduction delay in the accessory pathway suggests a different morphologic build up of this structure as compared to the A-V node (34). It does not exclude however the possibility of incorporation of specific conduction tissue in the accessory pathway (23,511).

PATTERNS OF V-A CONDUCTION

V-A conduction was observed in 98 patients during ventricular pacing. This means that nine patients with A-V conduction over both pathways during atrial pacing had no V-A

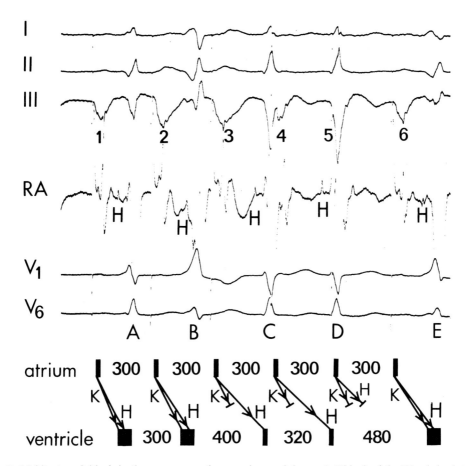

Fig. 2. Mobitz type 2 block in the accessory pathway and second degree A-V block of the Wenckebach type in the A-V nodal—His pathway. During regular pacing of the right atrium with a basic cycle length of 300 msec the first two atrial complexes are conducted to the ventricle over the accessory pathway. The third atrial complex is blocked in the accessory pathway. There is no change in the atrium to delta interval prior to the blocked beat, supporting Mobitz type 2 block in the accessory pathway. Atrial complexes 1 to 4 show a gradual increase in Atrium to His (H) interval, with the fifth atrial complex being blocked in the A-V node. This sequence indicates second degree A-V block of the Wenckebach type in the A-V node. The sixth atrial complex is conducted to the ventricle over both the accessory pathway and the A-V nodal-His pathway.

conduction over either pathway during ventricular pacing. In two patients however concealed retrograde penetration into the accessory pathway (see fig. 3) could be demonstrated. A similar example has been reported by Zipes et al. (960). The ERP_{AP} in A-V direction in nine patients without V-A conduction ranged from 210 to 480 msec.

Conduction over two pathways between atrium and ventricle will not only result in fused excitation of the ventricle during sinus or atrial rhythm, but also in fused excitation of the atrium during impulse formation originating in the ventricle (801).

Determination of the mode of activation of the atria during ventricular pacing in patients with the WPW syndrome is usually not possible from the surface ECG. As stressed by the group from Duke University (293) several simultaneously recorded intra-atrial leads (from right and left atrium or coronary sinus) are needed. When V-A conduc-

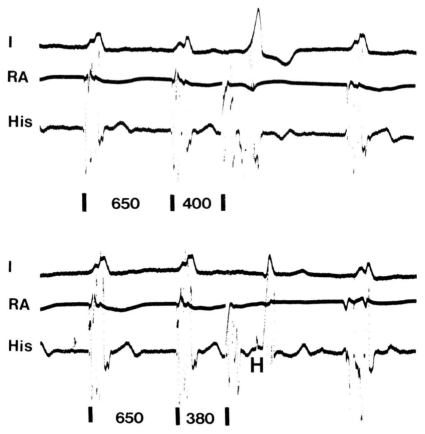

Fig. 3. 'Concealed' penetration into the accessory pathway during ventricular pacing in a patient with the WPW syndrome. No V-A conduction was seen during ventricular pacing with a frequency just above the sinus rate. However during simultaneous pacing of the right atrium and right ventricle with a basic cycle length of 650 msec it was found that atrial test stimuli given in the interval range 380 to 280 msec were conducted to the ventricle exclusively over the A-V node indicating that the preceding ventricular activation front resulting from the paced ventricular beat penetrated retrogradely into the accessory pathway, making it refractory for the atrial test stimulus. During atrial pacing without simultaneous ventricular pacing A-V conduction over the accessory pathway occurred up to the effective refractory period of the right atrium.

tion was studied by the single test stimulus method during ventricular pacing the following was found:

1. 66 patients showed either exclusive V-A conduction by way of the accessory pathway, V-A conduction through an accessory pathway with a shorter refractory period than the H-AV node pathway or identical refractory periods in both pathways. This decision was based upon one or more of the following findings during ventricular pacing using the single test stimulus method (911): 1. No increase in V-A conduction time following ventricular stimuli given with increasing prematurity. 2. Activation of left atrium, prior to, activation of atrium in His bundle lead. 3. A time relation between retrograde His bundle activation and retrograde atrial activation which was compatible with V-A conduction over the accessory pathway (either a short His to retrograde atrial activation

interval, or activation of the bundle of His synchronous with or following retrograde atrial activation).

2. In 12 patients the refractory period of the A-V node was shorter than that of the accessory pathway. In six patients V-A conduction over the node was followed at critical premature beat intervals by return of the impulse to the ventricle over the accessory pathway. In only one patient (905) this pattern was followed by sustained tachycardia with V-A conduction over the node and A-V conduction over the accessory pathway.

3. In 20 patients the pathway used during V-A conduction could not be determined with certainty.

V-A VERSUS A-V CONDUCTION OVER THE AP

In 27 patients it was possible to compare the length of the ERP of the accessory pathway in V-A direction with the ERP of the AP in A-V direction. In order to make this comparison it was required: a. that the basic pacing frequency during ventricular and atrial pacing during which the test stimuli were applied were the same; and b. that the ERP of both the right atrium and the right ventricle were shorter than that of the AP. In 24 patients the ERP of the AP was shortest in V-A direction. Possible explanations for this phenomenon include: 1. slowing in interventricular conduction following early ventricular premature beats with subsequent later arrival at the ventricular end of the AP and 2, differences in increase in latency time between ventricular and atrial stimuli on increasing the prematurity of the test pulse.

TACHYCARDIA AND THE WPW SYNDROME

According to different authors 12 to 80% of patients with WPW suffer from tachycardia (455) 94 out of our 107 patients had at least one electrocardiographically documented episode of tachycardia. The ECG diagnosis of their tachycardia is listed in table 3. Six more patients had a history of tachycardia but no attack was verified electrocardiographically.

During the stimulation study tachycardia other than atrial fibrillation or atrial flutter could be elicited in 83 patients. A classification of these tachycardias is given in table 4. Criteria used to differentiate between a tachycardia pathway comprising both the AP and the A-V node or one confined to the A-V node only are given in table 5. Atrial tachycardia included patients in whom atrial activation during tachycardia suggested sinus node reentrant tachycardia. In 15 patients the site of origin of tachycardia could not be determined.

Table 3.

Documented Atr. Fibrill.	20
Documented SVT	67
Documented Atr. Fibrill. + SVT	7

Table 4. Type Tachy initiated during electrical stimulation.

Atrial Tachycardia	2
AV nodal Tachycardia	8
CM Tachycardia incorporating AP	57
Ventricular Tachycardia	1
Undetermined	15

CM = circus movement
AP = accessory pathway

Table 5. Criteria for differentiation between a re-entry circuit confined to the A-V node and one incorporating the accessory pathway and the A-V node.

A. Positive criteria for re-entry in the A-V node.
  1. Activation of atrium before or simultaneous with ventricle in first and following beats of tachycardia after initiation of tachycardia by an atrial premature beat
  2. Gradual increase in V-A conduction time with appearance of a His bundle electrogram and pro rata increase in VH time following ventricular stimuli given with increasing prematurity
  3. Initiation of tachycardia following a similar pattern of V-A conduction as listed under 2)
  4. Persistence of tachycardia in spite of A-V block.

B. Positive criteria for incorporation of the accessory pathway in the tachycardia circuit.
  1. No increase in V-A conduction time following ventricular stimuli given with increasing prematurity
  2. Initiation of tachycardia following retrograde V-A conduction over the A-V node followed by A-V conduction over the accessory pathway
  3. Activation of left atrium during tachycardia prior to activation of atrium in His bundle lead
  4. Slowing in rate of tachycardia following bundle branch block to ventricle in which acc. pathway inserts
  5. V-A conduction time of induced ventricular stimulus during tachycardia equal to or less than V-A conduction time following tachycardia complex (A-Ae interval $\leq$ V-Ve interval)
  6. An A-Ae interval longer than V-Ve interval, but less than A-A interval, following an induced ventricular stimulus during tachycardia, with no effect of the ventricular stimulus on the antegrade His bundle electrogram
  7. Inability to initiate tachycardia or slowing of conduction in the tachycardia circuit outside the A-V node following drugs affecting the acc. pathway.

INITIATION OF A RE-ENTRANT TACHYCARDIA BY AN ATRIAL PREMATURE BEAT

In 56 patients a re-entrant tachycardia could be initiated by a single atrial premature beat. In 44 patients both the accessory pathway and the A-V node were incorporated in the tachycardia pathway. In two patients A-V conduction during tachycardia occurred over the accessory pathway. In the remaining 42 patients A-V conduction during tachycardia took place over the A-V node. In one patient the site of origin of the tachycardia which could be initiated by a single atrial premature beat was localized in the atrium, possibly the sinus node area (909). In another patient a ventricular tachycardia was elicited

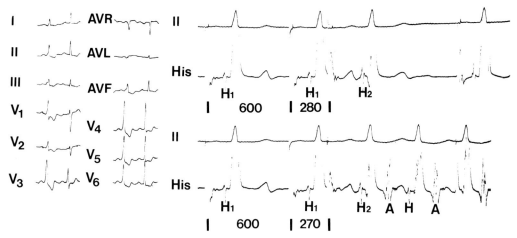

Fig. 4. Patient with 2 to 1 block in the accessory pathway during sinus rhythm with a frequency of 85/min (left pannel). During pacing of the right atrium with a frequency of 100/min (BCL 600 msec) A-V conduction occurred exclusively over the A-V node (right pannel). At a critical atrial premature beat interval (270 msec) a tachycardia was initiated.

by an atrial premature beat (906). In 10 patients (eight showing A-V conduction over the A-V node and two over the accessory pathway) the site of tachycardia could not be determined.

Six patients, in whom a tachycardia could be initiated by a single atrial premature beat showed an effective refractory period of their accessory pathway 80 to 400 msec longer than the longest premature beat interval able to initiate tachycardia. In all six patients the pattern of V-A conduction during ventricular pacing excluded the A-V node as the site of tachycardia (fig. 4 and 5). The finding of block in the accessory pathway at coupling intervals much longer than the tachycardia initiating coupling interval has been advanced as suggestive for A-V nodal re-entry (673a). Like Svenson et al. (800) we believe that initiation of tachycardia by an atrial premature beat at coupling intervals much shorter than the refractory period of the accessory pathway does not exclude the possibility of a tachycardia with V-A conduction over the accessory pathway.

INITIATION OF A RE-ENTRANT TACHYCARDIA BY A VENTRICULAR PREMATURE BEAT

In 42 patients a re-entrant tachycardia could be initiated by a single ventricular premature beat. In 23 patients the tachycardia initiating premature beat showed a V-A interval of the same length as seen during basic pacing. A circusmovement tachycardia with V-A conduction over the accessory pathway and A-V conduction over the A-V node was considered to be present in these patients. Five patients showed a gradual increase in V-A interval on increasing the prematurity of the test pulse. Based upon the criteria listed in table 5 however the accessory pathway had to be accepted as being part of the tachycardia circuit. In six patients a His bundle potential could be registered in between the tachycardia initiating ventricular premature beat and retrograde atrial activation. In

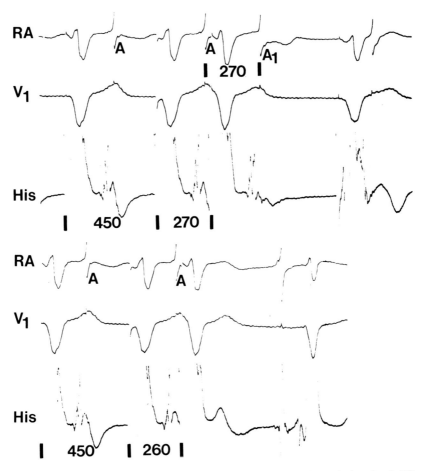

Fig. 5. Same patient as figure 4. During ventricular pacing with a basic cycle length of 450 msec V-A conduction occurred up to a premature beat interval of 270 msec. Note that there is no increase in V-A conduction time of the ventricular premature beat as compared to V-A time during basic pacing, indicating V-A conduction over the accessory pathway. These observations suggest that V-A conduction during tachycardia (fig. 4) occurred over the accessory pathway.

these patients both the time interval between the His bundle electrogram and retrograde atrial activation and the finding of concordant lengthening of the V-A interval on lengthening of the V-His interval were in agreement with the A-V node as the site of tachycardia. It is important to stress (as shown in fig. 6) that the finding of a His bundle electrogram in between the ventricular premature beat and the atrial electrogram does not proof that atrial activation is the consequence of retrograde atrial activation starting in the A-V node. In six patients the ventricular premature beat elicited re-entry at the ventricular level followed by tachycardia (227,909). In all six patients QRS configuration during tachycardia indicated ventricular activation starting over the A-V node—His axis. In two of them one or more of the criteria listed in table 5 were positive for incorporation of the accessory pathway in the tachycardia circuit. In the remaining four the pathway during tachycardia could not be elucidated.

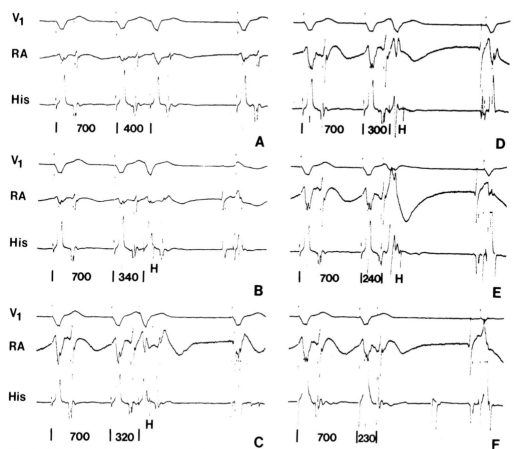

Fig. 6. V-A conduction following ventricular test stimuli given at different intervals. Note that in pannels A to C, without change in length of the V-A interval, His bundle activation moves towards atrial activation. As shown in pannel D and E the His bundle is activated without activation of the atrium. The absence of increase in V-A interval with the gradual increase in V-H interval suggests V-A conduction over an accessory pathway. The configuration of the atrial complex following the test stimulus in panels A to C suggests fusion following V-A conduction over both pathways.

In 22 patients a re-entrant tachycardia with A-V conduction over the A-V node—His pathway could be initiated both by a single atrial premature beat during atrial pacing and a single ventricular premature beat during ventricular pacing. In 16 of these patients, using the criteria listed in table 5, one could be certain that both the A-V node—His pathway (in A-V direction) and the accessory pathway (in V-A direction) were incorporated in the tachycardia circuit. This observation indicates that in these patients during atrial pacing, in order to initate a tachycardia, the ERP of the accessory pathway must have been longer than the ERP of the A-V node—His pathway, while the reverse must have been true during initiation of a tachycardia by a ventricular premature beat during ventricular pacing. Since the His bundle electrogram is usually not visible following the tachycardia initiating ventricular premature beat it was not possible to locate the exact site of block in the Purkinje—bundle branch—His bundle—A-V node axis.

Theoretically, increase in heart rate, by shortening the refractory period of the sub-nodal conduction system and by reducing differences in length of the refractory periods between the bundle branches, ventricular muscle and that part of the bundle branch–Purkinje system which has the longest refractory period (the 'gate') (573), would favour the A-V node to become the site of V-A block. It remains to be demonstrated whether the ability to initiate tachycardia at slow but not at fast ventricular pacing rates favours the subnodal conduction system as the site of V-A block at the time of initiation of tachycardia. Although examples have been reported of initiation of atrial tachycardia by a single ventricular premature beat (910) and of ventricular tachycardia by a single atrial premature beat (913) in patients with the A-V node—His pathway as their only connection between atrium and ventricle, initiation of tachycardia by a premature beat arising in another cardiac chamber will obviously be facilitated by the presence of an accessory A-V pathway. This is demonstrated in figures 7 and 8 where a single ventricular premature beat initiates an atrial tachycardia. As shown in figures 7 and 8 the sequence of atrial activation during tachycardia suggested re-entry in the sinus node area as the mechanism responsible for the arrhythmia.

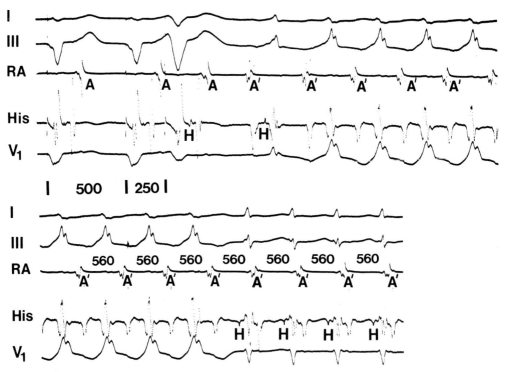

Fig. 7. Initiation of an atrial tachycardia by a single premature ventricular beat during ventricular pacing (upper pannel). As shown atrial activation during tachycardia occurs in cranio-caudal direction. The first ventricular complex during tachycardia shows activation of the ventricle over both the accessory pathway and the A-V node—His axis. Subsequent ventricular complexes show more pre-excitation. The lower pannel (which is a continuation of the upper pannel) shows a sudden change (without increase in A to delta interval) from A-V conduction over the accessory pathway to conduction over the A-V node only, indicating the occurrence of Mobitz type 2 block in the accessory pathway during atrial tachycardia. The sequence of atrial activation during tachycardia is compatible with an origin of the tachycardia in the sinus node area.

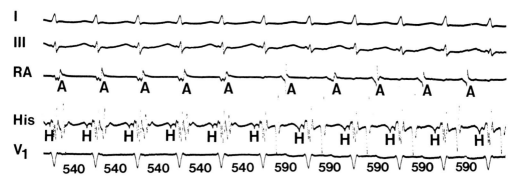

Fig. 8. Same patient as shown in figure 7. The tachycardia shown in the lower strip of fig. 7 changed one minute later (as shown in the middle of this figure) into a tachycardia of slower rate with a different direction of atrial activation (caudo-cranial). This sequence shows 'unmasking' of a circus movement tachycardia with V-A conduction over the accessory pathway on termination of a tachycardia of atrial origin.

THE ROLE OF A 'CONCEALED' A-V PATHWAY IN PATIENTS WITH RE-ENTRANT TACHYCARDIA

As discussed by Coumel, (chapter 24) evidence is accumulating that patients originally thought to suffer from paroxysmal A-V nodal re-entrant tachycardias are in fact using an accessory A-V pathway in V-A direction during tachycardia (150,598,960,782,911). In these patients no conduction over the accessory pathway can be demonstrated during atrial pacing. For therapeutic reasons it is of importance to identify these patients. Drugs like digitalis, which are beneficial in A-V nodal re-entrant tachycardia (912), may facilitate initiation and perpetuation of tachycardia using an accessory pathway in V-A direction by prolonging A-V nodal conduction time and delaying activation of the ventricular end of the accessory pathway. Procaine amide or quinidine may be more successful in these patients (vide infra).

ATRIAL FIBRILLATION AND WPW

In the normal heart the electrophysiologic properties of the A-V node protect the ventricle against high atrial rates during atrial flutter or atrial fibrillation. In patients with the WPW syndrome however the ventricular rate during atrial fibrillation will not only depend upon the properties of the A-V node but also upon those of the accessory pathway and the ventricle (table 6). In the presence of a short refractory period of the accessory pathway very high ventricular rates have been documented during atrial fibrillation (113,907a). Under these circumstances atrial fibrillation can be a life-threatening arrhythmia. Ventricular fibrillation developing from atrial fibrillation has been reported in both the human heart and the dog heart (6,81,118,206,526,827).

Twenty-seven of our patients had electrocardiographic documentation of paroxysmal atrial fibrillation. This incidence is higher than that of previously reported series

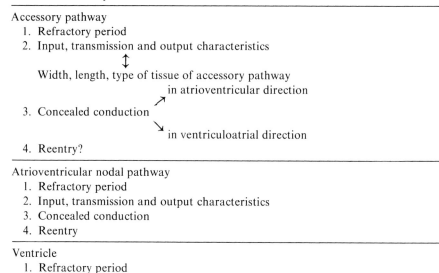

Table 6. Factors determining ventricular rate during atrial fibrillation in Wolff-Parkinson-White syndrome.

Accessory pathway
  1. Refractory period
  2. Input, transmission and output characteristics
      ↕
      Width, length, type of tissue of accessory pathway
                          ↗ in atrioventricular direction
  3. Concealed conduction
                          ↘ in ventriculoatrial direction
  4. Reentry?

Atrioventricular nodal pathway
  1. Refractory period
  2. Input, transmission and output characteristics
  3. Concealed conduction
  4. Reentry

Ventricle
  1. Refractory period

Table 7. Cardiac abnormalities, favouring the development of atrial fibrillation, found in 27 patients with WPW and atrial fibrillation.

Valvular Heart Disease	6
Cor. Heart Disease	3
Sick Sinus	3
No abnormality identifiable	15
	27

(455). As stressed however our material represents a selected group from patients showing a WPW electrocardiogram.

In only 12 patients a cardiac abnormality could be identified which might have contributed to the development of the arrhythmia (table 7). Ten of the 15 patients without an apparent cardiac cause for atrial fibrillation were under 40 years of age, seven under 30 years. This observation suggests that the presence of an accessory A-V pathway facilitates the initiation of atrial fibrillation. During the stimulation studies mechanisms of initiation of atrial fibrillation were observed which may be relevant for spontaneously occurring episodes of atrial fibrillation.

As shown in figure 9 atrial fibrillation may result from an early ventricular premature beat which is conducted over the accessory pathway to the atrium initiating the arrhythmia. Another mechanism is deterioration of a circus movement tachycardia into atrial fibrillation (fig. 10). Fourteen out of the fifteen patients without valvular heart disease, coronary artery disease or sick sinus syndrome, which might have contributed to the development of atrial fibrillation, had a left sided (WPW type A) accessory pathway.

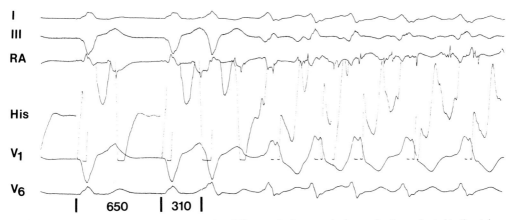

Fig. 9. A ventricular premature beat given after 310 msec during ventricular pacing is conducted to the atrium without increase in V-A conduction time as compared to V-A conduction during basic rhythm. The atrial activation front following the ventricular premature beat initiates atrial fibrillation.

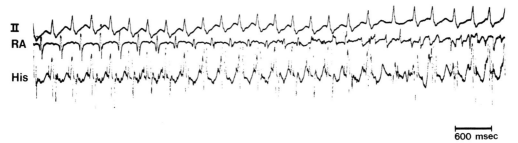

Fig. 10. Deterioration of a circus movement tachycardia into atrial fibrillation.

Future work (by echocardiographic and cineangiographic techniques) is needed to detect whether cardiomyopathy or abnormalities in function of the mitral valve apparatus subsequent to abnormal left ventricular activation may play a role in the genesis of atrial fibrillation.

As listed in table 6 several factors are of importance in determining the ventricular rate during atrial fibrillation in patients with the WPW syndrome (907a). There is however a definite relation between the length of the refractory period of the accessory pathway and ventricular frequency during atrial fibrillation (113,907a). This opens the possibility to identify those patients with the WPW syndrome who are at risk of having life-threatening high ventricular rates when atrial fibrillation occurs.

EFFECT OF DRUGS

The effect of several drugs on the electrophysiologic properties of both the accessory pathway and the A-V node—His pathway have been studied (522a, 672a, 782a, 906a, 911a, 914).

Table 8. Effect of drugs on refractory period and conduction velocity of the different parts of the heart in patients with the WPW syndrome.

	Atr.	AV node	His-Purkinje	Ventr.	Acc. P.
		Length of effective refractory period			
Digitalis	±	+	?	±	−
Procaine Amide	+	0	+	+	+
Quinidine	+	±	+	+	+
Ajmaline	+	0	+	+	+
Diphenylhydantoin	±	−	−	±	±
Atropine	0	−	?	0	0
Propranolol	±	+	?	±	0
Lidocaine	±	0	?	+	+
Verapamil	±	+	?	±	±
Amiodarone	+	+	+	+	+

+ = lengthened, − = shortened, 0 = no change, ± = inconsistent, ? = not known.

	Atr.	AV node	His-Purkinje	Ventr.	Acc. P.
		Conduction velocity			
Digitalis	±	−	?	±	?
Procaine Amide	−	±	−	−	?
Quinidine	−	±	−	−	?
Ajmaline	−	±	−	−	?
Diphenylhydantoin	±	+	0	+	?
Atropine	0	+	0	0	0
Propranolol	−	−	0	−	?
Lidocaine	−	±	?	±	?
Verapamil	0	−	0	0	?
Amiodarone	−	−	−	−	?

+ = increased, − = decreased, 0 = no change, ± = inconsistent, ? = not known.

During these studies it has become clear that although general conclusions can be made as to the acute effect of a certain drug on the electrophysiologic properties of the different parts of the tachycardia circuit (table 8) the outcome on the arhythmia in the individual patient can vary considerably. This is influenced by several factors.

1. Type of arrhythmias
A circus movement tachycardia using the accessory pathway may be terminated by a drug which impairs conduction over the accessory pathway like procaine amide. The same drug may not affect however a re-entrant tachycardia confined to the A-V node. This knowledge can also be used for determination of the tachycardia pathway (fig. 11).

2. Size of the re-entry circuit
When a re-entrant tachycardia is present the arrhythmia will stop when the product of the mean conduction velocity of the circulating wave and the mean refractory period of the different components of the tachycardia pathway exceeds the length of the tachycardia

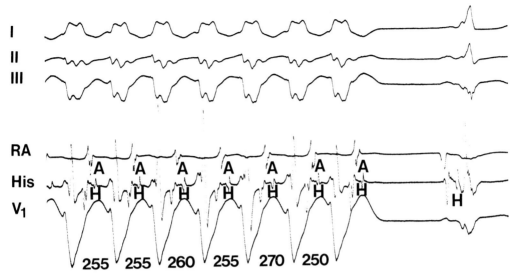

Fig. 11. Termination of tachycardia following injection of ajmaline. Note that the tachycardia ends with activation of the bundle of His, indicating block distal to this structure, possibly in view of QRS complex configuration, in the right bundle branch. This type of termination of tachycardia excludes intra-nodal re-entry and supports incorporation of the subnodal conduction system in the tachycardia circuit.

circuit (Mines, 1913 (552)). Most drugs however have a twofold action. On one hand benificial, (like prolongation of the length of the refractory period of components of the tachycardia circuit) on the other hand unfavourable (by slowing conduction of the circulatory wave). The net effect of the drug will depend upon the interplay of these changes in relation to the (unknown) size of the tachycardia circuit.

3. Dissimilar effects of drugs in A-V and V-A direction

The problem is further complicated by the observation that the effect of a drug on the properties of the accessory pathway in A-V direction may be quite different from that in V-A direction. This is illustrated in figures 12 and 13. Prior to ajmaline administration (fig. 12) an atrial premature beat given after 250 msec was blocked in the accessory pathway, conducted exclusively over the A-V node—His pathway and followed by tachycardia. The same sequence of events was seen following atrial premature beats given in the interval range 250 to 210 msec (the effective refractory period of the atrium). Application of the criteria listed in table 5 argued for incorporation of the accessory pathway in the tachycardia circuit. Following ajmaline (fig. 13) complete block occurred in the accessory pathway during atrial pacing. It was still possible however to initiate tachycardia by a single atrial premature beat. In fact the tachycardia zone had widened from 40 msec (250 to 210 msec) to 80 msec (310 to 230 msec).

The explanation for this unexpected finding was given during ventricular pacing. It was found that ajmaline in this patient had not affected the length of the refractory period of the accessory pathway in V-A direction! This example demonstrates that disappearance of the signs of pre-excitation during sinus rhythm following drug administration does not guarantee that the patient is cured from his circus movement tachycardia. A typical

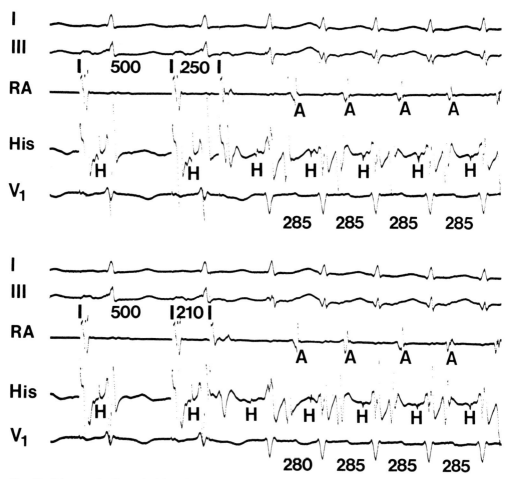

I

III

RA

His

V$_1$

I

III

RA

His

V$_1$

Fig. 12. Prior to ajmaline administration tachycardia can be initiated by an atrial premature beat in the premature beat interval range from 250 (upper pannel) to 210 msec (lower pannel).

example of a drug whose effect on circus movement tachycardia may be unfavourable is amiodarone (914). This drug usually lengthens the refractory period of all parts of the tachycardia circuit, however by concomitantly slowing conduction in the different components of the tachycardia pathway, perpetuation of the arrhythmia is frequently facilitated, be it at a slower rate.

4. Relation between drug effects following acute and chronic administration
Another problem in the study of the effect of drugs on arrhythmias in patients with the WPW syndrome is that usually they are administrated intravenously or intraatrially over a short period of time. This might result in pharmacodynamics different from those following chronic oral drug administration. This can be the reason for failure of therapy when the drug, which was found to be highly effective when given intravenously, is given orally. Stimulation studies correlating the effects following acute (intravenous) and

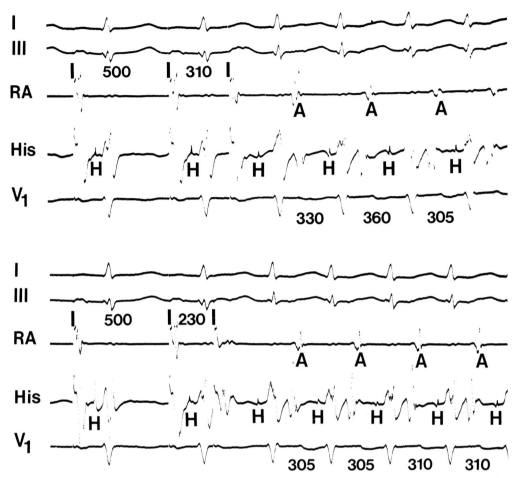

Fig. 13. Following 50 mg ajmaline intra-atrially there is complete block in the accessory pathway during basic atrial pacing. The zone of atrial premature beats able to initiate tachycardia however has increased from 40 (fig. 12) to 80 msec. Ventricular pacing in this patient revealed no effect of ajmaline on the accessory pathway in V-A direction.

chronic (oral) administration are needed to determine the relevance of the acute study for further oral treatment (912).

During studies following rapid intravenous administration it became apparent that the effect of several drugs lasted less longer than previously assumed (906a). This suggests that failure of oral drug administration might be caused by a too widely spaced dosage schedule. This stresses the use of long acting drug preparations, when available.

TREATMENT OF ARRHYTHMIAS IN THE WPW SYNDROME

The following points were found to be helpful in the treatment of patients with WPW suffering from arrhythmias.

1. Drug treatment should only be instituted when the arrhythmia interferes with the physical and/or psychological well being of the patient.
2. Factors which may contribute to the emergence of arrhythmias, like valvular heart disease, coronary heart disease, or sick sinus syndrome, should be identified, and when possible, corrected.
3. For prevention of the tachycardia initiating premature beat, quinidine, preferably given as a long acting preparation, is still the drug of choice.
4. Drug treatment during tachycardia should depend upon site of origin, type of tachycardia and electrophysiologic properties of the structures involved during tachycardia.

Frequently a stimulation study is needed to obtain this information. This should preferably be followed by evaluation of the effect of the drug which seems to be the most useful because of the outcome of the first part of the investigation. When needed the study should be repeated under chronic oral drug administration. Lengthening of the refractory period or block in the accessory pathway can usually be accomplished by procaine amide or ajmaline. Tachycardias based upon a circus movement incorporating the accessory pathway can usually be controlled by administration of these drugs.

The refractory period of the A-V node increases following digitalis, B blocking agents, verapamil and tensilon. Tachycardias confined to the A-V node should therefore be treated by the latter category of drugs.

When possible, long acting agents should be given to minimize changes in drug levels. If during atrial fibrillation or flutter a short refractory period of the accessory pathway is present acute control of the ventricular rate can usually be accomplished by intravenous procaine amide or ajmaline. Orally administrated amiodarone is very useful for long term control of the ventricular rate in patients with atrial fibrillation and a short refractory period of their accessory pathway. Possible dangers of digitalis therapy in atrial fibrillation and WPW have been discussed elsewhere (904a).

INDICATIONS FOR STIMULATION STUDIES IN THE PATIENT WITH THE WPW-SYNDROME

There is a definite indication for programmed electrical stimulation of the heart in:
1. patients with documented episodes of atrial fibrillation or atrial flutter with high ventricular rates. In these patients the length of the refractory period of the accessory pathway should be measured and the effect of drugs studied. In this way the most effective drug for lengthening of the refractory period of the accessory pathway can be identified. If lengthening of the refractory period of the accessory pathway cannot be accomplished by pharmacological means surgical interruption of the accessory pathway should be considered.
2. patients whose tachycardias cannot be controlled by drug therapy. In these patients the site of origin and mechanism of tachycardia should be determined. Thereafter, based upon the outcome of these studies, the most appropriate drug should be administrated and its effect tested. If no benificial effect can be demonstrated surgical interruption of the tachycardia circuit (132, 203a, 751, 874, 908a) or termination of

tachycardia by appropriately timed stimuli delivered by a chronically implanted pacemaker should be considered. As pointed out by Gallagher in chapter 32 also because of the possibility of more than one accessory pathway (419, 783) the stimulation study is essential in pre- and postoperative evaluation of the patient undergoing surgery of his tachycardia circuit. This also holds for the patient in whom for chronic interruption of his tachycardia, a pacemaker device is implanted.

Preferably, all patients with the WPW syndrome should be studied by programmed electrical stimulation of the heart. This will not only help us to establish a more appropriate drug regimen in patients symptomatic with tachycardia but also, by repeating the study over the years, give us the much needed information on the natural history of the WPW syndrome.

This is especially of importance in guiding the patient who is asymptomatic but has a short refractory period of the accessory pathway.

32

CORRELATION BETWEEN CATHETER ELECTROPHYSIOLO-GICAL STUDIES AND FINDINGS ON MAPPING OF VENTRICULAR EXCITATION IN THE W.P.W. SYNDROME

JOHN J. GALLAGHER, M.D., WILL C. SEALY, M.D., ANDREW G. WALLACE, M.D., AND JACKIE KASELL

The electrophysiological assessment (281,293) of a patient with Wolff-Parkinson-White syndrome is a multifaceted study which attempts to: 1. confirm the presence of pre-excitation; 2. identify the nature of the associated tachyarrhythmia; 3. confirm the participation of the accessory pathway in the tachyarrhythmia; 4. presumptively localize the site of the accessory pathway; 5. characterize the functional behavior of the accessory pathway; and 6. examine the effect of drugs or pacemaker therapy. The advent of surgical techniques (751) to interrupt accessory pathways (AP) as a treatment modality for the Wolff-Parkinson-White syndrome has made more apparent than ever the need to preoperatively localize the site(s) of the AP(s) and to implicate the participation of the latter in observed tachyarrhythmias. With such information one can then select optimal candidates for surgical intervention (lateral APs vs. septal APs) (292), identify the presence of multiple APS (81,148,419,511) or APs with unidirectional block (598, 821,960) and select the appropriate operative approach (thoracotomy vs. sternotomy). Importantly, electrophysiological studies of the type to be discussed can be carried out safely and systematically preoperatively, while the corresponding intra-operative investigations utilizing epicardial mapping are often hampered by limitations of time, poor patient tolerance of tachyarrhythmias while under general anesthesia as well as a number of technical problems which can arise.

Such preoperative electrophysiological studies provide several clues to the location of the AP: 1. Electrocardiograms recorded during pacing-induced maximal preexcitation are useful as a first approximation of the site of earliest epicardial activation, but do not always allow the fine discrimination required to distinguish septal from free wall APs (292–294). 2. The stimulus-delta interval is shortest and the degree of preexcitation maximal when atrial pacing is performed near the site of the AP [as compared with pacing other atrial sites at comparable cycle lengths (CL)] (192,293,824,825,902,903), 3. Increases in the V-A interval (> 30 msec) associated with the appearance of bundle branch block aberration, during supraventricular tachycardia (SVT) which utilizes the AP, localizes the AP to the ventricle exhibiting the bundle branch block pattern (150). 4. Efforts to localize the site of preexcitation have also included recordings from the ventricle during antegrade preexcitation. As noted by Frank (281), such attempts have been limited by difficulty in controlling the intraventricular catheter position and the inaccessibility of much of the ventricles (especially the left). Recordings of left ventriculograms from the coronary sinus have demonstrated early local activation during maximal preexcitation in patients with left lateral APs (470,823,873). 5. The sequence of retrograde atrial

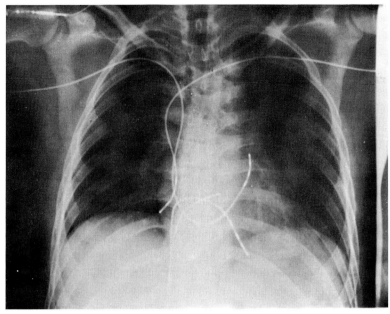

Fig. 1. Roentgenogram of the chest demonstrating the standard catheter positions used during electro-physiologic evaluation of the WPW syndrome. The catheters are positioned in the low lateral right atrium, the coronary sinus, the right ventricle and across the tricuspid valve.

activation has been utilized as a clue to the site of the AP (281, 293, 325, 800, 821, 903, 911, 960).

We will confine our remarks to the usefulness of retrograde atrial activation during SVT as a means of localizing the site of APs. The methodology described has been cor-related with intraoperative mapping studies in the last 24 of 34 patients operated on to date at the Duke University Medical Center for the Wolff-Parkinson-White syndrome.

We will first address ourselves to the methodology used and the results obtained in normal patients in order to lay the foundation for understanding the deviations from normal attending the presence of APs.

We routinely record simultaneous bipolar electrograms from the low lateral right atrium (RA), the low septal RA (via the His bundle catheter) and the medial and lateral left atrium (LA—via a coronary sinus catheter) (823 during SVT as well as during right (and at times left) ventricular stimulation (see fig. 1). A basic principle underlying all our studies is that proper assessment of the properties of conduction and refractoriness of accessory pathways necessitates stimulating and recording from sites as close as possible to the site of the AP. For this reason we attempt to make all our recordings as close as possible to the A-V ring, utilizing recording sites in the low right atrium, the low inter-atrial septum and the coronary sinus. Figure 2 represents the findings in normal patients and demonstrates initiation of retrograde atrial activation in the atrial septum with subsequent spread laterally to both atria (175, 529, 643, 800). More detailed recordings can be obtained from most of the circumference of the mitral valve by continuous record-ing of the coronary sinus catheter during withdrawal from a distal position back to the

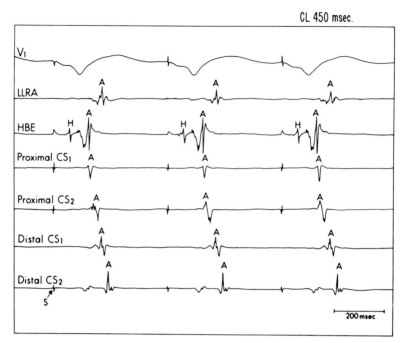

Fig. 2. The normal sequence of retrograde atrial activation during right ventricular pacing. Recordings from above down are ECG leads V_1, with bipolar electrograms recorded from the low lateral right atrium (LLRA), the His bundle electrogram (HBE), two bipolar electrograms recorded in the region of the os of the coronary sinus (proximal CS_1, CS_2) as well as two bipolar electrograms from the distal coronary sinus (distal CS_1 CS_2). A = atrial electrogram. H = His bundle. S = stimulus. During ventricular pacing from the apex at a cycle length of 450 msec, a retrograde His bundle deflection is observed on the HBE recording followed by near simultaneous activation of the low intra-atrial septum as recorded by the HBE and the os of the coronary sinus as recorded on the proximal CS_1. Atrial activation then spreads to the lateral right atrium and the lateral left atrium (as recorded on distal CS_2).

orifice. Detailed exploration of the circumference of the tricuspid valve has been heretofore limited by difficulty in accurate positioning of electrode catheters in stable reproducible positions within the right atrium. I have recently achieved some measure of success in obtaining these recordings by means of a bipolar electrode catheter[1] of my own design

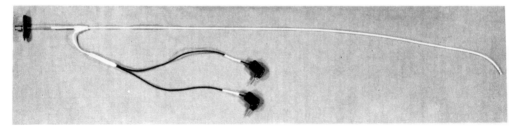

Fig. 3. Electrode catheter for intracavitary mapping of the atria. The #6 French catheter equipped with two tip electrodes is shown with the modified Brockenbrough needle inserted.

1. Catheter fabricated by Mr. Allen Tower of American Catheter Corp, Medford, N.J.

(fig. 3). The catheter has 2 electrodes mounted 2–3 mm apart at the tip of a luminal#6 French catheter, through which a long trochar is introduced fashioned after the traditional Brockenbrough needle. The tip of the latter has been made blunt to insure safety and is never extended beyond the tip of the electrode catheter. The catheter is advanced up the inferior vena cava and once inside the right atrium, can be rotated anteriorly and posteriorly as well as medially and laterally. Using the landmark of the foramen ovale and taking into account the oblique position of the tricuspid valve, we have evolved techniques to reproducibly record representative atrial sites near the level of the tricuspid valve.

An example of the normal sequence of retrograde atrial activation obtained by these combined methods is shown in figure 4. Septal activation recorded inferior and slightly anterior to the foramen by the modified Brockenbrough electrode catheter invariably corresponds well with local atrial septal activation as recorded by the His bundle catheter, while recording of activation of the postero-medial right atrium correlates well with activation recorded on the coronary sinus catheter at the point of withdrawal from the coronary sinus. In 10 normal patients studied to date, earliest retrograde atrial activation has been recorded on the low septal right atrium followed later by or simultaneous with activation of the os of the coronary sinus.

We have determined the sequence of retrograde atrial activation by epicardial map-

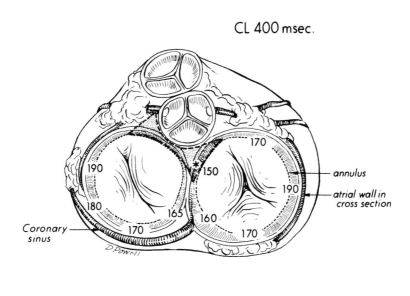

CL 400 msec.

* - BUNDLE of HIS

J.V. K60565

Fig. 4. Normal retrograde atrial activation during right ventricular pacing. A diagrammatic section through the heart at the level of the A-V valves is shown with the mitral valve on the left and the tricuspid valve on the right. Retrograde atrial activation time (measured relative to the onset of activation in the right ventricular apex) has been superimposed on the circumference of the A-V valves. In this patient earliest retrograde atrial activation occurs in the region of the His bundle followed shortly by activation of the os of the coronary sinus. Activation then spreads symmetrically to the lateral walls.

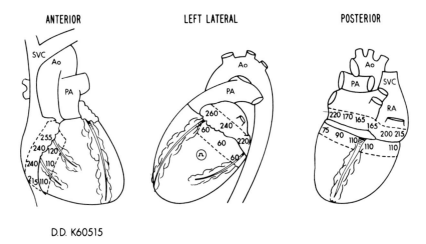

D.D. K60515

Fig. 5. Normal retrograde atrial activation determined by epicardial mapping. Schematic views of the anterior, left lateral, and posterior surfaces of the heart are shown. The left ventricle is being paced at a cycle length of 450 msec (⊓). The activation times around the base of the ventricles as well as the adjacent atrial points are shown. Note that retrograde atrial activation is initiated posteriorly in the region of the crux of the heart and spreads symmetrically to the right and left atrial appendages. See text for discussion.

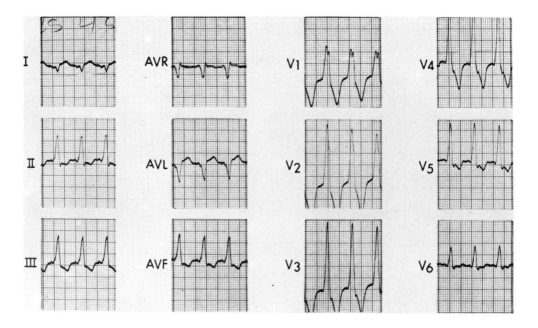

Fig. 6. Electrocardiogram of a patient with a left lateral accessory pathway recorded during left atrial pacing (via the coronary sinus) at a cycle length of 430 msec. Note the negative delta in I, aVL, V_4-V_6 and the positive delta in V_1-V_3.

ping in only a limited number of cases, generally after successful division of an AP (fig. 5). The findings have been consistent with that anticipated from the catheter studies, demonstrating symmetrical lateral spread from the region of the atrial septum at prolonged V-A intervals.

LEFT VENTRICULAR ACCESSORY PATHWAYS

Eight patients have been studied with LV accessory pathways with excellent correlation between preoperative and intra-operative studies. Figure 6 is the EKG of a 22 year old male who presented with ventricular fibrillation. During preoperative studies, SVT was precipitated easily (fig. 7,8) and was associated with early retrograde activation in the most distal portion of the coronary sinus, corresponding to the lateral left atrium. Left bundle branch block during SVT caused the V-A interval to prolong 35–40 msec. Epicardial mapping (fig. 9) demonstrated earliest activation during antegrade conduction at the margin of the left lateral A-V sulcus. Retrograde epicardial mapping (fig. 10) during left ventricular pacing demonstrated preexcitation of the left atrium at a site contiguous with the previously demonstrated site of antegrade preexcitation.

It should be noted that the coronary sinus does not complete the circumference of the mitral valve, leaving a 'blind' area unmapped anteriorly. In one patient thought to have

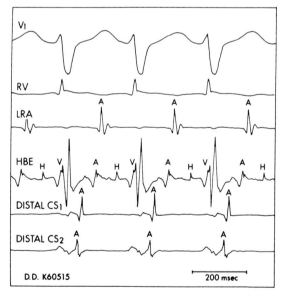

Fig. 7. Retrograde atrial activation during supraventricular tachycardia utilizing a left lateral accessory pathway (same patient as in figure 6). Recordings from above down are ECG leads V_1, with bipolar electrograms from the right ventricle (RV), the low lateral right atrium (LRA), the His bundle electrogram (HBE) and the lateral left atrium via electrograms recorded from the distal coronary sinus (CS_1, CS_2). A His bundle deflection precedes each normal QRS, followed by retrograde atrial activation with the earliest activation recorded from the lateral left atrium via the distal coronary sinus, with spread to the interatrial septum (as recorded by the HBE) and finally the low lateral right atrium.

CL 300 msec.

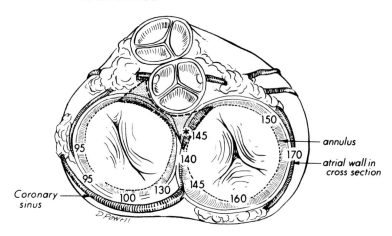

* - BUNDLE of HIS

D.D. K60515

Fig. 8. Composite sequence of retrograde atrial activation during SVT utilizing the left lateral accessory pathway (same patient as in figure 7). Note that retrograde atrial activity is earliest in the lateral left atrium and progressively spreads across the septum to the lateral right atrium.

a single accessory pathway located in the left lateral position by this technique, subsequent intraoperative mapping demonstrated multiple APs along the anterolateral portions of the mitral annulus.

RIGHT VENTRICULAR ACCESSORY PATHWAYS

Four patients with single right ventricular APs have been studied and again demonstrated excellent correlation between preoperative and intra-operative studies.

Figures 11 and 12 are EKGs in sinus rhythm and PAT respectively of a 15 year old girl who presented with intractable PAT and a cardiomyopathy. Electrophysiological study (fig. 13, 14) demonstrated abnormally early retrograde atrial activation in the anterolateral portion of the right atrium. Epicardial mapping was performed during SVT (fig. 15) and demonstrated earliest activation in the anterior RA. The later onset of earliest atrial activation measured by the catheter technique suggests that the atrial activity recorded by this technique was not as close to the annulus as that achieved by direct mapping from the epicardial surface, but still was a valid indication of the site of the AP.

SEPTAL ACCESSORY PATHWAYS

The dilemma presented by septal accessory pathways is illustrated by the following patient with a surgically proven AP in the anterior septum (fig. 16). During SVT, atrial activation is

PRE-INCISION   CL 450 msec.

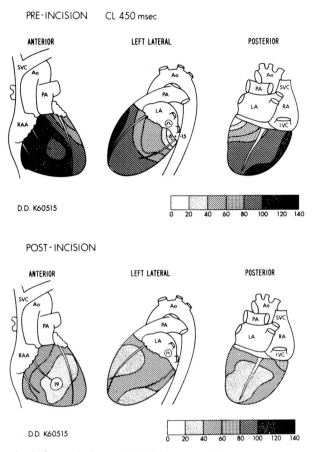

Fig. 9. Epicardial mapping before and after surgical division of a left lateral accessory pathway (same patient as in figure 8). During anomalous conduction, earliest epicardial activation occurs on the lateral left ventricle near the A-V ring 6 msec before the onset of the surface delta wave. The left atrium is being paced at a cycle length of 450 msec and the conduction time from the atrium opposite the earliest ventricular point to the ventricle measures 9 msec. Following division of the accessory pathway, a normal sequence of ventricular activation is observed.

initiated in the atrial septum following a short V-A interval, and subsequently spreads laterally to both atria (fig. 17). The sequence of atrial activation shown is compatible with retrograde participation of a septal AP but could just as likely result from a reentrant mechanism confined to the A-V node. The appearance of functional bundle branch block would not be expected to differentiate these two entities, since in the setting of septal accessory pathways, aberration does not change the V-A interval.

The *presence* of a septal AP may be suggested by the following observations: 1. the V-A conduction time should remain constant (taking into account intramyocardial conduction delay) during ventricular stimulation, irrespective of the cycle length of pacing or the prematurity of coupled ventricular extrasystoles during refractory period determinations (281, 293, 905), 2. V-A intervals during ventricular pacing at a CL comparable to that of observed tachycardia should be comparable to the V-A interval during spontaneous

(CL 450 msec)

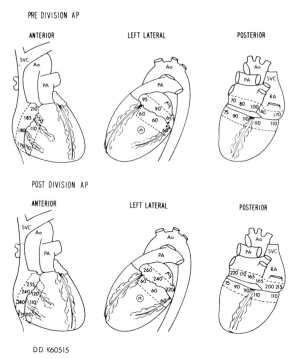

PRE DIVISION AP

ANTERIOR   LEFT LATERAL   POSTERIOR

POST DIVISION AP

ANTERIOR   LEFT LATERAL   POSTERIOR

D.D. K60515

Fig. 10. Retrograde epicardial mapping during left ventricular pacing in a patient with a left lateral accessory pathway. Prior to division of the accessory pathway, earliest retrograde atrial activation occurs in the lateral left atrium with progressive spread to the left and right atrial appendages. Following division of the accessory pathway, the earliest retrograde atrial activation occurs at a longer ventriculo-atrial conduction time and is situated in the atrium overlying the crux of the heart. (Same patient as in figure 9).

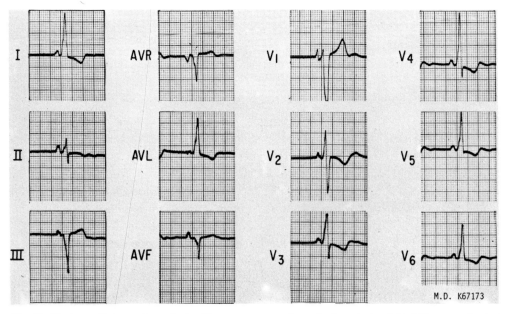

M.D. K67173

Fig. 11. Electrocardiogram of a patient with an accessory pathway in the anterior right A-V groove. See text for discussion.

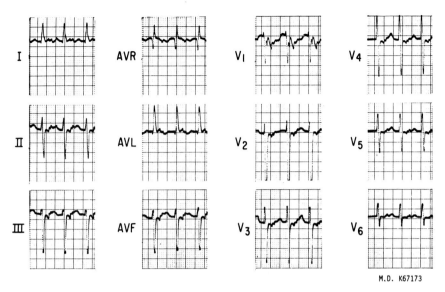

M.D. K67173

Fig. 12. Electrocardiogram recorded during supraventricular tachycardia in a patient with an accessory pathway in the right anterior A-V groove. See text for discussion.

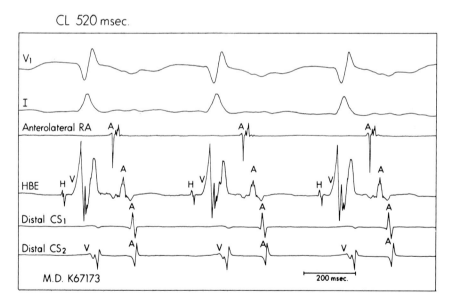

Fig. 13. Retrograde atrial activation during supraventricular tachycardia utilizing an accessory pathway in the right anterior A-V groove. Recordings from above down are standard ECG leads V_1 and lead I with bipolar electrograms recorded from the antero-lateral RA, the His bundle electrogram (HBE) and distal coronary sinus (CS_1, CS_2). Note that retrograde atrial activation is earliest in the anterolateral RA and spreads to the low medial RA (as recorded on the HBE) and then the lateral left atrium as recorded by the distal coronary sinus (CS_1, CS_2). This tachycardia varied clinically from rates of 120/minute to 170/min. Despite the slow rate of the tachycardia demonstrated, a junctional rhythm was excluded by the fact that the tachycardia could be started and stopped with single premature beats. (Same patient as in figure 11, 12).

PRE-OP PSVT – CL 400 msec

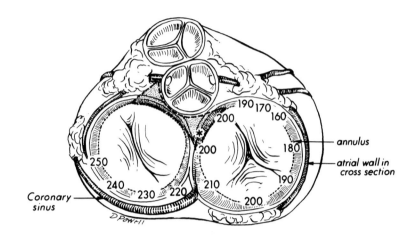

* - BUNDLE of HIS

M.D. K67173

Fig. 14. Composite of retrograde atrial activation in a patient with an accessory pathway in the right anterior A-V groove. Note that the earliest retrograde atrial activation occurs in the anterior RA with progressively later spread to the rest of the atria. (Same patient as in figure 13).

PSVT   CL 370 msec.

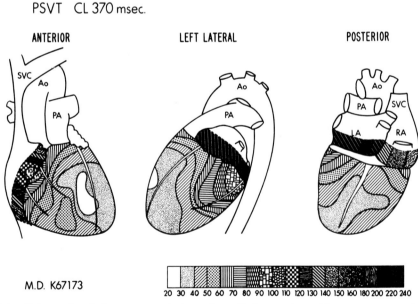

ANTERIOR   LEFT LATERAL   POSTERIOR

M.D. K67173

20 30 40 50 60 70 80 90 100 110 120 130 140 150 160 180 200 220 240

Fig. 15. Epicardial mapping during supraventricular tachycardia in a patient with an accessory pathway in the right anterior A-V groove. The epicardial map demonstrates a normal sequence of ventricular activation with earliest retrograde atrial activation occurring in the anterior right atrium with retrograde conduction time from the adjacent ventricle of 18 msec (same patient as in figure 14). Delayed activation is present over the anterolateral LV due to functional left anterior hemiblock.

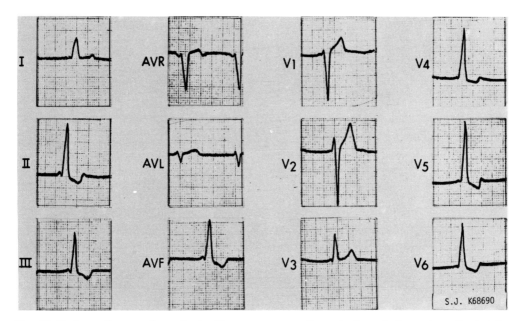

Fig. 16. Electrocardiogram of a patient with an accessory pathway in the anterior septum. See text for discussion.

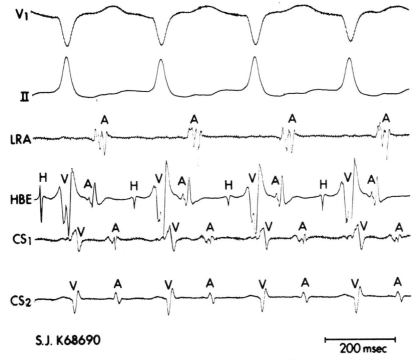

S.J. K68690   200 msec

Fig. 17. Retrograde atrial activation during supraventricular tachycardia in a patient with a septal accessory pathway. Recordings from above down are standard ECG leads V_1, lead II, low lateral right atrium (LRA), the His bundle electrogram (HBE) and distal coronary sinus electrograms (CS_1, CS_2). Note that the medial right atrium as recorded on the His bundle electrogram is earliest with retrograde spread to the lateral right and left atria. (Same patient as in figure 16.)

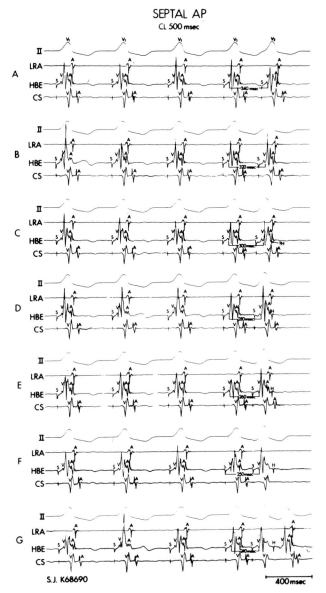

Fig. 18. Determination of retrograde refractory periods in a patient with a septal accessory pathway (Same patient as in figure 17). In panels A–G, recordings from above down are standard ECG lead II and bipolar electrograms from the low lateral right atrium (LRA), the His bundle electrogram (HBE) and the lateral left atrium via the coronary sinus (CS). The last four ventricular beats from a basic series of 8 paced beats at a cycle length of 500 msec are time-aligned (V_1-V_1) followed by a premature ventricular beat (V_2) which is introduced progressively earlier into diastole from panels A–G. Note that during the basic drive beats, the earliest retrograde atrial activation occurs on the low medial RA as recorded by the HBE followed by activation of the lateral right and left atrium. As V_2 is introduced progressively earlier in diastole, the V_2A_2 interval remains constant and with the same sequence of atrial activation. In panel D the His bundle deflection begins to be displaced from the ventricular electrogram and in panel E is clearly displaced later than the earliest retrograde atrial activity. In panel F, V_2 fails to propagate to the atrium. In panel G, the retrograde H_2 is followed by another ventricular response which in turn conducts retrogradely over the accessory pathway to the atrium. This represents the V_2V_3 phenomena described by Akhtar et al. (*Circulation* 50: 1150, 1974).

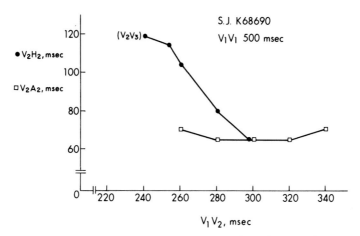

Fig. 19. Determination of the retrograde refractory period in a patient with a septal accessory pathway. This is a graphic representation of the refractory period determination shown in figure 18. On the vertical axis the V_2H_2 intervals as well as the V_2A_2 intervals are plotted against the V_1V_2 coupling intervals on the horizontal axis. Note that the V_2A_2 interval remains constant as the V_2H_2 interval becomes progressively longer.

tachycardia. 3. Ventricular premature depolarizations (VPDs) which induce tachycardia should be associated with V-A intervals comparable to those of control beats and have the same sequence of retrograde atrial activation as observed during tachycardia (293).

The above observations in our judgement, however, do not exclude enhanced retrograde A-V nodal conduction or the presence of dual A-V nodal pathways as the basis of the observed phenomena (190,593). Two further observations which favor the presence of an AP are: 1. the demonstration that early VPDs can conduct retrogradely to the atria with the 'septal' sequence of activation without intervening conduction over the His-A-V node (i.e. retrograde His appears after atrial depolarization—fig. 18,19); and 2. the demonstration that early VPDs can be induced during SVT which retrogradely preexcite the atria without disturbing the preceding His bundle deflection (598,821,960) (fig. 20). Both of these observations prove the *existence* of an AP, but do not per se prove its *participation* in the tachyarrhythmia. If the prematurely evoked atrial depolarization has a sequence of activation identical to that observed during tachycardia (fig. 17), this suggests participation of the AP in SVT.

We have correlated preoperative findings with intraoperative mapping in 10 cases of septal APs. Pacing at multiple atrial sites at comparable CLs did not have as marked an effect on the degree of preexcitation as found with more laterally situated APs. Likewise, the appearance of functional bundle branch block (right or left) during SVT did not significantly (i.e. > 30 msec) prolong the V-A interval. In patients with documented septal connections in the anterior septum or subjacent to the His bundle, activation of the medial RA tended to precede that of the os of the CS; with posterior septal connections, the os of the CS activated simultaneously with or earlier than activation of the medial RA. Representative findings in another documented case of septal preexcitation are shown in figures 21–24. The electrocardiogram (fig. 21) recorded during RA pacing at a CL of 350 msec demonstrated negative delta waves in leads II, III, F and V_1, sug-

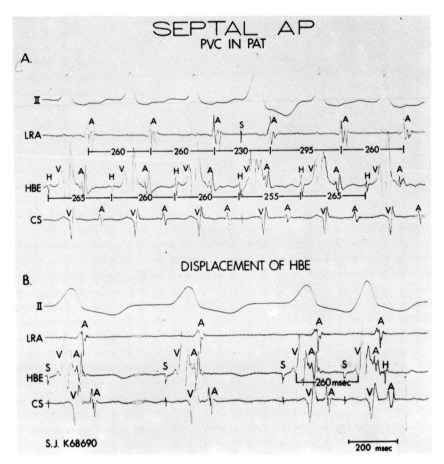

Fig. 20. Effect of premature ventricular beats during supraventricular tachycardia utilizing a septal accessory pathway (Same patient as in figure 19). In panel A, supraventricular tachycardia is present at a cycle length of approximately 260 msec. Note that retrograde atrial activation occurs earliest on the low medial RA as recorded by the HBE with spread to the lateral right and left atria. Note the relative constancy of the H-H intervals prior to the introduction of a ventricular premature beat. After the third beat of tachycardia, a premature ventricular beat is introduced which fails to disturb the antegrade His deflection. The latter occurs just before the premature stimulus and thus the A-V node-His system would be expected to be refractory to retrograde conduction from the premature ventricular beat. Despite this, the retrograde atrial activation following the premature ventricular beat occurs 30 msec earlier than expected, a finding which can be explained only by conduction over an accessory pathway. Note that the activation sequence of the prematurely evoked atrial depolarization has the same sequence as that observed during the tachycardia. For comparison, a panel selected from the retrograde refractory period determinations is shown in panel B. Following 3 ventricular paced beats at the basic driving cycle, a premature ventricular beat is introduced which conducts retrogradely with an identical sequence of atrial activation despite the appearance of a retrograde His deflection after the onset of retrograde atrial activation. (Same patient as in figure 19.)

gesting a site of earliest epicardial activation at the right side of the crux (281, 293, 294). Study of the sequence of retrograde atrial activation during SVT demonstrated earliest activation in the region of the os of the CS (fig. 22). Epicardial mapping (fig. 23) confirmed that the site of earliest epicardial activation was just to the right side of the crux. As with every case of septal AP studied to date, the earliest epicardial point occurred after

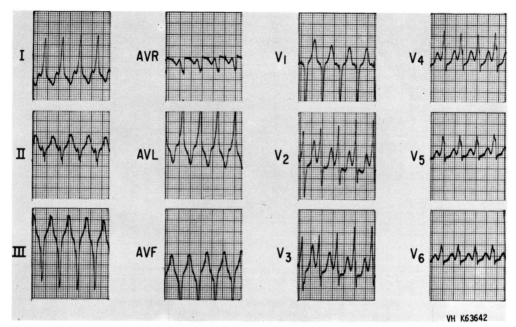

Fig. 21. Electrocardiogram of a patient with a posterior septal accessory pathway. The right atrium is being paced at a cycle length of 350 msec. 1:1 A-V conduction is present with negative delta waves in leads II, III and F and V_1 compatible with a site of epicardial breakthrough to the right of the crux.

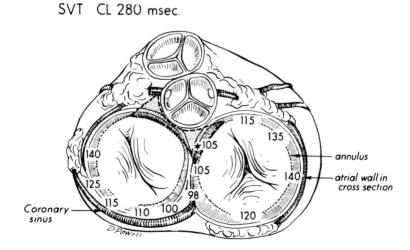

Fig. 22. Composite of the retrograde atrial activation sequence in a patient with a posterior septal accessory pathway (same patient as figure 21). Note that the earliest retrograde atrial activity is recorded in the region of the os the coronary sinus.

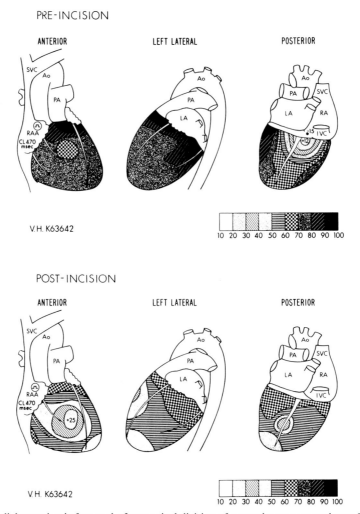

Fig. 23. Epicardial mapping before and after surgical division of a septal accessory pathway. The right atrial appendage is being paced at a cycle length of 470 msec. Prior to the division of the accessory pathway the earliest site of epicardial activation occurs 12 msec after the onset of the surface delta wave and is situated just to the right of the crux posteriorly. There is also an area of breakthrough in the anterior right ventricle resulting from conduction over the normal pathway. Following attempts at surgical division, the epicardial map transiently returned to a completely normal sequence of activation (Same patient as in figure 22.)

the onset of the surface delta wave (+12 msec) in contrast with the findings in lateral APs (right or left) where we are usually able to record epicardial data at or before the onset of the surface delta wave. Earlier activation in this patient could be recorded over the posterior superior aspect of the interventricular septum, where pressure abolished preexcitation. Retrograde mapping of the epicardium during right ventricular pacing demonstrated earliest retrograde activation over the region of the crux (fig. 24); subsequent recording of the orifice of the CS from inside during as episode of SVT while on cardiopulmonary bypass yielded a V-A interval of 100 msec, confirming the value obtained preoperatively by the catheter study. Dissection of the posterior septum, and the region of the CS

CL 430 msec.

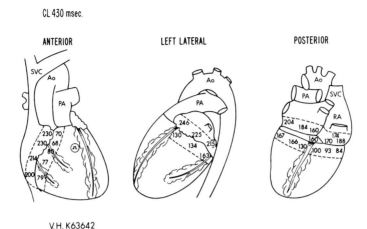

V.H. K63642

Fig. 24. Retrograde epicardial mapping during right ventricular pacing in a patient with a septal accessory pathway. (Same patient as in figure 23.) The sequence of retrograde activation is shown prior to division of the septal accessory pathway. Ventricles are being paced at a cycle length of 430 msec. The activation times at the base of the ventricles as well as the adjacent atrial points are shown. Note that earliest retrograde atrial activation occurs over the orifice of the coronary sinus as it turns inward near the interatrial septum. Following division of the accessory pathway (not shown) the ventriculo-atrial conduction time became markedly prolonged but the same relative sequence of activation was preserved.

orifice abolished preexcitation and the V-A interval became prolonged to 340 msec, associated with a similar activation sequence, suggesting that now retrograde conduction was via the A-V node. Unfortunately, preexcitation returned in this patient several hours postoperatively.

In one additional patient with a septal AP and Ebstein's anomaly of the tricuspid valve, an additional RV accessory pathway was correctly identified by the technique.

MULTIPLE ACCESSORY PATHWAYS

Thus far we have considered only single APs and the manner in which they modify the sequence of retrograde atrial activation. I would like to conclude by presenting a recently operated patient who was correctly diagnosed as having two free wall accessory pathways as well as abnormal A-V nodal physiology on the basis of the preoperative study (106, 874). This case most graphically demonstrates the techniques just described.

The patient was a 15 year old boy who presented with recurrent PAT and documented ventricular fibrillation. The electrocardiogram in sinus rhythm (fig. 25) demonstrated preexcitation with predominantly negative deflections in V_1. During left atrial pacing (fig. 26) via a patent foramen ovale (as well as via the coronary sinus) a pattern of preexcitation compatible with a left lateral free wall AP was evoked. Intracavitary recordings during sinus rhythm (fig. 27, panel A) demonstrated that left atrial activation occurred after the onset of the delta wave, and in addition, the LV electrogram recorded from the posterolateral left ventricular base via the CS catheter was late. Right atrial pacing up to a CL of 240 msec (fig. 27, panel B) resulted in 1:1 A-V conduction with a near

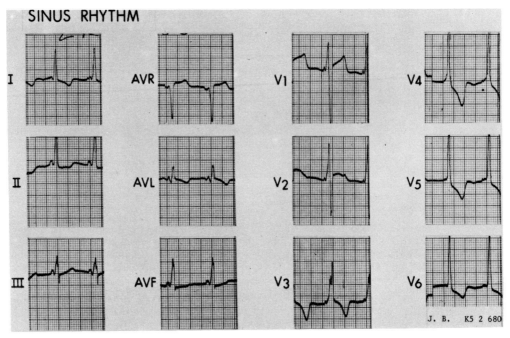

Fig. 25. Electrocardiogram during sinus rhythm from a patient with bilateral accessory pathways. See text for discussion.

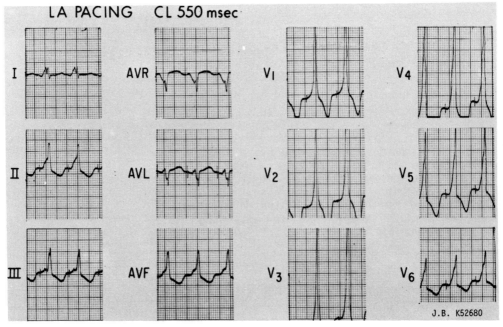

Fig. 26. Electrocardiogram recorded during left atrial pacing via a catheter across the foramen ovale in a patient with bilateral accessory pathways. Note that with left atrial pacing, a pattern of preexcitation is evoked which suggests a left lateral accessory pathway. (Same patient as in figure 25.)

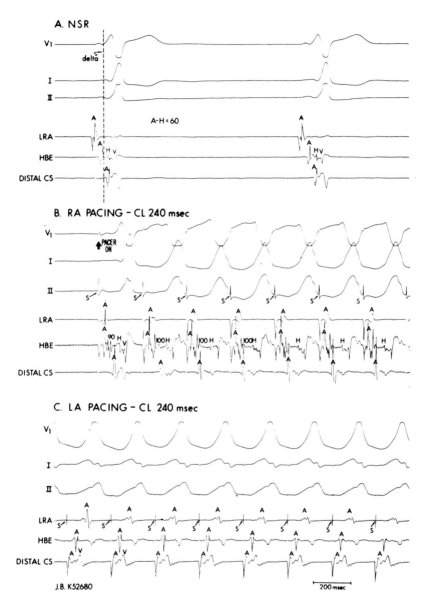

Fig. 27. Intracavitary recordings during normal sinus rhythm, right atrial and left atrial pacing in a patient with bilateral accessory pathways. In panels A–C recordings from above down in each panel are ECG leads V_1, I, II, with bipolar electrograms from the low lateral right atrium (LRA), the His bundle electrogram (HBE) and the lateral left atrium (distal CS). Note that during normal sinus rhythm (panel A) the His bundle depolarization occurs after the onset of the surface delta wave confirming the presence of preexcitation. Note that the activation of the lateral left atrium occurs after the onset of the delta wave. The A-H interval is at the lower limit of normal at 60 msec. In panel B, the right atrium is being paced at a cycle length of 240 msec. Following institution of pacing the A-H stabilizes at 100 msec. An rS pattern is present in V_1 and a His deflection occurs just after the onset of the delta wave. Atrial activation proceeds from the low lateral right atrium to the atrial septum and then to the left atrium. In panel C, the left atrium is being paced at a cycle length of 240 msec. Antegrade atrial activation now proceeds from the left atrium (via the distal CS) and spreads to the septum and the lateral right atrium. Note that the pattern of preexcitation is changed with a predominantly upright complex now present in V_1.

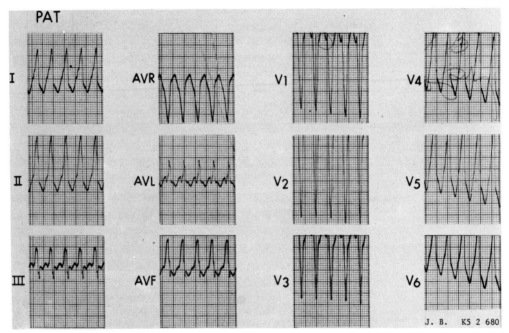

Fig. 28. Electrocardiogram recorded during supraventricular tachycardia in a patient with bilateral accessory pathways. (Same patient as in figure 27.) See text for discussion.

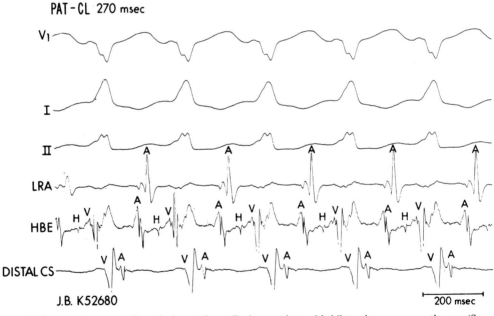

Fig. 29. Intracavitary recordings during tachycardia in a patient with bilateral accessory pathways. (Same patient as in figure 28.) Note that during tachycardia, retrograde atrial activation is initiated in the lateral left atrium (via the distal CS) and spreads to the atrial septum and the lateral RA indicating retrograde conduction over a left lateral accessory pathway. The QRS complexes are slightly anomalous and the H-V interval is short at 20–25 msec suggesting that antegrade conduction in the ventricle occurs over an additional accessory pathway as well as the normal conduction system.

constant A-H interval of 100 msec, and a rS pattern of preexcitation in V_1. With left atrial pacing at the same CL, the QRS became predominantly positive in V_2 and the LV electrogram now occurred in the delta wave (figure 27, panel C). This suggested the presence of two accessory pathways, one in the right and one in the left ventricle, and in addition, some 'enhanced' A-V nodal conduction.

During SVT (fig. 28,29), the QRS appeared to remain anomalous, resembling the pattern of preexcitation previously noted with RA pacing. The H-V interval remained short at 25 msec and the atrial activation sequence indicated retrograde participation of the left sided AP. We concluded from these findings that the tachycardia utilized the left sided pathway retrogradely, with activation returning to the ventricle over both the RV accessory pathway and the A-V node-His system, resulting in fusion. The presence of both APs was again demonstrated by ventricular stimulation (fig. 30). With LV pacing, the left sided AP was preferentially utilized; during straight RV pacing, retrograde atrial fusion was present with near synchronous atrial activation. Early VPDs, however, were noted to activate the antero-lateral RA slightly in advance of the septal RA. These findings were confirmed intraoperatively by epicardial mapping during sinus rhythm and left atrial pacing (fig. 31). Antegrade preexcitation was noted along the anterior right ventricular free wall as well as the lateral left ventricular free wall. Incision of the adjacent annuli of the tricuspid and mitral valves as shown in figure 32 completely abolished preexcitation as well as the ability to provoke tachyarrhythmias. Unfortunately, following cessation of cardiopulmonary bypass, the patient developed low output failure. He was supported by an intra-aortic balloon-assist device and intensive drug therapy but succumbed on the third postoperative day. Autopsy revealed a severe form of cardiomyopathy with massive concentric hypertrophy of the left ventricle predominantly with multiple areas of fibrosis suggestive of remote infarction. No residual connections were present on serial sections of the tricuspid and mitral annuli[2]. Serial section of the A-V node-His system revealed that the A-V node was situated more anterior in the septum than normal. A well developed muscular bundle was noted to insert in the posterior aspect of the A-V node but no fibers were found inserting directly into the His bundle (88).

In addition to localization and identification of the site of multiple accessory pathways (81,148,511), we have also utilized the technique effectively to localize the site of the AP in three patients with unidirectional anterograde block of AP, with retrograde conduction over the AP in SVT (821).

Studies of the type described permit accurate preoperative localization of free wall accessory pathways located anywhere on the circumference of the tricuspid valve and most of the circumference of the mitral valve. The necessity of providing effective input by stimulating and recording near the site of the AP is to be emphasized. Free wall APs are more accessible surgically and can be divided with a high degree of success (751, 874). Our studies further suggest that septal APs can be identified preoperatively. Elucidation of the exact topography of these pathways and development of more effective surgical techniques to interrupt them remains at the forefront of our present investigation.

---

2. We are grateful to Dr. Don Hackel for the histologic studies performed in this case.

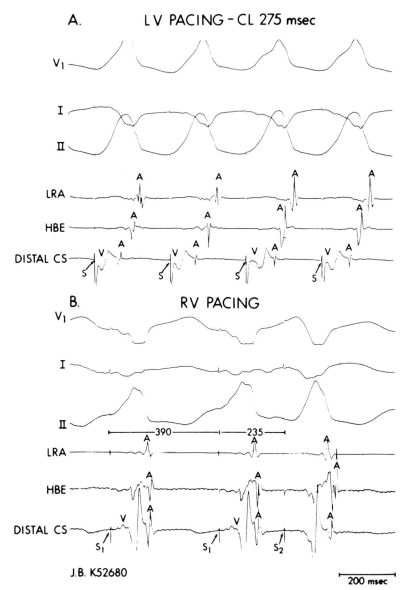

Fig. 30. Effect of left and right ventricular pacing in a patient with bilateral accessory pathways. (Same patient as in figure 29.) In panel A, the left ventricle is being paced at a cycle length of 275 msec. Note that retrograde atrial activation occurs with a short V-A interval comparable to that observed during tachycardia (fig. 29) and that the activation sequence spreads from lateral left atrium to lateral right atrium. In panel B, the right ventricle is being paced at a basic cycle length of 390 msec. Retrograde atrial activation sequences associated with these drive beats reveal almost synchronous depolarization of the left and right atria. Following the last two basic drive beats, however, a premature ventricular beat (S_2) is introduced. The lateral left atrium and the lateral right atrium activate at essentially the same V-A interval; however, activation of the low medial RA is delayed relative to the lateral right and left atrium suggesting that atrial fusion was present during the drive beats. This might have resulted from activation of the lateral RA by the right sided pathway, activation of the lateral LA by the left sided pathway and activation of the medial septum by the A-V node. It should be noted that the latter had demonstrated apparent enhanced conduction during antegrade studies. With the premature beat, delay presumably occurred in the A-V node delaying activation of the medial RA. An alternative explanation might be found in the phenomenon of intra-atrial delay.

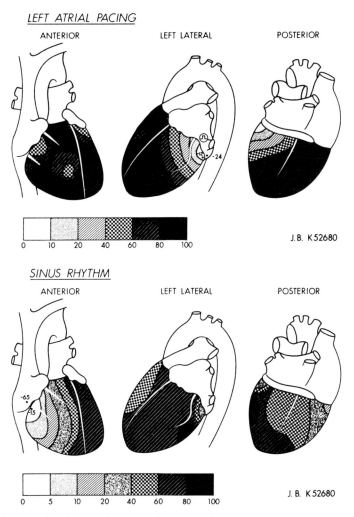

Fig. 31. Epicardial mapping during left atrial pacing and in sinus rhythm in a patient with bilateral accessory pathways. (Same patient as in figure 30.) Note that during left atrial pacing three areas of epicardial breakthrough are present, the earliest along the left lateral A-V groove with onset of ventricular activation 12 msec before the onset of the surface delta wave. A second breakthrough is present at the site of the second accessory pathway along the anterior right A-V groove and a third area is present over the lower anterior right ventricle due to activation over the normal conduction system. Epicardial mapping during sinus rhythm as shown in the lower panel demonstrates the earliest area of activation is in the right anterior A-V groove with ventricular activation 15 msec before the onset of the surface delta wave. A second area of breakthrough is present at the left lateral A-V groove at the site of the second accessory pathway. Fusion from the normal conduction system is no longer observed.

ACKNOWLEDGEMENTS

The authors gratefully acknowledge Mrs. Laura Cook, R.N., and Mr. Tom Novick for assisting with the patient studies, Mr. Don Powell for the artwork, Mr. Dave Huggett for the photographic reproductions and Mrs. Carolyn Jarrell for editing and typing the manuscript.

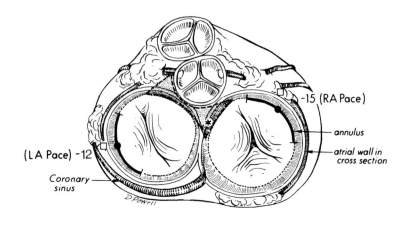

J.B. K52680   *- BUNDLE of HIS

Fig. 32. Schematic representation of the surgical incision in the mitral and tricuspid annuli required to ablate preexcitation due to the left and right sided accessory pathways. The clear square indicates the site of earliest epicardial activation. The dark bracketed bar on the annulus indicates the extent of the surgical incision. (Same patient as in figure 31.)

33

VENTRICULAR EXCITATION IN THE WOLFF-PARKINSON-WHITE SYNDROME

ANDREW G. WALLACE, M. D., WILL C. SEALY, M. D.,
JOHN J. GALLAGHER, M. D., AND JACKIE KASELL

In January of 1967 Professor Durrer and his colleagues from Amsterdam published the first report which described epicardial excitation of the ventricles in a patient with the Wolff-Parkinson-White syndrome (220). Eleven months later Howard Burchell and his colleagues from the Mayo Foundation presented a similar report. (99) In both of these early studies anomalous excitation of the right ventricle was noted with epicardial activation beginning in the region of the atrio-ventricular groove. The reports demonstrated the feasibility of localizing the site of an accessory bypass at surgery; and when coupled with the report by Durrer, Schoo, Schuilenburg and Wellens, (221) implicating the accessory pathway in reentrant tachycardia, led our group at Duke (132) to undertake studies which will be reported in part in this communication. In this chapter we will attempt to present our present view of ventricular excitation in the Wolff-Parkinson-White syndrome. Professor Wellens also asked that we include comments concerning the relation between the morphology of the QRS complex and activation data obtained at the time of surgery.

The material I will present is based upon 24 patients who have undergone successful surgical correction of the Wolff-Parkinson-White syndrome in the past 7 years. These patients constitute a subset, and fortunately a majority, of our total surgical experience with the Wolff-Parkinson-White syndrome at Duke University Medical Center. They were selected from the larger group because in these 24, separation of atrium from ventricle at the level of the annulus of the atrioventricular valves abolished the delta wave on surface electrocardiogram. Since anatomic material was not available for histologic study in any of these patients it is important to recognize at the outset our premise which underlies the conclusions to be presented; that is that the surgical procedure and the resultant normalization of the electrocardiogram and abolishment of arrhythmias constitute reasonable and adequate proof that a bypass tract did exist at the indicated sites.

Figure 1 presents, in diagrammatic form, a section at the level of the atrioventricular valves. The mitral valve is located to the left and the tricuspid valve to the right. Each solid circle depicts the site of presumed bypass tract based upon our best reconstruction of the location at which surgical separation of atrium from ventricle caused the delta wave to disappear from the surface electrocardiogram. From this evidence regarding the approximate location of bypass tracts four important conclusions follow. The first is that the sites of anatomic faults in the annulus are distributed widely and in our experience have been localized to essentially all portions of both the mitral and tricuspid rings with the exception of that portion of the mitral ring to which the anterior leaflet of the mitral valve inserts. Second, bypass tracts have been localized to those portions of the mitral and tricuspid

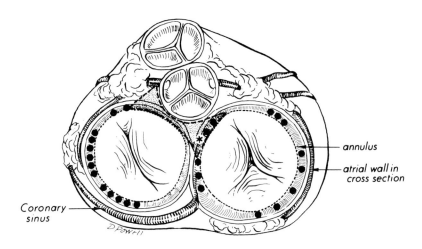

* - BUNDLE of HIS

Fig. 1. Section thru the heart at the level of the AV valves, mitral valve to the left, tricuspid valve to the right.
* = bundle of His. Each filled circle indicates the approximate location of an accessory AV connection
which was divided successfully by surgically techniques. See text for details.

annuli which join the free walls of the atrium and ventricle, but as well bypass tracts have
been located within the septal structures. Third, the bypass tracts responsible for the Wolff-
Parkinson-White syndrome in these patients were clearly accessory since they constituted
conducting bridges from atrium to ventricle which were separate from and in addition to

J.B. J95240

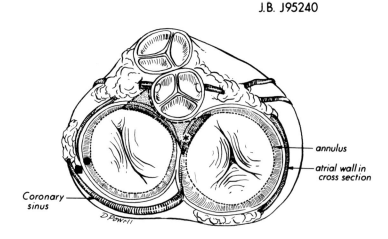

* - BUNDLE of HIS

Fig. 2. Diagramatic view of the area of earliest epicardial excitation (filled square) and the site at which
surgical separation of the atrium from ventricle abolished the delta wave (solid circle). See text for further
detail. Left lateral bypass.

the AV node and bundle of His. Finally, our data are consistent with the view that there may be more than 1 bypass tract in some patients with the Wolff-Parkinson-White syndrome since in 3 of these patients separate tracts were identified at the time of surgery.

Figure 2 is a diagrammatic localization of a bypass tract between the left atrium and the left ventricle in a lateral position of the mitral annulus. The black square indicates the area at which earliest epicardial excitation was demonstrated and the shaded dot in the mitral annulus indicates the site at which an incision which disarticulated the atrium from the ventricle abolish the delta wave on the surface electrocardiogram. Figure 3 presents an epicardial map demonstrating the sequence of ventricular epicardial excitation during sinus rhythm in this patient with a left-sided communication. The heart is viewed from anterior, left lateral and posterior projections along with the lead-2 electrocardiogram obtained at surgery. The time reference at the bottom illustrates the code used on the map for indicating timing of local epicardial excitation. You will note that the white area represents the earliest activation. Epicardial excitation was then divided into 6 intervals of 20 milliseconds each. In the lateral projection the white area on the ventricular surface adjacent to a marginal branch of the circumflex coronary artery indicates the point of earliest epicardial activation. The rapid component of the intrinsic deflection recorded from this area occurred 13 msec before the onset of the delta wave on the surface electrocardiogram. Activation then spread from this region to envelop the remaining portions of the left ventricle. This map also demonstrates that during sinus rhythm the QRS complex resulted from fusion. On the anterior surface of the right ventricle in the trabecular zone there was a circumscribed area of relatively early excitation which occurred between 40

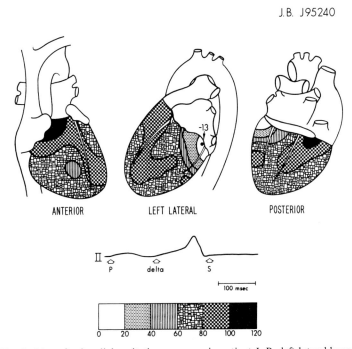

Fig. 3. Map of epicardial excitation sequence in patient J. B., left lateral bypass.

and 60 milliseconds after the onset of the delta wave. The right ventricle was activated almost entirely by an impulse arriving over the normal conduction system while the left ventricle was activated by the bypass tract with fusion noted both anterior and posterior in the regions of the interventricle groove.

Figure 4 is from the same patient. In the upper panels there are expanded left sagittal and posterior views demonstrating early epicardial excitation of the left ventricle adjacent to the atrioventricular groove. The lower panels illustrate the sequence of left atrial activation during paroxysmal supraventricular tachycardia in which the bypass tract was used for retrograde activation of the atrial chambers. During retrograde excitation of the atrium, the earliest point of atrial activation was in the lateral portion of the left atrium immediately above the ventricular area which had demonstrated anomalous pre-excitation during sinus rhythm. The impulse spread from this area to envelop the remaining portions of the left atrium. The figure demonstrates a feature common to all patients whom we have studied with laterally placed communications between the atrium and ventricle: there is a close anatomic correspondence between the area of early ventricular excitation during antegrade conduction over the bypass and the area of early atrial activation during retrograde conduction over the bypass tract.

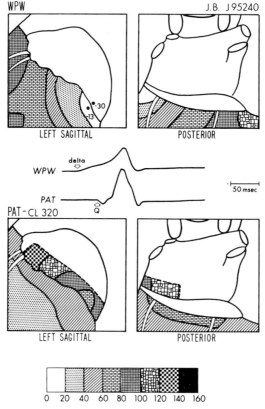

Fig. 4. Maps from patient JB with left lateral bypass, upper panels show ventricular excitation during sinus rhythm with antegrade conduction over bypass. Lower panels show retrograde excitation of left atrium during PAT. See text.

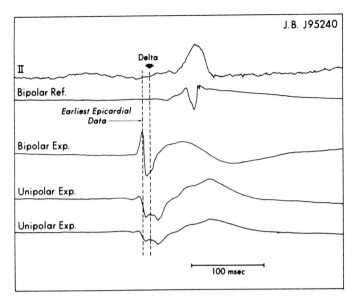

Fig. 5. EKG and electrograms from patient J. B. II = Lead II ECG. Note that rapid component of both uni-polar and bipolar electrograms from the area of earliest epicardial ventricular excitation preceed the onset of the delta wave on the ECG.

Figure 5 presents the electrocardiogram, bipolar epicardial reference, and the bipolar and unipolar derivatives of the signal recorded from the ventricular surface in the area of preexcitation. You will note that the rapid component of the intrinsic unipolar signal and its bipolar derivative occur 13 msec before the onset of the delta wave on the surface electrocardiogram. It has been our experience in all patients with lateral communications that epicardial excitation in the region of the bypass began at or before the onset of the earliest recorded body surface potential.

From the material I have presented so far, I would like to emphasize 4 points. The *first* is that during sinus rhythm, ventricular activation in most patients with left lateral bypass tracts result from fusion. The degree of preexcitation can be maximized and the degree of fusion minimized by pacing the atrium at a site close to the bypass tract. *Second,* when preexcitation is moderately or fully developed, the earliest area of epicardial excitation occurs adjacent to the AV-ring and this area of early excitation can be used as a first approximation to locate the bypass tract. *Third,* further localizing evidence can be obtained by either inducing reciprocating tachycardia or pacing the ventricle and then recording the sequence of atrial excitation during retrograde conduction over the bypass. *Finally,* the interval between atrial and ventricular excitation in the vicinity of the bypass tract is less than 40 msec and in some cases less than 20 msec. The earliest recorded ventricular excitation in the vicinity of the bypass tract is characteristically observed before the onset of the delta potential on traditional surface electrocardiographic leads.

Figure 6 is a diagrammatic illustration from a patient with a right lateral bypass tract. Again, the solid square indicates the area of earliest epicardial ventricular activation during sinus rhythm. The shaded dot in the annulus indicates the site at which the surgical incision interrupted the bypass tract and eliminated preexcitation. Figure 7 presents the

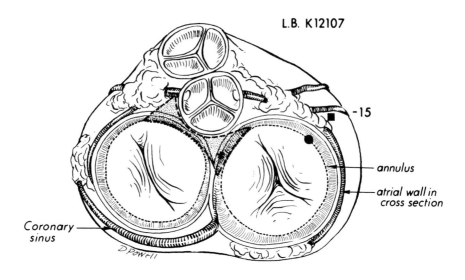

L.B. K12107

-15

annulus

atrial wall in
cross section

Coronary
sinus

* - BUNDLE of HIS

Fig. 6. Diagramatic illustration from patient LB with a right anterolateral bypass. Filled square = area of earliest epicardial ventricular excitation during sinus rhythm. Filled circle = area at which surgical separation of atrium from ventricle abolished delta wave.

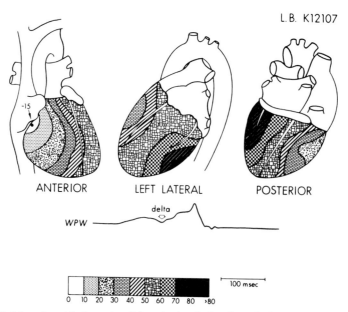

L.B. K12107

-15

ANTERIOR   LEFT LATERAL   POSTERIOR

delta

WPW

0   10   20   30   40   50   60   70   80 >80   100 msec

Fig. 7. Map of ventricular epicardial excitation during sinus rhythm in patient L. B.

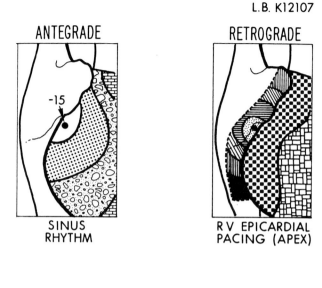

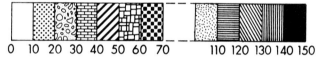

Fig. 8. Maps from patient L.B. Left panel shows ventricular excitation during sinus rhythm with antegrade conduction over the bypass. Right panel shows activation of the right atrium during ventricular pacing with retrograde conduction over bypass.

epicardial map from the patient whose bypass tract was identified diagrammatically in figure 6. The earliest area of epicardial ventricular excitation occurred adjacent to the annulus of the tricuspid valve and spread from this point over the epicardial surface. The sequence of epicardial excitation in this patient failed to demonstrate evidence of fusion. Thus, in this patient and in most patients with right lateral connections it has not been necessary to pace the atrium in the vicinity of the bypass tract to induce maximum preexcitation. Figure 8 presents an expanded view of the right atrial and ventricular epicardial activation during sinus rhythm with antegrade conduction over the bypass tract (left panel) and during retrograde activation over the bypass tract (right panel). Again, it can be noted that the earliest area of ventricular activation is adjacent to the right atrioventricular groove. During retrograde conduction over the bypass tract, the earliest area of atrial excitation was adjacent to the area of the bypass tract with atrial activation proceeding in a radial fashion away from the atrial insertion of the accessory bundle.

Figure 9 shows the electrocardiogram, bipolar reference tracing and the bipolar and unipolar derivatives of the electrogram recorded from the ventricular surface in the area of the presumed bypass tract. Again it should be noted that the rapid component of the intrinsic deflection on the unipolar tracing occurred 15 msec before the onset of the delta

EARLY AREA

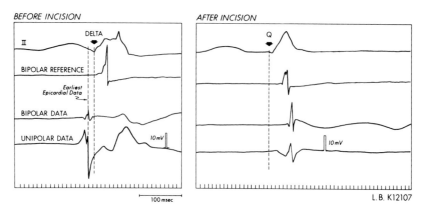

Fig. 9. ECG (lead II) and electrograms for patient L. B. Left panel before surgical separation of atrium from ventricle. Right panel after separation and abolishment of delta wave. Note on left panel that the rapid component of bipolar and unipolar data signals from the early area preceeds the delta wave.

wave on the surface electrocardiogram. From these observations it can be concluded that the criteria for localization of a laterally placed bypass tract in either the left or the right side of the heart are similar. These criteria include a demonstration of the earliest area of ventricular activation adjacent to the atrioventricular groove, an interval of less than 40 msec between atrium and ventricle adjacent to the bypass tract during either antegrade or retrograde conduction, ventricular activation which preceeds the onset of the surface

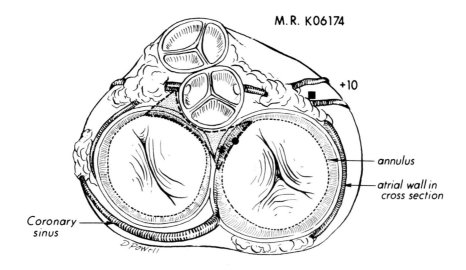

*- BUNDLE of HIS

Fig. 10. Diagramatic illustration from patient M12 with a septal bypass tract anterior to bundle of His. Filled square depicts site of earliest epicardial excitation of filled circle indicates region where separation of atrium from ventricle abolished the delta wave.

delta wave, and finally a high degree of correspondence between the site of earliest ventricular activation during antegrade conduction over the bypass tract and the site of earliest atrial activation during retrograde conduction over the bypass.

Figure 10 is a diagrammatic representation of the findings in a patient with an accessory bypass tract which was located within the septal structures, just a few mm anterior to the position of the His bundle. The black square indicates the area of earliest epicardial ventricular excitation in the region of the right ventricular outflow tract. The shaded dot in the annulus demonstrates the site of the incision which interrupted the bypass. In this patient, the incision was begun at the mid point of attachment of the anterior tricuspid leaflet. An incision at this point failed to interrupt anomalous ventricular excitation. The incision was then carried medially over the surface of the aorta and to a location just 2 to 3 mm anterior to the His bundle electrogram which was being monitored during the operation. At this point the delta wave disappeared from the electrocardiogram. Figure 11 shows the map of epicardial excitation from this patient with a bypass tract between the septal structures just anterior to the bundle of His. The earliest area of epicardial excitation was noted on the anterior projection adjacent to the atrioventricular ring near the right ventricular outflow tract. Activity spread from this point in a manner not dissimilar from that depicted in figure 7. However, it should be noted that the earliest area of epicardial ventricular excitation occurred 10 msec after the onset of the delta wave on the surface electrocardiogram. Figure 12 shows the electrocardiogram, the bipolar reference and the bipolar and unipolar derivatives of the electrogram recorded from the area of earliest ventricular excitation. The delay between the onset of the surface delta wave and the local ventricular electrogram should be noted as well as the low amplitude R-wave potential preceding the intrinsic deflection on the unipolar epicardial tracing.

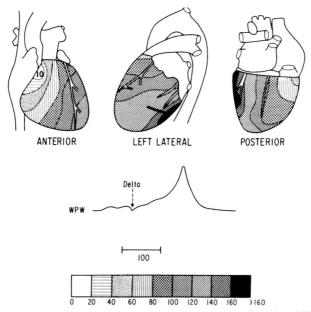

ANTERIOR   LEFT LATERAL   POSTERIOR

Delta

WPW

100

0   20   40   60   80   100   120   140   160   >160

Fig. 11. Sequence of epicardial ventricular excitation in patient MR.

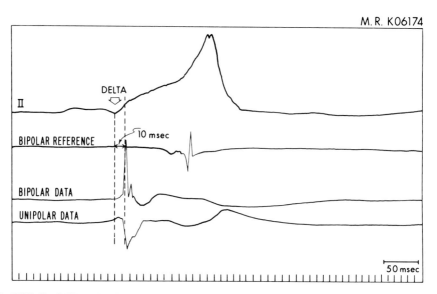

Fig. 12. ECG (lead II) and epicardial electrograms from patient MR. Note that the rapid components of the unipolar and bipolar data signals from the earliest area of epicardial breakthrough follow the onset of the delta wave on the ECG in this patient with a septal bypass.

Although Dr. Gallagher will present data in chapter 32 indicating several preoperative techniques we have utilized to identify septal tracts, the salient points at the time of direct studies of activation at surgery are indicated by this patient. They include that earliest epicardial excitation is in the vicinity of either the anterior or posterior interventricular groove, that earliest epicardial excitation is delayed with respect to the onset of the delta wave on surface leads and finally, the absence of a close anatomic and temporal correlation between the area of early epicardial ventricular excitation during antegrade conduction over the bypass and the area of earliest atrial excitation during retrograde conduction over the bypass.

Figure 13 presents a diagrammatic view of the heart from a patient with a septal bypass located posterior to the bundle of His and just beneath the orifice of the coronary sinus. The solid square indicates the earliest epicardial activation which was observed on the diaphragmatic surface of the right ventricle adjacent to the posterior interventricular groove. The shaded dot in the tricuspid annulus illustrates the site of the surgical incision which interrupted the bypass tract and abolished the delta wave. Figure 14 presents the epicardial map from this patient. The area of earliest ventricular excitation can be observed on the posterior projection adjacent to the interventricular groove on the right ventricular surface. This area of early excitation was noted 5 msec after the onset of the delta wave on the surface electrocardiogram and activation spread from this point to envelop the diaphragmatic surface of both the right and left ventricles. In this patient there was evidence of fusion during sinus rhythm with an early island of epicardial breakthrough 30 to 40 msec after the onset of the delta and visualized on the anterior surface in the trabecular zone.

T.E. K29605

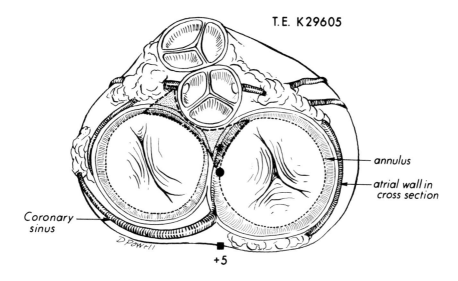

annulus
atrial wall in
cross section

Coronary sinus

+5

*- BUNDLE of HIS

Fig. 13. Diagramatic illustration from patient TE with a septal bypass posterior to the bundle of His. Filled square depicts site of earliest epicardial excitation and filled circle indicates region where separation of atrium from ventricle abolished the delta wave.

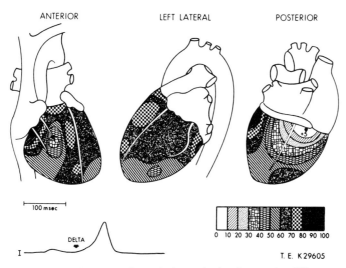

ANTERIOR   LEFT LATERAL   POSTERIOR

100 msec

DELTA

I

0 10 20 30 40 50 60 70 80 90 100

T. E. K29605

Fig. 14. Sequence of ventricular excitation from patient TE.

Figure 15 shows the electrocardiogram, epicardial reference and the bipolar and unipolar derivatives from the diaphragmatic surface of the right ventricle in the area of earliest epicardial excitation. The delay between the onset of the rapid component of the unipolar derivative and the onset of the delta wave, although small, was clearly evident. The criteria for recognizing a septal bypass tract at the time of surgery were equally applicable here with the earliest area of epicardial excitation occurring adjacent to the

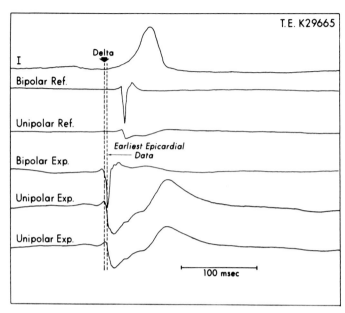

Fig. 15. ECG (lead I) and epicardial electrograms from patient TE. Note that the rapid components of the bipolar and unipolar electrograms recorded from the area of earliest epicardial excitation followed the onset of the delta wave by 5 msec in this patient with a septal bypass.

interventricular groove, a delay between the onset of the delta wave and the earliest area of epicardial excitation, and a wide interval between atrial and ventricular activation at this location.

Figure 16 illustrates some of the difficulties we have encountered in studying excitation in patients with bypass tracts in septum. The upper tracings are taken from a patient with a bypass tract located in the septal structures posterior to the bundle of His. During antegrade conduction, epicardial breakthrough occurred adjacent to the interventricular groove and just to the right of the septum. Activity occurred 5 msec after the onset of the surface delta wave. With right ventricular pacing and retrograde conduction over the bypass, the earliest area of atrial activation occurred in the same vicinity as epicardial ventricular activation during antegrade conduction. Furthermore, the interval between atrium and ventricle during regtograde excitation was only 32 msec. It was our impression, initially, that these data supported the view that the bypass tract was located in the free-wall structures. However, the subsequent surgical incision which interrupted the bypass tract was several centimeters from this location just beneath the orifice of the coronary sinus adjacent to the septal rather than the posterior leaflet of the tricuspid valve. It must be concluded from this observation that the nearly concurrent activation of the atrium and ventricle at this site, occurred not because the bypass tract was located in this vicinity but rather because these adjacent regions of atrium and ventricle were temporarily equidistant from the pacing site of the right ventricle but not in anatomic or electrical continuity. This is not a surprising observation, in retrospect, since in the vicinity of the crux the atrio-ventricular groove is quite deep and a bypass through the annulus of the tricuspid valve would be remote from any epicardial recording sites. The lower panel of figure 16

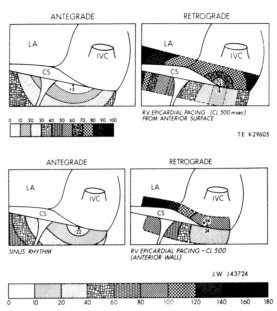

Fig. 16. Upper panels show excitation of the ventricle during antegrade conduction (left) and of the atria during retrograde conduction (right) from patient TE. Lower panels show excitation of the ventricles during antegrade conduction (left) and of the atria during retrograde conduction (right). See text for details.

provides additional evidence for this view. These are recordings from a patient who did have a bypass tract located in the annulus of the posterior tricuspid leaflet. During ante-grade conduction over the bypass tract, initial ventricular excitation occurred on the diaphragmatic surface of the right ventricle 22 msec before the onset of the delta wave on the surface electrocardiogram. During ventricular pacing with retrograde conduction over the bypass, the earliest area of atrial excitation occurred just above the subsequently identified bypass. However, the interval between activation at the ventricular end of the bypass and atrial activation at the atrial end of the bypass was 70 sec. Surgical division of the annulus from inside of the right atrium abolished the delta. Thus, we can be certain of the location of the bypass and that conduction was indeed taking place retrograde over the bypass tract. The 70 sec interval between ventricle and atrium at the site of the bypass is noteworthy. It is our current view that in the region of the curx such a long interval is still compatible with a free wall communication because the annulus is deep relative to epicardial recording sites and for that reason, atrial activation is delayed relative to input from the ventricular side because of the long path over which the impulse must travel.

ECG CORRELATIONS

At this point I would like to deviate from consideration of ventricular excitation and its use in localizing the bypass tract to an examination of the relation between the surface electrocardiogram and the site of the bypass tract. Figure 17 presents, in diagrammatic

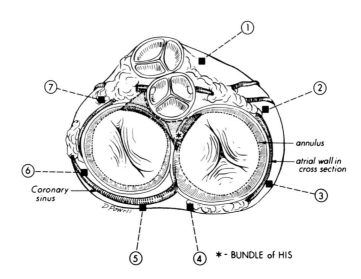

Fig. 17. Classification of regions of early epicardial excitation in the Wolff-Parkinson-White syndrome which appear to be recognizable by typical ECG presentations depicted in figure 18.

view, seven areas of *epicardial ventricular preexcitation* which we believe can be reasonably predicted on the basis of the surface electrocardiogram. The solid squares are actual sites at which epicardial excitation was observed in patients with the Wolff-Parkinson-White syndrome. Site *1* represents an area of early epicardial breakthrough in a patient with an anterior septal bypass. Sites *2* and *3* represent areas of early epicardial excitation in two patients with laterally placed communications between the right atrium and right ventricle. Sites *4* and *5* illustrate paraseptal areas of initial epicardial excitation in two patients with bypass tracts in posterior aspects of the tricuspid and mitral annulus respectively. Site *6* is illustrative of the area of the earliest epicardial breakthrough in a patient with a left lateral bypass tract, and site *7* from a patient with epicardial breakthrough on the anterior portion of the left ventricle just to the left of the anterior descending branch of the left coronary artter. Thus, positions *1* through *4* were characterized by early epicardial excitation of the right ventricle and cases *5* though *7* by early epicardial excitation of the left ventricle.

Figure 18 presents vectors characterizing the direction of the initial delta forces on the surface electrocardiograms from patients with epicardial breakthrough at the 7 positions noted above. The vectors described for positions 1 through 4 were from patients with epicardial excitation of the right ventricle and all had electrocardiograms which met criteria for Type B WPW. Vectors 1 and 2 were from patients with epicardial breakthrough on the anterior right ventricle in the regions of the pulmonary outflow tract and the right ventricle respectively. The delta forces were directed inferiorly and were essentially isoelectric in leads V1 and V2. Vectors 3 and 4 were from patients with epicardial breakthrough on the right ventricle, but at the acute margin and paraseptal regions of the diaphragmatic surface respectively. The vector describing the delta wave was more superiorly oriented and distinctly upright in leads V1 and V2, although the predominant QRS

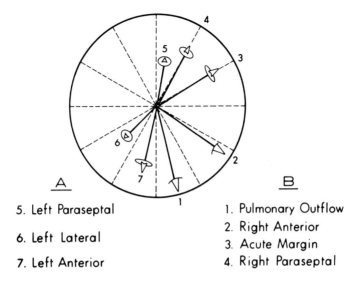

A

5. Left Paraseptal

6. Left Lateral

7. Left Anterior

B

1. Pulmonary Outflow
2. Right Anterior
3. Acute Margin
4. Right Paraseptal

Fig. 18. Position of the delta vector (first .04) corresponding to the areas of epicardial preexcitation shown in figure 17. See text for details.

deflection in anterior precordial leads was still negative. Vector 5 was from a patient with Type A WPW who had initial epicardial breakthrough at the paraseptal region on the diaphramatic surface of the left ventricle. The direction of the delta was predominantly superior and anterior with V1 nearly totally upright. Vector 6 was from a patient with a left lateral connection and epicardial breakthrough near the distal portion of the circumflex coronary artery. The delta vector was directed to the right, anterior and inferiorly. Vector 7 was from a patient with early excitation of the left ventricle near the bifurcation of the left main coronary artery. The delta vector was directed to the right, inferior and produced an upright force in lead V1. From this presentation, it can be concluded as suggested by Robert Frank in his thesis (281) that the initial forces describing the delta wave can be a useful first approximation of the *site of earliest epicardial excitation* in patients with the Wolff-Parkinson-White syndrome. While this is a useful approximation we think it is very important to identify certain limits of the electrocardiogram as a technique for predicting *the site of the bypass tract*. The correlations I have just illustrated were between the position of the delta vector and earliest area of epicardial excitation, *not* between the delta force and the location of the bypass tract. This is an important distinction I hope to illustrate further, together with other reservations we have about efforts to precisely locate the bypass tract on the basis of QRS morphology along.

Figure 19 lists our reservations about the reliability of predicting the site of the bypass tract from the morphology of the QRS complex on the surface electrocardiogram. Of the 34 patients who have undergone efforts at surgical correction of the Wolff-Parkinson-White syndrome at Duke, 19 have had significant associated cardiac abnormalities. Many of these conditions are characterized by alterations of the QRS complex even in the absence of the Wolff-Parkinson-White abnormality, thus suggesting the possibility that these conditions may modify the morphology of the QRS complex in the presence of

---

- Associated Abnormalities

- Septal versus Free Wall

- Two or More Pathways

- Delta Changes with Rate

- Simultaneous "P" and "Delta"

- Undirectional Block in Kent

Fig. 19. Limitations of the ECG (position of delta) in the recognitation of sites of bypass tracts.

anomalous excitation. Those conditions of particular note were the Ebstein's malformation of the tricuspid valve (6 patients) and cardiomyopathies with significant hypertrophy of the ventricles (5 patients). In more than one patient with the Ebstein's malformation we have observed bypass tracts which inserted into the atrialized portion of the ventricular chamber, and in whom the initial forces characterizing the delta wave did not accurately predict either the earliest area of epicardial right ventricular excitation or the location of the bypass tract. A *second* observed limitation is represented by those patients with communications within the septal structures. Our experience is now sufficient to indicate that in patients with a bypass located within the septum, posterior to the bundle of His, the initial epicardial excitation occurs at the crux in a manner which we cannot distinguish from excitation due to more peripherally located bypass tracts in the posterior portions of either the mitral or tricuspid annulus. The point of initial epicardial excitation can be identical and the sequence of ventricular excitation is remarkably similar in these two conditions. At least the gross morphology of the QRS complex is quite similar and cannot be adequately used to distinguish septal from free wall communications in the vicinity of the crux. This is perhaps the most significant limitation in our experience since it is critical to the surgical technique as well as the likelihood that surgical intervention will be successful in correcting the WPW abnormality.

A *third* limitation concerns those patients who have two or more bypass tracts located some distance apart. We have had at least three patients in whom we have recognized two bypass tracts of surgery. Initial epicardial excitation occurred in the vicinity of one of the bypass tracts but within 30 to 40 msec there was a second area of anomalous ventricular excitation due to wavefronts entering ventricle over the second bypass. The resulting epicardial activation sequence was complex and resulted from fusion of wavefronts arising from two anomalous bundles. The resulting QRS complex, while typical of the

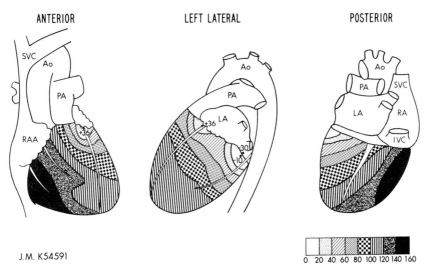

ANTERIOR   LEFT LATERAL   POSTERIOR

J.M. K54591

0 20 40 60 80 100 120 140 160

Fig. 20. Epicardial sequence of excitation during sinus in a patient with two (2) bypass tracts. One area of preexcitation appeared 10 msec prior to the delta wave adjacent to a marginal branch of the circumflex coronary artery. A second later area of preexcitation appeared subjacent to the anterior descending branch of the left coronary artery.

Wolff-Parkinson-White abnormality, was apparently distorted by these nearly simultaneous areas of annomolous activation in a manner which made the direction of the delta forces an inaccurate predictor of the site of either bypass. *Fourth*, we have observed several patients in whom the morphology of the delta wave changed during atrial pacing. In these instances the heart was paced at a site close to the bypass tract at a rate sufficient to produce a major degree of preexcitation as judged from both the surface electrocardiogram and that the His bundle potential was delayed until after the onset of the delta on the surface electrocardiogram. Despite this, when the rate of pacing was increased and sometimes only by a modest degree, the direction of the delta wave forces change significantly. We do not have an adequate explanation for this observation although it is not difficult to speculate on many potential causes for such an alteration. *Fifth*, we have observed both at the time of preoperative catheterization and at surgery that atrial excitation in the atrial chamber contralateral to the site of the bypass can be taking place for 20 to 50 msec after the onset of the delta wave on the surface electrocardiogram and after the initial area of ventricular excitation. This observation suggests that P wave activity which is occuring concurrently with the delta wave may distort the delta wave and this consideration is a major concern in those situations where the left atrium is enlarged.

   Finally, there is the extremely interesting group of patients who have a recurrent bouts of supraventricular tachycardia due to a reciprocating mechanism which utilizes a bypass tract, but in whom there is unidirectional (antegrade) block over the bypass tract such that the surface electrocardiogram never demonstrates the morphological characteristics of the WPW abnormality. We have seen two patients who clearly had such a mechanism and utilized a bypass tract for retrograde conduction from ventricle to atrium even though antegrade conduction over a bypass tract was never observed. We have also seen two patients postoperatively in whom the surgical intervention abolished antegrade conduction but failed to abolish retrograde conduction over the bypass tract. These patients clearly demonstrates a total lack of correlation between the delta wave and the location of a bypass tract. On the basis of these observations, we presently feel that the electrocardiogram, and more particularly QRS morphology in standard lead systems, cannot be used alone to reliably predict the site or sites of anatomic bypass tracts with the precision which is needed for operative intervention. In our view, preoperative physiological studies and detailed intraoperative mapping are essential to successful surgical intervention in the Wolff-Parkinson-White syndrome.

MYOCARDIAL INFARCTION

34

MECHANISMS OF ECTOPIC RHYTHM FORMATION DUE TO MYOCARDIAL ISCHEMIA: EFFECTS OF HEART RATE AND VENTRICULAR PREMATURE BEATS[1]

BENJAMIN J. SCHERLAG, Ph.D., RONALD R. HOPE, M.B., F.R.A.C.P.
DAVID O. WILLIAMS, M.B., MRCP, NABIL EL-SHERIF M.D., AND
RALPH LAZZARA, M.D.

INTRODUCTION

Almost 10 years ago when we started our investigations on arrhythmias due to myocardial ischemia, the prevailing concepts of ectopic impulse formation were based on the studies of Harris and his coworkers (340). After occlusion of the left anterior descending artery in the dog, ventricular premature beats, ventricular tachycardia and ventricular fibrillation were suddenly seen within the first few minutes (early phase) and then another period of similar arrhythmias was observed 24–48 hours later (late phase). Soon the idea of two phases of ventricular arrhythmias attracted the attention of clinicians. The pre-hospital phase of clinical, acute myocardial infarction with its sudden onset and high mortality seemed to be closely analogous to the early phase in the experimental setting. Whereas the ventricular arrhythmias seen in the coronary care unit were likened to the later phase of the experimental studies. Harris postulated (340, 343) that the mechanism and site of origin of both the early and late ventricular arrhythmias were related to rapidly discharging automatic foci arising at the borders of the ischemic or infarcted myocardium. Our aim was to test this hypothesis and clarify whether automaticity or reentry or both were the responsible mechanisms. Also, we attempted to test whether Purkinje or muscle tissue at the borders or within the ischemic or infarcted zones were the sites of origin of these arrhythmias. In keeping with the title of this report and on the basis of the relatively great interest in the prehospital phase arrhythmias, we will confine ourselves to the ventricular arrhythmias occurring during the early ischemic phase. Information regarding the later phase arrhythmias can be found elsewhere (82, 218, 226, 437, 474, 739).

METHODS

Adult mongrel dogs were anesthetized with sodium pentobarbital (30 mg/kg, IV). Under controlled ventilation the thorax was opened at the 4th intercostal space, and the heart was exposed via a pericardiotomy. The left atrial appendage was reflected and the left anterior descending coronary artery was exposed within 1–2 cm of its origin so that silk ligatures could be placed around the artery without ligation.

Two silver wires (diam 0.012 inches) were inserted into the distal portion of the right or left vago-sympathetic trunk (472). Vago-sympathetic trunk stimulation (0.05 msec, 20 Hz, 1–10 v) allowed reduction of the heart rate and assessment of the underlying

1. This work supported in part by NIH-NHLI Contract No. 72-2972-M.

ventricular automaticity. In addition, two fine stainless steel wires (diam 0.003 inches) were inserted by a 25-gauge hypodermic needle into the left atrial appendage. Atrial pacing (2 msec, 180–200 pulses/min, 2–10 v) was accomplished by stimulation delivered from an S88 Grass stimulator and SIU isolation unit.

To record from the specialized ventricular conduction tissue and regular ventricular muscle, both an electrode catheter (734) and plunge wire electrodes (735) were employed. A bipolar electrode catheter was inserted into the right and left common carotid artery and positioned at the aortic root for recording His bundle activation (738). In addition, plunge wire recordings from the heart were made using two fine Teflon-coated stainless steel wires (diam. 0.005 or 0.003 inches) for endocardial recordings. The wires were passed through 25 gauge needles $1\frac{1}{2}$ inches in length, bent back at the bevel of the needle to form small hooks. After plunging the electrodes through the left ventricular cavity, the needle could be removed thus allowing the wire hooks to engage the endocardium. The cut ends of the wire served as close bipolar recording electrodes (739). For subepicardial recordings similar plunge wires were placed just beneath the epicardium. Endocardial and subepicardial electrodes were positioned in the anterior left ventricular wall (perfused by the anterior descending coronary artery) and in the lateral or posterior left ventricular wall (not perfused by the anterior descending coronary artery). In later experiments recordings of the ischemic zone electrograms and the control zone electrograms were designed to obtain information from as large an area as possible within these zones. This was based on the finding that activation within the ischemic zone, during the first few minutes after coronary artery ligation, was markedly heterogeneous, so that close bipolar electrodes a few mm apart could record activation differences of 300 msec or more. Therefore a large multipolar paper electrode (379) was made with two separated silver wires (0.012 inches diam) which were threaded on to the surface of paper tape with 20 points exposed to create multiple bipolar contacts with an interpolar distance of 2–3 mm. The two wires were connected to pin jack terminals and the subsequent recording produced a 'composite' electrogram from the multiple exposed bipolar contacts. The paper electrode was positioned circumferentially over the surface of the ischemic area and secured by fine 6-0 sutures at each corner. In this position the electrode covered areas of almost simultaneous activation and during the control state recorded an electrogram which was very similar to those from close bipolar wires. The only detectable difference was a slight increase in duration seen in the composite electrogram (see fig. 6, CIZeg).

In addition to the electrograms, recordings were made from standard electrocardiographic leads. Electrical recordings were made at frequency limits between 0.1 and 2000 Hz and 40–200 Hz. Potentials were registered on an Electronics for Medicine oscillographic photographic recorder at paper speeds of 25, 50, 100 and 200 mm/sec. A peripheral vein was cannulated for administering drugs and a peripheral artery was cannulated for monitoring blood pressure by standard techniques.

PROCEDURES

Before ligation of the anterior descending coronary artery, control records were made during 1. atrial pacing at 200/min, and 2. vagal induced atrial arrest or complete atrioventricular (A-V) nodal block to determine the idioventricular escape rate. After one-stage ligation of the left anterior coronary artery, effects of atrial pacing were determined, and underlying ventricular automaticity was assessed at 2–5 min intervals up to 30 min after occlusion. In some cases, the effects of atrial pacing after 30 minutes up to 4 hours was used to test the susceptibility of the heart to ventricular arrhythmias.

VENTRICULAR PREMATURE STIMULATION

Ventricular premature stimulation was achieved with a medical system devices stimulator MK III. This unit was programmed to deliver an impulse (2 msec duration, 5–10 v) to the ventricle after every tenth atrial pacing stimuli. Stimulus intensity was kept constant in each dog but varied between experiments. Recordings were made before and during left anterior descending artery occlusion in sinus rhythm and during atrial pacing at 150 beats/min. If significant delays in the epicardial potentials in the ischemic zone were not apparent, higher atrial rates up to 200 beats/min were used. If arrhythmias occurred without apparent delay, alternate sites within the ischemic zone were selected for placement of bipolar recording pairs. During any spontaneous episode of ventricular tachycardia, the coupling interval of the initiating beat was determined. Five to 10 min were allowed to lapse between successive occlusions and analysis of the subsequent occlusive changes was only undertaken if the electrograms had returned to their normal control pattern recorded at the beginning of the experiment. It was found that no more than 5–6 occlusions could be performed before abnormalities persisted after the release of occlusion. The experiments were terminated by ventricular fibrillation to determine the greatest delay of epicardial potentials associated with the onset of this arrhythmia. Electrical defibrillation was not used. The atrial paced beat immediately preceding the extrasystole was also analyzed to indicate the progressive abnormalities of epicardial activation in the ischemic zone that occurred when the ventricles were activated along the normal atrioventricular pathways. In five dogs the coupling interval of the ventricular stimulus, (20% above threshold level), was adjusted in consecutive occlusions to fall early and late in diastole. Early diastole was defined as 5–10 msec after the point at which the stimulus was ineffective, i.e., within the T wave, and late diastole as 5–10 msec before the interval in which fusion complexes were produced.

PROCEDURE FOR STUDYING BRADYCARDIA DURING MYOCARDIAL ISCHEMIA

After placing the ligature around the anterior descending artery and placement of epicardial electrodes the left chest incision was closed and the animal turned. The right chest was opened at the 4th intercostal space and the right atrium and basal portions of the right ventricle were exposed through a pericardiotomy. The untied ligature around the coronary artery was brought to the right side and an occluding collar, consisting of a short length of polyethelene tubing was placed over both ends of the ligature so that subsequent occlusion of the vessel could be obtained by sliding the polyethelene collar down against

the left anterior descending artery. A plunge wire bipolar electrode was inserted into the
area of the His bundle in order to pace the heart from this site. The heart rate was slowed by
two methods: a. crushing the sinus node in order to induce low atrial or A-V nodal rhythms
at rates between 60–100 beats/min; b. induction of complete heart block with His bundle
or idioventricular rhythm at rates between 29–45 beats/min by injection of the A-V node with
0.1–0.3 cc formaldehyde (11). During left anterior descending artery occlusion, the occurrence of ventricular ectopic activity at various atrial paced rates from 40–310/min
was examined for periods up to 2–3 hours from the onset of coronary artery ligation.

RESULTS

Initially we confronted an important technical problem. Other investigators using the
one-stage ligation of the anterior descending artery in the dog reported great variability in
the incidence of arrhythmias within the first few minutes (786). In figure 1, taken from
our early studies, we found that atrial pacing at 200/min could be used to consistently
provoke the ventricular arrhythmias after coronary artery ligation, particularly when they
did not appear during normal sinus rhythm. With cessation of pacing or slowing of the
heart rate by vago-sympathetic stimulation, we could interrupt the ventricular arrhythmias
which occurred after coronary artery ligation. Table 1 summarizes our findings regarding
underlying ventricular automaticity during these early arrhythmias. Note that the idioventricular escape rate during the control state averaged 39 beats/min. During the first
20–30 minutes following coronary artery ligation the underlying automaticity as indicated
by the idioventricular rate was unchanged from control. With atrial pacing at 200 beats/
min ventricular arrhythmias were invariably produced during this interval and the rate of
these ventricular tachycardias averaged 275 beats/min.
  In regard to the site of origin of these ectopic rhythms, figure 2 shows electrical recordings from the endocardium and epicardium as well as standard ECG leads. His bundle recording and recordings from close bipolar wires in the endo- and epicardium in both the
normal and ischemic zones are shown. The magnified view of the endocardial potentials in

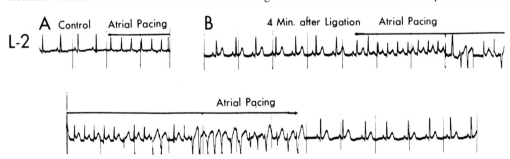

Fig. 1. Induction of ventricular arrhythmias by atrial pacing after acute coronary ligation. Lead II
(L-2) was recorded in the control state. Panel A shows normal sinus rhythm with left atrial pacing at 200/min.
In panel B four minutes after acute coronary artery ligation, ST and T wave changes are noted. Atrial pacing
at 200/min produces a progressive elevation of the ST segments until ventricular tachycardia occurs. Immediately after cessation of pacing there is reversion to sinus rhythm with abolition of ventricular tachycardia.
The interval between time lines was 1 second. (Reproduced by permission of *Amer. J. Physiol.* 219: 1665,
1970).

Table 1. Underlying ventricular escape rate in control hearts and within 20–30 minutes after coronary artery occlusion.

| Expt. No. | Control (beats/min) | | Ischemia (beats/min) | | |
	NSR	Idioventri-cular Rate	NSR	Idioventri-cular Rate	Ventricular Arrhythmia* Rate
1	152	41	158	43	300
2	148	37	138	38	260
3	180	68	168	65	220
4	111	39	108	35	240
5	162	51	168	52	330
6	88	26	91	29	240
7	148	10	131	12	260
8	163	36	158	38	300
9	109	45	107	42	320
Avg	140	39	139	39	275
±SD	29	15	27	14	40

NSR = heart rate during normal sinus rhythm
*Ventricular arrhythmias were observed during atrial pacing at 200 beats/min.

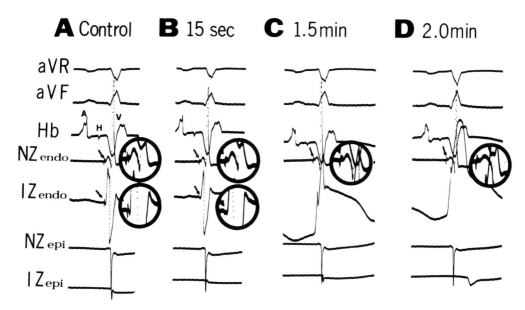

Fig. 2. Purkinje and muscle activation before and immediately after coronary artery ligation. Traces from above are ECG leads aVR and aVF, His bundle electrogram (Hb), close bipolar electrograms from the endocardium in the control or normal zone (NZ endo) and the ischemic zone (IZ endo) and close bipolar electrograms from the epicardium in the normal zone (NZ epi) and the ischemic zone (IZ epi). All electrograms were recorded with filter settings between 0.1–2000 Hz. The arrows and magnified inserts indicate the Purkinje activation in the endocardial zones (small sharp potentials preceding the larger endocardial muscle potential). See text for details. (Reproduced by permission of the American Heart Assn. *Circulat. Res.* 35: 372, 1974).

figure 2A indicate rapid deflections (arrows) which represent Purkinje tissue depolarization prior to endocardial muscle activation. During the first two minutes after coronary
artery occlusion (panels B through D) the following changes were noted: there was
marked reduction in the Purkinje potential in the ischemic zone with a dramatic alteration
of the ST segments of the endocardium muscle potential. In the epicardial potential of the
ischemic zone there was a gradual reduction of potential amplitude and delay of the epicardial potential (see panel D). No arrhythmias were seen at this time.

Figure 3 illustrates the onset of the ventricular arrhythmias that arose spontaneously
approximately $2\frac{1}{2}$ minutes after coronary artery ligation. The delay in the ischemic zone
epicardial potential continues in the first few beats and also shows marked fractionation.
The major components of the epicardial activation are delayed well beyond the QRS into
the ST segment and T wave (arrows). Delayed activation was very localized, since it occurred in the ST segment without any change of the QRS complex in the electrocardiogram. In panel B the occurrence of epicardial activation at the end of the T wave of the
second beat is associated with the abrupt onset of ventricular tachycardia which proceeded
to ventricular fibrillation. This documentation of such a sequence of events consistent
with a reentrant mechanism for malignant ventricular arrhythmias was seen four times in
our initial series of 20 dogs all of whom demonstrated ventricular tachycardia or ventricular fibrillation.

Figure 4 illustrates the effects of vagal stimulation causing slowing of the sinus rate
during the time when epicardial potentials in the ischemic zone showed marked diminution
and delay. In the first two sinus beats of figure 4 diminution and delay of epicardial potentials in the ischemic zone were evident and closely associated with the onset of ventricular
tachycardia (starred beats). Vagal stimulation initiated during ventricular tachycardia

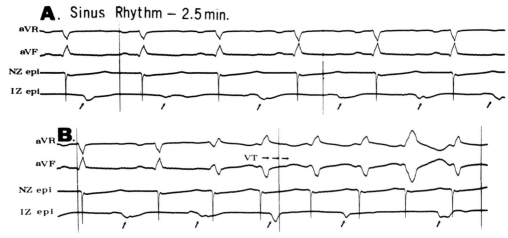

Fig. 3. Initiation of ventricular tachycardia (VT) associated with marked delay of localized epicardial activation.
Panels A and B are continuous records from figure 2 except for the His bundle recording and the endocardial
recordings which have been deleted for the sake of simplicity. It should be noted that epicardial delay in the
ischemic zone proceeded progressively without any change on the surface ECG. The occurrence of epicardial
activation at the end of the refractory period of the ventricles (second arrow in panel B) corresponded to
the onset of ventricular tachycardia which went on to ventricular fibrillation. The interval between time lines
equals 1 second. (Reproduced by permission of the American Heart Assn. *Circulat. Res.* 35: 372, 1974).

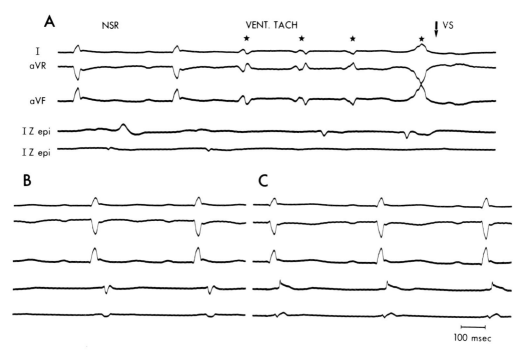

Fig. 4. Effect of vagal slowing of the heart rate on the epicardial activation in the ischemic zone. Traces from the top to the bottom are standard ECG leads I, aVR and AVF and two close bipolar epicardial electrograms in the ischemic zone (IZ epi). The slow, markedly delayed activation of epicardial sites in the ischemic zone during normal sinus rhythm (NSR) is shown in panel A. During normal sinus rhythm a multifocal ventricular tachycardia (starred beats) occurred. Vagal induced slowing of the heart rate (arrow) caused sinus rhythm to be restored. In panel B note the relative recovery of timing and configuration of the epicardial potentials in the ischemic zone and their closer association to each other and ventricular activation as seen on the standard ECG leads. In panel C the sinus rhythm stabilized 30 min after acute coronary artery ligation. Note the further recovery of the configuration upstroke and timing of the epicardial potentials in the ischemic zone. (Reproduced by permission of the American Heart Assn. *Circulat. Res.* 35: 372, 1974).

caused slowing of the sinus rate with some recovery of the amplitude and timing of the epicardial deflections (panel B). In panel C 20–30 min after acute left anterior descending coronary artery ligation, that is, after the cessation of the arrhythmic episodes, the epicardial potentials have further recovered amplitude and temporal relationship to the ventricular activation. These findings suggest a direct temporal relationship between the deterioration of the local epicardial potentials and the early ventricular arrhythmias. To further define this relationship, in 20 dogs the delay in epicardial activation in the ischemic zone was examined from the time of occlusion to the onset of ventricular arrhythmias and ventricular fibrillation. Figure 5 is a graphic representation of the relationship between the delay of ventricular activation in the ischemic epicardium and the occurrence of ventricular tachycardia or ventricular fibrillation or both. The former is represented on the ordinate and time on the abcissa. Zero is the onset of ischemia by coronary ligation. T represents the time of occurrence of ventricular tachycardia or ventricular fibrillation which averaged 4 minutes. However this was normalized in each dog and designated as T. The delay of the epicardial activation in several portions of the ischemic zone was

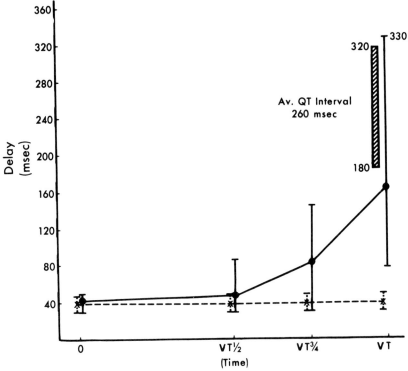

Fig. 5. Relationship between the delay of epicardial activation in recorded electrograms (ordinate) and the time of onset of ventricular tachycardia normalized in each of 20 dogs (VT, abscissa). The average time of onset of ventricular tachycardia was 4 min in absolute terms. The potentials from the ischemic epicardium (circles) show variable but significantly greater average delays that did the potentials from the non-ischemic epicardium (crosses). Note the marked variability of activation in the ischemic zone just prior to the onset of ventricular tachycardia when some recorded epicardial potentials showed delay of activation well beyond the end of the average QT interval (260 msec, range 180–330 msec). (Reproduced by permission of the American Heart Assn. *Circulat. Res.* 35: 372. 1974).

measured just before the onset of ventricular tachycardia (T) at 3/4 of this time and 1/2 of T. Compared to the activation of an epicardial electrogram outside the ischemic zone (broken line) there was progressive delay of epicardial activation measured from the onset of the QRS complex. It should be noted that as the delay increased, the variability of activation of local areas increased as indicated by the vertical bars. This corresponded to the finding of others (82,218,226) who also found that the ischemic or infarcted zone showed marked variability in its activation. In several instances delay of ventricular activation exceeded the average QT interval of 260 msec. The greatest delay seen was 330 msec. The occurrence of maximum delay in any given instance invariably preceded the onset of ventricular tachycardia and ventricular fibrillation.

VENTRICULAR PREMATURE STIMULATION

Several of our studies were undertaken to obtain information on a question which has received a great deal of attention recently, that is, the distinction between the so-called malignant and benign ventricular premature beat. We noted in our experiments that on many occasions the initial spontaneous ectopic beat that started ventricular tachycardia

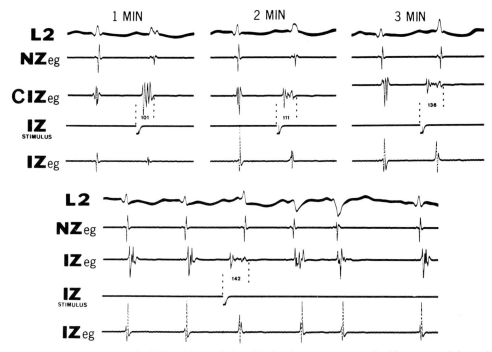

Fig. 6. Ventricular tachycardia initiated by an induced ischemic zone extrasystole. The top panel shows the induced ventricular extrasystole in the preceding atrial beat at 1, 2, and 3 minutes after occlusion. The lower panel was recorded at 3 min 20 sec. The composite ischemic zone electrogram (CIZ eg) demonstrates progressive delay of ventricular activation time (VAT) as measured from the earliest onset to the end of the latest recorded activity in all leads. VAT increased from 101 msec to 136 msec after 3 min and to 142 msec at the onset of arrhythmia. See text for details. (Reproduced by permission of American Heart Assn., *Circulation* 50: 1163, 1974).

leading to ventricular fibrillation was late-coupled. Before and after left anterior descending artery occlusion, electrical stimulation was delivered to the ventricle every tenth beat. In figure 6 the stimulus was delivered to the ischemic zone. Traces are similar to those before and show a standard electrocardiographic lead, lead II, electrograms from the epicardium in the control or normal zone, and three electrograms taken from three local sites in the ischemic zone (IZ). The latter includes a composite ischemic zone electrogram (CIZeg) recorded by a multiple contact bipolar electrode. (See composite electrogram described in Methods). At 1 min the recorded ischemic zone electrograms are beginning to show diminution of their potentials and fractionation as compared to the normal zone potential. The time from the stimulus to the end of activation as demarcated by the vertical broken lines is 101 msec. Note that the induced ventricular premature beat is late-coupled in relation to the basic rate which is seen in the panel below. Indeed the induced beat is almost a fusion beat. At 2 min and 3 min as the fractionation and delay increases in the sinus beats, there is a concomitant increase in the ventricular activation time of each induced ventricular ectopic beat until at 3 min repetitive ectopic beats result when the greatest delay in ventricular activation is observed, 142 msec.

In figure 7 another instance of this phenomenon is seen. The ectopic beat just prior to the onset of the arrhythmia is shown at the left. Ventricular activation time measured from the onset of the induced QRS to the latest ventricular activation recorded in the ischemic

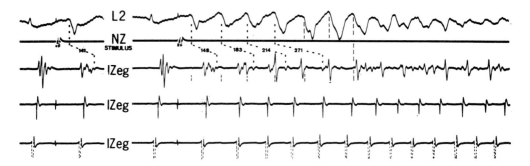

Fig. 7. Ventricular tachycardia initiated by a stimulus delivered to the normal zone (NZ). On the left, the sinus beat and extrasystole preceding the sequence on the right is shown with the ventricular activation time (VAT) during the extrasystole of 141 msec and no resulting arrhythmia. On the right, the tenth sinus beat following the preceding sequence is shown with a similar extrasystole delivered to the normal zone with the same coupling interval as on the left. The total VAT is 148 msec followed by ventricular tachycardia in which VAT progressively increases and ventricular fibrillation occurs. (Reproduced by permission of the American Heart Assn. *Circulation* 50: 1163, 1974).

zone electrogram was 141 msec. To the right 10 beats later the same stimulated beat in the presence of greater delay shown by the preceding sinus beat causes a longer ventricular activation time, 148 msec, leading to ventricular tachycardia with progressive increase in ventricular activation time and finally degenerating to ventricular fibrillation. These results indicated that the malignancy of a ventricular premature beat depends on the alteration of the activation of the heart, mainly fractionation and delay of epicardial activation. In addition the extrasystoles that initiated tachycardia and finally fibrillation had no specific relationship to the so-called vulnerable period. Extrasystoles were capable of producing arrhythmias irrespective of their diastolic coupling time and many examples of diastolic timing far removed from that part of the T wave which is classically considered to be vulnerable were seen. The relationship between the PR, Q-T, and coupling intervals of ectopic beats initiating ventricular tachycardia is shown in table 2. It was found that for both spontaneous ectopic beats and induced ectopic beats, the time from occlusion to onset of ventricular arrhythmias was consistently shorter when induced by early diastolic ectopic beats (3 min 38 sec, $\pm$ 51 sec average) than by late diastolic ectopic beats (4 min 25 sec, $\pm$ 53 sec average). This difference just bordered statistical significance, $p = 0.075$.

THE EFFECT OF BRADYCARDIA ON ECTOPIC RHYTHMS DUE TO MYOCARDIAL ISCHEMIA

Recently Epstein and his group (253) suggested that the accepted ideas regarding the potential dangers of bradycardia in acute myocardial infarction may be erroneous and that bradycardia with rates of 60/min or lower, uncomplicated by hypotension, may actually protect from malignant ventricular arrhythmias whereas increasing the rate with atropine may be deleterious. In one of our recent studies, the effect of heart rate over a wide range, viz., 40 beats/min to 300 beats/min, was obtained as described above (see Methods). In those dogs in whom complete heart block was induced with the subsequent occurrence of His bundle or idioventricular escape rates of less that 60 beats/min, there

Table 2. Relationship between R-R, Q-T, and coupling intervals of spontaneous and pacing-induced ventricular ectopic beats initiating ventricular tachycardia or ventricular fibrillation

Heart Rate (beats/min)	R-R (msec)	Q-T (msec)	CI (msec)
Spontaneous Ectopic Beats			
143	420	173	268
200	300	230	295
200	300	230	210
194	310	195	280
194	310	195	225
194	310	195	245
194	310	195	285
194	310	195	300
122	490	245	360
158	380	190	200
179	335	210	210
146	410	290	335
150	400	270	315
154	390	250	340
Induced Ectopic Beats			
211	280	195	235
158	380	270	280
157	385	290	340
194	310	195	255
158	380	275	300
194	310	195	260
194	310	195	280
164	365	255	340
158	380	270	350
174	345	240	240
150	400	260	300
146	410	290	335
164	365	255	340

CI = coupling interval

were no ventricular arrhythmias which occurred during the first hour or even up to 4 hours after coronary artery ligation. Concomitantly there was no fractionation or delay of epicardial potentials in the ischemic zone at these low rates. In figure 8 panel A the tracings at slow speed depict lead II and epicardial electrograms from the normal zone (NZeg) and ischemic zones (IZeg). Portions of the same record at faster paper speeds are shown in panel B below. Throughout the experiment, every 30–60 min, His bundle pacing at 200/min, as shown on the left side of the illustration, produced marked delay of the ischemic zone epicardial potential and in this case 2:1 block ensued prior to the onset of ventricular tachycardia. There was no appreciable change in the normal zone electrograms. The immediate cessation of pacing with marked slowing of the heart rate and resumption of His bundle rhythm caused a rapid return of the timing, amplitude and configuration of the ischemic zone epicardial electrogram. A reinstitution of 1:1 ventricular activation between

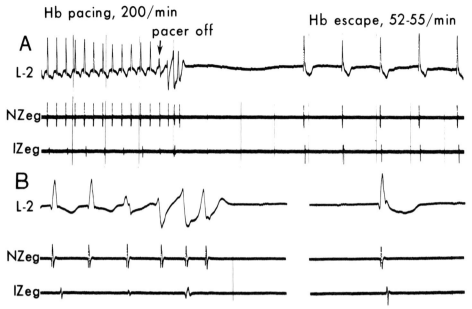

Fig. 8. Ventricular tachycardia induced by His bundle pacing in a dog with heart block. Tracings from above: lead II (L-2) ECG, normal zone electrogram (NZ eg) and ischemic zone electrogram (IZ eg). In panel A note that during His bundle pacing at 200/min the IZ eg electrogram shows 2:1 block in relation to the NZ eg prior to the onset of ventricular tachycardia. The immediate cessation of His bundle pacing (pacer off, arrow) allowed termination of ventricular tachycardia with a long asystole before a His bundle escape rhythm appears at a rate of 52–55/min. Note the rapid return of the timing, amplitude and configuration of the ischemic zone epicardial electrogram with a reinstitution of 1:1 conduction in the normal and ischemic zones. In panel B, the essential portions of the same sequence are shown at faster paper speed in order to contrast the effect on the IZ and NZ electrograms. The interval between time lines equals 1 second.

normal and ischemic zones with the coincident abolition of ventricular tachycardia was also observed at the slower heart rates (52–55/min). Thus, although the marked brady-cardia protected from the ventricular arrhythmias after coronary artery ligation the heart was vulnerable to the deleterious effects of rapid heart rates for a prolonged period of time.

Of importance as well was the finding that bradycardia itself, without untoward hypoten-sion, could be extremely hazardous in the first 2–4 hours after coronary artery occlusion. In figure 9, panel A standard lead II and electrograms from the ischemic and normal zones were recorded during sinus rhythm three hours after left anterior descending artery occlu-sion. During 1:1 conduction at a rate of 130/min, some delay of the epicardial activation in the ischemic zone can be seen in the composite electrogram (IZeg). A-V block and sinus slowing induced by vago-sympathetic stimulation shows two closely coupled ectopic beats, probably indicative of intermittent ectopic ventricular automaticity, followed by 2:1 A-V block at an effective ventricular rate of 44/min in panel B. One ectopic beat falling on the T wave induces ventricular fibrillation. Note the marked disperson in ventricular activation of the ischemic zone and normal zone in the ectopic beat and the very early activation in the ischemic zone of the post-ectopic beat. This activity occurs prior to the post-ectopic QRS complex in the standard lead electrocardiogram. The sequence of activation re-presents continuous activity consonant with a reentry mechanism leading to ventricular fibrillation. This phenomenon was not an isolated event but was seen in 15% of our experi-ments.

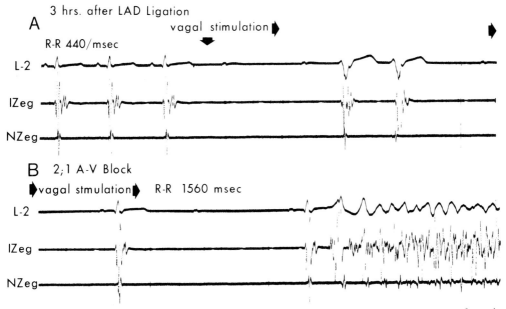

Fig. 9. Vagal mediated sinus slowing, unmasking ventricular premature beats with the occurrence of ventricular fibrillation. The traces are the same as those shown in the previous figure. In panel A during sinus rhythm,
1:1 conduction at a rate of 130/min is shown followed by sinus slowing and A-V block induced by vago-
sympathetic stimulation. The asystolic period is interrupted by two closely coupled ectopic beats followed by
2:1 A-V block at an effective ventricular rate of 44/min in panel B. One ectopic beat falling on the T wave of
the preceding sinus beat induces ventricular fibrillation. The interval between time lines equals 1 second.

Another interesting finding which bears on the role of heart rate in the induction of or
prevention of ectopic impulse formation during acute ischemia is shown in figure 10.
During the course of these bradycardia experiments we were able to determine the effect
of pacing over a wide range of heart rates on the occurrence of ectopic rhythms. In panels A
through F, a standard lead II electrocardiogram was recorded during low atrial rhythm
(after crushing the sinus node) at a rate of 70/min (panel A). At this time no ectopic beats
were seen. At a rate of 80 beats/min (panel B) ventricular tachycardia and premature
ventricular beats were consistently noted. In panel C at a heart rate of 115, utilizing His
bundle pacing, scattered ventricular beats were also noted. In panel D at a His bundle
pacing rate of 160/min no ectopic beats were seen. At a heart rate of 210/min (panel E)
ectopic beats appeared as fusion complexes. However at even faster rates (panel F 310/
min) no ectopic beats were seen during His bundle pacing. The indications of these findings
will be discussed below.

DISCUSSION

The first few minutes of ischemia in the dog heart presents a similar tendency towards serious
arrhythmia as reported clinically. The occurrence of ventricular fibrillation is markedly
enhanced by rapid heart rates (737). It seems likely that the human response to the crushing
chest pain associated with incipient myocardial infarction would lead to sympathetic discharge and increased heart rates. Although such data is lacking in man, in awake dogs

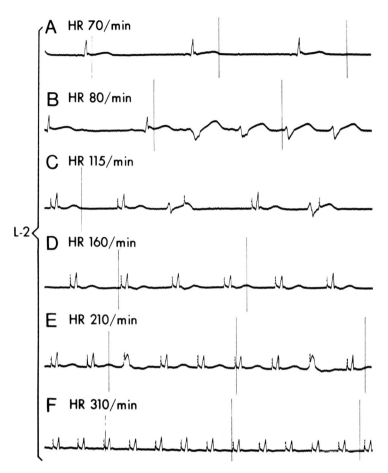

Fig. 10. The relationship between heart rate and the occurrence of ventricular ectopic beats during the first 30 min after coronary artery ligation. Lead II (L-2) is shown throughout. In panel A at rates of 70 or below no ventricular arrhythmias were seen; in panels B and C at rates between 80–120 bigeminy and ventricular tachycardia were noted. In panel D between heart rates of 120–180 no ventricular arrhythmias were observed but they did reappear at rates between 180–240/min (panel E). Again in panel F there was no ventricular ectopic activity between rates of 270–310/min. The interval between time lines equals 1 second.

subjected to coronary occlusion, heart rates increased as much as 50% within 1–2 minutes (438). This was associated with a 72% mortality due to ventricular fibrillation. Prehospital deaths associated with acute myocardial infarction have been reported in the range of 60–70% (140).

In regard to the mechanism of these very early arrhythmias, results from many experimental studies have provided data suggesting a reentry mechanism (156, 226, 295, 335, 732, 869). Studies from our laboratory (737) and others (437) indicate that immediately after occlusion of a major coronary vessel and for the first one to two hours, ventricular automaticity is essentially unchanged. Despite ventricular tachycardia at rates of 275/min underlying ventricular automaticity was unchanged from control rates which averaged 40 beats/min (see table 1). The fractionation and delay of electrical activation in ischemic muscle in our study is consonant with a reentrant mechanism. Certainly the degree of delay

of epicardial activation beyond the T wave, figures 3 and 4, meet the quantitative requirements of reentry (163). Instances of similar delays have been noted in ischemic (50, 82, 163)
and infarcted hearts. Due to the marked heterogeneity of activation the ischemic zone
(82, 218, 226, 739) the use of the multicontact bipolar electrogram (see Methods) allowed a
consistent demonstration of the direct relationship between rapid atrial pacing, epicardial
fractionation and delay and onset of ventricular tachycardia and fibrillation (fig. 3, 6, 6–9).

On the other hand, transient slowing of the heart rate by vagosympathetic trunk stimulation, cessation of atrial pacing during normal sinus rhythm or cessation of His bundle
pacing during heart block rapidly reversed the process and thus ameliorated the electrophysiological derangement which allowed supraventricular impulses to induce ventricular
arrhythmias. The benign or beneficial effects of bradycardia and the deleterious effects of
atropine induced heart rate increase has been the recent focus of much attention both
experimentally (253, 254) and clinically (530, 605). However, the use of atropine to increase
the heart rate particularly in the presence of bradycardia and hypotension secondary to
acute myocardial infarction appears to the effective therapy in many cases (487, 616). Our
findings confirm the difficulty in classifying bradycardia as completely beneficial or
completely detrimental. In our studies, transient bradycardia made it possible to terminate
many episodes of ventricular tachycardia, thus preventing the degeneration of this malignant rhythm into ventricular fibrillation, (fig. 1, 4, 8). However stable bradycardic rates
delayed the time during which the heart was vulnerable to the potentially dangerous effects
of rapid heart rates (see fig. 8).

In anesthetized dogs with average eart rates of 140/min (see table 1) it was consistently
found that within 30 min of acute coronary ligation, rapid heart rates (200/min) no longer
produced ischemic zone epicardial delay and fractionation and in turn no ventricular
arrhythmias occurred, (see fig. 4). However, in those dogs with stable bradycardia (below
60/min) transient speeding of the heart rate by His bundle pacing up to four hours after
coronary occlusion still introduced marked delay and fractionation in the ischemic zone
with subsequent appearance of ventricular tachycardia. During the later stages of ischemia,
bradycardia unmasked what appeared to be incipient automaticity which could cause
ventricular tachycardia and ventricular fibrillation due to the R on T phenomenon. An
example of this response is shown in figure 9. Of interest is the occurrence of "vagally"
mediated bradycardia and ventricular fibrillation. This finding corresponds to the same
association found in the early stages of acute myocardial infarction clinically (3). it is
markedly unlike the findings by Kerzner et al. (437) who found no instance of fibrillation in
all 34 dogs subjects to bradycardia during acute myocardial infarction. Epstein et al. (253,
254) indicated that vagal stimulation was a significant stabilizing influence on the ventricles
inhibiting ventricular fibrillation. The difference between our results, those seen clinically
on the one hand and the aforementioned experimental findings on the other hand may be
explained by the fact that the vago-sympathetic trunks were decentralized in the latter
experiments whereas they were intact in our studies. It seems likely that in the clinical
situation both parasympathetic and sympathetic influences play a role with the parasympathetic dominating the heart rate response. Corroborating this view are the findings of
VF during slow heart rates seen by Chadda et al. (120). These experiments used sinus node
clamping to slow the rate and the vagii were intact.

The occurrence of ischemia-induced ventricular arrhythmias during stable versus transient bradycardia revealed that the relationship between heart rate and the occurrence of arrhythmia is not a simple matter. Chadda et al. (120) showed that at stable heart rates between 110/min–150/min the frequency of ventricular arrhythmias after coronary artery ligation was much reduced compared to those occurring between rates of 69/min–90/min or higher rates of 180 min–200/min. Our present data confirms and extends these findings since at stable spontaneous or paced rates below 60–70/min no ventricular arrhythmias were seen after ischemia. However, between rates of 70–140/min ventricular arrhythmias including ventricular tachycardia were consistently noted. Pacing the heart at rates between 140–180/min again showed the minimal occurrence of ventricular premature beats or ventricular tachycardia whereas at rates of 180–240/min arrhythmias were prevalent. Interestingly, at rates between 270–310/min the occurrence of arrhythmias was again significantly decreased. A multiform response involving a reentrant mechanism similar to this has been described by Wit et al. (930,931) and its relation to arrhythmias due to ischemia has been pointed out (933). In the latter studies by Wit et al., a systematic delineation of the reentrant circuit and determination of the sites of unidirectional block were defined providing strong evidence for a reentry mechanism (930,931). In the present studies the degree of delay necessary for reentry has been consistently shown. However the delineation of the reentrant circuit and site of the unidirectional block have not been defined. It cannot be denied that the possibility of transient automaticity or automaticity triggered by a single depolarizing impulse of supraventricular origin could account for the ventricular arrhythmias (164,165).

The relationship between the experimentally induced ventricular arrhythmias as a result of coronary artery ligation and its mechanisms may not be directly transferable to the clinical situation. We realize that the induction of ischemia is a result of ligation of vessels in an essentially normal mongrel dog heart, whereas the occurrence of acute myocardial infarction in the clinical situation is usually preceded by a long history of progressive atherosclerosis. Thus, the basic researcher is forced to uncover parallelisms between the two situations, i.e., experimental and clinical, which are suggestive of similar etiologies, mechanisms and responses and similar sequences of events. For example, during the initial stages of myocardial ischemia in our studies, it was found that ventricular ectopic beats falling early or late in diastole can induce tachycardia and fibrillation. This would appear to be at variance with previous experimental and clinical evidence. However, similar observations have been made in the clinical setting (571,790). Recently a systematic clinical study of deSoyza et al. (198) showed that early coupled ectopic ventricular beats initiated ventricular tachycardia less frequently than similar beats occurring beyond the T wave of preceding beats in the first 24 hours of acute myocardial infarction. These findings are also consonant with previous experimental findings since extension of the vulnerable period as a result of ischemia has been postulated (554).

The demonstration of marked delay of local activation induced by coronary artery ligation clearly focuses attention on the electrophysiological alterations caused by ischemia rather than on the occurrence of an early (malignant VPB) or late coupled (benign VPB) ventricular premature beats. If these mechanisms are operative in clinical settings of acute myocardial infarction, the potential malignancy of all ventricular ectopic beats regardless of their diastolic timing, must be suspected.

SUMMARY

The electrophysiological derangements induced by acute myocardial ischemia were studied in anesthetized dogs subjected to coronary artery ligation. Using electrocardiograms, local endocardial and epicardial electrograms and His bundle recordings, activation of Purkinje and regular muscle were monitored during the first few minutes up to three to four hours after occlusion. Underlying ventricular automaticity was assessed by vagal induced atrial arrest. The ventricular arrhythmias occurring in the first few minutes were unrelated to underlying automaticity, were provoked by rapid atrial pacing and abolished by transient slowing of the heart rate. A consistent prodromal sign of these early ventricular arrhythmias was the fractionation and delay (up to 330 msec) of epicardial potentials in the ischemic zone consonant with a reentrant mechanism for the ectopic impulse formation. In other experiments spontaneous or induced ventricular ectopic beats which caused ventricular tachycardia or ventricular fibrillation were analyzed during atrial pacing at 150–200 beats/min. These arrhythmias always followed the progressive delay and fractionation of the ischemic zone potentials. Ventricular tachycardia was repeatedly produced by ectopic beats with late diastolic coupling (fusion beats). The malignant characteristic of ventricular ectopic beats occurring in acute ischemia appeared to be related more to abnormalities of underlying ventricular activation than to the coupling of the premature beats.

In another series of 15 anesthetized dogs myocardial ischemia was instituted by coronary artery occlusion for a period of three to four hours. The effects of a wide range of heart rates (40/min to 300/min) were studied either by inducing complete heart block to achieve heart rates below 60/min and His bundle pacing or by crushing the sinus node to slow the heart rate and utilizing atrial pacing to increase it. At rates below to beats/min no ventricular arrythmias were seen for a period up to four hours after coronary artery ligation. Concomitantly, there was no fractionation or delay of epicardial potentials in the ischemic zone at these low rates. Throughout these experiments, His bundle pacing at 200/min produced marked delay of the ischemic zone epicardial potentials prior to the onset of ventricular tachycardia. Cessation of pacing with marked slowing of the heart rate caused resumption of His bundle or idioventricular rhythm and a rapid return of the timing, amplitude and configuration of the ischemic zone epicardial electrograms. During periods of stable pacing at heart rates between 40–300/min, the occurrence of ventricular ectopic beats showed a consistent but multiphasic relationship to heart rate. At rates below 70/min, between 120–150/min and 270–310/min, there were few if any ectopic beats. At rates between 70–120/min, 180–240/min ventricular premature beats, ventricular tachycardia and fusion beats were frequent.

ACKNOWLEDGEMENT

We gratefully acknowledge the assistance of Mr. Edward J. Berbari in the statistical evaluation of our study. We also thank Mr. Jorge Rodriguez, Dr. Joseph Herbstman, Messrs. Israel Dingle and David Young, Jr. for their technical assistance, and Mrs. Marie Ellis for her aid in the preparation of the manuscript.

35

OBSERVATIONS DURING ELECTRICAL STIMULATION OF THE HEART IN PATIENTS WITH SINUS BRADYCARDIA FOLLOWING ACUTE MYOCARDIAL INFARCTION

HEIN J. J. WELLENS, M.D., HENK J. M. DOHMEN, M.D., AND K. I. LIE, M.D.

Approximately 10% of patients admitted to hospital because of acute myocardial infarction show sinus bradycardia (3,420,503,605).

Most authors consider increase in vagal tone responsible for this phenomenon (398,955). Other suggested mechanisms (see table 1) include ischemia of the sinus node and infarction of the sinus node area (390,401). If increased vagal tone is responsible for the sinus bradycardia one would expect depressed function of both the sinus and the A-V node during the phase of bradycardia. This article reports the outcome of electrophysiologic studies on sinus and A-V nodal function during sinus bradycardia following acute myocardial infarction. From Febr. 1972 to May 1974, 800 patients were consecutively admitted to our coronary care unit with a proven myocardial infarction.

When sinus bradycardia was defined as a sinus rate of less than 60 per minute and patients with pre-existing bradycardia, and patients receiving β blocking agents and/or digitalis were excluded, 103 patients showed sinus bradycardia (an incidence of 12,8%) (503).

Out of this group ten consecutively admitted patients with sinus bradycardia were studied. The mean hospital arrival time was 4 hours. Eight were males, two females. Ages ranged fom 52 to 79 years. In nine patients the infarct was localized on the infero-posterior wall. One patient had an anterior wall infarction. The highest SGOT value (from samples taken every 6 hours) varied from 70 to 192 u/1 (upper limit of normal 20 u/1).

The study was performed 4 to 20 hours after the onset of acute myocardial infarction. In eight patients within ten hours after onset. Using the Seldinger technique three catheters were passed through the femoral veins. Two (bipolar) catheters were positioned high in the right atrium, close to the entrance of the superior caval vein. One catheter was used for bipolar atrial stimulation. The other for registering a bipolar intra-atrial electrogram.

Table 1. Possible mechanisms for sinus bradycardia following acute myocardial infarction.

1. Neuroreflexes (reflexly mediated sympathetic inhibition or parasympathetic stimulation)
2. Coronary chemoreflexes (vagally mediated)
3. Oxygen conserving ('diving') reflex
4. Humoral (non-neural) reflexes (P_H, enzymes, potassium etc)
5. Infarction or ischemia of the sinus node and/or surrounding atrium.

The third (bipolar) catheter was positioned in the region of the bundle of His, to record to His bundle electrogram.

The sinus node recovery time (SRT (587)), and corrected sinus node recovery time (CSRT (587)), were determined during sinus rhythm by way of the single atrial test stimulus method. Thereafter the same measurements were made following rapid atrial stimulation during one minute at increasing rates up to 160/min. Sinus node recovery time (SRT) was defined as the interval between the atrial test stimulus or last atrial paced complex to the succeeding atrial electrogram of sinus origin. The corrected SRT (CSRT) was defined as the recovery interval in excess of the average sinus cycle length (SRT minus the average of at least five sinus cycles) (587).

Normal values of SRT given in the literature vary from 958 msec ± 149 msec, to less than 1400 msec (248,521,522,587,670).

For our study the latter value was accepted as upper limit of normal. As upper limit of normal for the CSRT was used a value of 525 msec. (587). Following cessation of rapid stimulation at increasing atrial pacing rates the longest pause found was used for determination of the SRT and CSRT.

The effective refractory period of the A-V node was measured by way of the single atrial test stimulus method during sinus rhythm and during atrial pacing at a frequency just above the sinus rate. The effective refractory period of the A-V node (ERP_{AVN}) was defined as the longest atrial premature beat interval at which conduction did not propagate to the His bundle. A value of 370 msec was accepted as the upper limit of normal for the ERP_{AVN} (191). Also the atrial pacing rate at which Wenckebach type A-V block developed was determined. In seven patients these tests of sinus and A-V node function were repeated following the intra-atrial administration of 1 mg of atropine. All patients had normal sinus rates, when they were discharged from the coronary care unit.

Table 2. Sinus node recovery time and corrected sinus node recovery time following a single atrial test stimulus during sinus rhythm.

Pat.	P-P msec	S.R.T. msec	C.S.R.T. msec	Max. depr. %
1	1100	1200–1310	100–210	119
2	1140	1240–1340	100–210	115
3	1020	1130–1240	110–220	125
4	1080	1050–1270	0–90	119
5	1070	1080–1220	10–150	114
6	1220	1290–1350	70–130	110
7	1100	1160–1320	60–120	119
8	1200	1250–1320	50–120	110
9	1180	1210–1330	30–150	112
10	1140	1210–1440	40–300	125

P-P = the interval between two successive sinus beats.
SRT = sinusnode recovery time;
CSRT = corrected sinusnode recovery time.

SINUS NODE FUNCTION

During sinus rhythm, following a single atrial test stimulus given with increasing prematurity up to the refractory period of the right atrium, all patients showed a normal range
of sinus node recovery times and corrected sinus node recovery times (table 2). All but one
patient showed a type II response (793) to atrial test stimuli, suggesting that at a certain premature beat interval the sinus node pacemaker was invaded, discharged and reset.

In eight patients the SRT and CSRT were determined after rapid atrial pacing at increasing rates (table 3). Only one patient showed prolongation of his SRT (to 1780 msec)
and CSRT (to 610 msec).

Of the seven patients receiving atropine six increased their sinus rate by 27 to 60% of
their original value. They also showed shortening of their SRT, but no significant change
in their CSRT. In one patient atropine administration did not result in any change in sinus
rate, SRT and CSRT.

A-V NODAL FUNCTION

During sinus bradycardia all patients showed normal values for their A-H and H-V
intervals. In only four patients the effective refractory period of the A-V node could be
measured during sinus rhythm. The value varied from 300 to 360 msec. They can be considered to be within the normal range for the cardiac frequencies present (746, 793).

In six patients the ERP$_{AVN}$ could not be measured because A-V conduction was present
up to the effective refractory period of the right atrium. The ERP of the right atrium
varied from 230 to 450 msec. Similar observations were made during pacing of the atrium
at a frequency just above that of the sinus node.

In nine patients the atrial pacing rate at which Wenckebach type second degree A-V
block occurred was determined. Values varied from 100 to 160/min.

Table 3. Sinus node recovery time and corrected sinus node recovery time following
rapid atrial pacing.

Pat.	P-P msec	S.R.T. msec	C.S.R.T. msec
1	1100	1200	100
2	1140	1500	360
3	1020	1250	230
4	1080	1250	170
5	1070	1780	610
6	1220	—	—
7	1100	—	—
8	1200	1180	20
9	1180	1310	130
10	1140	1420	300

Same abbreviations as in table 2.

In three patients Wenckebach type of block became manifest at rates from 100 to 120/min.

Following atropine the ERP of the A-V node could be measured in all seven patients receiving the drug, indicating that the increase in heart rate resulted in marked shortening of the ERP of the right atrium enabling determination of the ERP of the A-V node.

Following atropine the ERP_{AVN} ranged from 240 to 310 msec. After atropine administration Wenckebach type second degree block occurred at atrial pacing rates above 150/min.

DISCUSSION

Within the limitations of our present methods for evaluation of sinus node function in man (907) our data indicate that during sinus bradycardia following acute myocardial infarction, only one patient showed moderate prolongation of his SRT and CSRT following atrial pacing at increasing pacing rates. One other patient showed a type I response to atrial test stimuli during sinus rhythm suggesting the possibility of sino-auricular entrance block or intraatrial block. This patient also showed a high atrial stimulation threshold (more than 10 m AMP) and did not increase his sinus rate following atropine administration. In view of the normal A-V nodal function in this patient these observations suggest the possibility of an ischemic lesion of the sinus node and surrounding atrium. Although atrial activation progressed in a high-low direction, the inability to influence the atrial rate by atropine suggests that in this patient atrial impulse formation may have occurred outside the sinus node area.

As far as A-V nodal function was concerned only three patients showed some depression, based upon the observation of the development of a Wenckebach type A-V block at atrial pacing rates below 120/min.

If a marked increase in vagal tone would have been responsible for the sinus bradycardia in our patients, one would have expected to find more depression in both sinus and A-V nodal function. It is not possible however to exclude some degree of enhanced vagal tone. It is not known, whether lengthening of the sinus node recovery time or impairment of A-V nodal conduction occur at the same level of vagal activity, which leads to sinus bradycardia.

Ischemia of the sinus node area has been advanced as a possible cause of sinus bradycardia following acute myocardial infarction (390,401). Billette et al. (73) could produce sinus slowing in the dog heart by acutely impeding blood supply to the sinus node. It seems unlikely that ischemia or infarction of the sinus node is a frequent cause for sinus bradycardia following acute myocardial infarction. In man, the sinus node artery arises with about equal frequency from the right coronary artery and the left coronary artery and from the anterior third, rather than the distal third (401).

Kennel and Titus (433) demonstrated, in the human heart, anastomoses between the sinus node and other branches of the same parent artery or branches of the opposite coronary artery. Sinus bradycardia following acute myocardial infarction however shows preference for inferiorly located infarcts, while the peak SGOT value is usually compatible with a small to moderately sized infarct suggesting a rather distal obstruction of a single coronary artery (503). Also the increase in rate of the sinus node following administration of atropine in nine of our ten patients seem to argue against ischemia of the sinus node. It is of interest that one patient showed no change in sinus rate following atropine. The possibility of ischemic damage to the sinus node and right atrium was further supported by the finding of a markedly elevated right atrial stimulation threshold. Further work is needed to evaluate the value of these observations as indicators for an ischemic lesion of the sinus node area.

Our observations suggest that neither markedly enhanced vagal tone nor ischemia of the sinus node can be considered as the mechanism responsible for sinus bradycardia following acute myocardial infarction in the majority of patients seen in the coronary care unit showing this phenomenon. It is important to stress however that the patients studied represent a group in which sinus bradycardia is present more than two hours after the acute myocardial infarction. The outcome of our studies cannot be transposed to patients showing sinus bradycardia occurring immediately after onset of myocardial infarction. The observations by Adgey et al. (3) suggest that during this phase of infarction in view of the high incidence of both sinus bradycardia and A-V nodal conduction disturbances, vagal mechanisms may play a much more important role.

36

A-V NODAL BLOCK IN ACUTE MYOCARDIAL INFARCTION

ALFRED C. TANS, M.D. AND K. I. LIE, M.D.

The mechanism, clinical course and prognosis of conduction disturbances following acute myocardial infarction are closely related to the blood supply of the specific conduction system and the site of infarction (449,603,667,703,799). Conduction disturbances in the A-V node are usually associated with acute inferior myocardial infarction (424,667,703) presumably due to occlusion proximal to the origin of the A-V nodal artery. This artery is in 90% of cases a branch of the right coronary artery (401). The usual precursor of complete intranodal block in association with acute inferior myocardial infarction is type I second degree A-V block (449,603,703). The escape pacemaker during complete intranodal block is located just below the node (667) and usually produces an acceptable and dependable frequency (449,603,703). In contrast, conduction disturbances in the bundle branches are usually associated with acute anteroseptal infarction (424,449,603,667,703,799), presumably following occlusion proximal to the origin of the septal branches of the left anterior descending artery (401). Bifascicular block is the usual precursor of complete infranodal block complicating acute anteroseptal infarction (603,667,703). During complete infranodal block the escape pacemaker that emerges from the peripheral Purkinje-system is unstable and has a slow rate (424). The conduction disturbances in the bundle branch system will be discussed in the next chapter. Therefore in this chapter we will only consider conduction disturbances located in the A-V node. The generally accepted indications for atropine or pacemaker therapy in A-V block complicating acute inferior myocardial infarction are: 1. Stokes-Adams attacks; 2. a low ventricular rate (< 50/min); 3. powerfailure; and 4. bradycardia dependent ventricular arrhythmias (424,607,703). However, whether pacemaker therapy of A-V conduction disturbances following acute inferior myocardial infarction has contributed to a significant decrease in mortality remains to be clarified (283,469,603,607,704). The purpose of this chapter is therefore to evaluate the clinical setting and factors influencing the prognosis of a hundred patients with high degree A-V block in the setting of acute inferior myocardial infarction. From these data we will try to outline the indications for pacemaker therapy.

MATERIAL AND METHODS

Inferior myocardial infarction included inferior and/or posterior infarction, with or without lateral involvement. High degree A-V block was defined as the presence of second or third degree A-V block occurring via a type I mechanism lasting for at least half an hour. The presence and degree of power failure at the time of onset and following the episode of high degree A-V block was noted. Severe power failure was defined as pulmonary oedema or shock (a systolic blood pressure of less than 90 mmHg, peripheral vascular constriction and an altered sensorium).

The diagnosis of cardiogenic shock was made if patients with shock had an urine output of less than 20 cc per hour during the subsequent clinical course. Atropine was administered or pacemaker therapy was instituted according to the previously mentioned indications.

INCIDENCE AND MORTALITY

Four hundred and sixty nine patients admitted consecutively to the coronary care unit because of acute inferior myocardial infarction were studied. Of these 100 (21%) had high degree A-V block (table 1). The mean age of the patients with high degree A-V block was higher (65 years) than of those without high degree A-V block (p < 0.01).

The mean peak SGOT was significantly higher in the patients with high degree A-V block (141 I.U.) than in those without A-V block (90 I.U.). High degree A-V block in acute inferior myocardial infarction was associated with a higher hospital mortality, since 23 of the 100 patients with high degree A-V block died (23%), compared to 33 of the 369 patients without A-V block.

These differences were even significant (p < 0.01) if both subgroups were matched for age. The cause of death in the patients with A-V block was primarily power failure: of the 23 deaths 14 died of cardiogenic shock and four of congestive heart failure.

ELECTROCARDIOGRAPHIC COURSE OF HIGH DEGREE A-V BLOCK

The maximal degree of A-V block did not influence the immediate prognosis: eight of 31 patients (25%) with second degree A-V block only died, compared to 15 of 69 (22%) with third degree A-V block. Second degree A-V block was registered in 61 patients (table 2). In 41 of these first degree A-V block was noticed prior to the onset of second degree A-V

Table 1. Incidence, age, sex, mean peak SGOT and mortality.

	all patients with I.M.I.	patients without A-V block	patients with high degree A-V block
No	469	369	100
Mean age (yr)	63	62	65
Sex — male	341	264	77
Sex — female	128	105	23
Mean peak SGOT (I.U.)	100	90	141
Mortality (%)	12	9	23

Table 2. ECG prior to and following second degree A-V block

	No			No
1 → 2	41 ⎫		→ 3	30
Normal PR → 2	5 ⎬ 61		→ 1	26
On admission 2	15 ⎭		→ †	5

1. = first degree A-V block, 2. = second degree A-V block.
3. = third degree A-V block.

block, whilst in the 20 others it was the first manifestation of the A-V conduction disturbance in the coronary care unit. Five patients died during second degree A-V block. Of the 30 patients with second degree A-V block, who progressed to third degree A-V block, four died during the episode of third degree A-V block. In the 26 others three died after A-V conduction was restored.

Table 3. ECG prior to and following third degree A-V block.

	No			No
1 → 2 → 3	19		→ 2	42
2 → 3	11	69	→ 1	21
Normal PR → 3	8		→ †	6
On admission 3	31			

1. = first degree A-V block, 2. = second degree A-V block,
3. = third degree A-V block.

In 39 patients third degree A-V block was the first manifestation of conduction disturbances in the coronary care unit (table 3). Fourty-two patients returned to 1:1 A-V conduction through a phase of second degree A-V block, 21 patients returned directly to 1:1 A-V conduction and six patients died during third degree A-V block.

All survivors of high degree A-V block were discharged from the hospital with 1:1 A-V conduction.

Table 4. Onset of third degree A-V block.

	No	Mortality
on admission	31	9
0–6 hours	7	1
6–12 hours	3	0
12–24 hours	5	1
24–72 hours	10	3
≧ 3 days	13	1

TIME OF ONSET OF THIRD DEGREE A-V BLOCK (TABLE 4)

In 31 patients the third degree A-V block was already present on admission; the hospital arrival time in 26 of these was less than six hours and in only one more than 24 hours. Seventeen of these 31 patients had a Stokes-Adams attack and/or syncope prior to admission. Third degree A-V block developed in 45 patients (65%) within 24 hours after onset of symptoms and in 81% within three days. The latest time of onset of A-V block we observed was the fifth day of infarction.

Table 5. Duration of third degree A-V block.

	No	Mortality
≤ 6 hours	19	6
6–12 hours	9	3
12–24 hours	12	2
24–72 hours	7	2
≥ 3 days	22	2

DURATION OF THIRD DEGREE A-V BLOCK (TABLE 5)

Duration of third degree A-V block varied from half an hour to nine days. In 19 patients (28%) the duration was less than 6 hours, in 40 (58%) less than 24 hours and in 22 patients (32%) more than three days.

POWER FAILURE AND THIRD DEGREE A-V BLOCK

Controversy exists as to whether A-V block contributes to a higher mortality or merely reflects an inferior infarction with a poor prognosis (449, 607, 704). We therefore studied the degree of power failure at the time of onset of the third degree A-V block (table 6). Severe power failure was present in 27 patients, 25 of these being in shock. Because an urine output of less than 20 cc per hour is obligatory for the diagnosis of cardiogenic shock, one cannot establish this diagnosis at the very time of onset of third degree A-V block. In 20 of the 25 patients the shock was found to be reversible after pacing was started. Seventeen of these 20 patients had a ventricular rate of less than 50 beats per minute.

Table 6. Degree of power failure at time of onset of third degree A-V block.

	No	Mortality
Severe — shock — reversible	20	3
Severe — shock — irreversible	5	5
Severe — pulmonary edema	2	0
Mild or absent	42	7

In five patients the shock did not respond to pacemaker therapy; all died in true cardio-genic shock. In 13 patients of the 20 with reversible shock, the third degree A-V block was present on admission; 11 of these 13 had a Stokes-Adams attack or syncope prior to admission. In four of five patients with irreversible shock the third degree A-V block was present on admission; all four had a Stokes-Adams attack prior to admission. Three of five patients with irreversible shock had a ventricular rate of less than 50 beats per minute.

FREQUENCY AND QRS WIDTH OF ESCAPE RHYTHM DURING THIRD DEGREE A-V BLOCK

Neither frequency (table 7), nor width (table 8) of the escape rhythm was of prognostic significance. An escape rhythm with widened (more than 0,12 sec) QRS complexes was observed in 27 patients. They all had narrow QRS complexes in the conducted beats. These widened QRS complexes had a left bundle branch block configuration in five patients, a right bundle branch block configuration in 18 and both LBBB and RBBB in four patients. In patients with widened complexes the mortality was even lower than that of patients with narrow QRS complexes, although this was not statistically significant. The mechanism of these widened QRS complexes have been described before (500).

RATE AND SITE OF ORIGIN OF SUPRANODAL RHYTHM DURING THIRD DEGREE A-V BLOCK

Fifty-four patients had a sinus rhythm at the time of onset of the third degree A-V block. The sinus rate did not influence mortality. However when the supranodal rhythm was not a sinus rhythm but atrial fibrillation, the mortality was higher: six of 15 patients (40%) with

Table 7. Escape frequency during third degree A-V block.

Beats/min.	No	Mortality	PM
≤ 30	6	3	5
30–40	24	4	17
40–50	22	3	20
50–60	12	4	8
60–70	3	1	1
≥ 70	2	0	1

PM = pacemaker therapy.

Table 8. QRS width during third degree A-V block.

	No	%	Mortality No	%
Narrow	42	61	11	26
Widened	27	39	4	15

Table 9. Management of high degree A-V block and mortality.

	No	None	Atropine	Atropine + PM	PM
Second degree	31	16	3	6	6
Mortality	8	6	0	1	1
Third degree	69	13	4	14	38
Mortality	15	1	2	2	10

PM = pacemaker therapy.

atrial fibrillation died, compared to nine of 54 patients (16%) with sinus rhythm (p < 0.001).

TREATMENT

The majority of patients, especially those with third degree A-V block, were treated with a temporary pacemaker (table 9). In 20 of 27 patients treated with atropine, the beneficial effects were small or too short lasting, and a pacemaker had to be inserted. The mortality rate of patients who were paced was not higher than that of those who were not paced.

ROLE AND INDICATIONS OF PACEMAKER THERAPY

This study demonstrates that patients with high degree A-V block complicating acute inferior myocardial infarction have more extensive myocardial damage, a higher incidence of power failure and a higher mortality rate than those with inferior myocardial infarction without A-V block. These differences could be attributed to the following factors.

Firstly for inferior myocardial infarction to be complicated by A-V block it may require a more proximal occlusion of the right coronary artery so as to involve the A-V nodal artery.

Secondly the conduction disorder itself may contribute to the development of power failure or extention of infarction. The present data indicates that even patients with high degree A-V block who were asymptomatic and had an acceptable ventricular rate (of whom only a few were paced) had a higher mortality rate than those without A-V block.

This suggests that in this subgroup of patients the poorer prognosis is due to extensive myocardial damage associated with the A-V block rather than directly to the conduction disorder itself.

On the other hand a considerable percentage of our patients (80%) with severe power failure seem to profit from cardiac pacing, the mortality rate in patients who were paced being not higher than that of patients who were not paced.

The majority of our patients with a low ventricular escape frequency and A-V block of long duration were paced and the mortality in these patients was equal to that of patients with A-V block with an acceptable escape rate or A-V block of short duration of whom only a few were paced.

These findings suggest that there is a subset of patients with acute inferior myocardial infarction complicated by high degree A-V block in whom the conduction disorder contributes to the deterioration of clinical condition and/or further extension of infarction. We are aware that we as well as others (283, 703, 704) do not have hard data to establish this statement. It is in our view unethical to determine the true natural history of symptomatic high degree A-V block complicating acute inferior myocardial infarction by withholding pacemaker therapy in such patients. Therefore it is necessary to evaluate the effect of cardiac pacing on left ventricular function in patients with high degree A-V block complicating acute inferior myocardial infarction who are either symptomatic or have a low ventricular rate.

In summary this study reveals that A-V block in acute inferior myocardial infarction may occur in association with an extensive myocardial infarction but also can contribute to the development of power failure or to further extension of infarction. Only in the latter situation may pacemaker therapy influence the natural course and reduce hospital mortality. However from the present data we cannot delineate a subset of patients with symptomatic high degree A-V block who might profit from pacemaker therapy. In view of the absence of such data we would recommend pacemaker insertion in all patients with high degree A-V block complicating acute inferior myocardial infarction who are either symptomatic or have a low ventricular rate ($<$ 50 per minute).

37

BUNDLE BRANCH BLOCK AND ACUTE MYOCARDIAL INFARCTION

K. I. LIE, M.D., HEIN J. WELLENS, M.D., AND REINIER M. SCHUILENBURG, M.D.

When bundle branch block (BBB) complicates acute myocardial infarction, the site of infarction is usually anteroseptal (41,306,319,383,604,726). During complete infranodal block the escape pacemaker that emerges from the peripheral Purkinje system (385,667) is unstable and has a slow rate (41,306).

Bifascicular block is the usual precursor of complete infranodal block complicating acute anteroseptal infarction (41,307,501). Prophylactic pacing has been recommended in these circumstances primarily in order to prevent Stokes Adams attacks (41,501). It does not influence the mortality rate significantly since the majority of these patients die as a consequence of pump failure due to the extensive myocardial damage (307,501). However, in some individual cases this procedure might be life-saving (41,606).

Early diagnosis and recognition of bifascicular block following acute myocardial infarction is often hampered by the following factors. Firstly in 40–83% of reported cases (41,306,319,383,604,726) BBB is already present on admission and may reflect preexistent disorders in the conducting system. Often in these cases a previous electrocardiogram has not been recorded or is not readily available for comparison.

Secondly bifascicular block may be difficult to diagnose since in acute myocardial infarction factors other than a hemiblock can also alter the frontal QRS axis (478).

It is the purpose of this chapter to present new information on the characteristics, clinical setting and prognosis of both acquired and preexistent BBB following acute myocardial infarction.

On the basis of this information we will discuss the management of BBB in acute myocardial infarction.

INCIDENCE AND CHARACTERISTICS OF ACQUIRED AND PREEXISTENT BBB

In an attempt to determine the true incidence of acquired and of preexistent BBB in acute myocardial infarction we tried to obtain previously recorded electrocardiograms of those patients presenting with a BBB pattern on admission. BBB was considered to be a consequence of infarction if it developed after admission or if the conduction disorder was not present on an electrocardiogram taken within six months prior to admission. Of the 1200 patients who were consecutively admitted because of an acute myocardial infarction 106 (9.6%) had acquired BBB and 42 (3.8%) a preexistent conduction disorder in the bundle branch system. In 30 others ($2\frac{1}{2}$%) we could not determine whether the BBB

Table 1.

	RBBB	LBBB	Preexistent BBB	No BBB
Total no	73	33	42	1052
Incidence	6.6%	3%	3.8%	86.6%
Mean age	63.1	64.4	70.4	63.8
Male	54	24	27	765
Female	19	9	15	287
Localization:				
Inferior	3	25	14	496
Anteroseptal	70	2	5	195
Anterior	0	6	8	326
Undetermined	0	0	15	35
Mortality	71%	21%	28%	14%
Complete infranodal block	18	0	1	0

was a consequence of the presenting infarction. The latter patients were excluded from this study.

Table 1 shows the clinical data of patients with acquired and preexistent BBB and those without BBB. Patients with preexistent BBB had a higher mean age (p < 0.01) than either those with acquired BBB or those without BBB. Seventy-five percent of patients with preexistent BBB were 70 years of age or older compared to 30% of patients with acquired BBB. As reported previously (501) we found in patients with acquired BBB a marked association between the type of BBB and site of infarction. By contrast in patients with preexistent right bundle branch block (RBBB) there was no predilection for the site of infarction (table 2). In our patients with preexistent left bundle branch block (LBBB) the site of infarction could not be determined in 62% of cases. The development of complete infranodal block was observed in 18 patients with acquired RBBB. All these patients had acute anteroseptal infarction and showed a bifascicular block pattern before progressing to complete infranodal block. By contrast, none of the patients with acquired LBBB and only one patient with preexistent BBB developed complete infranodal block.

The mortality rate in patients with acquired RBBB was more than three times as high as in patients with acquired LBBB. This difference could be attributed to the site of infarction associated with the type of BBB (501). In addition anteroseptal infarction complicated by RBBB has a higher mortality than anteroseptal infarction without RBBB (501) because

Table 2. Preexistent bundle branch block in acute myocardial infarction.

	No	Mean age	M	F	Localization				A-V block	Mortality	
					I	A	AS	U		No	%
RBBB	18	70.3	12	6	8	6	4	0	0	6	33
LBBB	24	70.4	15	9	6	2	1	15	1	6	25
No preexistent BBB > 59 year	737	69.3	495	242	309	216	170	42		169	23

it requires a more proximal occlusion of the left descending anterior artery. Since the mortality rate of patients with preexistent BBB could be influenced by differences in age, the clinical data of these patients were compared to that of patients without BBB who were matched for age and sex (table 2). It then appeared that a preexistent BBB was not associated with a significantly higher mortality rate.

The present data in patients with preexistent BBB are in conflict with those of Gann et al. (297), who found a higher mortality rate and a higher incidence of progression into complete A-V block. However the mean age of their patients with preexistent BBB was 75 years and the mortality rate was not compared with that of patients without BBB matched for age. Moreover they did not mention whether the complete block was intranodal or infranodal.

Our data indicate that only patients with acquired RBBB are at risk of developing of complete infranodal block. However only 50% of our patients with acquired RBBB developed the conduction disturbance after admission. In the other 50% a previous electrocardiogram was usually not readily available. Moreover in 28% of patients with BBB on admission no electrocardiogram was recorded within six months prior to admission. This stresses the importance of evaluating those factors which might help early identification of patients with an acquired BBB from those having preexistent BBB. In addition to the previously mentioned factors such as patient age and site of infarction, the QRS configuration in VI also helps in differentiating acquired from preexistent RBBB (table 3). Sixty of 70 patients with acquired RBBB and acute anteroseptal infarction had QR complexes in V_1 during the first 24 hours of admission whereas 16 of 18 patients with preexistent RBBB had either a qR pattern or trifasic QRS patterns in V_1.

The two patients with a preexistent RBBB and a QR pattern in VI each had previous anteroseptal infarction. Therefore the above listed characteristics are probably more valuable in patients with a first attack than in those with a recurrent infarct.

ACQUIRED BBB-PATTERN OF DEVELOPMENT, CLINICAL SETTING AND PROGNOSIS

RBBB with or without hemiblock

Since only three patients with acquired RBBB had inferior myocardial infarction and none of these three progressed into complete infranodal A-V block the discussion will be confined to the pattern of development, clinical setting and prognosis of RBBB in association with acute anteroseptal infarction. The incidence of RBBB (with or without

Table 3. Characteristics of acquired vs preexistent RBBB.

	Acquired	Preexistent
Age	≦ 70	> 70
Site of infarct	Anteroseptal	No preference
QRS in V1	QR	qR rSR RsR rsR

Table 4. Incidence of RBBB in anteroseptal infarction and its relation to mortality.

| | Incidence | | Mean | M | F | Mortality | |
	No	%	age			No	%
All pts with AS infarct	272	100	63.2	195	77	98	36
Pts with RBBB	70	26	63.1	52	18	52	74
Pts without RBBB	202	74	62.9	143	59	46	23

Table 5. Incidence of type of RBBB and relation to mortality and complete infranodal block.

| | Incidence | | Mortality | | Complete block | infra-nodal |
	No	%	No	%	No	%
RBBB	22	32	15	68	0	0
RBBB + LAH	31	44	21	68	10	32
RBBB + LPH	17	24	15	88	8	47

hemiblock) in 272 patients with acute anteroseptal infarction was 26% (table 4). The mortality rate in patients with RBBB was more than three times as high as in those without RBBB, (both groups were comparable with respect to age and sex). The various types of conduction disturbances that were observed in acute anteroseptal infarction are presented in table 5. Although patients with RBBB and left posterior hemiblock had a higher mortality than in other subgroups and a higher incidence of progression to complete infranodal block than those with RBBB and left anterior hemiblock, these differences were not statistically significant. Prior to complete infranodal block all patients showed bifascicular block. As previously reported (501) patients with RBBB of short duration (< 6 hours) and patients with RBBB of delayed onset (24 hours, after infarction) tended not to progress to complete infranodal block (table 6 and 7).

The pattern of development of RBBB was registered in 10 patients during continuous tape recording. Development of incomplete RBBB occurred in 5 over a period ranging from several minutes to 2 hours. This was followed later by the sudden onset of complete RBBB

Table 6. Duration of RBBB in relation to mortality and complete infranodal block.

	No	Mortality	Complete infranodal block
1–6 hours	10	1	0
6–24 hours	6	3	1
1–6 days	4	4	2
pers until discharge	6	0	1
pers until death	44	44	14

Table 7. Onset of RBBB in relation to mortality and complete infranodal block.

Onset of RBBB	No	Mortality		Complete infrandol block	
		No	%	No	%
Within 24 hours of infarction	55	45	82	17	31
After 24 hours of infarction	15	7	47	1	7

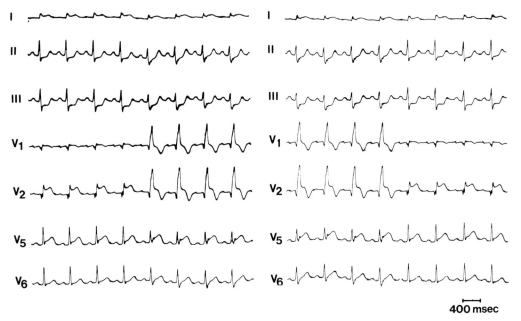

Fig. 1. Acute anteroseptal infarction with incomplete RBBB (left panel). Sudden onset of a complete RBBB pattern without change in the preceding RR intervals. Note the concomitant leftward shift or frontal QRS axis. Several hours later the complete RBBB pattern disappeared within one beat (right panel).

occurring within one beat. No change in the preceding RR intervals was observed prior to the onset of complete RBBB (fig. 1).

In the other five complete RBBB developed without passing through a phase of incomplete RBBB and occurred within one beat without change in length of the preceding cardiac cycle (fig. 2). In nine of the ten patients the onset of complete RBBB was associated with a concomitant shift of the frontal QRS axis to the left (fig. 2). The range of these left axis shift varied from 10 to 30 degrees.

In only one patient was a concomitant right axis deviation observed at the time of sudden onset of RBBB. In those patients in whom RBBB was transient the complete RBBB pattern disappeared within one beat (fig. 1). These observations on the development of RBBB suggest that the conduction disorder is located in the proximal right bundle. Recent observations by Schuilenburg et al. (745) also favor this concept in that selective stimulation

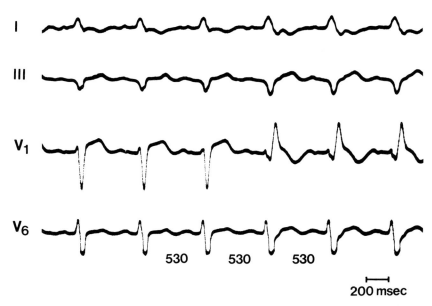

Fig. 2. Sudden onset of complete RBBB without change in the preceding RR intervals. Note the concomitant leftward shift of frontal QRS axis.

with a bipolar catheter 1 cm distal to the His bundle area resulted in normalization of QRS without RBBB pattern. Stimulation after advancing the catheter another 1 cm distally resulted in a QRS complex with a complete LBBB pattern. This suggest that the disappearance of RBBB during stimulation 1 cm distal to the His bundle area was caused by overriding of the zone of block in the proximal right bundle.

Diagnosis of hemiblock in acute myocardial infarction may be hampered by two factors which influence the frontal QRS axis under these circumstances. Firstly the frontal QRS axis in transmural myocardial infarction may change to a direction away from the leads showing QS complexes i.e. away from site of infarction. Secondly in nontransmural myocardial infarction the frontal QRS axis may shift toward the site of infarction as a consequence of intramural conduction block near the site of infarction with delayed activation of this area forming QR complexes. In an attempt to evaluate the nature of true hemiblock complicating acute myocardial infarction, we observed the pattern and degree of changes in frontal QRS axis in 12 patients with acute anteroseptal infarction who had on admission non-aberrant conduction and subsequently developed complete infranodal block after a phase of bifascicular block.

As shown in figure 3 all patients who developed RBBB with left anterior hemiblock had a left axis deviation of at least $-60°$ and a change of frontal QRS axis of 60° or more prior to the development of complete infranodal block. Patients who developed RBBB with left posterior hemiblock showed an axis of $+90°$ or more and a rightward shift of frontal QRS axis of 60° or more before they progressed to complete infranodal block. These data suggest that the classical criteria for diagnosis of hemiblock as far as deviation of frontal QRS axis is concerned should probably be corrected by a factor of 30° to the left, in acute anteroseptal infarction.

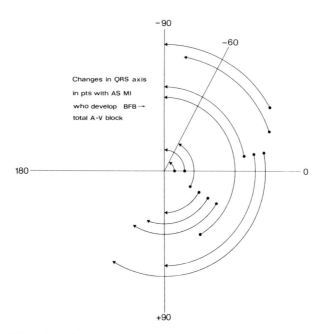

Fig. 3. QRS Axis shift in frontal plane in patients with anteroseptal myocardial infarction who develop bifascicular block followed by total AV block.

A possible explanation is that in acute anteroseptal infarction the frontal QRS axis usually already shifts to a horizontal position (fig. 3) presumably due to loss of forces in the apical area.

We also observed that the classical initial QRS patterns (689) of hemiblock are often not present if hemiblock complicates acute anteroseptal infarction (fig. 4). This could possibly be attributed to the fact that the infarction involves into the areas of early activation by the anterior or posterior fascicle of the left bundle, resulting in an absent initial r wave if the hemiblock occurs contralateral to the infarcted area. Although these data revealed that the classical criteria for diagnosis of hemiblock in acute anteroseptal infarction are often not present, we think that other new characteristics might be of help in these circumstances. First of all a left or right ward shift of 60° or more in the frontal QRS plane favors the diagnosis of hemiblock as a consequence of acute anteroseptal infarction. Secondly if a hemiblock pattern is already present on admission the diagnosis of acquired hemiblock in acute anteroseptal infarction should be considered of the frontal QRS axis in $-60°$ or less or $+90°$ or more.

In contrast to the development of RBBB, patients with acquired hemiblock showed a gradual shift of QRS axis over periods ranging from 1–12 hours. In our patients who developed bifascicular block after admission we either observed both the hemiblock preceding the RBBB and the reverse (fig. 4 and 5). The latter type of development of bifascicular block has clinical importance because patients with an initial pattern of monofascicular RBBB might develop later bifascicular block and even progress into complete infranodal block.

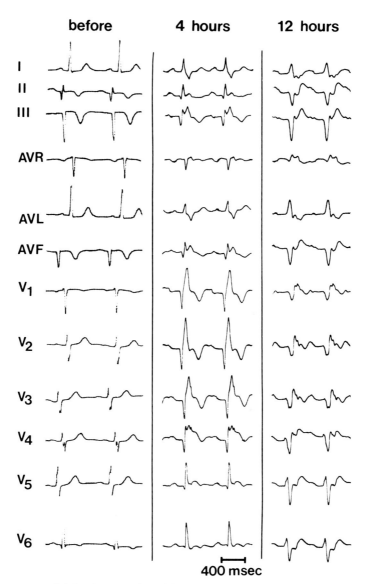

Fig. 4. Acute anteroseptal infarction complicated by complete RBBB (middle panel). Eight hours later a leftward shift of frontal QRS axis to −70° has occurred (right panel). Note that the classical initial QRS patterns of left anterior hemiblock are not present.

Bifascicular block complicating acute anteroseptal infarction is the usual precursor of complete infranodal block (71, 307, 501). We have previously reported (501) that the H-V interval under these circumstances was of value in identifying a subgroup of patients who are at immediate high risk of developing complete infranodal block.

At present we have performed a His bundle study in 30 patients with bifascicular block complicating acute myocardial infarction and these data (table 8) are in agreement with our previously reported experience (501). In contrast the P-R interval was of limited value

1 h.   **2 h.**   **3 h.**   **8 h.**

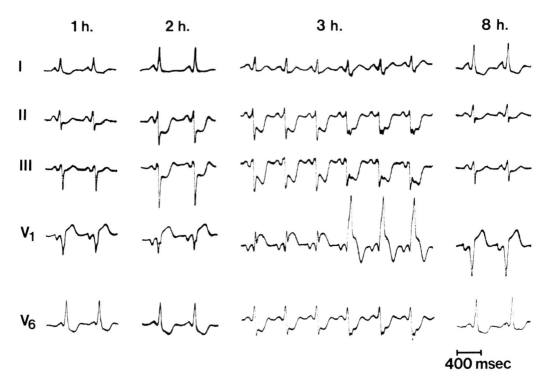

Fig. 5. Development of bifascicular block with left anterior hemiblock preceding the right bundle branch block.

Table 8. H-V interval in patients with bifascicular block and relation to infranodal block.

H-V interval	No of patients	Progression into complete infranodal block
Normal	14	1
Prolonged	16	12

in predicting both prolonged H-V interval or progression to complete infranodal block (501).

Eighteen of 48 patients (37%) with bifascicular block complicating acute anteroseptal infarction progressed to complete infranodal block. In only two patients was Mobitz II second degree A-V block registered prior to complete infranodal block (fig. 6). The onset of complete infranodal block varied from 8 hours to 3 days post onset of infarction. The latter finding suggests that if bifascicular block complicates acute anteroseptal infarction, development of complete infranodal block after the 3rd day is unlikely.

LBBB

Table 9 shows the incidence of rate dependent acquired LBBB and its relation to site of infarction. The majority of patients with acquired LBBB had bradycardia dependent

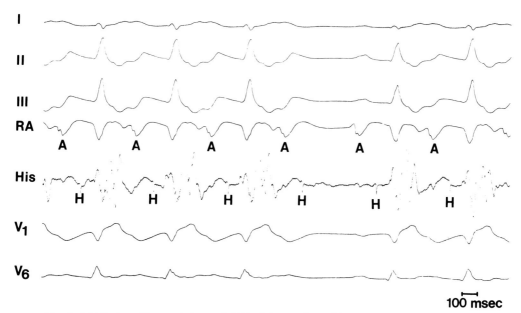

Fig. 6. Mobitz type II second degree A-V block in a patient with acute anteroseptal infarction.

LBBB which occurred during high degree intranodal block in association with acute inferior myocardial infarction (500). A rate dependent LBBB was not associated with a poor prognosis. The number of patients in whom LBBB was presumably not rate dependent is too small in order to draw conclusions concerning its prognostic significance.

MANAGEMENT OF BBB IN ACUTE MYOCARDIAL INFARCTION

Our data reveals that patients with acquired LBBB and preexistent RBBB or LBBB seldom progress into complete infranodal block.

We therefore feel that prophylactic pacing in these subgroups of patients is not necessary. On might consider careful electrocardiographic monitoring in those patients with preexistent RBBB and acute inferior myocardial infarction or those with preexistent LBBB in whom there might be electrocardiographic evidence of anteroseptal

Table 9. Rate dependency and mortality of LBBB complicating acute myocardial infarction.

	No	Localization			Mortality	
		I	A	AS	No	%
All pts with LBBB	33	25	6	2	7	21
Rate dependent:						
—Phase 3	1	1			0	0
—Phase 4	20	20			4	20
—Phase 3 and 4	3	1	1	1	0	0
Not rate dependent	9	3	5	1	3	33

infarction, since these subgroups of preexistent BBB are theoretically at higher risk for development of complete infranodal block.

In patients with RBBB on admission who fulfill the characteristics of acquired RBBB we would advise frequent 12 lead electrocardiographic monitoring if the frontal QRS axis ranges between $-60°$ and $+90°$. On the other hand we would recommend prophylactic pacing if these patients show a frontal QRS axis of $-60°$ or less or $+90°$ or more especially if the H-V interval is prolonged (table 10).

If the facilities to record the His bundle electrogram are not available, we would recommend prophylactic pacing under these circumstances irrespective of the P-R interval. The same procedure should be followed in patients with acute anteroseptal infarction who develop RBBB within 24 hours of infarction which last for at least 6 hours.

Table 10. Management of pts with RBBB on admission within 3 days of AS infarction with QR in V1 or with RBBB which developed <24 hours of admission and which lasted for at least 6 hours.

A. *Axis $+90°$ to $-60°$*

Observation with frequent 12 lead
ECG monitoring

B. *Axis $\geq +90°$ or $\leq -60°$*

HBE recording:
Prophylactic pacing if HV prolonged

If no HBE recording:
Prophylactic pacing irrespective of PR

BIBLIOGRAPHY ON THE CONDUCTION SYSTEM

1. Abella, J. B., Teixiera, O. Misra, K., Hastreiter, A., Changes of atrioventricular conduction with age in infants and children. *Am J Cardiol* 30: 876, 1973.
2. Abramson, D. L., Margolin, S., Purkinje conduction network in the myocardium of the mammalian ventricle. *J Anat* 70: 250, 1936.
3. Adgey, A. A. I., Mulholland, H. C., Geddes, J. S., Keegan, D. A. J., Pantridge, J. F., Incidence, significance and management of early bradyarrhythmias complicating acute myocardial infarction. *Lancet* 2: 1097, 1968.
4. Adrian, E. D., Lucas, K., On the summation of propagated disturbances in nerve and muscle. *J Physiol* 44: 68, 1912.
5. Agha, A. S., Castellanos, A., Wells, D., Ross, M. D., Befeler, B., Myerburg, R. J., Type I, type II and type III gap in bundle branch conduction. *Circulation* 47: 325, 1973.
6. Ahlinger, S., Granath, A., Holmer, S., Wolff-Parkinson-White syndrom med paroxysmalt atrieflimmer overgaende i ventrikelflimmer. *Nord Med* 70: 1336, 1963.
7. Akhtar, M., Damato, A. N., Caracta, A. R., Batsford, W. P., Vargas, G., Lau, S. H., Unmasking and conversion of gap phenomenon in the human heart. *Circulation* 49: 624, 1974.
8. Akhtar, M., Damato, A. N., Caracta, A. R., Batsford, W. R., Lau, S. H., The gap phenomenon during retrograde conduction in man. *Circulation* 49: 811, 1974.
9. Akhtar, M., Damato, A. N., Batsford, W. P., Ruskin, J. N., Ogunkelu, J. B., Vargas, G., Demonstration of re-entry within the His-Purkinje system in man. *Circulation* 50: 1150, 1974.
10. Akhtar, M., Damato, A. N., Caracta, A. R., Batsford, W. R., Josephson, M. E., Lau, S. H., Electrophysiologic effects of atropine on atrioventricular conduction studied by His bundle electrogram. *Am J Cardiol* 33: 333, 1974.
11. Akhtar, M., Damato, A. N., Batsford, W. P., Ruskin, J. N., Ogunkelu, J. B., A comparative analysis of antegrade and retrograde conduction patterns in man. *Circulation* 52: 766, 1975.
12. Allessie, M. A., Bonke, F. I. M., Schopman, F. J. G., Circus movement in rabbit atrial muscle as a mechanism of tachycardia II. The role of nonuniform recovery of excitability in the occurrence of unidirectional block, as studied with multiple microelectrodes. *Circulation Res* in press.
13. Allessie, M. A., Bonke, F. I. M., Schopman, F. J. G., Circus movement in rabbit atrial muscle as a mechanism of tachycardia. *Circulation Res* 33: 54, 1973.
14. Amer, N. S., Stuckey, J. H. Hoffman, B. F., Cappeletti, R. R., Domingo, R. T., Activation of the interventricular septal myocardium studied during cardiopulmonary bypass. *Am Heart J* 59: 224, 1960.
15. Amory, D. W., West, T. C., Chronotropic response following direct stimulation of the isolated sinoatrial node: A pharmacologic evaluation. *J Pharmacol Exp Ther* 137: 14, 1962.
16. Anderson, G. J., Greenspan, K.. Bandura, J. P., Fisch, C., Asynchrony of conduction within the canine specialized Purkinje fiber system. *Circulation Res* 27: 691, 1970.
17. Anderson, G. J., Greenspan, K., Fisch, C., Bayley, J. C., Electrophysiologic studies on Wenckebach structures below the atrioventricular junction. *Am J Cardiol* 30: 232, 1972.
18. Anderson, P. A. W., Rogers, M. C., Canent, R. V., Spach, M. S., Atrioventricular conduction in secundum atrial septal defects. *Circulation* 48: 27, 1973.
19. Anderson, R. H., Latham, R. A., The cellular architecture of the human atrioventricular node, with a note on its morphology in the presence of a left superior vena cava. *J Anat* 109: 443, 1971.
20. Anderson, R. H., Histologic and histochemical evidence concerning the presence of morphologically distinct cellular zones within the rabbit atrioventricular node. *Anat Rec* 173: 7, 1972.
21. Anderson, R. H., The disposition, morphology and innervation of cardiac specialized tissue in the guinea pig. *J Anat* 111: 453, 1972.
22. Anderson, R. H., The disposition and innervation of atrioventricular ring specialized tissue in rats and rabbits. *J Anat* 113: 197, 1972.

23. Anderson, R. H., Taylor, I. M., Development of atrioventricular specialized tissue in human heart. *Brit Heart J* 34: 1205, 1972.

24. Anderson, R. H., Thaper, M. K., Arnold, R., Jones, R. S., Study of conducting tissue in a case of ventricular pre-excitation. *Brit Heart J* 35: 566, 1973.

25. Anderson, R. H., Bouton, J., Burrow, C. T., Smith, A., Sudden death in infancy: a study of cardiac specialized tissue. *Brit Med J* 2: 135, 1974.

26. Anderson, R. H., Ashley, G. T., Growth of the Cardiovascular System 1) Anatomical development. In: *Scientific foundations of pediatrics*, edited by Davies J, Dobbing J, Heinemann, London, 1974.

27. Anderson, R. H., Arnold, R., Thaper, M. K., Jones, R. S., Hamilton, D. I., Cardiac specialized tissue in hearts with an apparently single ventricular chamber (Double inlet left ventricle). *Am J Cardiol* 33: 96, 1974.

28. Anderson, R. H., Becker, A. E., Arnold, R., Wilkinson, J. L., The conducting tissues in congenitally corrected transposition. *Circulation* 50: 911, 1974.

29. Anderson, R. H., Bouton, J., Burrow, C., Smith, A., Sudden death in infancy. A study of the cardiac specialized tissue. *Brit Med J* 2: 135, 1974.

30. Anderson, R. H., Davies, M. J., Becker, A. E., Atrioventricular ring specialized tissue in the normal heart. *Europ J Cardiol* 2: 219, 1974.

31. Anderson, R. H., Janse, M. J., van Capelle, F. J. L., Billette, J., Becker, A. E., Durrer, D., A combined morphological and electrophysiological study of the atrioventricular node of the rabbit heart. *Circulation Res* 35: 909, 1974.

32. Anderson, R. H., Becker, A. E., Wenink, A. C. G., Janse, M. J., The development of the cardiac specialized tissue. Chapter this book. 1975.

33. Anderson, R. H., Becker, A. E., Brechenmacher, C., Davies, M. J., Rossi, L., The human atrioventricular junctional area—a morphologic study of the atrioventricular node and bundle. *Europ J Cardiol* 3: 11, 1975.

34. Anderson, R. H., Becker, A. E., Brechenmacher, C., Davies, M. J., Rossi, L., Ventricular pre-excitation. A proposed nomenclature for its substrates. *Europ J Cardiol* 3: 27, 1975.

35. Anderson, R. H., Becker, A. E., Wilkinson, J. L., Morphogenesis of bulboventricular malformations IV Univentricular hearts. In preparation.

36. Angelakos, E. T., Fuxe, K., Torchiana, M. L., Chemical and histochemical evaluation of the distribution of catecholamines in the rabbit and guinea pig hearts. *Acta Physiol Scand* 59: 184, 1963.

37. Arbel, E., Sasyniuk, B. I., Moe, G. K., Super-

normal ventricular conduction in the dog heart. (Abstract) *Fed Proc* 30: 553, 1971.

38. Aronson, R. S., Cranefield, P. F., The effect of resting potential on the electrical activity of canine cardiac Purkinje fibers exposed to Na-free solution or to ouabain. *Pfluegers Arch* 347: 101, 1974.

39. Aschoff, L., Referat über die Herzstörungen in ihren Beziehungen zu den spezifischen Muskelsystems des Herzens. *Verh dtsch path Ges* 14: 3, 1910.

40. Ashman, R., Gouaux, J. L., Reflex inhibition of the human heart: Complete A-V block and parasystole. *Proc Soc Exp Biol Med* 37: 25, 1937.

41. Atkins, J. N., Leshin, S. J., Blomqvist, G., Mullins, C. B., Ventricular conduction blocks and sudden death in acute myocardial infraction. *New Eng J Med* 288: 281, 1973.

42. de Azevedo, I. M., Watanabe, Y., Dreifus, L. S., Electrophysiologic antagonism of quinidine and bretylium tosylate. *Am J Cardiol* 33: 633, 1974.

43. de Azevedo, I. M., Dreifus, I. S., Watanabe, Y., Electrophysiologic effects of a new ester of ajmaline 17-mono chloroacetyl ajmaline hydrochloride (MCAA). *Europ J Cardiol* 2/3: 321, 1975.

44. Bacaner, M. B., Quantitative comparison of bretylium with other antifibrillatory drugs. *Am J Cardiol* 21: 504, 1968.

45. Bachmann, G., The inter-auricular time interval. *Am J Physiol* 41: 309, 1916.

46. Bailey, J. C., Anderson, G. J., Pippenger, D., Fisch, C., Re-entry within the isolated canine bundle of His. Possible mechanism for reciprocal rhythm. *Am J Cardiol* 32: 808, 1973.

47. Baird, J. A., Robb, J. S., Study, reconstruction, and gross dissection of the atrioventricular conducting system of the dog heart. *Anat Rec* 108: 747, 1950.

48. Bandura, J. P., Brody, D. A., Microelectrode study of alternating responses to repetitive premature excitation in canine Purkinje fibers. *Circulation Res* 34: 406, 1974.

49. Barry, A., Pattern, B. M., The structure of the adult heart, In: *Pathology of the heart and blood vessels*, edited by Gould S. E., Thomas, Springfield, Ill. 3rd Ed, 1968, p. 123.

50. Baschiere, L., Palagi, L., Puletti, M., Experimental study of the pathogenesis of ventricular extrasystoles. *Cardiologia* 50: 366, 1967.

51. Bassingthwaighte, J. B., Reuter, H., Calcium movements and excitation-contraction coupling in cardiac cells. In: *Electrical phenomena in the heart*, edited by de Mello W. C., Acad Press, New York and London, 1972, p. 353.

52. Beccari, E., Latenziamento dell'ajmalina *Il Farmaco* 18: 65, 1963.

53. Becker, A. E., Middelhoff, CJEM, unpublished observations.
54. Becker, R. A., Acher, A. M., Erickson, R. V., Ventricular excitation in experimental left bundle branch block. *Am Heart Journal* 55: 547, 1958.
55. Behnke, O., Zelander, T., Preservation of inter-cellular substances by the cationic dye alcian blue in preparative procedures for electron microscopy. *J Ulstrastruc Res* 31: 424, 1970.
56. Bekheit, S., Murtagh, J. G., Morton, P., Flet-cher, E., Effect of lidocaine on conduction system of human heart. *Brit Heart J* 35: 305, 1973.
57. Bekheit, S., Morton, P., Murtagh, J. G., Fletcher, E., Comparison of sinoventricular conduction in children and adults using bundle of His electrograms. *Brit Heart J* 35: 507, 1973.
58. Bencosme, S. A., Berger, J. M., Specific granules in mammalian and non-mammalian vertebrate cardiocytes. In: *Meth Achievm Exp Path.* Vol. 5. Bajusz, E., Jasmin, G., Eds. Basel, 1971, p. 173.
59. Benitez, D., Mascher, D., Alanis, J., The electri-cal activity of the bundle of His. The fast and slow inward currents. *Pfluegers Arch* 345: 61, 1973.
60. Bennett, G., Leblond, C. P., Haddad, A., Migra-tion of glycoprotein from the golgi apparatus to the surface of various cell types as shown by radioautography after labeled fucose injection into rats. *J Cell Biol* 60: 258, 1974.
61. Bennett, H. S., Morphological aspects of extra-cellular polysaccharides. *J Histochem Cytochem* 11: 14, 1963.
62. Benninghof, A., Über die Beziehungen des Reitsleitungssystem und der papillarmuskeln zu der Konturfasern des Herzschlauses. *Anat Anz* 57: 185, 1923.
63. Berger, J. M., Rona, G., Functional and fine structural heterogeneity of atrial cardiocytes. In *Meth Achievm Exp Path.* Vol. 5. Bajusz, E., Jasmin G., Eds. Basel, 1971, p. 540.
64. Berger, W. K., Correlation between the Ultra-structure and function of intercellular contacts. In: *Electrical phenomena in the heart*, edited by de Mello, W. C., Acad. Press, New York and London, 1972, p. 63.
65. Berkman, N. L., Lamb, L. E., The Wolff-Parkinson-White electrocardiogram. A follow-up of five to twenty-eight years. *New Engl J Med* 278: 492, 1968.
66. Bigger, J. T. jr. Bassett, A. L., Hoffman, B. F., Electrophysiological effects of diphenylhydan-toin on canine Purkinje fibers. *Circulation Res* 22: 221, 1968.
67. Bigger, J. T. jr, Schmidt, D. H., Kutt, H., Re-lationship between the plasma level of diphenyl-hydantoin sodium and its cardiac antiarrhythmic effects. *Circulation* 38: 363, 1968.
68. Bigger, J. T. jr, Goldreyer, B. N., The mechan-ism of supraventricular tachycardia. *Circulation* 42: 673, 1970.
69. Bigger, J. T. jr, Mandel, W. J., Effect of lido-caine on conduction in canine Purkinje fibers and the ventricular muscle-Purkinje fiber junction. *J Pharmacol Exp Ther* 172: 239, 1970.
70. Bigger, J. T. jr, Mandel, W. I., Effect of lido-caine on the electrophysiological properties of ventricular muscle and Purkinje fibers. *J Clin Invest* 49: 63, 1970.
71. Bigger, J. T. jr, Jaffe, C. C., The effect of bretyl-ium tosylate on the electrophysiologic properties of ventricular muscle and Purkinje fibers. *Am J Cardiol* 27: 82, 1971.
72. Bigger, J. T. jr: Arrhythmias and antiarrhythmic drugs *Adv Int Med* 18: 251, 1972.
73. Billette, J., Elharrar, V., Porlier, G., Nadeau, R. A., Sinus slowing produced by experimental ischemia of the sinus node in dogs. *Am J Cardiol* 31: 331, 1973.
74. Billette, J., Janse, M. J., van Capelle, F. J. L., Anderson, R. H., Touboul, P., Durrer, D., Cycle length dependent properties of AV nodal activation in rabbit heart. To be published.
75. Birchfield, R. I., Menefee, E. E., Bryant, G. D. N., Disease of the sinoatrial node associated with bradycardia, asystole, syncope, and paroxysmal atrial fibrillation. *Circulation* 16: 20, 1957.
76. Bissett, J. K., Thompson, A. J., de Soyza, N., Murphy, M. L., Atrioventricular conduction in patients with short PR intervals and normal QRS complexes. *Brit Heart J* 35: 123, 1973.
77. Blair, D. M., Davies, F., Observations on the conducting system of the heart. *J Anat* 69: 303, 1935.
78. Blondeau, M., Lenègre, J., Bloc atypique de la branche droite. *Masson Ed. Paris*, 1970.
79. de Boer, S., On the fibrillation of the heart. *J Physiol* 54: 400, 1921.
80. Bogusch, G., Investigations on the fine structure of Purkinje fibers in the atrium of the avain heart. *Cell Tiss Res* 150: 43, 1974.
81. Boineau, J. P., Moore, E. N., Evidence for propagation of activation across an accessory atrio-ventricular connection in types A and B pre-excitation. *Circulation* 41: 375, 1970.
82. Boineau, J. P., Cox, J. L., Slow ventricular activation in acute myocardial infarction. A source of re-entrant premature ventricular contractions. *Circulation* 48: 702, 1973.
83. Bojson-Møller, F., Tranum-Jensen, J., On nerves and nerve endings in the conducting system of

the moderator band (septomarginal trabecula). *J Anat* 108: 387, 1971.

84. Bojsen-Møller, F., Tranum-Jensen, J., Rabbit heart nodal tissue, sinuo-atrial ring bundle and atrioventricular connexions defined as a neuromuscular system. *J Anat* 112: 367, 1972

85. Bonke, F. I. M., Bouman, I. N., Van Rijn, H. E., Change of cardiac rhythm in the rabbit after an atrial premature beat. *Circulation Res* 24: 533, 1969.

86. Bonke, F. I. M., Bouman, I. N., Schopman, F. J. G., Effect of an early atrial premature beat on activity of the sinoatrial node and atrial rhythm in the rabbit. *Circulation Res* 29: 704, 1971.

87. Boyd, J. D., Development of the heart. In: Handbook of Physiology. Section 2: Circulation Vol. 3: 2511, 1965 Ed. by Hamilton W. F. American Physiological Society, Washington.

88. Brechenmacher, C., Laham, J., Iris, L., Gerbaux, A., Lenègre, J., Etude histologique des voies anormales de conduction dans un syndrome de Wolff-Parkinson-White et dans un syndrome de Lown-Ganong-Levine. *Arch Mal Coeur* 67: 507, 1974.

89. Brodsky, S. I., Mirowski, M., Krovetz, J., Rowe, R. D., Recording of His bundle and other potentials in children. *J. Pediatr* 79: 61, 1971.

90. Bronowski, J., Science and human values. Perennial Library, Harper and Row, Pub. 1972, p. 13.

91. Brooks, C., Mc.C., Hoffman, B. F., Suckling, E. E., Excitability of the heart. Grune and Stratton, New York, 1955.

92. Brooks, C. Mc.C., Lu, H. H., The sinoatrial pacemaker of the heart. Springfield, Ill. 1972.

93. Brown, G. L., Eccles, J. C., Action of a single vagal volley on the rhythm of the heart beat. *J Physiol* 82: 211, 1934.

94. Brusca, A., Rosettani, E., Activation of the human fetal heart *Am Heart J* 86: 79, 1973.

95. Bryson, A. L., Parisi, A. F., Schechter, E., Wolfson, S., Life-threatening ventricular arrhythmias induced by exercise. Cessation after coronary bypass surgery. *Am J Cardiol* 32: 995, 1973.

96. Burch, G. E., Wajszzuk, W. J., Cronvich, J. A., Spread of activation in the anterolateral papillary muscle of the left ventricle of the dog under normal and pathologic conditions. *Am Heart J* 79: 769, 1970.

97. Burchell, H. B., Essex, H. E., Pruitt, R. D., Studies on the spread of excitation through the ventricular myocardium: The ventricular septum. *Circulation* 6: 161, 1952.

98. Burchell, H. B., Sturm, R. E., Electroshock hazards. *Circulation* 35: 227, 1967.

99. Burchell, H. B., Frye, R. L., Anderson, M. W., McGoon, D. C., Atrioventricular and ventriculoatrial excitation in Wolff-Parkinson-White Syndrome (Type B): Transitory ablation at surgery. *Circulation* 36: 663, 1967.

100. Burchell, H. B., Meredith, J., Management of cardiac tachyarrhythmias with cardiac pacemakers. *Ann N Y Acad Sci* 167, 546, 1969.

101. Camerini, F., Baldi, N., Gori, P., Martinoli, E., Ajmaline in the prognosis of bifascicular blocks. *Giornale Ital Cardiologia* 3: 880, 1973.

102. Cannom, D. S., Goldreyer, B. N., Damato, A. N., Evidence for a 'gate' in the distal human ventricular specialized conduction system. (Abstract) *Circulation* 44 (suppl. II): II–148, 1971.

103. Cannon, F., Sjostrand, T., The occurrence of a positive afterpotential in the ECG in different physiological and pathological conditions. *Acta med Scand* 146: 191, 1953.

104. van Capelle, F. J. L., Janse, M. J., Varghese, P. J., Freud, G. E., Mater, C., Durrer, D., Spread of excitation in the atrioventricular node of isolated rabbit hearts studied by multiple microelectrode recording. *Circulation Res* 31: 602, 1972.

105. van Capelle, F. J. L., Janse, M. J., Influence of geometry on the shape of the propagated action potential. This volume.

106. Caracta, A. R., Damato, A. N., Gallagher, J. J., Josephson, M. E., Varghese, P. J., Lau, S. H., Westura, E. E., Electrophysiologic studies in the syndrome of short P-R interval, normal QRS complex. *Am J Cardiol* 31: 245, 1973.

107. Caracta, A. R., Damato, A. N., Josephson, M. E., Gallagher, J. J., Ricciutti, M., Lau, S. H., Electrophysiology of diphenylhydantoin. *Circulation* 47: 1234, 1973.

108. Carmeliet, E., Vereecke, J., Adrenaline and the plateau phase I of the cardiac action potential. Importance of Ca^{++}, Na^+ and K^+ conductance. *Pfluegers Arch* 313: 300, 1969.

109. Carmeliet, E., VanBogaert, P. P., Strontium action potentials in cardiac Purkinje fibers. *Arch Int Physiol et Biochem* 77: 134, 1969.

110. Castellanos, A., Genesis of bidirectional tachycardia. *Am Heart J* 61: 733, 1961.

110a. Castellanos, A., Jr, Chapunoff, E., Castillo, C. A., Maytin, O., Lemberg, L., His bundle electrogram in two cases of Wolff-Parkinson-White (pre-excitation) syndrome. *Circulation* 41: 399, 1970.

111. Castellanos, A., Castillo, C. A., Agha, A. S., Tessler, M., His bundle electrograms in patients with short P-R intervals, narrow QRS complexes, and paroxysmal tachycardias. *Circulation* 43: 667, 1971.

112. Castellanos, A., Iyengar, R., Agha, A. S.,

Castillo, C. A., Wenckebach phenomenon within the atria. *Brit Heart J* 34: 1121, 1972.

113. Castellanos, A., Myerburg, R. J., Craparo, K., Befeler, B., Agha, A. S., Factors regulating ventricular rates during atrial flutter and fibrillation in pre-excitation (Wolff-Parkinson-White) syndrome. *Brit Heart J* 35: 811, 1973.

114. Castellanos, A., Befeler, B., Myerburg, J., Pseudo A. V., block produced by concealed extrasystoles arising below the bifurcation of the His bundle. *Brit Heart J* 36: 457, 1974.

115. Castellanos, A., Sung, R. I., Cunha, D., Myerburg, R. J., His bundle recordings in paroxysmal atrioventricular block produced by carotid sinus massage. *Brit Heart J* 36: 487, 1974.

116. Castillo, C. A., Castellanos, A., Retrograde activation of the His bundle during intermittent paired ventricular stimulation in the human heart. *Circulation* 42: 1079. 1970.

117. Castillo, C. A., Castellanos, A., Retrograde activation of the His bundle in the human heart. *Am J Cardiol* 27: 264, 1971.

118. Castillo-Fenoy, A., Goupil, A., Offenstadt, G., Syndrome de Wolff-Parkinson-White et mort subite. *Ann Med Interne* (Paris) 124: 871, 1973.

119. Cervoni, P., Ellis, C. H., Mazwell, R. A., The antiarrhythmic action of bretylium in normal reserpine-pretreated and chronically denervated dog hearts. *Arch Int Pharmacodyn* 190: 91, 1971.

120. Chadda, K. D., Banka V., Helfant, R. H., Rate dependent ventricular ectopia following acute coronary occlusion: The concept of an optimal antiarrhythmic heart rate. *Circulation* 49: 654, 1974.

121. Challice, C. E., Studies on the microstructure of the heart. I. The sino-atrial node and the sino-atrial ring bundle. *J Roy Micr Soc* 85: 1, 1966.

122. Challice, C. E., Functional morphology of the specialized tissues of the heart. *Meth Achievm Exp path* 5: 121, 1971.

123. Challice, C. E., Virágh, S., The embryologic development of the mammalian heart. In: *Ultrastructure of the mammalian heart*. Challice, C. E., Virágh, S., eds. Acad Press New York and London, 1973, p. 91.

124. Cheng, Y. P., The ultrastructure of the rat sinoatrial node. *Acta Anat Nipponica* 46: 339, 1971.

125. Childers, R. W., Merideth, J., Moe, G. J., Supernormality in Bachmann's bundle: An *in vivo* and *in vitro* study. *Circulation Res* 22: 363, 1968.

126. Childers, R. W., Arnsdorf, M. E., de la Fuente, D. L., Sinus nodal echoes. *Am J. Cardiol* 31: 220, 1973.

127. Childers, R. W., Supernormality. *Cardiovasc Clin* 5: 136, 1973.

128. Chuaqui, B., Lupenpräparatorische Darstellung der Ausbreitungs-züge des Sinusknotens. *Virchows Arch* (Path Anat) 356: 141, 1972.

129. Chaqui, B., Zur histogenese des AV-Knotens beim Menschen. *Basic Res in Card* 68: 266, 1973.

130. Chung, K. Y., Walsh, T. J., Massie, E., Double ventricular parasystole. *Am Heart J* 67: 162, 1964.

131. Chung, K. Y., Walsh T. J., Massie, E., Combined atrial and ventricular parasystole. *Am J Cardiol* 16: 462, 1965.

132. Cobb, F. R., Blumenschein, S. D., Sealy, W. C., Boineau, J. P., Wagner, G. S., Wallace, A. G., Successful surgical interruption of the bundle of Kent in a patient with Wolff-Parkinson-White syndrome. *Circulation* 38: 1018, 1968.

133. Cohen, H. C., Gozo, E. G., Pick, A., Ventricular tachycardia with narrow QRS complexes (left posterior fascicular tachycardia). *Circulation* 45: 1035, 1972.

134. Cohen, H. C., Langendorf, R., Pick, A., Intermittent parasystole; mechanism of protection. *Circulation* 48: 761, 1973.

135. Cohen, L., Diphenylhydantoin sodium (dilantoin) in: Donoso E, Ed. Drugs in Cardiology Part I. Stratton Intercontinental Medical Book Corp, New York, 1975, p. 49.

136. Cohen, S. I., Lau, S. H., Scherlag, B. J., Damato, A. N., Alternate patterns of premature ventricular excitation during induced atrial bimeminy. *Circulation* 39: 819, 1969.

137. Cohen, S. I., Smith, I. K., Aroesty, J. M., Voukydis, P., Morkin, E., Concealed retrograde conduction in complete atrioventricular block. *Circulation* 50: 496, 1974.

138. Cohn, A. E., A case of bradycardia with postmortem examination. *Heart* 3: 23, 1911.

139. Colborn, G. L., Carsey, E. jr, Electron microscopy of the sino-atrial node of the squirrel monkey (saimiri Sciureus) *J Mol Cell Cardiol* 4: 525, 1972.

140. Cooper, T., First Annual Report of the Director of the National Heart and Lung Institute. *DHEW Publicat* (NIH) 74–514: 36, 1974.

141. Copenhaver, W. M., Heteroplastic transplantation of the sinus venosus between two species of amblystomas. *J Exp Zool* 100: 203, 1945.

142. Copenhaver, W. M., Truex, R. C., Histology of the atrial portion of the cardiac conduction system in man and other mammals. *Anat Rec* 114: 601, 1952.

143. Coraboeuf, E., Otsuka, M., L'action des solutions hyposodiques sur les potentials cellulaires de tissu cardiaque de mammiferes. *CR Acad Sci* 243: 441, 1956.

144. Corrado, G., Levi, R. J., Nau, G. J., Rosenbaum, M. B., Paroxysmal atrioventricular block related

to phase 4 bilateral bundle branch block. *Am J Cardiol* 33: 553, 1974.

145. Cough, O. A., Cardiac aneurysm with ventricular tachycardia and subsequent excision of aneurysm. *Circulation* 20: 251, 1955.

146. Coumel, Ph., Motté, G., Gourgon, R., Fabiato, A., Slama, R., Bouvrain, Y., Les tachycardies supra-ventriculaires en dehors du syndrome de W.P.W. *Arch Mal Coeur* 63: 35, 1970.

147. Coumel, Ph., Fabiato, A., Waynberger, M., Motté, G., Slama, R., Bouvrain, Y., Bradycardia-dependent atrio-ventricular block. Report of two cases of AV-block elicited by premature beats. *J. Electrocardiol* 4: 168, 1971.

148. Coumel, Ph., Waynberger, M., Fabiato, A., Slama, R., Aigueperse, J., Bouvrain, Y., Wolff-Parkinson-White syndrome: Problems in evaluation of multiple accessory pathways and surgical therapy. *Circulation* 45: 1216, 1972.

149. Coumel, Ph., Waynberger, M., Les tachycardies par rythme réciproque au cours du syndrôme de W.P.W. Physiopathologie et traitement. *Coeur Med Intern* 11: 77, 1972.

150. Coumel, Ph., Attuel, P., Reciprocating tachycardia in overt and latent pre-excitation: Influence of functional bundle branch block on the rate of the tachycardia. *Europ J Cardiol* 1: 423, 1974.

151. Coumel, Ph., Supraventricular tachycardias. In: *Fundamentals of cardiac arrhythmias*, Goodwin & Krikler Ed. W. B. Saunders Comp Ltd Publ, London 1975, p. 62.

152. Coumel, Ph., Junctional reciprocating tachycardias. The permanent and paroxysmal forms of A-V nodal reciprocating tachycardias. *J Electrocardiology* 8: 79, 1975.

153. Coumel, Ph., Barold, S. S., Mechanism of supraventricular tachycardia. In: His bundle electrocardiography and clinical electrophysiology. Ed. by Narula OS, F. A. Davis, Philadelphia, 1975, p. 203.

154. Coumel, Ph., Attuel, P., Localization of the circus movement during reciprocating tachycardia in WPW syndrome. In: His bundle electocardiography and clinical electrophysiology. Ed. by Narula OS, F. A. Davis, Philadelphia, 1975, p. 343.

155. Coumel, Ph., Attuel, P., Motté, G., Slama, R., Bouvrain, Y., Les tachycardies jonctionnelles paroxystiques. Evaluation du point de jonction inférieur du circuit de ré-entrée. Démembrement des soi-disant rythmes réciproques intra-nodaux. *Arch Mal Coeur* (in press).

156. Cox, J. L., Daniel, T. M., Sabiston, D. C., Boineau, J. P., De-synchronized activation in myocardial infarction. A re-entry basis. (Abstract). *Circulation* 39: (suppl. III)III-63, 1969.

157. Cox, W. V., Robertson, H. R., The effect of stellate ganglionectomy on the cardiac function of intact dogs. *Am Heart J* 12: 285, 1936.

158. Cranefield, P. E., Hoffman, B. E., Siebens, A. A., Anodal excitation of cardiac muscle. *Am J Physiol* 190: 383, 1957.

159. Cranefield, P. E., Hoffman, B. E., Paes de Carvalho, A., Effects of acetylcholine on single fibers of the atrioventricular node. *Circulation Res* 7: 19, 1959.

160. Cranefield, P. E., Klein, H. O., Hoffman, B. E., Conduction of the cardiac impulse. I. Delay, block and one-way block in depressed Purkinje fibers. *Circulation Res* 28: 199, 1971.

161. Cranefield, P. E., Hoffman, B. E., Conduction of the cardiac impulse: II. Summation and inhibition. *Circulation Res* 28: 220, 1971.

162. Cranefield, P. F., Wit, A. L., Hoffman, B. E., Conduction of the cardiac impulse. III. Characteristics of very slow conduction. *J Gen Physiol* 59: 227, 1972.

163. Cranefield, P. F., Wit, A. L., Hoffman, B. F., Genesis of cardiac arrhythmias. *Circulation* 47: 190, 1973.

164. Cranefield, P. F., Ventricular fibrillation. *New Engl J Med* 289: 732, 1973.

165. Cranefield, P. F., Wit, A. L., Sustained rhythmicity in cardiac fibers with slow response activity triggered by propagated action potentials. *Circulation* (Abstract) 50 (Suppl.III) III–97, 1974.

166. Cranefield, P. F., Aronson, R. S., Wit, A. L., Effect of verapamil on the normal action potential and on a calcium dependent slow response of canine cardiac Purkinje fibers. *Circulation Res* 34: 204, 1974.

167. Cranefield, P. F., Aronson, R. S., Initiation of sustained rhythmic activity by single propagated action potentials in canine cardiac Purkinje fibers exposed to sodium-free solution or to ouabain. *Circulation Res* 34: 477, 1974.

168. Cranefield, P. F., The conduction of the cardiac impulse; The slow response and cardiac arrhythmias. Futura Publ Co Mt Kisco, N.Y., 1975.

169. Cushny, A. R., Matthews, S. A., On the effects of electrical stimulation of the mammalian heart. *J Physiol* 21: 213, 1897.

170. van Dam, R. Th., Durrer, D., Strackee, J., van der Tweel, L. H., The excitability cycle of the dog's ventricle determined by anodal, cathodal and bipolar stimulation. *Circulation Res* 4: 196, 1956.

171. van Dam, R. Th., Moore, E. N., Hoffman, B. F., Initiation and conduction of impulses in partially depolarized cardiac fibers. *Am J Physiol* 204: 1133, 1963.

172. Van Dam, R. Th., Janse, M. J., The effect of changes in rate and rhythm on the refractory

period of the ventricular myocardium and specialized conducting system on the canine heart. In: *Research in Physiology*, edited by Kao FF, Kaizumi K, Vassalle M. Aulo Gaggi, Bolongna, 1971.

173. Damato, A. N., Lau, S. H., Helfant, R. H., Stein, E., Patton, R. D., Scherlag, B. J., Berkowitz, W. D., A study of heart block in man using His bundle recording. *Circulation* 39: 297, 1969.

174. Damato, A. N., Lau, S. H., The clinical value of the electrogram of the conducting system. *Progr Cardiovasc Dis* 13: 119, 1970.

175. Damato, A. N., Lau, S. H., Bobb, G. A., Studies on ventriculo-atrial conduction and the re-entry phenomenon. *Circulation* 41: 423, 1970.

176. Damato, A. N., Varghese, P. J., Lau, S. H., Gallagher, J. J., Bobb, G. A., Manifest and concealed re-entry. A mechanism of AV nodal Wenckebach phenomenon. *Circulation Res* 30: 283, 1972.

177. Damato, A. N., Varghese, P. J., Caracta, A. R., Akhtar, M., Lau, S. H., Functional 2:1 A-V block within the His-Purkinje system. Simulation of type II second-degree A-V block. *Circulation* 47: 534, 1973.

178. Davies, F., The conducting system of the vertebrate heart. *Brit Heart J* 4: 66, 1942.

179. Davies, F., Francis, E. T. B., The conducting system of the vertebrate heart. *Biol Rev* 21: 173, 1946.

180. Davies, M. J., Morphology of the conduction system. In: Davies, M. J., Pathology of the conducting tissue of the heart, New York 1971.

181. Davies, M. J., Pomerance, A., Quantitative study of ageing changes in the human sinoatrial node and internodal tract. *Brit Heart J* 34: 150, 1972.

182. Davis, L. D., Temte, J. V., Electrophysiological actions of lidocaine on canine ventricular muscle and Purkinje fibers. *Circulation Res* 24: 639, 1969.

183. Davis, L. D., Effect of changes in cycle length on diastolic depolarization produced by ouabain in canine Purkinje fibers. *Circulation Res* 32: 206, 1973.

184. Dawes, G. S., Sudden death in babies. Physiology of the fetus and newborn. *Am J Cardiol* 22: 469, 1968.

185. D'Cruz, I. A., Cohen, H., Pick, A., Langendorf, R., Mechanisms of electrical alternans in left and in right bundle block: Early or late phases of refractoriness in the bundle branch system (Abstract). *Am J Cardiol* 35: 131, 1975.

186. De la Fuente, D., Jedlicka, J., Moe, G. K., Time course of vagal effects on S-A and A-V nodes (Abstract). *Fed Proc* 28: 269, 1969.

187. De la Fuente, D., Sasyniuk, B. I., Moe, G. K., Conduction through a narrow isthmus in isolated canine atrial tissue. A model of the WPW syndrome. *Circulation* 46, 803, 1971.

188. Demoulin, J. C., Kulbertus, H. E., Histopathological examination of concept of left hemiblock. *Brit Heart J* 34: 807, 1972.

189. Demoulin, J. C., Simar, L. J., Kulbertus, H. E., Quantitative study of left bundle branch fibrosis in left anterior hemiblock. A stereological approach. *Am J Cardiol*: in press.

190, Denes, P., Wu, D., Dhingra, R. C., Chuquimia, R., Rosen, K. M., Demonstration of dual A-V nodal pathways in patients with paroxysmal sypraventricular tachycardia. *Circulation* 48: 549, 1973.

191. Denes, P., Wu, D., Dhingra, R., Pietras, R. J., Rosen, K. M., The effects of cycle length on cardiac refractory periods in man. *Circulation* 49: 32, 1974.

192. Denes, P., Wyndham, C. R. C., Dhingra, R. C., AmatyLeon, E., Levitsky, S., Rosen, K. M., Prediction of anomalous pathway location in patients with WPW syndrome using atrial pacing at multiple sites. (Abstract) *Circulation* 50 (III): 222, 1974.

193. Denes, P., Wu, D., Rosen, K. M., Demonstration of dual A-V pathways in a patient with Lown-Ganong-Levine syndrome. *Chest* 65: 343, 1974.

194. Denes, P., Dhingra, R. C., Rosen, K. M., Electrophysiologic evidence for dual A-V nodal pathways in man. In: His bundle electrocardiography and clinical electrophysiology, edited by Narula O. S., F. A. Davis, Philadelphia, 1975.

195. Denes, P., Wu, D., Dhingra, R. C., Amat. y Leon, F., Wyndham, C. R. C., Rosen, K. M., Dual A-V nodal pathways. *Brit Heart J*: 37: 1069, 1975.

196. Denes, P., Wyndham, C. R. C., Wu, D., Rosen, K. M., 'Supernormal conduction' of a premature impulse utilizing the fast pathway in a patient with dual A-V nodal pathways. *Circulation*: 51:811, 1975.

197. Denes, P., Wyndham, C., Wu, D., Kosowsky, B., Hall, R., Cooley, D., Rosen, K. M., Intractable paroxysmal tachycardia due to a concealed retrogradely conducting Kent Bundle. Demonstration by epicardial mapping and cure of tachycardia by surgical interruption of the His bundle. Submitted for publication.

198. DeSoyza, N., Bissett, J. K., Kane, J. J., Murphy, M., Doherty, J. E., Ectopic ventricular prematurity and its relationship to ventricular tachycardia in acute myocardial infarction in man. *Circulation* 50: 529, 1974.

199. Dhingra, R. C., Rosen, K. M., Rahimtoola, S. H., Wenckebach periods with repetitive block: Evaluation with His bundle recording. *Am Heart J* 86: 444, 1973.

200. Doer, R. W., Die Morphologie des Reitzleitung-systems, ihre Orthologie und Pathologie. In Rhythmusstörungen des Herzens. Ed. by Spang K, Thieme, Stuttgart, 1957, p. 19.

201. Downar, E., Waxman, M., This volume.

202. Dreifus, L. S., Watanabe, Y., Sirlin, N., Katz, M., Potassium and the action of quinidine. J Lab Clin Med 60: 870, 1962.

203. Dreifus, L. S., Josipovic, V., Effects of pro-pranolol on A-V transmission (Abstract). Fed Proc 27: 226, 1968.

203a. Dreifus, L. S., Nichols, H., Morse, D., Watanabe, Y., Truex, R., Controle of recurrent tachycardia of Wolff-Parkinson-White syndrome by surgical ligature of the A-V bundle. Circulation 38: 1030, 1968.

204. Dreifus, L. S., Watanabe, Y., Cardanas, N., Newer antiarrhythmic drugs. Cardiovasc Clin 1: 3, 1969.

205. Dreifus, L. S., Watanabe, Y., Current status of diphenylhydantoin. Am Heart J 80: 709, 1970.

206. Dreifus, L. S., Haiat, R., Watanabe, Y., Arriaga, J., Reitman, N., Ventricular fibrilla-tion: a possible mechanism of sudden death in patients with the Wolff-Parkinson-White syndrome. Circulation 43: 520, 1971.

207. Dreifus, L. S., Watanabe, Y., Clinical correlates of the electrophysiologic action of digitalis on the heart. Drug treatment 2: 179, 1972.

208. Dreifus, L. S., Filip, Z., Sexton, L., Watanabe, Y., Electrophysiological and clinical effects of a new antiarrhythmic agent: Disopyramide. (Abstract). Am J. Cardiol 31: 129. 1973.

209. Dreifus, L. S., Kimbiris, D., Wellens, H.J., Sinus bradycardia and atrial fibrillation associated with Wolff-Parkinson-White syndrome (Ab-stract). Circulation 48: (suppl. IV) IV-17, 1973.

210. Dreifus, L. S., de Azevedo, I. M., Watanabe, Y., Electrolyte and drug interaction. Am Heart J 88: 95, 1974.

211. Dreifus, L. S., de Azevedo, I. M., Dreifus, H. N., Watanabe, Y., Interaction of procaine amide and lidocaine. (Abstract). Circulation 50: III-170, 1974.

212. Dreifus, L. S., Electrophysiology of Norpace. Angiology 26: 111, 1975.

213. DuBrow, I. W., Fischer, E. A., Amat y Leon, F., Denes, P., Wu, D., Rosen, K. M., Hastreiter, A. R., Comparison of cardiac refractory periods in children and adults. Circulation 51: 485, 1975.

214. Dudel, J., Trautwein, W., Elektrophysiologische Messungen zur Strophanthinwirkung am Herzmuskel. Arch Exp Pathol 232: 393, 1958.

215. Dudel, J., Rüdel, R., Excitatory sodium current in cooled Purkinje fibers. Pfluegers Arch 315: 136, 1970.

216. Van Durme, J. P., Bogaert, M. G., Rosseel, M. T., Effectiveness of aprindine, procaine amide, and quinidine in chronic ventricular dysrhythmias. (Abstract). Circulation 50: III-248, 1974.

217. Durrer, D., Formijne, P., van Dam, R. T., Büller, J., van Lier, A., Meyler, F. L., Electro-cardiogram in normal and some abnormal conditions. Am Heart J 61: 303, 1961.

218. Durrer, D., van Lier, A., Büller, J., Epicardial and intramural excitation in chronic myocardial infarction. Am Heart J 68: 765, 1964.

219. Durrer, D., Roos, J. P., Büller, J., Spread of excitation in canine and human heart. In: Electrophysiology of the Heart. Taccardi, B., Marchetti, G., Ed. Pergamon, Oxford, 1965.

220. Durrer, D., Roos, J. P., Epicardial excitation of the ventricles in a patient with Wolff-Parkinson-White syndrome (type B). Circulation 35: 15, 1967.

221. Durrer, D., Schoo, L., Schuilenburg, R. M., Wellens, H. J. J., The role of premature beats in the initiation and termination of supraventri-cular tachycardia in the Wolff-Parkinson-White syndrome. Circulation 36: 644, 1967.

222. Durrer, D., Electrical aspects of human cardiac activity: A clinical physiological approach to excitation and stimulation. Cardiovasc Res 2: 1, 1968.

223. Durrer, D., van Dam, R. T., Freud, G. E., Meijler, F. L., Roos, J. P., Excitation of the human heart. In: Electrical activity of the heart. Charles C. Thomas, Springfield Ill. 1969, p. 53.

224. Durrer, D., van Dam, R. T., Freud, G. E., Janse, M. J., Meijler, F. L., Arzbaecher, R. C., Total excitation of the isolated human heart. Circula-tion 41: 899, 1970.

225. Durrer, D., Schuilenburg, R. M., Wellens, H. J. J., Pre-excitation revisited. Am J Cardiol 25: 690, 1970.

226. Durrer, D., van Dam, R. T., Freud, G. E., Janse, M. J., Re-entry and ventricular arrhythmias in local ischemia and infarction of the intact dog heart. Proc K. of Nedrl Akad van Wetensch. Amsterdam, Series C 73: 321, 1971.

227. Durrer, D., Wellens, H. J. J., The Wolff-Parkin-son-White syndrome: anno 1973. Europ J Cardiol 1: 347, 1974.

228. Easly, R. M. jr, Goldstein, S., Sino-atrial syn-cope. Am J Med 50: 166, 1971.

229. Eccles, J. C., Hoff, H. E., The rhythm of the heart beat. I. Location, action potential, and electrical excitability of the pacemaker, Proc Roy Soc Lond Series B 115: 307, 1934.

230. Eccles, J. C., Hoff, H. E., The rhythm of the heart beat. II. Disturbances of rhythm produced by late premature beats. Proc Roy Soc Lond Series B 115: 327, 1934.

231. Eccles, J. C., Hoff, H. E., The rhythm of the heart beat. III. Disturbances of rhythm produced by early premature beats. *Proc Roy Soc Lond Series B* 115: 352, 1934.

232. Ecker, R. R., Mullins, C. B., Grammer, J. C., Control of intractable ventricular tachycardia by coronary revascularization. *Circulation* 44, 666, 1971.

233. Ehinger, B., Falck, B., Persson, H., Sporrong, B., Adrenergic and cholinesterase-containing neurons of the heart. *Histochemie* 16: 197, 1968.

234. Ehinger, B., Falck, B., Stenevi, U., Adrenergic and nonadrenergic valvular nerves of the heart. *Exp* 25: 742, 1969.

235. Einthoven, W., Le telecardiogramme. *Arch Int Physiol* 4: 132, 1906.

236. Elizari, M. V., Estudio histopatologico del sistema de conduccion en cuatro casos de miocarditis cronica chagasica. VII Congresso Arg Cardiol. Buenos Aires (quoted by Rosenbaum MB, Elizari MV, Lazzari JO. 1968, réf) 2 1967.

237. Elizari, M. V., Lazzari, J. O., Rosenbaum, M. B., Phase-3 and phase-4 intermittent left anterior hemiblock: Report of first case in the literature. *Chest* 62: 673, 1972.

238. Elizari, M. V., Greenspan, K., Fisch, C., Electrophysiological mechanism of aberrant conduction of premature beats (Abstract). *Circulation* 46: (suppl. II) 28, 1972.

239. Elizari, M. V., Greenspan, K., Fisch, C., Exposure of the canine proximal A-V conducting system for electrophysiological studies. *J Appl Physiol* 34: 538, 1973.

240. Elizari, M. V., Lazzari, J. O., Rosenbaum, M. B., Phase 3 and phase 4 intermittent left bundle branch block occurring spontaneously in a dog: Correlation with histological study of the conducting system. *Europ J Cardiol* 1: 95, 1973.

241. Elizari, M. V., Nau, G. J., Levi, R. J., Lazzari, J. O., Halpern, M. S., Rosenbaum, M. B., Experimental production of rate dependent bundle branch block in the canine heart. *Circulation Res* 34: 730, 1974.

242. Elizari, M. V., Novakovsky, A., Quinteiro, R., Levi, R. J., Lazzari, J. O., Rosenbaum, M. B., The experimental evidence for the role of phase 3 and phase 4 block in the genesis of disturbances in atrioventricular conduction. Chapter this book.

243. El-Said, G., Rosenberg, H. S., Mullins, C. E., Hallman, G. L., Cooley, D. A., McNamara, D. G., Dysrhythmias after Mustard's operation for transposition of the great arteries. *Am J Cardiol* 30: 526, 1972.

244. El-Sherif, N., Tachycardia and bradycardia-dependent bundle branch block after acute myocardial ischemia. *Brit Heart J.* 36: 291, 1974.

245. El-Sherif, N., Scherlag B. J., Lazzara R: Conduction disorders in the canine proximal His-Purkinje system following acute myocardial ischemia. I. The pathophysiology of intra-His bundle block. *Circulation* 49: 837, 1974.

246. El-Sherif, N., Scherlag, B. J., Lazzarra, R., Hope, H., Williams, D. O., Samet, Ph., The pathophysiology of tachycardia-dependent paroxysmal atrioventricular block after acute myocardial ischemia: Experimental and clinical observations. *Circulation* 50: 515, 1974.

247. Emberson, J. W., Challice, C. E., Studies on the impulse conducting pathways in the atrium of the mammalian heart. *Am Heart J* 79: 653, 1970.

248. Engel, T. R., Schaal, S. F., Digitalis in the sick sinus syndrome. The effects of digitalis in sino-atrial automaticity and atrioventricular conduction. *Circulation* 48: 1201, 1973.

249. Engelman, T. W., Ueber den Ursprung der Herzbewegung und die physiologischen Eigenschaften der grossen Herznerven des Frosches. *Archiv f d ges Physiol* 65: 109, 1896.

250. Engstfeld, G., Antoni, H., Fleckenstein, A., Die Restitution der Erregungsfortleitung und Kontraktionskraft des K^+-gelahmten Frosch und Saugertiermyokards durch Adrenalin. *Pfluegers Arch* 273: 145, 1961.

251. Entman, M. L., Estes, E. H., Hackel, D. B., The pathologic basis of the electrocardiographic pattern of parietal block. *Am Heart J* 74: 202, 1967.

252. Eppinger, H., Rothberger, J., Wien-Klin Wochenschrift 22: 1091, 1909.

253. Epstein, S. E., Redwood, D. R., Smith, E. R., Atropine and acute myocardial infarction. *Circulation* 45: 1273, 1972.

254. Epstein, S. E., Goldstein, R. E., Redwood, D. R., Kent, K. M., Smith, E. R., The early phase of acute myocardial infarction, Pharmacologic aspects of therapy. *An Int Med* 78: 918, 1973.

255. Eraut, D., Shaw, D. B., Sinus bradycardia. *Brit Heart J* 33: 742, 1971.

256. Erickson, R. V., Scher, A. M., Becker, R. A., Ventricular excitation in experimental bundle-branch block. *Circulation Res* 5: 5, 1957.

257. Esmond, W. G., Moulton, A., Cowley, R. A., Attar, A., Blair, E., Peripheral ramification of the cardiac conducting system. *Circulation* 27: 732, 1963.

258. Eyster, J. A. E., Evans, J. S., Sino-auricular heart block. *Arch of Internal Med* 16: 832, 1915.

259. Fabiato, A., Coraboeuf, E., Facteurs cellulaires de desynchronization electrique ventriculaire: Etude sur le coeur isolé de lapin dans des conditions de perfusion normale et de depolarization parielle. *J Physiol* (Paris) 61: 277, 1969.

260. Fatt, P., Ginsborg, B. L., The ionic requirements

for the production of action potentials in crustacean muscle fibers. *J Physiol* 142: 516, 1958.

261. Fawcett, D. W., McNutt, N. S., The ultrastructure of the cat myocardium. I. Ventricular papillary muscle. *J Cell Biol* 42: 1, 1969.

262. De Felice, L. J., Challice, C. E., Anatomical and ultrastructural study of the electrophysiological atrioventricular node of the rabbit. *Circulation Res* 24: 457, 1969.

263. Ferrer, M. I., The sick sinus syndrome in atrial disease. *JAMA* 206: 645, 1968.

264. Ferrer, M. I., The sick sinus syndrome. *Circulation* 48: 635, 1973.

265. Ferrier, G. R., Saunders, J. H., Mendez, C., A cellular mechanism for the generation of ventricular arrhythmias by acetylstrophanthidin. *Circulation Res* 32: 600, 1973.

266. Ferrier, G. R., Dresel, P. E., Role of the atrium in determining the functional and effective refractory periods and the conductivity of the atrioventricular transmission system. *Circulation Res* 33: 375, 1973.

267. Ferrier, G. R., Moe, G. K., Effect of calcium on acetylstrophanthidin-induced transient depolarizations in canine Purkinje tissue. *Circulation Res* 33: 508, 1973.

268. Ferrier, G. R., Dresel, P. E., Relationship of the functional refractory period to conduction in the atrioventricular node. *Circulation Res* 35: 204, 1974.

269. Finlay, M., Anderson, R. H., The development of cholinesterase activity in the rat heart. *J Anat* 117: 239, 1974.

270. Fisch, C., Steinmetz, E. F., Fasola, A. F., Martz, B. L., Effect of potassium and 'toxic' doses of digitalis on the myocardium. *Circulation Res* 7: 424, 1959.

271. Fisch, C., Chevalier, R. B., Intermittent atrial parasystole. *Circulation* 22: 1149, 1960.

272. Fisch, C., Zipes, D. P., McHenry, P. L., Rate dependent aberrancy. *Circulation* 48: 714, 1973.

273. Fleckenstein, A., Specific inhibitors and promotors of calcium action in the excitation-contraction coupling of heart muscle and their role in the prevention of production of myocardial lesions. In: *Calcium and the heart*, New York, Academic Press, 1971, p. 135.

274. Fleischmann, P., Interpolation of atrial premature beats of infra-atrial origin due to concealed A-S conduction. *Am Heart J* 66: 309, 1963.

275. Flensted-Jensen, E., Wolff-Parkinson-White syndrome. A long term follow-up of 47 cases. *Acta Med Scand* 186: 65, 1969.

276. Fontaine, G., Frank, R., Bonnet, M., Cabrol, C., Guiraudon, G., Methode d'étude experimentale et clinique des syndromes de Wolff-Parkinson-White et d'ischemie myocardique par cartographie de la depolarisation ventriculaire épicardique. *Coeur et Med Int* 12: 105, 1973.

277. Fontaine, G., Frank, R., Guiraudon, G., Vedel, J., Grosgogeat, Y., Cabrol, C., Surgical treatment of resistant reentrant ventricular tachycardia by ventriculotomy: a new application of epicardial mapping. *Circulation* 50 suppl. III, 319, 1974.

278. Fontaine, G., Guiraudon, G., Frank, R., Gerbaux, A., Cousteau, J. P., Barillon, A., Gay, J., Cabrol, C., Facquet, J., La cartographie epicardique et le traitement chirurgical par simple ventriculotomie de certaines tachycardies ventriculaires rebelles par reentree. *Arch Mal Coeur* 68: 113, 1975.

279. Foster, P. R., Zipes, D. P., King, R. M., Nicoll, A. D., Fasola, A. F., Suppression of ouabain-induced arrhythmias with aprindine HCl. *Clin Res* 22: 595A, 1974.

280. Foster, P. R., Elharrar, V., Zipes, D. P., Accelerated ventricular escapes produced with barium and strontium. *Clin Res*: in press.

281. Frank, R., Apport des investigations endocaitaires et des cartographies epicardiques dans l'étude des syndromes de pre-excitation ventriculaire. Thèse pour le doctorat en Medicine. *Ed. Medicals et universitaires*, Paris 1974.

282. Freud, G. E., van Capelle, F. J. L., Bosveld, J. E., A tenfold microelectrode for multiple synchronous intracellular recordings. *J Appl Physiol* 31: 305, 1971.

283. Friedberg, C. K., Cohen, H., Donoso, E., Advanced heart block as a complication of acute myocardial infarction. Role of pacemaker therapy. *Progr Cardiovasc Dis* 10: 466, 1968.

284. Friedberg, H. D., Concealed extrasystoles. *Am J Cardiol* 24: 283, 1969.

285. Friedman, P. L., Stewart, J. R., Fenoglio, J. J. Jr, Wit, A. L., Survival of subendocardial Purkinje fibers after extensive myocardial infarction in dogs. *In vitro* and *in vivo* correlations. *Circulation Res* 33: 597, 1973.

286. Friedman, P. L., Stewart, J. R., Wit, A. L., Spontaneous and induced cardiac arrhythmias in subendocardial Purkinje fibers surviving extensive myocardial infarction in dogs. *Circulation Res* 33: 612, 1973.

287. Frink, R. J., James, T. N., Normal blood supply to the human His bundle and proximal bundle branches. *Circulation* 47, 8, 1973.

288. Gallagher, J. J., Damato, A. N., Varghese, P. J., Lau, S. H., Localization of an area of maximum refractoriness or 'gate' in the ventricular specialized conduction system in man. *Am Heart J* 84: 310, 1972.

289. Gallagher, J. J., Damato, A. N., Caracta, A. R.,

Varghese, P. J., Josephson, M. E., Lau, S. H., Gap in A-V conduction in man. Types I and II. *Am Heart J* 85: 78, 1973.

290. Gallagher, J. J., Damato, A. N., Varghese, P. J., Lau, S. H., Manifest and concealed reentry. A mechanism of A-V nodal Wenckebach in man, *Circulation* 47: 752, 1973.

291. Gallagher, J. J., Ticzon, A. R., Wallace, A. G., Kasell, J., Activation studies following experimental hemiblock in the dog. *Circulation Res* 35: 752, 1974.

292. Gallagher, J. J., Miller, H. C., Svenson, R. H., Wallace, A. G., Sealy, W. C., Recognition of septal atrioventricular (A-V) accessory pathways in the Wolff-Parkinson-White syndrome. Circulation 50: (II) 57, 1974.

293. Gallagher, J. J., Gilbert, M., Svenson, R. H., Sealy, W. C., Kasell, J., Wallace, A. G., Wolff-Parkinson-White syndrome. The problem, evaluation and surgical correction. Circulation 51: 83, 1975.

294. Gallagher, J. J., Svenson, R. H., Sealy, W. C., Wallace, A. G., The Wolff-Parkinson-White syndrome and the preexcitation dysrrhythmias; Medical and surgical management. *Med Clin N America*, in press.

295. Gambetta, M., Childers, R. W.. Initial electrophysiologic disturbance in experimental myocardial infarction (Abstract). *Ann Intern Med* 70: 1076, 1969.

296. Gambetta, M., Childers, R. W., Rate-dependant right precordial Q waves: Septal focal block. *Am J Cardiol* 32: 196, 1973.

297. Gann, D., Balachandran, P. K., El-Sherif, N., Samet, P., Prognostic significance of chronic versus acute bundle branch block. *Chest* 67: 298, 1975.

298. García, H., Rosenbaum, M. B., El 'efecto fuello' en los bloqueos intermitentes de rama. *Rev Argentina de Cardiol* 40: 75, 1972.

299. Gelband, H., Steeg, C. N., Bigger, J. T. jr, Use of massive doses of procaine amide in the treatment of ventricular tachycardia in infancy. *Ped* 48: 110, 1971.

300. Gerlis, L. M., Anderson, R. H., Becker, A. E., Complete heart block as a consequence of atrionodal discontinuity. *Brit Heart J* 37: 345, 1975.

301. Gettes, L. S., Surawicz, B., Shiue, J. C., Magnitude of ventricular transmembrane action and resting potential during development of intraventricular conduction disturbances in rabbit heart: Effects of high and low K^+ and quinidine. *Fed Proc* 21: 134, 1962.

302. Gettes, L. S., The electrophysiologic effects of antiarrhythmic drugs. *Am J Cardiol* 28: 526, 1971.

303. Gianelly, R., Von Der Groeben, J. O., Spivack,

A. P., Harrison, D. C., Effect of lidocaine on ventricular arrhythmias in patients with coronary heart disease. *New Engl J Med* 277: 1215, 1967.

304. Gibbs, C. L., Johnson, E. A., Effect of changes in frequency of stimulation upon rabbit ventricular action potential. *Circulation Res* 9: 165, 1961.

305. Gillette, P. C., El-Said, G. M., Sivarajan N., Mullins, C. E., Williams, R. L., McNamara, D. G., Electrophysiological abnormalities after Mustard's operation for transposition of the great arteries. *Brit Heart J* 36: 186, 1974.

306. Godman, M. J., Lassers, B. W., Julian, D. G., Complete bundle branch block complicating acute myocardial infarction. *New Engl J Med* 282: 237, 1970.

307. Godman, M. J., Alpert, B. A., Julian, D. G., Bilateral bundle branch block complicating acute myocardial infarction. *Lancet* II: 345, 1971.

308. Goldreyer, B. N., Bigger, J. T., Ventriculoatrial conduction in man. *Circulation* 41: 935, 1970.

309. Goldreyer, B. N., Bigger, J. T. jr, The site of reentry in paroxysmal supraventricular tachycardia in man. *Circulation* 43: 15, 1971.

310. Goldreyer, B. N., Damato, A. N., The essential role of atrioventricular conduction delay in the initiation of paroxysmal supraventricular tachycardia. *Circulation* 43: 679, 1971.

311. Goldreyer, B.N., Damato, A. N., Sinoatrial-node entrance block. *Circulation* 44: 789, 1971.

312. Goldreyer, B. N., Gallagher, J. J., Damato, A. N., The electrophysiologic demonstration of atrial ectopic tachycardia in man. *Am Heart J* 85: 205, 1973.

313. Goodfriend, M. A., Barold, S. S., Tachycardia-dependent and bradycardia-dependent Mobitz II atrioventricular block within the bundle of His. *Am J Cardiol* 33, 908, 1974.

314. Goodman, D., Van der Steen, A. B. M., Van Dam, R. Th., Endocardial and epicardial activation pathways of the canine right atrium. *Am J Physiol* 220: 1, 1971.

315. Goodman, D. J., Rossen, R. M., Cannon, D. S., Rider, A. K., Harrison, D. C., Effect of digoxin on atrioventricular conduction: Studies in patients with and without autonomic innervation *Circulation* 51: 251, 1975.

316. Goss, C. M., The physiology of the embryonic mammalian heart before circulation. *Am J Physiol* 137, 146, 1942.

317. Gossrau, R., Ueber das Reizleitungssystem der Vögel. Histochemische und elektronenmikroskopische Untersuchungen. *Histochemie* 13: 111, 1968.

318. Gouaux, J. L., Ashman, R., Auricular fibrilla-

tion with aberration simulating ventricular paroxysmal tachycardia. *Am Heart J* 34: 366, 1947.

319. Gould, L., Venkatamaman, K., Mohammad, N., Prognosis of right bundle branch block in acute myocardial infarction. *JAMA* 219: 502, 1972.

320. Graham, A. F., Miller, D. C., Stinson, E. B., Daily, P. O., Fogarty, T. J., Harrison, D. C., Surgical treatment of refractory life-threatening ventricular tachycardia. *Am J Cardiol* 32: 909, 1973.

321. Grant, R. P., Left axis deviation. *Mod Concepts Cardiovasc Dis* 27: 437, 1958.

322. Greenspan, K., Anderson, G. J., Fisch, C., Electrophysiologic correlate of exit block. *Am J Cardiol* 28: 197, 1971.

323. Greenspan, K., Steinberg, M., Holland, D., Freeman, A. R., Electrophysiologic alterations in cardiac dysrhythmias: Antiarrhythmic effects of aprindine (Abstract). *Am J Cardiol* 33: 140, 1974.

324. Grohmann, H. W., Theisen, K., Jahrmarker, H., Wechselnde atrio-ventriculare überleitungszeit bei der Vorhofstimulation des menschlichen Herzens. *Klin Wschr* 49: 367, 1971.

325. Grolleau, R., Dufoix, R., Puech, P., Latour, H., Les tachycardies par rythme réciproque au cours du syndrôme de W.P.W. Physio-pathologie et traitement. *Arch Mal Coeur* 63, 74, 1970.

326. Grolleau, R., Puech, P., Latour, H., Cabasson, J., Robin, J. M., Baissus, C., Gilbert, M., Les dépolarisations Hissiennes ectopiques non progagées. *Arch Mal Coeur* 65: 1069, 1972.

327. Guérot, Cl., Coste, A., Valère, P. E., Tricot, R., L'épreuve à l'ajmaline dans le diagnotic des blocs auriculoventriculaires paroxystiques. *Arch Mal Coeur* 66: 1241, 1973.

328. Guérot, Cl., Valère, P. E., Castillo-Fenoy, A., Tricot, R., Tachycardie par ré-entrée de branche à branche. *Arch Mal Coeur* 67: 1, 1974.

329. Guiraudon, G., Frank, R., Fontaine, G., Intérêt des cartographies dans le traitement chirurgical des tachycardies ventriculaires rebelles récidivantes. *Nouv Presse Med* 3: 273, 1974.

330. Gupta, P. K., Haft, J. L., Retrograde ventriculo-atrial conduction in complete heart block. Studies with His bundle electrography. *Am J Cardiol* 30, 408, 1972.

331. De Haan, R. L., Development of pacemaker tissue in the embryonic heart. *Ann N Y Acad Sci* 127: 7, 1965.

332. Hagemeijer, F., Lown, B., Effect of heart rate on electrically induced repetitive responses in the digitalized dog. *Circulation Res* 27: 333, 1970.

333. Hagiwara, S., Nakajima, S., Differences in Na and Ca spikes as examined by application of tetrodotoxin, procaine and manganese ions. *J Gen Physiol* 49: 793, 1966.

334. Han, J., Malozzi, A. N., Moe, G.K. Sino-atrial reciprocation in the isolated rabbit heart. *Circulation Res* 22: 355, 1968.

335. Han, J., Mechanisms of ventricular arrhythmias associated with myocardial infarction. *Am J Cardiol* 24: 800, 1969.

336. Han, J., Goel, B. G., Hanson, C. S., Reentrant beats induced in the ventricle during coronary occlusion. *Am Heart J* 80: 778, 1970.

337. Han, J., The concept of reentrant activity responsible for ectopic rhythm. *Am J Cardiol* 28: 253, 1971.

338. Han, J., Ventricular ectopic activity in myocardial infarction. In: Cardiac arrhythmias, edited by Han, J., Charles, C., Thomas Pub, Springfield Ill., 1972, p. 171.

339. Han, J., Goel, B. G., Yoon, M. S., Rogers, R., Effect of procaine amide and lidocaine on ventricular automaticity and re-entry during acute coronary occlusion. *Am J Cardiol* 34: 171, 1974.

340. Harris, A. S., Rojas, A. G., The initiation of ventricular fibrillation due to coronary occlusion. *Exp Med & Surg* 1: 105, 1943.

341. Harris, A. S., Matlock, W. P., The effects of anoxemic anoxia in excitability conduction and refractoriness of mammalian cardiac muscle. *Am J Physiol* 150: 493, 1947.

342. Harris, A. S., Delayed development of ventricular ectopic rhythms following experimental coronary occlusion. *Circulation* 1: 1318, 1950.

343. Harris, A. S., Potassium and experimental coronary occlusion. *Am Heart J* 71: 797, 1966.

344. Harrison, L. A., Wittig, J., Wallace, A. G., Adrenergic influence on the distal Purkinje system of the canine heart. *Circulation Res* 32: 329, 1973.

345. Hashimoto, K., Moe, G. K., Transient depolarizations induced by acetylstrophanthidin in specialized tissue of dog atrium and ventricle. *Circulation Res* 32, 618, 1973.

346. Hashimoto, K., Kubota, K., Positive chronotropic effect of ouabain in the excised and blood-perfused canine SA node preparation of the dog. *Naunyn-Schmiedeberg's Arch Pharmacol* 281: 357, 1974.

347. Hauswirth, O., Noble, D., Tsien, R. W., The mechanism of oscillatory activity at low membrane potentials in cardiac Purkinje fibers. *J Physiol* 200: 255, 1969.

348. Hawley, R. L., Pryor, R., Quantitative and electrocardiographic correlation of the conduction system of the heart (Abstract). *Am J Cardiol* 15: 132, 1965.

349. Hayashi, K., An electron microscope study

on the conduction system of the cow heart. *Jap Circ J* 26: 765, 1962.

350. Hayashi, S., Electron microscopy of the heart conduction system of the dog. *Arch Histol Jap* 33: 67, 1971.

351. Hayden, W. G., Hurley, E. J., Rytand, D. A., The mechanism of canine atrial flutter. *Circulation Res* 20: 496, 1967.

352. Hecht, H. H., Normal and abnormal transmembrane potentials of the spontaneously beating heart. *Am New York Acad Sc* 65: 700, 1957.

353. Hecht, H. H., Kossmann, C. E., Childers, R. W., Langendorf, R., Lev, N., Rosen, K. M., Pruitt, R. D., Truex, R. C., Uhley, H. N., Watt, T. B., Atrioventricular and intraventricular conduction.—revised nomenclature and concepts. *Am J Cardiol* 31: 232, 1973.

354. Helfant, R. H., Scherlag, B. I., Damato, A. N., The electrophysiological properties of diphenylhydantoin sodium as compared to procaine amide in the normal and digitalis-intoxicated heart. *Circulation* 36: 108, 1967.

355. Hering, H. E., Die myoerithischen Unregelmassigkeiten des Herzens. *Prag Med Wochenschr* 26: 7 and 23, 1901.

356. Hewlett, A. W., Digitalis heart block. *JAMA* 48: 47, 1907.

357. Hibbs, R. G., Ferrans, V. J., An ultrastructural and histochemical study of the rat atrial myocardium. *Am J Anat* 124: 251, 1969.

358. Hirschfelder, A. D., Eyster, J. A. E., Extrasystoles in the mammalian heart. *Am J Physiol* 18: 222, 1907.

359. Hodgkin, A.L., Katz, B., Ionic currents underlying activity in the giant axon of the squid. *J Physiol* 108: 37, 1949.

360. Hodgkin, A. L., Huxley, A. F., A quantitative description of membrane current and its application to conduction and excitation in nerve. *J Physiol* 117: 500, 1952.

361. Hoff, H. E., Nahum, L. H., The supernormal period in the mammalian ventricle. *Am J Physiol* 124: 591, 1938.

362. Hoffman, B. F., Suckling, E. E., Effect of heart rate on cardiac membrane potentials and the unipolar electrogram. *Am J Physiol* 179: 123, 1954.

363. Hoffman, B. F., The action of quinidine and procaine amide on single fibers of dog ventricle and specialized conducting system. *An Acad Brasil Cienc* 29: 365, 1958.

364. Hoffman, B. F., Paes De Carvalho, A., Mello, W. C., Cranefield, P. F., Electrical activity of single fibers of the atrioventricular node. *Circulation Res* 7: 11, 1959.

365. Hoffman, B. F., Cranefield, P. F., Stuckey, J. H.,

Amer, N. S., Cappelletti, R. R., Domingo, R. T., Direct measurement of conduction velocity in the insitu specialized conducting system of the mammalian heart. *Proc Soc Exp Biol Med* 102: 55, 1959.

366. Hoffman, B. F., Cranefield, P. F., Electrophysiology of the heart. McGraw Hill Book Co, New York, 1960.

367. Hoffman, B. F., Cranefield, P. F., Stuckey, J. H., Concealed conduction. *Circulation Res* 9: 194, 1961.

368. Hoffman, B. F., Electrical activity of the atrioventricular node. In: The specialized tissue of the heart. Ed Paes De Carvalho A, Elsevier, Amsterdam 1961.

369. Hoffman, B. F., Moore, E. N., Sbuckey, T. H., Cranefield, P. F., Functional properties of the atrioventricular conduction system. *Circulation Res* 13: 308, 1963.

370. Hoffman, B. F., Singer D. H., Effects of digitalis on electrical activity of cardiac fibers. *Progr Cardiovasc Dis* 7: 226, 1964.

371. Hoffman, B. F., Electrophysiology of heart muscle and the genesis of arrhythmias. In: Mechanism and therapy of cardiac arrhythmias. Ed. Dreifus L, Likoff W, New York, 1966.

372. Hoffman, B. F., Bigger, J. T. jr, Antiarrhythmic drugs. In: Drills Pharmacology in Medicine, DiPalma JR, ed. 4th ed. McGraw Hill Book Co Inc, New York, 1971, p.824.

373. Hoffman, B. F., Effects of digitalis on electrical activity of cardiac membranes. In: Basic and clinical pharmacology of digitalis, ed. by Marks BH, Weissler AM, Springfield, Charles C. Thomas, Publisher 1972, p. 118.

374. Hoffman, B. F., Rosen, M. R., Wit, A. L., Electrophysiology and pharmacology of cardiac arrhythmias III. The cause and treatment of cardiac arrhythmias. *Am Heart J* 89: 115, 1975.

375. Hogan, P. M., Daves, L. D., Electrophysiological characteristics of canine atrial plateau fibers. *Circulation Res* 28: 62, 1971.

376. Hogan, P. M., Wittenberg, S. M., Klocke, E. J., Relationship of stimulation frequency of automaticity in the canine Purkinje fiber during ouabain administration. *Circulation Res* 32: 377, 1973.

377. Holsinger, J. W., Wallace, A. G., Sealy, W. C., The identification and surgical significance of the atrial internodal conduction tracts. *Ann Surg* 167: 447, 1968.

378. Holzmann, M., Scherf, D., Ueber Electrocardiogramme mit verkürzter Vorhof-Kammer-Distanz und positiven P-Zacken. *Zeitschr f klin Med* 121: 404, 1932.

379. Hope, R. R., Williams, D. O., El-Sherif, N.,

Lazzara, R., Scherlag, B. J., The efficacy of anti-arrhythmic agents during acute myocardial iscemia and the role of heart rate. *Circulation* 50: 507, 1974.

380. Hoshi, T., Matsuda, K., Excitability cycle of cardiac muscle examined by intracellular stimulation. *Jap J Physiol* 12: 433, 1962.

381. Howse, H. D., Ferrans, V. J., Hibbs, R. G., A comparative histochemical and electron microscopic study of the surface coatings of cardiac muscle cells. *J Mol Cell Cardiol* 1: 157, 1970.

382. Hudson, R. E. B., The human conducting-system and its examination. *J Clin Path* 16: 492, 1963.

383. Hunt, D., Sloman, G., Bundle branch block in acute myocardial infarction. *Brit Med J* 1: 85, 1969.

384. Hunt, D., Sloman, G., Westlake, O., Ventricular aneurysmectomy for recurrent tachycardia. *Brit Heart J* 31, 264, 1969.

385. Hunt, D., Lie, J. T., Vohra, J., Sloman, G., Histopathology of heart block complicating acute myocardial infarction. Correlation with His bundle electrogram. *Circulation* 48: 1252, 1973.

386. Huxley, A. F., Can a nerve propagate a sub-threshold disturbance. *J Physiol* 148: p. 80, 1959.

387. Imaneshi, S., Surawicz, B., Effects of lidocaine and verapamil on slow channel-dependent automatic depolarization in depolarized guinea pig ventricular myocardium. *Am J Cardiol* 35: 145, 1975.

388. Isaacson, R., Titus, J. L., Merideth, J., Feldt, R. H., McGoon, D. C., Apparent interruption of atrial conduction pathways after surgical repair of transposition of great arteries. *Am J Cardiol* 30: 533, 1972.

389. James, T. N., Morphology of the human atrio-ventricular node, with remarks pertinent to its electrophysiology. *Am Heart J* 62, 756, 1961.

390. James, T. N., Myocardial infarction and atrial arrhythmias. *Circulation* 24: 761, 1961.

391. James, T. N., Anatomy of the human sinus node. *Anat Rec* 141: 109, 1961.

392. James, T. N., Anatomy of the sinus node of the dog. *Anat Rec* 143: 251, 1962.

393. James, T. N., The connecting pathways between the sinus node and the A-V node and between the right and left atrium in the human heart. *Am Heart J* 66: 498, 1963.

394. James, T. N., Nadeau, R. A., The Mechanism of action of quinidine on the sinus node studies by direct perfusion through its artery. *Am Heart J* 67: 804, 1964.

395. James, T. N., Anatomy of the sinus node, A-V node and os cordis of the beef heart. *Anat Rec* 153: 361, 1965.

396. James, T. N., Sherf, L., Fine, G., Morales, A. R., Comparative ultrastructure of the sinus node in man and dog. *Circulation* 34: 139, 1966.

397. James, T. N., Spence, C. A., Distribution of cholinesterase within the sinus node and A-V node of the human heart. *Anat Rec* 155: 151, 1966.

398. James, T. N., Cardial innervation: Anatomic and pharmacologic relations. *Bull New York, Acad Med* 43: 1041, 1967.

399. James, T. N., Anatomy of the cardiac conduction system in the rabbit. *Circulation Res* 20: 638, 1967.

400. James, T. N., Sudden death in babies: New observations in the heart. *Am J Cardiol* 22: 479, 1968.

401. James, T. N., The coronary circulation and conduction system in acute myocardial infarction. *Progr Cardiovasc Dis* 10: 410, 1968.

402. James, T. N., Pathogenesis of arrhythmias in acute myocardial infarction. *Am J Cardiol* 24: 791, 1969.

403. James, T. N., Cardiac conduction system: fetal and post-natal development. *Am J Cardiol* 25: 213, 1970.

404. James, T. N., Sherf, L., Specialized tissues and preferential conduction in the atria of the heart. *Am J Cardiol* 28: 414, 1971.

405. James, T. N., Sherf, L., P waves, atrial depolarization and pacemaking site. In: Advances in electrocardiography, edited by Schlant RC, New York, 1972.

406. James, T. N., Marshall, M. L., Craig, M. W., The subitaneis mortibus. VII. Disseminated intra-vascular coagulation and paroxysmal atrial tachycardia. *Circulation* 50: 395, 1974.

407. Janse, M. J., van der Steen, A. B. M., van Dam, R. T., Durrer, D., Refractory period of dogs ventricular myocardium following sudden changes in frequency. *Circulation Res* 24: 251, 1969.

408. Janse, M. J., Influence of the direction of the atrial wave front on A-V nodal transmission in isolated hearts of rabbits. *Circulation Res* 25: 439, 1969.

409. Janse, M. J., Van Capelle, F. J. L., Freud, G. E., Durrer, D., Circus movement within the A-V node as a basis for supraventricular tachycardia as shown by multiple micro-electrode recording in the isolated rabbit heart. *Circulation Res* 28: 403, 1971.

410. Janse, M. J., Anderson, R. H., Specialized internodal atrial pathways—fact or fiction? *Europ J Cardiol* 2: 117, 1974.

411. Janse, M. J., Anderson, R. H. Van Capelle, F. J. L., Durrer, D., A combined electro-physiological and anatomical study of the human fetal heart. *Am Heart J*: in the press.

412. Jensen, R. A., Katzung, B. G., Electrophysiological actions of diphenylhydantoin on rabbit atria. *Circulation Res* 26: 17, 1970.

413. Jewett, P. H., Leonard, S. D., Sommer, J. R., Chicken cardiac muscle: Its elusive extended junctional sarcoplasmic reticulum and sarcoplasmic reticulum fenestrations. *J Cell Biol* 56: 595, 1973.

414. Johnson, E. A., The effects of quinidine, procaine amide and pyrilamine on the membrane resting and action potential of guinea pig ventricular muscle fibers. *J Pharmacol & Exp Therap* 117: 237, 1956.

415. Johnson, E. A., McKinnon, M. G., The differential effect of quinidine and pyrilamine on the myocardial action potential at various rates of stimulation. *J Pharmacol & Exp Therap* 120: 460, 1957.

416. Jonas, E. A., Kosowsky, B. D., Ramaswamy, K., Complete His-Purkinje block produced by carotid sinus massage: Report of a case. *Circulation* 50: 192, 1974.

417. Josephson, M. E., Caracta, A. R., Ricciutti, M. A., Lau, S. H., Damato, A. N., Correlation of electrophysiological properties of procaine amide with plasma levels in man (Abstract). *Circulation* 46: 681, 1972.

418. Josephson, M. E., Seides, S. E., Battsford, W. P., Weisfogel, G. M., Akhtar, M., Caracta, A. R., Lau, S. H., Damato, A. N., The electrophysiological effects of intramuscular quinidine on the atrioventricular conducting system in man. *Am Heart J* 87: 55, 1974.

419. Josephson, M. E., Caracta, A. R., Lau, S. H., Alternating type A and type B Wolff-Parkinson-White syndrome. *Am Heart J* 87: 363, 1974.

420. Julian, D. G., Valentine, P. A., Miller, G. G., Disturbances of rate, rhythm, and conduction in acute myocardial infarction: a prospective study of 100 consecutive unselected patients with the aid of electrocardiographic monitoring. *Am J Med* 37: 915, 1964.

421. Kabela, E., The effects of lidocaine on potassium efflux from various tissues of the heart. *J Pharmacol & Exp Ther* 184: 611, 1973.

422. Kao, C. Y., Hoffman, B. F., Graded and decremental response in heart muscle fibers. *Am J Physiol* 194: 187, 1958.

423. Kastor, J. A., Spear, J. F., Moore, E. N., Localization of ventricular irritability by epicardial mapping: origin of digitalis induced unifocal tachycardia from left ventricular Purkinje tissue. *Circulation* 45: 952, 1972.

424. Kastor, J. A., Atrioventricular block. *New Engl J Med* 292: 462, 1975.

425. Katz, L. N., Pick, A., Clinical electrocardiography. Part I: The Arrhythmias. *Lea & Febiger*, Philadelphia, 1956.

426. Kaufmann, R., Rothberger, C. J., Beitrag zur Kenntnis der Enstehungsweise extrasystolischer Allorhythmien. *Ztschr f d ges exp Med* 5: 349, 1917.

427. Kaufman, R., Rothberger, C. J., Die Uebergang von Kammer-Allorhythmien in Kammer-Arrhythmie in klinischen Fällen von Vorhof-flattern, Alternans der Reisleitung. *Ztschr f d ges exp Med* 57: 600, 1927.

428. Kawamura, K., Electron microscope studies on the cardiac conduction system of the dog. II. The sinoatrial and atrioventricular nodes. *Jap Circ J* 25: 973, 1961.

429. Kawamura, K., James, T. N., Comparative ultrastructure of cellular junctions in working myocardium and the conduction system under normal and pathologic conditions. *J Molec Cell Cardiol* 3: 31, 1971.

430. Keith, A., Flack, M. W., The auriculo-ventricular bundle of the human heart. *Lancet* 1: 101, 1906.

431. Keith, A., Flack, M. W., The form and nature of the muscular connections between the primary divisions of the vertebrate heart. *J Anat Physiol* 41, 171, 1907.

432. Keith, A., The Hunterian lectures on malformations of the heart. *Lancet* 2: 359, 1909.

433. Kennel, J. A., Titus, J. C., The vasculature of the human sinus node. *Mayo Clin Proc* 47: 556, 1972.

434. Kent, A. F. S., Researches on the structure and function of the mammalian heart. *J. Physiol* 14: 233, 1893.

435. Kent, K. M., Epstein, S. E., Cooper, T., Jacobowitz, D. M., Cholinergic innervation of the canine and human ventricular conducting system: Anatomic and electrophysiologic correlation. *Circulation* 50: 948, 1974.

436. Kerin, H., Schwartz, H., Wenckebach phenomenon within the atria. *J Electrocardiol* 8: 61, 1975.

437. Kerzner, J., Wolf, M., Kosowsky, B. D., Lown, B., Ventricular ectopic rhythms following vagal stimulation in dogs with acute myocardial infarction. *Circulation* 47: 44, 1973.

438. Khan, M. I., Hamilton, J. T., Manning, G. W., Early arrhythmias following experimental coronary occlusion in conscious dogs and their modification by beta-adrenoceptor blocking drugs. *Am Heart J* 86: 347, 1973.

439. Kim, S., Baba, N., Atrioventricular node and Purkinje fibers of the guinea pig heart. *Am J Anat* 132: 339, 1971.

440. King, R. M., Zipes, D. P., Nicoll, B. de, Linderman, J., Suppression of ouabain-induced ventricular ectopy with verapamil and reversal with calcium (Abstr.) *Am J Cardiol* 33: 148, 1974.

441. Kinoshita, S., Wenckebach phenomenon of

entrance block in intermittent parasystole. *Chest* 66: 530, 1974.

442. Kirk, J. E., Kvorning, S. A., Sinus bradycardia: a clinical study of 515 consecutive cases. *Acta Med Scand Suppl* 266: 625, 1952.

443. Kisch, B., Zucker, G., Sinoauricular block and retrograde auricular conduction in a case of permanent complete heart block. *Am Heart J* 23: 20, 1942.

444. Klein, H. O., Cranefield, P. F., Hoffman, B. F., Effect of extrasystoles on idio-ventricular rhythm. *Circulation Res* 30: 651, 1970.

445. Klein, H. O., Singer, D. H., Hoffman, B. F., Effects of atrial premature systoles on sinus rhythm in the rabbit. *Circulation Res* 32: 480, 1973.

446. Klein, H. O., Lebson, R., Cranefield, P. F., Hoffman, B. F., Effect of extra-systoles on idio-ventricular rhythms—clinical and electrophysiological correlation. *Circulation* 47: 758, 1973.

447. Kleinsorge, H., Gaida, P., Behavior of the serum level after intravenous injections of ajmaline. *Klin Wschr* 40: 149, 1962.

448. Kline, E. M., Conn, J. W., Rosenbaum, F. F.; Variations in AV and VA conduction dependent upon the time relations of auricular and ventricular systole: the supernormal phase. *Am Heart J* 17: 524, 1939.

449. Kostuk, W. J., Beanlands, D. S., Complete heart block associated with acute myocardial infarction. *Am J Cardiol* 26: 380, 1970.

450. Krongrad, E., Steeg, C. N., Waldo, A. L., Gersony, W. M., The response of the atrioventricular specialized conduction system to rapid atrial stimulation in children. *Ped Res* 7: 229, 1973.

451. Kugler, J. H., Parkin, J. B., Continuity of Purkinje fibers with cardiac muscle. *Anat Rec* 126: 335, 1956.

452. Kulbertus, H. E., The concept of left hemiblocks revisited. A histopathological and experimental study. *Adv in Cardiol* 14: 126, 1975.

453. Kulbertus, H. E., de Leval-Rutten, E., Casters, P., Variations of aberrant ventricular conduction. A vectorcardiographic study (in print).

454. Kunin, A. S., Surawicz, B., Sims, E. A., Decrease in serum potassium concentrations and appearance of cardiac arrhythmias during infusion of potassium with glucose in potassium-depleted patients. *New Engl J Med* 266: 228, 1962.

455. Laham, J., Le syndrome de Wolff-Parkinson-White. Maloine SA, Paris, 1969.

456. Langendorf, R., Mehlman, J. S., Blocked (nonconducted) A-V nodal premature systoles imitating first and second degree heart block. *Am Heart J* 34: 500, 1947.

457. Langendorf, R., Ventricular premature systoles

with postponed compensatory pause. *Am Heart J* 46: 401, 1953.

458. Langendorf, R., Pick, A., Mechanism of intermittent bigeminy. II. Parasystole, and parasystole or reentry with conduction disturbance. *Circulation* 11: 431, 1955.

459. Langendorf, R., Pick, A., Concealed conduction. Further evaluation of a fundamental aspect of propagation of the cardiac impulse. *Circulation* 13: 381, 1956.

460. Langendorf, R., Lesser, M. E., Plotkin, P., Levin, B. D., Atrial parasystole with interpolation. Observations on prolonged sinoatrial conduction. *Am Heart J* 63: 649, 1962.

461. Langendorf, R., Pick, A., Edelist, A., Katz, I. N., Experimental demonstration of concealed A-V conduction in the human heart. *Circulation* 32, 386, 1965.

462. Langendorf, R., Pick, A., Parasystole with fixed coupling. *Circulation* 35: 304, 1967.

463. Langendorf, R., Pick, A., Artificial pacing of the human heart. *Am J Cardiol* 28: 516, 1971.

464. Langendorf, R., Cohen, H., Gozo, E. G., Observations on second degree atrio-ventricular block, including new criteria for the differential diagnosis between type I and type II block. *Am J Cardiol* 29: 111, 1972.

465. Langendorf, R., Pick, A., Manifestations of concealed reentry in the atrioventricular junction. *Europ J Cardiol* 1/1: 11, 1973.

466. Langendorf, R., Pick, A., First degree sino-atrial block (Abstract). *Circulation* 49–50: (Suppl. III) III–81, 1974.

467. Langendorf, R., Pick, A., Concealed intraventricular conduction in the human heart. Recent advances in ventricular conduction. *Adv. Cardiol* 14: 40 (Karger, Basel), 1975.

468. Laslett, E. E., Syncopal attacks, associated with prolonged arrest of the whole heart. *Quart J Med* 2: 347, 1909.

469. Lassers, B. W., Julian, G. D., Artificial pacing in management of complete heart block complicating acute myocardial infarction. *Brit Med J* 2: 142, 1968.

470. Latour, H., Puech, P., Electrocardiographie endocavitaire. *Masson Edit.*, Paris, 1957.

471. Lau, S. H., Damato, A. N., Berkowitz, W. D., Patton, R. D., A study of atrioventricular conduction in atrial fibrillation and flutter in man using His bundle recordings. *Circulation* 40: 71, 1969.

472. Lazzara, R., Scherlag, B. J., Robinson, M. J., Samet, P., Selective in situ parasympathetic control of the canine sinoatrial and atrioventricular nodes. *Circulation Res* 32, 393, 1973.

473. Lazzara, R., Yeh, B. K., Samet, P., Functional transverse interconnections within the His

bundle branches. *Circulation Res* 32: 509, 1973.

474. Lazzara, R., El-Sherif, N., Scherlag, B. J., Electrophysiological properties of canine Purkinje cells in 1-day-old myocardial infarction. *Circulation* Res 33: 722, 1973.

475. Lazzara, R., Scherlag, B. J., El-Sherif, N., Transmembrane potentials in the His bundle after coronary occlusion (Abstract). *Am J Cardiol* 33: 150, 1974.

476. Lazzara, R., Yeh, B. K., Samet, P., Functional anatomy of the canine left bundle branch. *Am J Cardiol* 33: 623, 1974.

477. Lazzara, R., Personal communication.

478. Leachman, R. D., Angelini, P., Lufschanowski, R., Electrocardiographic signs of infarction masked by coexistent contra-lateral hemiblock. *Chest* 62: 542, 1972.

479. Legato, M. J., Langer, G. A., The subcellular localization of calcium ion in mammalian myocardium. *J. Cell Biol* 41: 401, 1969.

480. Legato, M. J., Ultrastructural characteristics of the rat ventricular cell grown in tissue culture, with special reference to sarcomerogenesis. *J Mol Cell Cardiol* 4: 299, 1972.

481. Lenfant, J., Mironneau, J., Gargouil, Y. M., Galand, G., Analyse de l'activité électrique spontanée de centre de l'automatisme cardiaque de lapin par les inhibiteurs de permeabilities membranaires. *CR Acad Sci* (D) (Paris) 266: 901, 1968.

482. Lev, M., Widran, J., Erickson, E. E., Method for the histopathologic study of the atrioventricular node, bundle and branches. *Arch Pathol* 52: 73, 1951.

483. Lev, M., Ageing changes in the human sinoatrial node. *J Gerontol* 9: 1, 1954.

484. Lev, M., The architecture of the conduction system in congenital heart disease. I. Common AV orifice. *Arch Pathol* 65: 174, 1958.

485. Lev, M., The conduction system. In: Pathology of the heart and blood vessels, edited by Gould SE, Springfield, Ill. 1968, p. 185.

486. Lev, M., Fox, S. M., Bharati, S., Rosen, K. M., Langendorf, R., Pick, A., Mahaim fibers as a basis for a unique variety of pre-excitation. *Am J Cardiol* 35, 152, 1975.

487. Levin, H. J., Pre-hospital management of acute myocardial infarction. *Am J Cardiol* 24: 826, 1969.

488. Levine, S., Observations on sino-auricular heart block. *Arch of Internal Med* 17: 153, 1916.

489. Levites, R., Haft, J. L., Significance of first degree heart block (prolonged P-R interval) in bifascicular block. *Am J Cardiol* 34: 259, 1974.

490. Levy, M. N., Ng, M., Martin, P., Zieske, H.; Sympathetic and parasympathetic interactions upon the left ventricle of the dog. *Circulation Res*

19: 5, 1966.

491. Levy, M. N., Leed, M. H., Zieske, H., A feedback mechanism responsible for fixed coupling in parasystole. *Circulation Res* 31: 846, 1972.

492. Lewis, T., Paroxysmal tachycardia, the result of ectopic impulse formation. *Heart 1*: 262, 1909.

493. Lewis, T., Galvanometric curves yielded by cardiac beats generated in various areas of the auricular musculature. *Heart 2*: 23, 1910.

494. Lewis, T. Certain physical signs of myocardial involvement *Brit Med J* 7: 484, 1913.

495. Lewis, T., White, P. D., The effects of premature contractions in vagotomised dogs, with especial reference to atrioventricular rhythm. *Heart 5*: 335, 1913.

496. Lewis, T., Rothshild, M. A., Excitatory process in the dog's heart: II. Ventricles. *Phil Trans R Soc Land* (Biol) 204: 181, 1915.

497. Lewis, T., Feil, H. S., Stroud, W. D., Observations upon flutter and fibrillation: II. Nature of auricular flutter. *Heart 7*: 191, 1920.

498. Lewis, T., Master, A. M., Observations upon conduction in the mammalian heart. A-V conduction. *Heart 12*: 209, 1925.

499. Lichstein, E., Chadda, K. D., Gupta, P. K., Atrioventricular block with lidocaine therapy. *Am J Cardiol* 31: 277, 1973.

500. Lie, K. I., Wellens, H. J., Schuilenburg, R. M., Durrer, D., Mechanism and significance of widened QRS complexes during complete A-V block in acute inferior myocardial infarction. *Am J Cardiol* 33: 833, 1974.

501. Lie, K. I., Wellens, H. J., Schuilenburg, R. M., Becker, A. E., Durrer, D., Factors influencing prognosis of bundle branch block complicating acute anteroseptal infarction: the value of His bundle recordings. *Circulation* 50: 935, 1974.

502. Lieberman, M., Kootsey, J. M., Johnson, E. A., Sawanobori, T., Slow conduction in cardiac muscle. *Biophys J* 13: 37, 1973.

503. Liem, K. L., Lie, K. I., Louritdz, W. I., Durrer, D., Wellens, H. J. J., Prognostic significance of sinusbradycardia complicating acute myocardial infarction. Submitted for publication.

504. Lindsay, A. E., Schamroth, L., Atrioventricular junctional parasystole with concealed conduction imitating second degree atrioventricular block. *Am J Cardiol* 31: 397, 1973.

505. Los, J. A., Embryology. In: *Ped Cardiol*, edited by Watson H, Lloyd-Luke London, 1968, p. 1.

506. Louvros, N., Costeas, F., Syrimbeis S., 'Upper' A-V nodal parasystole. *Cardiologia* 53: 365, 1968.

507. Lown, B., Electrical reversion of cardiac arrhythmias. *Brit Heart J* 29: 469, 1967.

508. Lu, H., Lange, G., Brooks, C. Mc. C., Factors controlling pacemaker action in cells of the sinoatrial node. *Circulation Res* 17: 460, 1965.

509. Lu, H., Brooks, C. Mc. C., Role of calcium in cardiac pacemaker cell action. *Bull N Y Acad Med* 45: 100, 1969.

510. Lubbers, W. J., Losekoot, T. G., Anderson, R. H., Wellens, H. J. J., Paroxysmal supraventricular tachycardia in infancy and childhood. *Europ J Cardiol* 2: 91, 1974.

511. Lumel, A. V., Significance of annulus fibrosus of heart in relation to AV conduction and ventricular activation in cases of Wolff-Parkinson-White syndrome. *Brit Heart J* 34: 1263, 1972.

512. Mack, I., Langendorf, R., Katz, I. N., The supernormal phase of recovery of conduction in the human heart. *Am Heart J* 34: 374, 1947.

513. Mackenzie, J., Pulsations in the veins, with the description of a method for graphically recording them. *J. Path Bacteriol* 1: 53, 1892.

514. Mackenzie, J., The venous and liver pulses and the arrhythmic contractions of the cardiac cavities. *J Path Bacteriol* 2: 84, 1894.

515. Mackenzie, J., The cause of heart irregularity in influenza. *Brit Med J* 2: 1411, 1902.

516. Mahaim, I., Winston, M. R., Recherches d'anatomie comparée et de pathologie expérimentale sur les connexions hautes du faisceau de His-Tawara. *Cardiologia* 5: 189, 1941.

517. Mahaim, I., Kent's fibers and the AV paraspecific conduction through the upper connection of the bundle of His-Tawara. *Am Heart J* 33, 651, 1947.

518. Mall, E. P., On the development of the human heart. *Am J Anat* 13: 249, 1912.

519. Maloy, N. C., Arrants, J. E., Sowell, B. E., Left ventricular aneurysm with recurrent ventricular arrhythmias. *New Engl J Med* 285, 662, 1971.

520. Mandel, W. J., Danzig, R., Hayakawa, H., Lown-Ganong-Levine syndrome. A study using His bundle electrogram. *Circulation* 44: 696, 1971.

521. Mandel, W. J., Hayakawa, H., Danzig, R., Marcus, H. S., Evaluation of sinotrial node function in man by overdrive suppression. *Circulation* 44: 59, 1971.

522. Mandel, W. J., Hayakawa, H., Allen, H. N., Danzig, R., Kermaier, A. J., Assesment of sinus node function in patients with the sick sinus syndrome. *Circulation* 46: 761, 1972.

522a. Mandel, W. J., Laks, M., Obayasi, K., Clifton, J., Electrophysiologic features of the WPW syndrome: modification by procainamide (Abstract). *Circulation* 48: suppl. 4, 195, 1973.

523. Mandel, W. J., Obayashi, K., Laks, M. M., Overview of the sick sinus syndrome. *Chest* 66: 223, 1974 (editorial).

524. Mandel, W. J., Laks, M. M., Fink, B., Obayashi, K., Comparative electrophysiologic features of the WPW syndrome in the pediatric and adult patient. *Am J Cardiol* 33: 155, 1974.

525. Marriott, H. J. L., Myerburg, R. J., The cardiac arrhythmias. In: Hurst J. W., Logue R. B. (Eds.): The Heart 3rd ed. McGraw-Hill, N. Y., 1974.

526. Martin-Noel, P., Denis, B., Grunwald, D., Buisson Mme, Deux cas mortels de syndrome de Wolff-Parkinson-White. *Arch Mal Coeur* 63: 1647, 1970.

527. Mascher, D., Peper, K., Zwei Einwärtskomponenten des Membranstromes in Myokard. *Pfluegers Arch* 307: 32, 1969.

528. Massing, G. K., Liebman, J., James, T. N., Cardiac conduction pathways in the infant and child. *Cardiovasc Clin* 4: 27, 1973.

529. Massumi, R. A., Sabin, R. K., Tawakkol, A. A., Rios, J. C., Jackson, H., Time sequence of right and left atrial depolarization as a guide to the origin of the P waves. *Am J Cardiol* 24: 28, 1969.

530. Massumi, R. A., Mason, D. T., Amsterdam, E. A., DeMaria, A., Scheinman, M. M., Zelis, R., Ventricular fibrillation and tachycardia after intravenous atropine for treatment of bradycardia. *New Engl J Med* 287, 366, 1972.

531. Mazzoleni, A., Johnson, D., Fletcher, E., Class, R. N., Concealed conduction in left bundle of His. *Brit Heart J* 34: 365, 1972.

532. McCans, J. L., Brenman, F. J., Chiong, M. A., Parker, J. O., Effects of ouabain and diphenylhydantoin on myocardial potassium balance in man. *Am J Cardiol* 31: 320, 1973.

533. McCans, J. L., Lindenmayer, G. E., Munson, R. G., Evans, R. W., Schwartz, A., A dissociation of positive staircase (Bowditch) from ouabain-induced positive inotropism. *Circulation Res* 35: 439, 1974.

534. McNutt, N. S., Fawcett, D. W., The ultrastructure of the cat myocardium. II. Atrial muscle. *J Cell Biol* 42: 46, 1969.

535. McWilliams, J. A., Fibrillar contraction of the heart. *J Physiol* 8: 296, 1887.

536. McWilliams, J. A., On the rhythm of the mammalian heart. *J Physiol* 9: 167, 1888.

537. Medrano, G. A., Brenes, C. P., De Micheli, A., Sodi-Pallares D: El bloqueo simultaneo de las subdivisiones anterior y posterior de la rama izquierda del haz de His (bloqueo bifascicular). Y su associacion con bloqueo de la rama derecha (bloqueo trifascicular). *Arch Inst Cardiol Mex* 40: 752, 1970.

538. Meilhac, B., Le Pailleur, C., Heulin, A., Vacheron, A., Guize, L., Di Matteo, J., Intérêt de la stimulation auriculaire et des épreuves pharmaco-dynamiques dans le diagnostic des syncopes à électrocardiogramme normal. *Arch Mal Coeur* 67: 775, 1974.

539. De Mello, W. C., Membrane lipids and cardiac electrogenensis. In: Electrical phenomena in the

heart. De Mello W. C., ed. Acad Press New York & London, 1972, p. 89.

540. Mendez, C., Mendez, R., The action of cardiac glycosides on the refractory period of heart tissues. *J Pharmacol Exp Ther* 107: 24, 1953.

541. Mendez, C., Gruhzit, C. C., Moe, G. K., Influence of cycle length upon refractory period of auricles, ventricles and A-V node in the dog. *Am J Physiol* 184: 287, 1956.

542. Mendez, C., Han, J., Moe, G. K., A comparison of the effects of epinephrine and vagal stimulation upon the refractory periods of the A-V node and the bundle of His. *Naunyn-Schmiedebergs Arch Exp Path u Pharmak* 248: 99, 1964.

543. Mendez, C., Han, J., Garcia de Jalon, P. D., Moe, G. K., Some characteristics of ventricular echoes. *Circulation Res* 16: 526, 1965.

544. Mendez, C., Moe, G. K., Demonstration of a dual A-V conduction system in the isolated rabbit heart. *Circulation Res* 19: 378, 1966.

545. Mendez, C., Moe, G. K., Some characteristics of transmembrane potentials of AV nodal cells during propagation of premature beats. *Circulation Res* 19, 993, 1966.

546. Mendez, C., Mueller, W. J., Merideth, J., Moe, G. K., Interaction of transmembrane potentials in canine Purkinje fibers and at Purkinje fiber-muscle junctions. *Circulation Res* 24: 361, 1969.

547. Mendez, C., Mueller, W. J., Urquiaga, X., Propagation of impulses across the Purkinje fiber-muscle junctions in the dog heart. *Circulation* 26: 135, 1970.

548. Merideth, J., Mendez, C., Mueller, W. J., Moe, G. K., Electrical excitability of atrioventricular nodal cells. *Circulation Res* 23: 69, 1968.

549. Van Mierop, L. H. S., Discussion in the proceedings of the conduction development conference. U. S. Government Printing Office, Washington D. C., 1969, p. 128.

550. Mignone, R. J., Wallace, A. G., Ventricular echoes: Evidence for dissociation of conduction and reentry within the A-V node. *Circulation Res* 19: 638, 1966.

551. Miller, H. C., Strauss, H. C., Measurement of sinoatrial conduction time by premature atrial stimulation in the rabbit. *Circulation Res* 35: 935, 1974.

552. Mines, G. R., On dynamic equilibrium in the heart. *J Physiol* 46: 349, 1913.

553. Mines, G. R., On circulating excitations in heart muscles and their possible relation to tachycardia and fibrillation. *Trans Soc Can* 4: 43, 1914.

554. Moe, G. K., Wegria, R., Wiggers, C. J., Comparison of the vulnerable periods and fibrillation thresholds of normal and idioventricular beats. *Am J Physiol* 133: 651, 1941.

555. Moe, G. K., Preston, J. B., Burlington, H.,

Physiologic evidence for dual A-V transmission system. *Circulation Res* 4: 357, 1956.

556. Moe, G. K., On the multiple wavelet hypothesis of atrial fibrillation. *Arch Intern Pharmacodyn Thes* 140: 183, 1962.

557. Moe, G. K., Rheinboldt, W. C., Abilskov, J. A., A computer model of atrial fibrillation. *Am Heart J* 67: 200, 1964.

558. Moe, G. K., Abildskov, J. A. Mendez, C., An experimental study of concealed conduction. *Am Heart J* 67: 338, 1964.

559. Moe, G. K., Mendez, C., Han, J., Aberrant A-V impulse propagation in the dog heart. A study of functional bundle branch block. *Circulation Res* 16: 261, 1965.

560. Moe, G. K., Mendez, C., The physiologic basis of reciprocal rhythm *Prog Cardiovas Dis* 8: 461, 1966.

561. Moe, G. K., Childers, R. W. Merideth, J., An appraisal of 'supernormal' A-V conduction. *Circulation* 38: 5, 1968.

562. Mönckeberg, J. G., Zur entwicklungsgeschichte des Atrioventrikular-systems. *Verh dtsch Path Ges* 16: 228, 1913.

563. Mönckeberg, J. G., Das spezifische Muskelsystem im Menschlichen Herzern. *Ergebn allg Path Anat* 19: 328, 1921.

564. Montiel, M. M., Muscular apparatus of the mitral valve in man and its involvement in left sided cardiac hypertrophy. *Am J Cardiol* 26: 341, 1970.

565. Moore, E. N., Hoffman, B. F., Patterson, J. H., Stuckey, J. H., Electrocardiographic changes due to delayed activation of the wall of the right ventricle. *Am Heart J* 68: 347, 1964.

566. Moore, E. N., Preston, J. B., Moe, G. K., Duration of transmembrane action potentials and functional refractory periods of canine false tendons and ventricular myocardium: Comparisons in single fibers. *Circulation Res* 17: 259, 1965.

567. Moore, E. N., Experimental electrophysiological studies on avian hearts. *Ann. N Y Acad Sci* 127: 127, 1965.

568. Moore, E. N., Microelectrode studies on concealment of multiple premature atrial responses. *Circulation Res* 18: 660, 1966.

569. Moore, E. N., Bloom, M., Method for intracellular stimulation and recording using a single microelectrode. *J Appl Physiol* 27: 734, 1969.

570. Moore, E. N., Spear, J. E., Experimental studies on the facilitation of AV conduction by ectopic beats in dogs and rabbits. *Circulation Res* 29: 29, 1971.

571. Mounsey, P., Intensive coronary care—Arrhythmias after acute myocardial infarction. *Am J Cardiol* 20, 475, 1967.

572. Myerburg, R. J., Stewart, J. W., Hoffman, B. F., Electrophysiological properties of the canine peripheral AV conducting system. *Circulation Res* 26, 361, 1970.

573. Myerburg, R. J., Gelband, H., Hoffman, B. F., Functional characteristics of the gating mechanism in the canine A-V conducting system. *Circulation Res* 28: 136, 1971.

574. Myerburg, R. .J., The gating mechanism in the distal A-V conducting system. *Circulation* 43: 955, 1971.

575. Myerburg, R. J., Nilsson, K., Gelband, H., Physiology of canine intraventricular conduction and endocardial excitation. *Circulation Res* 30: 217, 1972.

576. Myerburg, R. J., Nilsson, K., Gelband, H., Castellanos, A., Befeler, B., Comparison of anatomy and physiology of canine and primate left ventricular conducting systems. *Clin Res* 21: 83, 1973.

577. Myerburg, R. J., Nilsson, K., Castellanos, A., Gelband, H., The mechanism of ventricular endocardial excitation. In: *Cardiac Arrhythmias*, edited by Dreifus LS, Likoff W, Grune & Stratton, New York, 1973, p. 181.

578. Myerburg, R. J., Gelband, H., Castellanos, A., Befeler, B., Balanced and unbalanced propagation in the division of the canine left bundle branch system. *Clin Res* 21: 440, 1973.

579. Myerburg, R. J., Nilsson, K., Befeler, B. Castellanos, A., Gelband, H., Transverse spread and longitudinal dissociation in the distal A-V conducting system. *J Clin Invest* 52: 885, 1973.

580. Myerburg, R. J., Gelband, H., Hoffman, B. F., Confinement of premature impulses in functional compartments of regions of the A-V conducting system. *Cardiovasc Res* 7: 69, 1973.

581. Nadas, A. S., Fyler, D. C., Pediatric Cardiology. *W. B. Saunders C Phil*, 1972.

582. Nagumo, J., Arimoto, S., Yoshizawa, S., An active pulse transmission line simulating nerve axon. *Proc Inst Radio Eng* 50: 2061, 1962.

583. Nakhjavan, E. K., Morse, D. P., Nichols, H. T., Emergency aortocoronary bypass treatment of ventricular tachycardia due to ischemic heart disease. *JAMA* 216: 2138, 1971.

584. Narahashi, T., Moore, J. W., Scott, W., Tetrodotoxin blockade of sodium conductance increase in lobster giant axons. *J Gen Physiol* 47: 965, 1964.

585. Narula, O. S., Scherlag, B. J., Samet, P., Javier, R. P., Atrioventricular block. Localization and classification by His bundle recordings. *Am J Med* 50: 146, 1971.

586. Narula, O. S., Atrioventricular conduction defects in patients with sinus bradycardia. *Circulation* 44: 1096, 1971.

587. Narula, O. S., Samet, P., Javier, R. P., Significance of the sinus-node recovery time. *Circulation* 45: 140, 1972.

588. Narula, O. S., Runge, M., Samet, P., Second degree Wenckebach type AV block due to block within the atrium. *Brit Heart J* 34: 1127, 1972.

589. Narula, Q. S., Wolff-Parkinson-White syndrome: A review. *Circulation* 47: 872, 1973.

590. Narula, O. S., Conduction disorders in the A-V transmission system. In: *Cardiac Arrhythmias*, edited by Dreifus L. S., Likoff W., Grune & Stratton, New York, 1973.

591. Narula, O. S., Wenckebach type I and type II atrioventricular block (revisited). *Cardiovasc Clin* 6 (3), 137, 1974.

592. Narula, O. S., Sinus node re-entry: a mechanism for supraventricular tachycardia. *Circulation* 50: 114, 1974.

593. Narula, O. S., Retrograde pre-excitation. Comparison of antegrade and retrograde conduction intervals in man. *Circulation* 50: 1129, 1974.

594. Narula, O. S., Current concepts of atrioventricular block. In: His bundle electrocardiography and clinical electrophysiology, edited by Narula, O.S., F. A. Davis, Philadelphia, 1975, p. 139.

595. Narula, O. S., Intraventricular conduction defects. In: His bundle electrocardiography and clinical electrophysiology, edited by Narula, O. S., F. A. Davis, Philadelphia, 1975, p. 177

596. Neidergerke, R., Orkand, R. K., The dependence of the action potential of the frog's heart on the external and intracellular sodium concentration. *J Physiol* 84: 312, 1966.

597. Netter, F. H., The Ciba collection of medical illustrations. *The Heart* 5: 13, 1969.

598. Neuss, H., Schlepper, M., Thormann, J., Analysis of reentry mechanisms in three patients with concealed Wolff-Parkinson-White syndrome. *Circulation* 51: 75, 1975.

599. Nilsson, E., Sporrong, B., Electron microscopic investigation of adrenergic and non-adrenergic axons in the rabbit SA-node. *Z Zellforsch* 111: 404, 1970.

600. Noble, D., A modification of the Hodgkin-Huxley equations to Purkinje-fibre action and pacemaker potentials. *J Physiol* 160: 317, 1962.

601. Noble, D., Tsien, R. W., The kinetics and rectifier properties of the slow potassium current in cardiac Purkinje fibers. *J Physiol* 195: 185, 1968.

602. Noble, D., Tsien, R. W., Outward membrane currents activated in the plateau range of potentials in cardiac fibers. *J Physiol* 200: 205, 1969.

603. Norris, R. M., Heart block in posterior and anterior myocardial infarction. *Brit Heart J* 31: 352, 1969.

604. Norris, R. M., Croxson, M. S., Bundle branch

block in acute myocardial infarction. *Am Heart J* 79, 728, 1970.

605. Norris, R. M., Mercer, C. J., Yeates, S. E., Sinus rate in acute myocardial infarction. *Brit Heart J* 34: 901, 1972.

606. Norris, R. M., Mercer, C. J., Croxson, M. S., Conduction disturbances due to anteroseptal infarction and their treatment by endocardial pacing. *Am Heart J* 84: 560, 1972.

607. Norris, R. M., Mercer, C. J., Significance of idioventricular rhythms in acute myocardial infarction. *Progr Cardiovasc Dis* 16: 455, 1974.

608. Obayashi, K., Hayakawa, H., Mandel, W. J., Inter-relationships between external potassium concentration and lidocaine: effects on canine Purkinje fiber. *Am Heart J* 80: 221, 1975.

609. Orinius, E., Pre-excitation. Studies on criteria, prognosis and heredity. *Acta Med Scand* (Suppl) 465, 1966.

610. Orsos-Pécs, Ein intramuraler Sehnenstrang des rechter Vorhofes. *Verh Dtsch Path Ges* 14: 98, 1910.

611. Paes de Carvalho, A., Mello, W. C., Hoffman, B. F., Electrophysiological evidence for specialized fiber types in rabbit atrium. *Am J Physiol* 196: 483, 1959.

612. Paes de Carvalho, A., de Almeida, D. F., Spread of activity through the atrioventricular node. *Circulation Res* 8: 801, 1960.

613. Paes de Carvalho, A., Cellular electrophysiology of the atrial specialized tissues. In: The specialized tissues of the heart, edited by Paes de Carvalho, Amsterdam, 1961.

614. Paes de Carvalho, A., Hoffman, B. F., De Paula Carvalho, M., Two components of the cardiac action potential: I. Voltage-time course and the effect of acetylcholine on atrial and nodal cells of the rabbit heart. *J Gen Physiol* 54, 607, 1969.

615. Pamintuan, J. C., Dreifus, L. S., Watanabe, Y., Comparative mechanism of antiarrhythmic agents. *Am J Cardiol* 26: 512, 1970.

616. Pantridge, J. F., Adgey, A. A. J., Pre-hospital coronary care. *Am J Cardiol* 24: 666, 1969.

617. Pappano, A. J., Calcium-dependent action potentials produced by catecholamines in guinea pig atrial muscle fibers depolarized by potassium. *Circulation Res* 27: 379, 1970.

618. Paritzky, Z., Obayashi, K., Mandel, W. J., Atrial tachycardia secondary to sinoatrial node reentry. *Chest* 66: 526, 1974.

619. Patten, B. M., The development of the sino-ventricular conduction system. *Univ Mich Med Bull* 22: 1, 1956.

620. Paulay, K. L., Varghese, J. P., Damato, A. N., Atrial rhythms in response to an early atrial premature depolarization in man. *Am Heart J* 85, 323, 1973.

621. Paulay, K. L., Varghese, P. I., Damato, A. N., Sinus node re-entry: an in vivo demonstration in the dog. *Circulation Res* 32: 455, 1973.

622. Paulay, K. L., Weisfogel, G. M., Damato, A. N., Sinus nodal reentry. *Am J Cardiol* 33: 617, 1974.

623. Pearson, R. S. B., Sinus bradycardia with cardiac asystole. *Brit Heart J* 7: 85, 1945.

624. Petitier, H., Polu, J., Dodinot, B., Sommelet, P., Mathieu, P., Faivre, G., Tachycardie ventriculaire irreductible traitement par electro-coagulation après localisation du foyer. *Arch Mal Coeur* 64: 331, 1971.

625. Pick, A., Langendorf, R., A case of reciprocal beating with evidence of repetitive and blocked re-entry of the cardiac impulse. *Am Heart J* 40: 13, 1950.

626. Pick, A., Langendorf, R., Katz, L. N., Depression of cardiac pacemakers by premature impulses. *Am Heart J* 41: 49, 1951.

627. Pick, A., Parasystole. *Circulation* 8: 251, 1953.

628. Pick, A., Langedorf, R., Katz, L. N., The supernormal phase of atrioventricular conduction. I. Fundamental mechanism. *Circulation* 26: 388, 1962.

629. Pick, A., Langendorf, R., Recent advances in the differential diagnosis of A-V junctional arrhythmias. *Am Heart J* 76: 553, 1968.

630. Pick, A., Mechanism of cardiac arrhythmias: From hypothesis to physiologic fact. *Am Heart J* 86: 249, 1973.

631. Pick, A., Langendorf, R., Jedlicka, J., Exit block. *Cardiovasc Clin* 5(3): 113, 1974.

632. Pick, A., Personal communication.

633. Posner, P., Lambert, C., Miller, B. L., Effect of verapamil on ^{42}K transport in canine cardiac Purkinje fibers (Abstract). *Am J Cardiol* 35: 163, 1975.

634. Van Praagh, R., Corsini, L., Cor triatriatum: pathologic anatomy and a consideration of morphogenesis based on 13 postmortem cases and a study of normal development of the pulmonary vein and atrial septum in 83 human embryos. *Am Heart J* 78: 379, 1969.

635. Prakash, R., The heart and its conducting system in the common Indian fowl. *Proc Nat Inst Sci India* 22B: 22, 1956.

636. Preston, J. B., McFaddens, Moe, G. K., Atrioventricular transmission in young mammals. *Am J Physiol* 197: 236, 1959.

637. Pruitt, R. D., Essex, H. E., Burchell, H. B., Studies on the spread of excitation through ventricular myocardium. *Circulation* 3: 418, 1951.

638. Pryor, R., Blount, S. C., The clinical significance of true left axis deviation. Left intraventricular blocks. *Am Heart J* 72: 391, 1966.

639. Przybylski, J., Chiale, P. A., Quiteiro, R., Elizari,

M. V., Rosenbaum, M. B., The occurrence of phase 4 block in the anomalous bundle of patients with the Wolff-Parkinson-White system. *Europ J of Cardiol:* in press.

640. Puech, P., Slama, R., Grolleau, R., Motte, G., Dufoix, R., Balmes, P., L'activation auriculaire rétrograde dans les blocs auriculo-ventriculaires de haut degré. *Acta Cardiologica* 25: 443, 1970.

641. Puech, P., Grolleau, R., Latour, H., Cabasson, J., Robin, J. M., Baissus, C. I., Gilbert, M., Diagnostic des blocs tronculaires hisiens par l'enregistrement endocavitaire et la stimulation du faisceau de His. *Arch Mal Coeur* 65: 315, 1972.

642. Puech, P., Grolleau, R., L'activité du faisceau de His normale et pathologique. *Ed. Sandoz,* Paris, 1972.

643. Puech, P. The P wave: Correlation of surface and intraatrial electrograms. *Cardiovasc Clin* 6 (1): 43, 1974.

644. Puech, P., Grolleau, R., Cabasson, J., Baissus, C., Di Biase, M., Les blocs auriculoventriculaires unidirectionel. *Arch Mal Coeur* 67: 1241, 1974.

645. Puech, P., Atrioventricular block: The value of intracardiac recordings. In: *Fundamentals of cardiac arrhythmias,* edited by Krikler D. Saunders, London, 1975.

646. Purkinje, J. E., Mikroskopisch-neurologische Beobachtungen. *Arch Anat Physiol Wissenschaftliche Med* 12: 281, 1854.

647. Rambourg, A., Leblond, C. P., Electron microscope observations on the carbohydrate-rich cell coat present at the surface of cells in the rat. *J Cell Biol* 32: 27, 1967.

648. Reid, P. R., Varghese, J. P., Electropharmacology of aprindine HCl (Abstract). *Circulation* 50: III-200, 1974.

649. Reiffel, J. A., Bigger, J. T. jr, Kontam, M. A., The relationship between sinoatrial conduction time and sinus cycle length during spontaneous sinus arrhythmia in adults. *Circulation* 50: 924, 1974.

650. Reiser, J., Freeman, A. R., Greenspan, K., Aprindine—a calcium mediated antidysrhythmic. *Fed Proc* 33, 476, 1974.

651. Retzer, R., Some results of recent investigations on the mammalian heart. *Anat Rec* 2: 149, 1908.

652. Reuter, H., The dependence of slow inward current in Purkinje fibers on the extracellular calcium concentration. *J Physiol* 192: 479, 1967.

653. Reuter, H., Divalent cations as charge carries in excitable membranes. *Prog Biophys Mol Biol* 26: 1, 1973.

654. Ritter, E. R., Intractable ventricular tachycardia due to ventricular aneurysm with surgical cure.

Ann Int Med 71: 1155, 1969.

655. Robb, J. S., Kaylor, C. T., The A-V conduction system in the heart of the guinea pig. *Proc Soc Exp Biol Med* 59: 92, 1945.

656. Robb, J. S., Kaylor, C. T., Turman, W. G., A study of specialized heart tissue at various stages of development of the human fetal heart. *Am J Med* 5: 324, 1948.

657. Robb, J. S., Petrie, R., Expansions of the atrioventricular system in the atria. In: The specialized tissues of the heart, edited by Paes de Carvalho A, Amsterdam, 1961.

658. Robb, J. S., Comparative basic cardiology. New York, Grune & Stratton, 1964.

659. Robb, J. S., Comparative histology of the atrio-ventricular connecting system. In: Comparative basic cardiology, edited by Robb J. S., New York, 1965.

660. Roberts, N., Olley, P., Kidd, B. S. L., Effect of drugs on the atrioventricular conduction system in children. *Clin Res* 19: 761, 1971.

661. Roberts, N., Olley, P., His bundle electrogram in children: Statistical correlation of the atrioventricular conduction times in children with their age and heart rate. *Brit Heart J* 34: 1099, 1972.

662. Roberts, N., Olley, P., His bundle recordings in children with normal hearts and congenital heart disease. *Circulation* 45: 295, 1972.

663. Roberts, N. K., Heath, M. J., The maturation of the action potential of the rat papillary muscle. *Circulation* 50: III-83, 1974.

664. Rodriguez, M. L., Sodi-Pallares, D., The mechanism of complete and incomplete bundle branch block. *Am Heart J* 44: 715, 1952.

665. Rogers, M. C., Willerson, J. T., Goldblatt, A., Smith, T. W., Serum digoxin concentrations in the human fetus, neonate and infant. *New Engl J Med* 287: 1010, 1972.

666. Rosati, R. A., Alexander, J. A., Schaal, S. E., Influence of diphenylhydantoin on electrophysiological properties of the canine heart. *Circulation Res* 21: 757, 1967.

667. Rosen, K. M., Loeb, H. S., Chuquinia, R., Sinno, M. Z., Rahimtoola, S. H., Gunnar, R. M., Site of the heart block in acute myocardial infarction. *Circulation* 42: 925, 1970.

668. Rosen, K. M., Lau, S. H., Weiss, M. R., Damato, A. N., The effect of lidocaine on atrioventricular and intraventricular conduction in man. *Am J Cardiol* 25: 1, 1970.

669. Rosen, K. M., Rahimtoola, S. H., Gunnar, R. M., Pseudo A-V block secondary to premature nonpropagated His bundle depolarizations. Documentation by His bundle electrocardiography. *Circulation* 42: 367, 1970.

670. Rosen, K. M., Loeb, H. S., Sinno, M. Z., Rahim-

toola, S. H., Gunnar, R. M., Cardiac conduction in patients with symptomatic sinus node disease. *Circulation* 43: 836, 1971.

671. Rosen, K. M., Loeb, H. S., Gunnar, R. N., Rahimtoola, S. H., Mobitz type II block without bundle branch block. *Circulation* 44: 1111, 1971.

672. Rosen, K. M., Evaluation of cardiac conduction in the catheterization laboratory. *Am J Cardiol* 30: 701, 1972.

672a Rosen, K. N., Barwolf, C., Ehsani, A., Rahimtoola, S. H., Effects of lidocaine and propanolol on the normal and anomalous pathways with pre-excitation. *Am J Cardiol* 30: 801, 1972.

673. Rosen, K. M., Dhingra, R. C., Loeb, H. S., Rahimtoola, S. H., Chronic heart block in adults. *Arch Intern Med* 131: 663, 1973.

673a. Rosen, K. M., A-V nodal re-entrance: an unexpected mechanism of paroxysmal tachycardia in patients with pre-excitation. *Circulation* 47: 1267, 1973.

674. Rosen, K. M., Mehta, A., Miller, R. A., Demonstration of dual atrioventricular nodal pathways in man. *Am J Cardiol* 33: 291, 1974.

675. Rosen, M. R., Hoffman, B. F., Mechanisms of action of antiarrhythmic drugs. *Circulation Res* 32: 1, 1973.

676. Rosen, M. R., Gelband, H., Hoffman, B. F., Correlation between effects of ouabain on the canine electrocardiogram and transmembrane potentials of isolated Purkinje fibers. *Circulation* 47: 65, 1973.

677. Rosen, M. R., Gelband, H., Merker, C., Hoffman, B. E., Mechanisms of digitalis toxicity: Effects of ouabain on phase 4 of canine Purkinje fiber transmembrane potentials. *Circulation* 47: 681, 1973.

678. Rosen, M. R., Ilvento, J. P., Merker, C., The electrophysiological basis for the suppression of cardiac arrhythmias by verapamil (Abstract). *Am J Cardiol* 33: 166, 1974.

679. Rosen, M. R., Ilvento, J., Gelband, H., Merker, C., Effects of verapamil on electrophysiologic properties of canine cardiac Purkinje fibers. *J Pharmacol Ex Ther* 189: 414, 1974.

680. Rosen, M. R., Vulliemoz, Y., Hodess, A., Verosky, M., Hordorff, A., Effects of ouabain on the electrophysiologic properties of newborn, puppey and adult canine Purkinje fibers. *Circulation* 50: III–210, 1974.

681. Rosen, M. R., Wit, A. L., Hoffman, B. F., Electrophysiology and pharmacology of cardiac arrhythmias. IV. Cardiac antiarrhythmic and toxic effects of digitalis. *Am Heart J* 89: 391, 1975.

682. Rosen, M. R., Hoffman, B. F., Wit, A. L., Electrophysiology and pharmacology of cardiac arrhythmias. V. Cardiac antiarrhythmic effects of lidocaine. *Am Heart J* 89: 526, 1975.

683. Rosen, M. R., Hordorff, A. J., Hodess, A. M., Verosky, M., Vulliemoz, Y., Ouabain-induced changes in electro-physiologic properties of neonatal, young and adult canine cardiac Purkinje fibers. *J Pharm Exp Ther*: in press

684. Rosenbaum, F. R., Levine, S. A., Auricular standstill: Its occurrence and significance. *Am J Med Sci* 198: 774, 1939.

684a. Rosenbaum, F. F., Hecht, H. H., Wilson, F. N., Johnston, F. D., Potential variations of the thorax and the esophagus in anomalous atrioventricular excitation (Wolff-Parkinson-White syndrome). *Am Heart J* 29: 281, 1945.

685. Rosenbaum, M. B., Lepeschkin, E., The Effect of ventricular systole on auricular rhythm in auriculoventricular block. *Circulation* 11: 240, 1955.

686. Rosenbaum, M. B., Elizari, M. V., Lazzari, J. O., Los Hemibloqueos. *Paidos Buenos Aires*, 1968.

687. Rosenbaum, M. B., Elizari, M. V., Lazzari, J., The mechanism of bidirectional tachycardia. *Am Heart J* 78: 4, 1969.

688. Rosenbaum, M. B., Elizari, M. V., Lazzari, J. O., Nau, G. J., Levi, R. J., Halpern, S., Intraventricular trifascicular blocks. *Am Heart J* 78: 450, 1969.

689. Rosenbaum, M. B., The hemiblocks: Diagnosis criteria and clinical significance. *Mod Conc Cardiovasc Dis* 39: 141, 1970.

690. Rosenbaum, M. B., Elizari, M. V., Lazzari, J. O., The hemiblocks. *Tampa Tracings*, Oldsmar, Fla, 1970.

691. Rosenbaum, M. B., Elizari, M. V., Mechanism of intermittent bundle branch block and paroxysmal atrioventricular block. *Postgraduate Med* 53: 87, 1973.

692. Rosenbaum, M. B., Elizari, M. V., Lazzari, J. O., Halpern, M. S., Nau, G. I., Levi, R. J., The mechanism of intermittent bundle branch block. Relationships to prolonged recovery, hypopolarization and spontaneous diastolic depolarization. *Chest* 63: 666, 1973.

693. Rosenbaum, M. B., Elizari, M. V., Levi, R. I., Nau, G. I., Paroxysmal atrioventricular block related to hypopolarization and spontaneous diastolic depolarization. *Chest* 63: 678, 1973.

694. Rosenbaum, M. B., Elizari, M. V., Lazzari, J. O., Halpern, M. S., Nau, G. J., Levi, R. I., The physiological basis of intermittent bundle branch block. In: Second Symposium on Cardiac Arrhythmias, edited by Dreifus LS, Likoff W, Grune & Stratton, New York and London, 1973, p. 349.

695. Rosenbaum, M. B., A new clinical and experimental model for studying the effects of anti-

arrhythmic drugs upon automaticity and conduction. *Acta Cardiol Suppl* 18: 289, 1974.

696. Rosenbaum, M. B., Elizari, M. V., Chiale, P., Levi, R. J., Nau, G. I., Halpern, M. S., Lazzari, J. O., Novakovsky, A., Relationship between increased automaticity and depressed conduction in the main intraventricular conduction fascicles of the human and canine heart. *Circulation* 49: 818, 1974.

697. Rosenblueth, A., Garcia Ramos, J., Studies on flutter and fibrillation. II. The influence of artificial obstacles on experimental auricular flutter. *Am Heart J* 33: 677, 1947.

698. Rosenbluuth, A., Ventricular 'echoes'. *Am J Physiol* 195: 53, 1958.

699. Rossi, L., Histopathologic features of cardiac arrhythmias. *Milan* 1969.

700. Rossi, L., Sistema di conduzione trifascicolari ed emiblocchi di branca sinistra. Considerazioni anatomiche ed istopatologiche. *G Ital Cardiol* 1: 55, 1971.

701. Rostgaard, J., Behnke, O., Fine structural localization of adenine nucleoside phosphatase activity in the sarcoplasmic reticulum and the T system of rat myocardium. *J Ultrastruc Res* 12: 579, 1965.

702. Rothberger, C. J., Winterberg, H., Experimentelle Beiträge zur Kenntnis der Reitzleitungstörungen in den Kammern des Säugetierherzens. *Z Ges Exp Med* 5: 264, 1917.

703. Rotman, M., Wagner, G. S., Wallace, A. G., Bradyarrhythmias in acute myocardial infarction. *Circulation* 45: 703, 1972.

704. Rotman, M., Wagner, G. S., Waugh, R. A., Significance of high degree atrioventricular block in acute posterior myocardial infarction. *Circulation* 47: 257, 1973.

705. Rougier, O., Vassort, G., Garnier, D., Gargouil, Y. M., Coraboeuf, E., Existence and role of a slow inward current during the frog atrial action potential. *Pfluegers Arch* 308: 91, 1969.

706. Rubenstein, J. J., Schulman, C. L., Yurchak, P. M., DeSanctis, R. W., Clinical spectrum of the sick sinus syndrome. *Circulation* 46: 5, 1972.

707. Runge, M., Samet, P., Narula, O. S., Accomodation of A-V nodal (A-H) conduction time in man. *Circulation* 46: (Suppl II) 214, 1972.

708. Runge, M., Narula, O. S., 'Fatigue' phenomenon in the His Purkinje system (HPS). *Circulation* 48: (Suppl IV) 102, 1973.

709. Rushton, W. A. H., Initiation of the propagated disturbance. *Proc R Soc* 124: 210.

710. Ryan, M. J., Tmete, J., Lown, B., Evaluation of a new antiarrhythmic agent, disopyramide phosphate (Abstract). *Circulation* 49 & 50: (Suppl 1) 1–79, 1974.

711. Saetersdal, T. S., Mykleburst, R., Justesen, N. P. B., Ultrastructural localization of calcium in the pigeon papillary muscle as demonstrated by cytochemical studies and X-ray microanalysis. *Cell Tiss Res* 155: 57, 1974.

712. Sanabria, T., Recherches sur la differenciation du tissu nodal et connecteur du coeur des mammiferes. *Arch de Biol* 47: 1, 1936.

713. Sanna, G., Arcidiacono, R., Chemical ventricular defibrillation of the human heart. *Am J Cardiol* 32: 982, 1973.

714. Sano, T., Yamagishi, S., Spread of excitation from the sinus node. *Circulation Res* 16: 423, 1965.

715. Sano, T., Iida, W., Yamagishi, S., Changes in the spread of excitation from the sinus node induced by alternations in extracellular potassium. In: Electrophysiology and ultrastructure of the heart, editors Sano, T., Mizuhira, V., Matsuda, K., Grune & Stratton, Inc. New York, 1967, p. 127.

716. Sano, T., Suzuki, F., Sato, S., Lida, Y., Mode of action of new anti-arrhythmic agents. *Jap Heart J* 9: 161, 1968.

717. Sansum, W. D., Extrasystoles in the mammalian heart caused by stimulation of the Keith-Flack node. *Am J Physiol* 30: 421, 1912.

718. Sasyniuk, B. I., Dresel, P., The effect of diphenylhydantoin on conduction in isolated blood perfused hearts. *J Pharmacol Exp Ther* 161: 191, 1968.

719. Sasyniuk, B. I., Mendez, C., A mechanism for reentry in canine ventricular tissue. *Circulation Res* 28: 3, 1971.

720. Schamroth, L., Marriott, H. J. L., Concealed ventricular extrasystoles. *Circulation* 27: 1043, 1973.

721. Schamroth, L., Sinus parasystole. *Am J Cardiol* 3, 434, 1967.

722. Schamroth, L., Yoshonis, K. F., Mechanisms in reciprocal rhythm. *Am J Cardiol* 24: 224, 1969.

723. Schamroth, L., The disorders of cardiac rhythm. *Blackwell Pub Oxford & Edinburgh*, 1971.

724. Schamroth, L., Surawicz, B., Concealed interpolated A-V junctional extrasystoles and A-V junctional parasystole. *Am J Cardiol* 27: 703, 1971.

725. Schamroth, L., Krikler, D. M., Garrett, C., Immediate effects of intravenous verapamil in cardiac arrhythmias. *Brit Med J* 224: 73, 1972.

726. Scheinman, M., Brenman, B. S., Clinical and anatomical implications of intraventricular conduction blocks in acute myocardial infarction. *Circulation* 46: 753, 1972.

727. Scher, A. M., Young, A. C., Malmgren, A. L., Paton, R. R., Spread of electrical activity through the wall of the ventricle. *Circulation Res* 1: 539, 1953.

728. Scher, A. M., Young, A. C., Malmgren, A. L.,

Erickson, R. V., Activation of the interventricular septum. *Circulation Res* 3: 56, 1955.

729. Scherf, D., Kyung-Hi-Choi, Bahadori, A., Orphanos, R. P., Parasystole. *Am J Cardiol* 27: 527, 1963.

730. Scherf, D., Cohen, J., The atrioventricular node and selected cardiac arrhythmias. Grune & Stratton, New York, 1964.

731. Scherf, D., Bornemann, C., Tachycardias with alternation of the ventricular complexes. *Am Heart J* 74: 667, 1967.

732. Scherlag, B. J., Helfant, R. H., Damato, A. N., Electrophysiological basis of ventricular arrhythmias induced by acute coronary ligation in dogs (Abstract). *Circulation* 38: (Suppl VI) 6–173, 1968.

733. Scherlag, B., Helfant, R. H., Damato, A. N., The contrasting effects of diphenylhydantoine and procaine amide on A-V conduction in the digitalis-intoxicated and the normal heart. *Am Heart J* 75: 200, 1968.

734. Scherlag, B. J., Helfant, R. H., Damato, A. N., Catheterization technique for His bundle stimulation and recording in the intact dog. *J Appl Physiol* 25: 425, 1968.

735. Scherlag, B. J., Kosowsky, B. D., Damato, A. N., Technique for ventricular pacing from the His bundle of the intact heart. *J Appl Physiol* 25: 584, 1968.

736. Scherlag, B. J., Lau, S. H., Helfant, R. H., Berkowitz, W. D., Stein, E., Damato, A. N., Catheter technique for recording His bundle activity in man. *Circulation* 39: 13, 1969.

737. Scherlag, B. J., Helfant, R. H. Haft, J. T., Damato, A. N., Electrophysiology underlying ventricular arrhythmias due to coronary ligation. *Am J Physiol* 219: 1665, 1970.

738. Scherlag, B. J., Abelleira, J. L., Samet, P., Electrode catheter recordings from the His bundle and left bundle in the intact dog. In: Research in Physiology, edited by Kao F. F., Koizumi K., Vassalle M., Aulo Gaggi, Bologna, 1973, p. 223.

739. Scherlag, B. J., El-Sherif, N., Hope, R. R., Lazzara, R., Characterization and localization of ventricular arrhythmias resulting from myocardial ischemia and infarction. *Circulation Res* 35: 372, 1974.

740. Schmitt, F. O., Erlanger, J., Directional differences in the conduction of the impulse through heart muscle and their possible relation to extrasystolic and fibrillary contractions. *Am J Physiol* 87: 326, 1928.

741. Schreurs, A. W., Selij, A. P. L., Allessie, M. A., Bonke, F. I. M., A concentrically and radially adjustable holder for ten microelectrodes. *Pflüg Arch* 346: 167, 1974.

742. Schuilenburg, R. M., Durrer, D., Ventricular echo beats in the human heart elicited by induced ventricular premature beats. *Circulation* 40: 337, 1969.

743. Schuilenburg, R. M., Durrer, D., Further observations on the ventricular echo phenomenon elicited in the human heart. Is the atrium part of the echo pathway? *Circulation* 45: 629, 1972.

744. Schuilenburg, R. M., Durrer, D., Rate-dependency of functional block in the human His bundle and bundle branch-Purkinje system. *Circulation* 48: 526, 1973.

745. Schuilenburg, R. M., Lie, K. I., Durrer, D., Localization of the block in patients with acute anteroseptal infarction and complete right bundle branch block. *Circulation* 50: Suppl. IV, 3, 245, 1974.

746. Schuilenburg, R. M., Observations on atrioventricular conduction in man using intracardiac electrocardiography and stimulation. Swado Offset B. V. Amsterdam, 1974.

747. Schuilenburg, R. M., Durrer, D., Problems in the recognition of conduction disturbances in the His bundle. *Circulation* 51: 68, 1975.

748. Schutz, E., Physiologie des Herzens. Springer, Berlin, 1958.

749. Scott, T. M., The ultrastructure of ordinary and Purkinje cells of the fowl heart. *J Anat* 110: 259, 1971.

750. Sealy, W. C., Wallace, A. G., Surgical treatment of Wolff-Parkinson-White syndrome. *J Thor Cardiovasc Surg* 68: 757, 1974.

751. Sealy, W. C., Wallace, A. G., Ramming, K. P., Gallagher, J. J. Svenson, R. H., An improved operation for the definitive treatment of the Wolff-Parkinson-White syndrome. *Annals Thoracic Surg* 17: 107, 1974.

752. Seifen, E., Schaer, H. Marshall, J. M., Effect of calcium on the membrane potentials of single pacemaker fibers and atrial fibers in isolated rabbit atria. *Nature* 202: 1223, 1964.

753. Seipel, L., Breithardt, A., Both, A., Loogen, F., Messung der sinuatrialen leitungszeit mittels vorzeitiger Vorhof-stimulation beim Menschen. *Dtsch Med Wsch* 99: 1895, 1974.

754. Sherf, L., James, T. N., A new electrocardiographic concept: synchronized sinoventricular conduction. *Dis Chest* 55: 127: 1969.

755. Shigenobu, K., Kamiyama, A., Takagi, K., Membrane effects of pronethalol on the mammalian heart muscle fiber. *Jap Heart J* 7: 494, 1966.

756. Shigeto, N., Irisawa, H., Slow conduction in the atrioventricular node of the cat: A possible explanation. *Experientia* 28: 1442, 1972.

757. Short, D. S., The syndrome of alternating bradycardia and tachycardia. *Brit Heart J* 16: 208, 1954.

758. Simpson, F. O., Rayns, D. G., Ledingham, J. M., The ultrastructure of ventricular and atrial myocardium. In: Ultrastructure of the mammalian heart, edited by Challice C.E., Virágh S., Academic Press, New York & London, 1973, p. 1.

759. Sims, B. A., Pathogenesis of atrial arrhythmias. *Brit Heart J* 34: 336, 1972.

760. Singer, D. H., Lazzara, R., Hoffman, B. F., Interrelationship between automaticity and conduction in Purkinje fibers. *Circulation Res* 21: 537, 1967.

761. Singer, D. H., Ten Eick, R. E., De Boer, A., Electrophysiological correlates of human atrial tachyarrhythmias. In: *Cardiac Arrhythmias*, edited by Dreifus L. S., Likoff W., New York, 1973.

762. Singer, D. H., Parameswaran, R., Drake, F. T., Meijers, S. N., De Boer, A. A., Ventricular parasystole and re-entry: Clinical-electrophysiological correlations. *Am Heart J* 88: 79, 1974.

763. Singh, B. N., A study of the pharmacological actions of certain drugs and hormones with particular reference to cardiac muscle. *Ph D thesis*, Oxford University, 1971.

764. Singh, B. N., Explanation for the discrepancy in reported cardiac electrophysiological actions of diphenylhydantoin and lignocaine. *Brit J Pharmacol* 41: 385, 1971.

765. Singh, B. N., Vaughn Williams, E. M., Effect of alternating potassium concentration on the action of lidocaine and diphenylhydantoin on rabbit atrial and ventricular muscle. *Circulation Res* 29: 286, 1971.

766. Singh, B. N., Comparative mechanisms of antiarrhythmic agents. *Am J Cardiol* 28: 240, 1971.

767. Singh, B. N., Hauswirth, O., Comparative mechanisms of action of antiarrhythmic drugs. *Am Heart J* 87: 367, 1974.

768. Slama, R., Foucault, J. P., Bouvrain, Y., Le traitement d'urgence des trouble du rythme cardiaque par l'ajmaline intraveineuse. *Press Med* 71: 2250, 1963.

769. Sodi-Pallares, D., Rodriguez, M. I., Chait, L. O., Zuchermann, R., Activation of the interventricular septum. *Am Heart J* 41: 569, 1951.

770. Soloff, I. A., Fewell, J. W., Supernormal phase of ventricular excitation in man: Its bearing on the genesis of ventricular premature systoles and a note on atrioventricular conduction. *Am Heart J* 59: 869, 1960.

771. Sommer, J. R., Johnson, E. A., Cardiac muscle. Comparative study of Purkinje fibers and ventricular fibers. *J Cell Biol* 36: 497, 1968.

772. Sommer, J. R., Johnson, E. A., Cardiac muscle: A comparative ultrastructural study with special reference to frog and chicken hearts. *Z Zellforsch* 98, 437, 1969.

773. Sommer, J. R., Johnson, E. A., Comparative ultrastructure of cardiac cell membrane specializations. A review. *Am J Cardiol* 25: 184, 1970.

774. Spach, M. S., Huang, S. N., Armstrong, S. I., Canent, R. V., jr., Demonstration of peripheral conduction system in human hearts. *Circulation* 28: 333, 1963.

775. Spach, M. S., King, T. D., Barr, R. C., Boaz, D. E., Morrow, M. N., Herman-Giddens, S., Electrical potential distribution surrounding the atria during depolarization and repolarization in the dog. *Circulation Res* 24: 857, 1969.

776. Spach, M. S., Lieberman M., Scott, J. C., Barr, R. C., Johnson, E. A., Kootsey, J. M., Excitation sequences of the atrial septum and AV node in isolated hearts of the dog and rabbit. *Circulation Res* 29: 156, 1971.

777. Spach, M. S., Barr, R. C., Serwer, G. S., Johnson, E. A., Kootsey, J. M., Collision of excitation waves in the dog Purkinje system. *Circulation Res* 29: 499, 1971.

778. Spear, J. F., Moore, E. N., Influence of brief vagal and stellate nerve stimulation on pacemaker activity and conduction within the atrioventricular conduction system of the dog. *Circulation Res* 32: 27, 1973.

779. Spear, J. F., Moore, E. N., Supernormal excitability and conduction in the His-purkinje system of the dog. *Circulation Res* 35: 782, 1974.

780. Spear, J. F., Moore, E. N., The effect of changes in rate and rhythm on supernormal excitability in the isolated Purkinje system of the dog. A possible role in re-entrant arrhythmias. *Circulation* 50: 1144, 1974.

781. Spurrell, R. A. J., Sowton, E., Deuchar, D. C., Ventricular tachycardia in four patients evaluated by programmed electrical stimulation of heart and treated in two patients by surgical division of anterior radiation of left bundle-branch. *Brit Heart J* 35: 1014, 1973.

782. Spurrell, R. A. J., Krikler, D. M., Sowton, E., Retrograde invasion of the bundle branches producing aberration of the QRS complex during supraventricular tachycardia studied by programmed electrical stimulation. *Circulation* 50: 487, 1974.

782a. Spurrell, R. A. J., Krikler, D. M., Sowton, E., Effects of verapamil on electrophysiological properties of anomalous atrioventricular connection in Wolff-Parkinson-White syndrome. *Brit Heart J* 36: 256, 1974.

783. Spurrell, R. A. J., Krikler, D. M., Sowton, E., Problems concerning assessment of anatomical site of accessory pathway in Wolff-Parkinson-White syndrome. *Brit Heart J* 37: 127, 1975.

784. Starmer, C. F., Whalen, R. E., McIntosh, H. D.,

Hazards of electrical shock in cardiology. *Am J Cardiol* 14: 537, 1964.

785. Steffens, T. G., Intermittent parasystole due to entrance block failure. *Circulation* 44: 442, 1971.

786. Stephenson, S. E., Cole, R. K., Parrish, T. F., Bauer, F. M., Johnson, I. T., Kochtitzky, M., Anderson, J. S. jr., Hibbitt, L. L., McCarty, J. E., Young, E. R., Wilson, J. R., Meiers, H. N., Meador, C. K., Ball, C. O. T., Meneely, R., Ventricular fibrillation during and after coronary artery occlusion. *Am J Cardiol* 5: 77, 1960.

787. Stern, S., Synergistic action of propranolol with quinidine. *Am Heart J* 72: 569, 1966.

788. Stern, S., Conversion of chronic atrial fibrillation to sinus rhythm with combined propranolol. *Am Heart J* 74: 170, 1967.

789. Stern, S., Treatment and prevention of cardiac arrhythmias with propranolol and quinidine. *Brit Heart J* 33: 522, 1971.

790. Stock, J. P. P., In Diagnosis and treatment of Cardiac arrhythmias. Ed. 2, Butterworth and Co., London, 1970, p. 241.

791. Strauss, H. C., Bigger, J. T. jr., Bassett, A. L., Actions of diphenylhydantoin on the electrical properties of isolated rabbit and canine atria. *Circulation Res* 23: 463, 1968.

792. Strauss, H. C., Bigger, J. T. jr., The electrophysiological properties of the rabbit sinoatrial perinodal fibers. *Circulation Res* 31: 490, 1972.

793. Strauss, H. C., Saroff, A. L., Bigger, J. T. jr., Giardina, E. G. V., Premature atrial stimulation as a key to the understanding of sinoatrial conduction in man. *Circulation* 47: 86, 1973.

794. Strauss, H. C., Bigger, J. T., jr., Saroff, A. L., Giardina, E. G. V., Electrophysiologic evaluation of sinus node function in patients with sinus bradycardia. Submitted for publication.

795. Stuckey, J. H., Hoffman, B. F., Kottmeier, P. K., Fishbone, H., Electrode identification of the conducting system during open heart surgery. *Surg Forum* 9: 202, 1959.

796. Stutz, H., Feigelson, E., Emerson, J., Bing, R. J., The effect of digitalis (cedilanid) on the mechanical and electrical activity of extracted and nonextracted heart muscle preparations. *Circulation Res* 2: 555, 1954.

797. Sugiura, M., Okada, R., Hiraoka, K., Ohkawa, S., Histological studies on the conduction system in 14 cases of right bundle branch block associated with left axis deviation. *Jap Heart J* 10: 121, 1969.

798. Surawicz, B., Electrolytes and the electrocardiogram. *Am J Cardiol* 12: 656, 1963.

799. Sutton, R., Davies, M., The conduction system in acute myocardial infarction complicated by heart block. *Circulation* 38: 987, 1968.

800. Svenson, R. H., Gallagher, J. J., Sealy, W. C.,

Wallace, A. G., An electrophysiologic approach to the surgical treatment of the Wolff-Parkinson-White syndrome. *Circulation* 49: 799, 1974.

801. Svenson, R. H., Miller, H. C., Gallagher, J. J., Wallace, A. G., Ventriculo-atrial conduction and atrial fusion in the Wolff-Parkinson-White syndrome. *Circulation* 50: (Suppl. III) 3–58, 1974.

802. Tanaka, H., Katanazako, H., Uemura, H., Toyama, Y., Kanehisa, J., Amatatsu, K., Ventriculo-atrial conduction in complete atrio-ventricular block due to AH block. *Jap Heart J* 15: 1, 1974.

803. Taussig, H., On the technique for the demonstration of the specialized tissue in the heart. *J Tech Meth Bull Intern Assoc Med Museums* 13: 85, 1934.

804. Tawara, S., Das Reitzleitungssystem des Saügetierherzens. Gustav Fischer, Jena 1906.

805. Taylor, I. M., Anderson, R. H., Cholinesterase and the atrioventricular node and bundle in the human fetus up to midterm. *J Histochem Cytochem* 21: 464, 1973.

806. Teague, S., Collins, S., Wu, D., Denes, P., Rosen, K., Arzbaecher, R., Quantitative description of the normal A-V nodal conduction curve in man. Submitted for publication.

807. Terry, F. H., Wennemark, J. R., Brody, D. A., Numerical simulation of conduction in blocked Purkinje tissue. *Circulation Res* 31: 53, 1972.

808. Thaemert, J. C., Fine structure of neuromuscular relationship in the mouse heart. *Anat Rec* 163: 575, 1969.

809. Thaemert, J. C., Atrioventricular node innervation in ultrastructural three dimensions. *Am J Anat* 128: 239, 1970.

810. Thaemert, J. C., Fine structure of the atrioventricular node as viewed in serial sections. *Am J Anat* 136: 43, 1973.

811. Thind, G. S., Blackmore, W. S., Zinsser, H. F., Ventricular aneurymectomy for the treatment of recurrent ventricular tachycardia. *Am J Cardiol* 27: 690, 1971.

812. Thorel, C., Vorläufige Mitteilung über eine besondere Muskel-verbindung zwischen der Cava superior und den Hisschen Bündeln. *Münch med Wschr* 56: 2159, 1909.

813. Thorel, C., Über den Aufbau des Sinusknotens und seine Verbindung mit der Vena Cava superior und den Wenckebachschen Bündel. *Münch med Wschr* 57: 183, 1910.

814. Thornell, L. E., Evidence of an imbalance in synthesis and degradation of myofibrillar proteins in rabbit Purkinje fibers. *J Ultrastruc Res* 44: 85, 1973.

815. Thornell, L. E., Sjöström, M., Ribosomes and Polyribosomes in heart muscle. *J Ultrastruc Res* 44: 439, 1973.

816. Thornell, L. E., Distinction of glycogen and ribo-

some particles in cow Purkinje fibers by enzymatic digestion en bloc and in sections. *J Ultrastruc Res* 47: 153, 1974.

817. Thyrum, P., Inotropic stimuli and systolic transmembrane calcium flow in depolarized guinea pig atria. *J. Pharmacol Exp Ther* 188: 166, 1974.

818. Ticzon, A. R., Strauss, H. C., Gallagher, J. J., Wallace, A. G., Sinus node function in the intact dog heart evaluated by premature atrial stimulation and atrial pacing. *Am J Cardiol* 35: 492, 1975.

819. Titus, J. L., Daugherty, G. W., Edwards, J. E., Anatomy of the normal human atrioventricular conduction system. *Am J Anat* 113: 407, 1963.

820. Todd, T. W., The specialized tissue of the heart. In: Special cytology, edited by Cowdry E. V., Vol. II, New York, 1932.

821. Tonkin, A. M., Gallagher, J. J., Svenson, R. H., Wallace, A. G., Sealy, W. C., Antegrade block in accessory pathways with intact retrograde conduction in reciprocating tachycardia. *Europ J Cardiol* 3: 143, 1975.

822. Torii, H., Electron microscope observations of the S-A and A-V nodes and the Purkinje fibers of the rabbit. *Jap Circ J* 26: 39, 1962.

823. Torresani, J., Amichot, J. L., Picard, J. P., Jouve, A., Acquisitions recente dans les techniques d'explorations electrocardiographiques des cavités cardiaques. *Arch Mal Coeur* 62: 193, 1969.

824. Touboul, P., Tessier, Y., Magrina, J., Clement, C., Delahaye, J. P., His bundle recording and electrical stimulation of atria in patients with Wolff-Parkinson-White syndrome type A. *Brit Heart J* 34: 623, 1972.

825. Touboul, P., Clement, C., Porte, J., Chulliat, J. C., Bons, J. P., Delahaye, J. P., Etude comparée des effets de la stimulation auriculaire gauche et droite dans le syndrome de Wolff-Parkinson-White. *Arch Mal Coeur* 66: 1027, 1973.

826. Touboul, P., Janse, M. J., Billette, J., van Capelle, F. J. L., Durrer, D., Evidence for several levels of block within the A-V node following premature atrial stimuli as shown by multiple microelectrode recording in the isolated rabbit heart (Abstract). *Am J Cardiol* 33: 173, 1974.

827. Touche, M., Jouvet, M., Touche, S., Fibrillation ventriculaire au cours d'un syndrome de Wolff-Parkinson-White. Réduction par choc électrique externe. *Arch Mal Coeur* 59: 1122, 1966.

828. Tranum-Jensen, J., Bojsen-Møller, E., The ultrastructure of the sinuatrial ring bundle and of the caudal extension of the sinus node in the right atrium of the rabbit heart. *Z Zellforsch* 138: 97, 1973.

829. Tranum-Jensen, J., This volume.

830. Trautwein, W., Uchizono, K., Electron microscopic and electrophysiologic study of the pacemaker in the sino-atrial node of the rabbit heart. *Z Zellforsch Mikrosk Anat* 61: 96, 1963.

831. Trautwein, W., Membrane currents in cardiac muscle fibers. *Physiol Rev* 53: 793, 1973.

832. Truex, R. C., Copenhaver, W. M., Histology of the moderator band in man and other mammals with special reference to the conducting system. *Am J Anat* 80: 173, 1947.

833. Truex, R. C., Curry, J. L., Smythe, M. Q., Visualization of the Purkinje network of the beef heart. *Anat Rec* 118: 723, 1954.

834. Truex, R. C., Bishof, J. K., Hoffman, E. L., Accessory atrioventricular muscle bundles of the developing human heart. *Anat Rec* 131: 45, 1958.

835. Truex, R. C., Comparative anatomy and functional considerations of the cardiac conducting system. In: The specialized tissues of the heart, edited by Paes de Carvalho A., W. C. de Mello and B. F. Hoffman. Amsterdam, 1976, p. 22.

836. Truex, R. C., Smythe, M. Q., Recent observations on the human cardiac conduction system, with special considerations of the atrioventricular node and bundle. In: Electrophysiology of the heart, edited by Taccardi B., New York, 1965.

837. Truex, R. C., Smythe, M. Q., Comparative morphology of the cardiac conduction tissue in animals. *Ann N Y Acad Sci* 127: 19, 1965.

838. Truex, R. C., Anatomical considerations of the human atrioventricular junction. In: Mechanisms and therapy of cardiac arrhythmias, edited by Dreifus L. S., New York, 1966.

839. Truex, R. C., Impulse formation and conduction in the atrioventricular junction. Anatomical considerations of the human atrioventricular junction. In: Mechanisms and therapy of cardiac arrhythmias, edited by Dreifus L., Likoff W., Grune & Stratton, New York & London, 1966, p. 333.

840. Truex, R. C., Smythe, W. Q., Reconstruction of the human atrioventricular node. *Anat Rec* 158: 11, 1967.

841. Truex, R. C., Smythe, M. Q., Taylor, M. J., Reconstruction of the human sinoatrial node. *Anat Rec* 159: 371, 1967.

842. Truex, R. C., Anatomy related to atrioventricular block. *Cardiovasc Clin* 2, Arrhythmias 1, 1970.

843. Truex, R. C., Myocardial cell diameters in primate hearts. *Am J Anat* 135: 269, 1972.

844. Truex, R. C., Anatomy of the specialized tissues of the heart. In: Cardiac arrhythmias, edited by Dreifus, L. S., New York, 1973.

845. Truex, R. C., Structural basis of atrial and ventricular conduction. *Cardiovasc Clin* 6, 1, 1974.

846. Truex, R. C., Belej, R., Ginsberg, L. M., Hartman, R. L., Anatomy of the ferret heart:

An animal model for cardiac research. *Anat Rec* 179: 411, 1974.

847. Uhley, H. N., Rivkin, L. M., Visualization of the left branch of the human atrioventricular bundle. *Circulation* 20: 419, 1959.

848. Uhley, H. N., Rivkin, L. M., Peripheral distribution of the canine A-V conduction system. *Am J Cardiol* 5: 688, 1960.

849. Uhley, H. N., Some controversy regarding the peripheral distribution of the conduction system. *Am J Cardiol* 30: 919, 1972.

850. Valdes-Dapena, M. A., Green, M., Basavanand, N., Catherman, R., Truex, R. C., Myocardial conduction system in sudden death in infancy. *New Engl J Med* 289: 1179, 1973.

851. Vassalle, M., Karis, J., Hoffman, B. F., Toxic effects of ouabain on Purkinje fibers and ventricular muscle fibers. *Am J Physiol* 203: 433, 1962.

852. Vassalle, M., Analysis of cardiac pacemaker potential by means of a "voltage clamp" technique. *Am J Physiol* 210: 1334, 1966.

853. Vassalle, M., Electrogenic suppression of automaticity in sheep and dog Purkinje fibers. *Circulation Res* 27: 361, 1970.

854. Vassalle, M., Carpentier, R., Hyperpolarizing and depolarizing effects of norepinephrine in cardiac Purkinje fibers. In: Research in physiology, edited by Kao F. F., Koizumi K., Vassalle, M., Aulgo Gaggi, Bologna, 1971, p 373.

855. Vassort, G., Rougier, O., Garnier, D., Sauviat, M. P., Coraboeuf, E., Gargouil, Y. M., Effects of adrenaline on membrane inward currents during the cardiac action potential. *Pfluegers Arch* 309: 70, 1969.

856. Vedoya, R., Parasystolia. Buenos Aires, Aniceto Lopez, 1944.

857. Venerose, R. S., Seidenstein, J. H., Stuckey, J. H., Hoffman, B. E., Activation of subendocardial Purkinje fibers and muscle fibers of the left septal surface before and after left bundle branch block. *Am Heart J* 63: 346, 1962.

858. Vereecke, J., Carmeliet, E., Sr action potentials in cardiac Purkinje fibers. I. Evidence for a regenerative increase in Sr conductance. *Pfleugers Arch* 322: 60, 1971.

859. Vereecke, J., Carmeliet, E., Sr action potentials in cardiac Purkinje fibers. II Dependence in the Sr conductance on the external Sr concentration and Sr-Ca antagonism. *Pfluegers Arch* 322: 73, 1971.

860. Virágh, S., Porte, A., Le noeud de Keith et Flack et les différentes fibres auriculaires du coeur du rat. Etude au microscopie optique et électronique. *C R Acad Sci* (Paris) 251: 2086, 1960.

861. Virágh, S., The fine structure of the conducting system and the force producing muscle of the

heart. *Thesis* (in Hungarian), Budapest, 1969.

862. Virágh, S., Porte, A., Structure fine du tissue vecteur dans le coeur du rat. *Zeitschr Zellforsch* 55: 263, 1969.

863. Virágh, S., Porte, A., The fine structure of the conducting system of the monkey heart (Macaca mulatta) I. The sino-atrial node and the internodal connections. *Z Zellforsch* 145: 191, 1973.

864. Virágh, S., Porte, A., On the impulse conducting system of the monkey heart. II. The atrioventricular node and bundle. *Z Zellforsch* 145: 363, 1973.

865. Virágh, S., Challice, C. E., Origin and differentiation of cardiac muscle cells in the mouse. *J Ultrastruc Rec* 42: 1, 1973.

866. Virágh, S., Challice, C. E., The impulse generation and conduction system of the heart. In: Ultrastructure in biological systems. edited by Dalton A. J., Challice C. E., Vol 6, Ultrastructure of the mammalian heart, New York, 1973, p. 43.

867. Vismara, L. A., Mason, D. T., Amsterdam, R. A., Disopyramide phosphate: Clinical efficacy of a new oral antiarrhythmic drug. *Clin Pharmacol Ther* 16: 330, 1974.

868. de Vries, P. A., Saunders, J. B. C. M., Development of the ventricles and spiral outflow tract in the human heart. *Contr Embryol* 37: 89, 1962.

869. Waldo, A. L., Kaiser, G. A., Castany, R. J., Hoffman, B. E., Study of arrhythmias associated with acute myocardial infarction (Abstr.). *Circulation* 38 (Suppl VI) 6–200, 1968.

870. Waldo, A. L., Vitikainen, K. J., Kaiser, G. A., Malm, J. R., Hoffman, B. F., The P wave and P-R interval: Effects of the site of origin of atrial depolarization. *Circulation* 42: 653, 1970.

871. Waldo, A. L., Karp, B. B., Kouchoukos, N. T., McLean, W. A. H., Massing, G. K., James, T. N., Electrophysiological delineation of the left bundle branch in man (Abstract). *Am J Cardiol* 33: 176 1974.

872. Wallace, A. G., Sarnoff, S. L., Effects of cardiac sympathetic nerve stimulation on conduction in the heart. *Circulation Res* 14: 86, 1964.

873. Wallace, A. G., Boineau, J. P., Davidson, R. M., Sealy, W. C., Wolff-Parkinson-White syndrome. A new look. *Am J Cardiol* 28: 509, 1971.

874. Wallace, A. G., Sealy, W. C., Gallager, J. I., Svenson, R. H., Strauss, H. C., Kasell, J., Surgical correction of anomalous left ventricular preexcitation: Wolff-Parkinson-White (type A). *Circulation* 49: 206, 1974.

875. Walls, E. W., The development of the specialized conducting tissue in the human heart. *J Anat* 81: 93, 1947.

876. Watanabe, Y., Dreifus, L. S., McGarry, T. F., Likoff, W., Electrophysiologic antagonism of

potassium and antiarrhythmic agents. *Circulation* 26: 799, 1962.

877. Watanabe, Y., Dreifus, L. S., Likoff, W., Electrophysiologic antagonism and synergism of potassium and antiarrhythmic agents. *Am J Cardiol* 12: 702, 1963.

878. Watanabe, Y., Antagonism and synergism of potassium and antiarrhythmic agents, In: Electrolytes and cardiovascular diseases, edited by Bajusz E., S. Karger A. G., Basel, 1965, p 86.

879. Watanabe, Y., Dreifus, L. S., Inhomogeneous conduction in the A-V node: A model for reentry. *Am Heart J* 70: 505, 1965.

880. Watanabe, Y., Dreifus, L. S., Electrophysiologic effects of digitalis on A-V transmission. *Am J Physiol* 211: 1461, 1966.

881. Watanabe, Dreifus, L. S., Second degree atrioventricular block. *Cardiovasc Res* 1: 150, 1967.

882. Watanabe, Y., Dreifus, L. S., Interactions of quinidine and potassium on atrioventricular transmission. *Circulation Res* 20: 434, 1967.

883. Watanabe, Y., Dreifus, L. S., Sites of impulse formation within the atrioventricular junction of the rabbit. *Circulation Res* 22: 717, 1968.

884. Watanabe, Y., Josipovic, V., Dreifus, L. S., Electrophysiological mechanism of bretylium tosylate (Abstract). *Fed Proc* 28: 270, 1969.

885. Watanabe, Y., Effects of electrolytes and antiarrhythmic drugs on atrioventricular conduction, In: Symposium on cardiac arrhythmias, edited by Sandoe E, Flensted-Jensen E, Oleson KH, Sodertalje, Sweden, 1970.

886. Watanabe, Y., Dreifus, L. S., Interactions of lanatoside C and potassium on atrioventricular conduction in rabbits. *Circulation Res* 27, 931, 1970.

887. Watanabe, Y., Reassesment of parasystole. *Am Heart J* 81: 451, 1971.

888. Watanabe, Y., Dreifus, L. S., Levels of concealment in second degree and advanced second degree A-V block. *Am Heart J* 84: 330, 1972.

889. Watanabe, Y., Dreifus, L. S., Electrophysiological effects of magnesium and its interactions with potassium. *Cardiovasc Res* 6: 79, 1972.

890. Watanabe, Y., de Azevedo, I. M., Dreifus, L. S., Electrophysiologic antagonism of quinidine and bretylium tosylate (Abstract). *Circulation* 45/46: (Suppl 2) 40, 1972.

891. Watanabe, A. M., Besch, H. R. jr, Subcellular myocardial effects of verapamil and D$_{600}$: Comparison with propranolol. *J Pharm Exp Ther* 191: 241, 1974.

892. Watanabe, A. M., Besch, H. R. jr, Cyclic adenosine monophosphate modulation of slow calcium influx channels in guinea pig hearts. *Circulation Res* 35: 316, 1974.

893. Watt, T. B., Murao, Pruitt, R. D., Left axis deviation induced experimentally in a primate heart. *Am Heart J* 69: 642, 1965.

894. Watt, T. B., Pruitt, R. D., Electrocardiographic findings associated with experimental arborization block in dogs. *Am Heart J* 69: 642, 1965.

895. Watt, T. B., Freud, G. F., Durrer, D., Pruitt, R. D., Left anterior arborization block combined with right bundle branch block in canine and primate hearts. *Circulation Res* 22: 57, 1968.

896. Weibel, E. R., Kistler, G. S., Scherle, W. E., Practical stereological methods for morphometric cytology. *J Cell Biol* 30: 23, 1966.

897. Weidmann, S., The effect of the cardiac membrane potential on the rapid availability of the sodium carrying system. *J Physiol* 127, 213, 1955.

898. Weidmann, S., Effects of calcium ions and local anesthetics on electrical properties of Purkinje fibers. *J Physiol* 129: 568, 1955.

899. Weidmann, S., Elektrophysiolgie der Herzmuskelfaser. Hans Huber Medical Publisher, Bern, 1956, p 42.

900. Weidmann, S., Electrophysiology. *Am Rev Physiol* 36: 155, 1974.

901. Wellens, H. J. J., Durrer, D., Supraventricular tachycardia with left aberrant conduction due to retrograde invasion into the left bundle branch. *Circulation* 38: 474, 1968.

902. Wellens, H. J. J., Schuilenburg, R. M., Durrer, D., Electrical stimulation of the heart in patients with Wolff-Parkinson-White syndrome type A. *Circulation* 43: 99, 1971.

903. Wellens, H. J. J., Electrical stimulation of the heart in the study and treatment of tachycardias. Stenfert Kroese, Leiden, 1971.

904. Wellens, H. J. J., Schuilenburg, R. M., Durrer, D., Electrical stimulation of the heart in patients with ventricular tachycardia. *Circulation* 46: 216, 1972.

904a. Wellens, H. J. J., Durrer, D., Effect of digitalis on atrioventricular conduction and circus-movement tachycardias in patients with Wolff-Parkinson-White syndrome. *Circulation* 47: 1229, 1973.

904b. Wellens, H. J. J., Durrer, D., Combined conduction disturbances in two A-V pathways in patients with Wolf-Parkinson-White syndrome. *Europ J Cardiol* 1: 23, 1973.

905. Wellens, H. J. J., Durrer, D., Patterns of ventriculo-atrial conduction in the Wolff-Parkinson-White syndrome. *Circulation* 49: 22, 1974.

906. Wellens, H. J. J., Lie, K. L., Durrer, D., Further observations on ventricular tachycardia as studied by electrical stimulation of the heart. Chronic recurrent ventricular tachycardia and

ventricular tachycardia during acute myocardial infarction. *Circulation* 49: 647, 1974.

906a. Wellens, H. J. J., Durrer, D., Effect of procaine amide, quinidine and ajmaline on the Wolff-Parkinson syndrome. *Circulation* 50: 114, 1974.

907. Wellens, H. J., Durrer, D., Contribution of atrial pacing to understanding of the genesis of arrhythmias. In: Complex electrocardiography, edited by Fisch C. *Cardiovasc Clin* 6: 26, 1974.

907a. Wellens, H. J. J., Durrer, D., Relation between refractory period of the accessory pathway and ventricular frequency during atrial fibrillation in patients with Wolff-Parkinson-White syndrome. *Am J Cardiol* 33, 178, 1974.

908. Wellens, H. J. J., Preferential conduction in the atrium. Something special? *Europ J Cardiol* 2: 113, 1974.

908a. Wellens, H. J. J., Janse, M. J., van Dam, R. Th., van, Capelle, E. J. L., Meijne, N. G., Mellink, H. M., Durrer, D., Epicardial mapping and surgical treatment in Wolff-Parkinson-White syndrome type A. *Am Heart J* 86: 69, 1975.

909. Wellens, H. J. J., Contribution of cardiac pacing to our understanding of the Wolff-Parkinson-White syndrome. *Brit Heart J* 37: 231, 1975.

910. Wellens, H. J. J., Unusual examples of re-entrant supraventricular tachycardia. *Circulation* 51: 997, 1975.

911. Wellens, H. J. J., Durrer, D., The role of an accessory atrioventricular pathway in reciprocal tachycardia. Observations in patients with and without the Wolff-Parkinson-White syndrome *Circulation* 52: 58, 1975.

911a. Wellens, H. J. J., Effect of drugs on Wolff-Parkinson-White syndrome. In: His bundle electrocardiography, and clinical electrophysiology edited by Narula O. F. A. Davis, Philadelphia, 1975, p. 367.

912. Wellens, H. J. J., Liem, K. L., Düren, D. R., Lie, K. I., Effect of digitalis on re-entrant A-V nodal tachycardia in man. *Circulation* 52: 779, 1975.

913. Wellens, H. J. J., Pathophysiology of ventricular tachycardia in man. *Arch Int Med* 135: 473, 1975.

914. Wellens, H. J. J., Bär, F., Wesdorp, J., Dohmen, H. I. M., Düren, D. R., Durrer, D. Effect of amiodarone in the Wolff-Parkinson-White syndrome. Submitted for publication.

915. Wenckebach, K. F., Ueber die Dauer der compensatorischen Pause nach Reizung der Vorkammer des Säugethierherzens. *Archiv für Anat und Physiol* (Physiol Abth) 57, 1903.

916. Wenckebach, K. F., Arrhythmia of the heart. A physiological and clinical study. Translated by T. Snowball. William Green and Sons, Edinburgh and London, 1904.

917. Wenckebach, K. F., Beitrage zur Kenntnis der

Menschlichen Herztätigkeit. *Archiv für Anat und Physiol* (Physiol Abth) 297, 1906.

918. Wenink, A. C. G., Some details on the final stages of heart septation in the human embryo. Thesis. Leiden Drukkerij Luctor et Emergo, 1971.

919. Wenink, A. C. G., La formation du septum membranaceum dans le coeur humain. Bull de l'Assoc des Anat 58: 1127, 1974.

920. Wenink, A. C. G., Considerations from studies of human embryos relative to the development of the cardiac conduction system. *J Anat* submitted for publication.

921. Wennemark, J. R., Ruesta, V. J., Brody, D. A., Microelectrode study of delayed conduction in the canine right bundle branch. *Circulation Res* 23: 753, 1968.

922. West, T. C., Amory, D. W., Single fiber recording of the effects of quinidine at atrial and pacemaker sites in the isolated right atrium of the rabbit. *J Pharmacol Exp Ther* 130: 183, 1960.

923. Williams, D., Treatment of epilepsy with sodium diphenylhydantoinate. *Lancet* 2: 678, 1939.

924. Wilson, EN, Macleod, A. G., Barker, P. S., The order of ventricular localization in human bundle branch block. *Am Heart J* 7: 305, 1932.

925. Wit, A. L., Weiss, M. D., Berkowitz, W. D., Rosen, K. M., Steiner, C. Damato, A. N., Patterns of atrioventricular conduction in the human heart. *Circulation Res* 27: 345, 1970.

926. Wit, A. L., Weiss, M. B., Berkowitz, W. D., Rosen, K. M., Steiner, C., Damato, A. N., Patterns of atrioventricular conduction in the human heart. *Circulation Res* 27: 345, 1970.

927. Wit, A. L., Damato, A. N., Weiss, M. B., Steiner, C., Phenomenon of the gap in atrioventricular conduction in the human heart. *Circulation Res* 27: 679, 1970.

928. Wit, A. L., Steiner, C., Damato, A. N., Electrophysiologic effects of bretylium tosylate on single fibers of the canine specialized conducting system and ventricle. *J Pharmacol Exp Ther* 173: 344, 1970.

929. Wit, A. L., Goldreyer, B. N., Damato, A. N., In vitro model of paroxysmal supraventricular tachycardia. *Circulation* 43: 862, 1971.

930. Wit, A. L., Hoffman, B. E., Cranefield, P. F., Slow conduction and reentry in the ventricular conducting system: I. Return extrasystole in canine Purkinje fibers. *Circulation Res* 30: 1, 1972.

931. Wit, A. L., Cranefield, P. F., Hoffman, B. F., Slow conduction and reentry in the ventricular conducting system: II. Single and sustained circus movement in networks of canine and bovine Purkinje fibers. *Circulation Res* 30: 11, 1972.

932. Wit, A. L., Fenoglio, J. J. jr, Wagner, B. M., Bassett, A. L., Electrophysiological properties of cardiac muscle in the anterior mitral valve leaflet and the adjacent atrium in the dog— Possible implications for the genesis of atrial dysrhythmias. *Circulation Res* 32: 731, 1973.

933. Wit, A. L., Cranefield, P. F., Atropine and acute myocardial infarction. Letter to the Editor. *Circulation* 47: 1397, 1973.

934. Wit. A. L., Rosen, M. R., Hoffman, B. F., Electrophysiology and pharmacology of cardiac arrhythmias. II. Relationship of normal and abnormal electrical activity of cardiac fibers to the genesis of arrhythmias. A. Automaticity. *Am Heart J* 88: 515, 1974.

935. Wit, A. L., Rosen, M. R., Hoffman, B. F., Electrophysiology and pharmacology of cardiac arrhythmias. II. Relationship of normal and abnormal electrical activity of cardiac fibers to the genesis of arrhythmias B. Reentry. Section 1. *Am Heart J* 88: 664, 1974.

936. Wit, A. L., Rosen, M. R., Hoffman, B. G., Electrophysiology and pharmacology of cardiac arrhythmias. II. Relationship of normal and abnormal electrical activity of cardiac fibers to the genesis of arrhythmias B. Re-entry. Section 2. *Am Heart J* 88: 798, 1974.

937. Wit, A. L., Cranefield, P. F., Effect of verapamil on the sinoatrial and atrioventricular nodes of the rabbit and the mechanism by which it arrests re-entrant atrioventricular nodal tachycardia. *Circulation Res* 35: 413, 1974

938. Wit, A. L., Cranefield, P. F., Verapamil inhibition of the slow response; A mechanism for its effectiveness against reentrant A-V nodal tachycardia. *Circulation* 50: 3–146, 1974.

939. Wit, A. L., Friedman, P. L., Basis for ventricular arrhythmias accompanying myocardial infarction. *Arch Int Med* 135: 459, 1975.

940. Wit. A. L., Cranefield, P. E., Triggered activity in cardiac muscle fibers of the Simian mitral valve. *Circulation Res* (submitted).

941. Wittenberg, S. M., Streuli, E., Klocke, F. J., Acceleration of ventricular pacemakers by transient increases in heart rate in dogs during ouabain administration. *Circulation Res* 26: 705, 1970.

942. Wittig, J., Harrison, I. A., Wallace, A. G., Electrophysiological effects of lidocaine on distal Purkinje fibers of canine heart. *Am Heart J* 86: 69, 1973.

943. Wolferth, C. C., The so-called supernormal recovery phase of conduction in heart muscle. *Am Heart J* 3: 706, 1928.

944. Wolferth, C. C., Wood, E. C., The mechanism of production of short P-R intervals and prolonged QRS. Hypothesis of an accessory pathway of auriculoventricular conduction (bundle of Kent). *Am Heart J* 8: 297, 933.

945. Woodbury, L. A., Hecht, H. H., Effects of cardiac glycosides upon electrical activity of single ventricular fibers of the frog heart, and their relation to the digitalis effect of the electrocardiogram. *Circulation* 6: 172, 1952.

946. Wu, D., Denes, P., Dhingra, R., Rosen, K., Nature of gap phenomenon in man. *Circulation Res* 34: 682, 1974.

947. Wu, D., Denes, P., Dhingra, R., Khan, A., Rosen, K. M., The effects of propranolol on induction of A-V nodal reentrant paroxysmal tachycardia. *Circulation* 50: 665, 1974.

948. Wu, D., Denes, P., Wyndham, C., Amat y Leon, E., Dhingra, R. C., Rosen, K. M., Demonstration of dual A-V nodal pathways utilizing a ventricular extra-stimulus in patients with A-V nodal reentrant paroxysmal supraventricular tachycardia (Abstr.). *Clin Res.* 23: 215, 1975.

949. Wu, D., Amat y Leon, F., Denes, P., Dhingra, R. C., Pietras, R. I., Rosen, K. M., Demonstration of sustained sinus and atrial reentry as a mechanism of paroxysmal supraventricular tachycardia. *Circulation* 51: 234, 1975.

950. Wu, D., Wyndham, C., Amat Y Leon, E., Denes, P., Dhingra, R. C. Rosen, K. M., The effects of ouabain on induction of A-V nodal reentrant paroxysmal supraventricular tachycardia. *Circulation* 52: 201, 1975.

951. Wu, D., Denes, P., Dhingra, R., Pietras, R. J., Rosen, K. M., New manifestation of dual A-V nodal pathways. *Europ J Card* 2: 459, 1975.

952. Wu, D., Denes, P., Dhingra, R. C., Wyndham, C., Rosen, K. M., Determinants of fast and slow pathway conduction in patients with dual A-V nodal pathways. *Circulation Res* 36: 782, 1975.

953. Yamagishi, S., Effect of tetrodotoxin on the pacemaker action potential of the sinus node. *Proc Jap Acad* 42: 1194, 1966.

954. Yamauchi, A., Ultrastructure of the innervation of the mammalian heart. In: Ultrastructure of the mammalian heart, edited by Challice CE, Virágh S, Acad Press, New York & London, 1973, p 127.

955. Zipes, D. P., The clinical significance of bradycardic rhythm in acute myocardial infarction. *Am J Cardiol* 24: 814, 1969.

956. Zipes, D. P., The contribution of artificial pacemaking to understanding the pathogenesis of arrhythmias. *Am J Cardiol* 28: 211, 1971.

957. Zipes, D. P., Mendez, C., Moe, G. K., Evidence of summation and voltage dependency in rabbit atrioventricular nodal fibers. *Circulation Res* 32: 170, 1973.

958. Zipes, D. P., Mendez, C., Action of mangenese ions and tetrodotoxin on A-V nodal transmem-

brane potentials in isolated rabbit hearts. *Circulation Res* 32: 447, 1973.

959. Zipes, D. P., Fischer, J. C., Effects of agents which inhibit the slow channel on sinus automaticity and atrioventricular conduction in the dog. *Circulation Res* 34: 184, 1974.

960. Zipes, D. P., DeJoseph, R. L., Rothbaum, D. A., Unusual properties of accessory pathways. *Circulation* 49: 1200, 1974.

961. Zipes, D. P., Arbel, E., Knope, R. F., Moe, G. K., Accelerated ventricular escape rhythms

caused by ouabain intoxication. *Am J Cardiol* 33: 248, 1974.

962. Zipes, D. P., Nobel, R. J., Carmichael, R. T., Rowell, H., Fasola, A. F., Relations between aprindine concentration heart rate, ischemia, and ventricular fibrillation in dogs (Abstract). *Am J Cardiol* 35: 179, 1975.

963. Zipes, D. P., Knope, R. E., Mendez, C., Moe, G. K., The site of functional right bundle branch block in the intact canine heart, *Adv Cardiol* in press.

INDEX OF SUBJECTS